The British
Medical Association

NEW FAMILY
DOCTOR
HOME ADVISER

The British Medical Association

NEW FAMILY DOCTOR
HOME ADVISER

BMA Consulting Medical Editor
DR MICHAEL PETERS

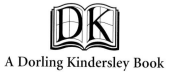

A Dorling Kindersley Book

LONDON, NEW YORK, MUNICH, MELBOURNE, AND DELHI

BRITISH MEDICAL ASSOCIATION

CHAIRMAN OF COUNCIL Mr James Johnson
TREASURER Dr David Pickersgill
CHAIRMAN OF THE REPRESENTATIVE BODY Dr Michael Wilks

BMA CONSULTING MEDICAL EDITOR

Dr Michael Peters MB BS

DORLING KINDERSLEY

SENIOR MANAGING EDITOR Martyn Page
PROJECT EDITOR Katie John
SENIOR ART EDITOR Ian Spick
DTP DESIGNER Julian Dams
PICTURE RESEARCH Samantha Nunn
PRODUCTION CONTROLLER Elizabeth Cherry
PUBLISHING DIRECTOR Corinne Roberts

DK INDIA

MANAGER Aparna Sharma
PROJECT EDITOR Dipali Singh
EDITOR Aekta Jerath
PROJECT ART EDITOR Kavita Dutta
DTP COORDINATOR Pankaj Sharma
DTP OPERATOR Harish Aggarwal

The British Medical Association New Family Doctor Home Adviser provides information on a wide range of medical topics, and every effort has been made to ensure that the information in this book is accurate. The book is not a substitute for expert medical advice, however, and you are advised always to consult a doctor or other health professional for specific information on personal health matters. Never disregard expert medical advice or delay in seeking advice or treatment due to information obtained from this book. The naming of any product, treatment, or organization in this book does not imply endorsement by the BMA, BMA Consulting Medical Editor, other consultants or contributors, or publisher, nor does the omission of any such names indicate disapproval. The BMA, BMA Consulting Medical Editor, consultants, contributors, and publisher do not accept any legal responsibility for any personal injury or other damage or loss arising from any use or misuse of the information and advice in this book.

First published in Great Britain in 1986 by Dorling Kindersley Limited, London
First published in paperback in 1989, reprinted 1990
Second edition 1992, reprinted 1992, 1994, 1995, 1996, 1997
Third edition 2001
Fourth edition 2006

Published in the United Kingdom by Dorling Kindersley Limited
80 Strand, London WC2R 0RL
A Penguin Company

2 4 6 8 10 9 7 5 3 1

A CIP catalogue record for this book is available from the British Library.

ISBN 1-4053-1266-1

Colour reproduction by Colourscan, Singapore
Printed and bound by Star Standard, Singapore

see our complete catalogue at
www.dk.com

FOREWORD

Medicine is constantly evolving. An increasing amount of information is available in books and magazines and on the internet, and people are more aware of health matters today than ever before. It is sometimes difficult, however, to know where to go for reliable advice on everyday problems or on new developments in healthcare. The *Family Doctor Home Adviser* is designed as a guide to many of the most common health issues.

The bulk of this book consists of flow charts to help you analyse symptoms of illness. It helps you to think the same way as your own doctor in trying to determine the cause of a symptom. The charts lead you from one main symptom to any associated problems and then to the possible cause or causes. Once you have found a likely cause, the chart gives advice on whether you can take action yourself or whether to obtain medical aid. It gives self-help measures or over-the-counter remedies where appropriate; alternatively, if you need medical attention, the chart indicates the degree of urgency in seeking it.

The introductory section, "Your Body and Health", outlines how your body works and how to keep it healthy. The "Professional Healthcare" section describes the checks and examinations that you may receive from your GP; it also outlines some common diagnostic procedures that you may undergo when in hospital. At the end of the book, the "Useful Addresses" section directs you to sources of further information and support.

The book includes the latest thinking on a range of health matters. On one hand, it incorporates new official guidelines on childhood immunizations and on the planned national screening programme for colorectal cancer. On the other, it also includes practical advice on issues such as dealing with fever in children and breast-feeding correctly.

Inevitably, the *Family Doctor Home Adviser* is no substitute for specific, personally tailored advice from your own doctor. I believe, however, that the information given here will provide you with a firm basis for managing your own and your family's health.

DR MICHAEL PETERS
BMA CONSULTING MEDICAL EDITOR

CONTENTS

HOW TO USE THIS BOOK

The first part of this book gives background information on how the body works and how to keep it healthy, and outlines procedures that healthcare professionals might use to assess symptoms. The second, major part consists of 150 question-and-answer symptom charts, which help you determine the possible cause of a symptom and work out what to do yourself. The book concludes by listing useful sources of further health information.

Your body and health

You will find general information about the body and health in this highly illustrated section, which is divided into four parts. Your Body shows how major body systems function, and also covers pregnancy, birth, and child development. In Healthy Living, you can find out how to stay healthy and minimize the risks of common disorders. What to expect when you see your doctor and other healthcare professionals is covered in Professional Healthcare. Finally, Medical Tests covers procedures that doctors may use to diagnose and assess disorders.

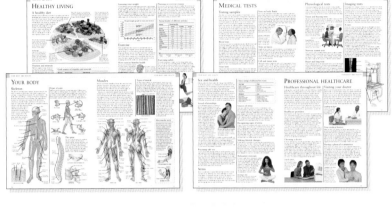

Symptom charts

The Symptom Charts are grouped according to age and/or sex – there are charts for children of different ages, charts for all adults, and charts specifically for men and women. The charts help you find a possible cause of many symptoms that may affect you or your child and tell you what steps you should take, whether the action involves professional help or self-help. At the beginning of the section, there are detailed instructions on how to use the charts, along with a "chartfinder" to help you find the most appropriate chart for a particular symptom.

Useful addresses

The Useful Addresses section lists support groups for different conditions and sources for additional health information. Addresses, telephone numbers, and online sites are given for each organization.

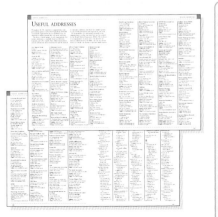

Finding information

You can find the information that you need from this book in several ways:

CONTENTS LISTS The comprehensive contents (pp.6–7) lists every symptom chart as well as the main headings in the other sections of the book. In addition, at the start of each group of charts, there is a contents list of the charts in that group.

CHARTFINDER The symptom-by-symptom chartfinder (p.44) alphabetically lists all the symptoms and can direct you to the appropriate chart.

CROSS-REFERENCES Throughout the book, there are cross-references to take you to pages with further information.

INDEX If you still cannot find what you need, the index (pp.289–296) covers every subject within the book.

YOUR BODY & HEALTH

Understanding how your body works and how to look after yourself are essential if you want to stay healthy. This section starts by explaining the structure and function of the major body systems. It then looks at how you can modify your lifestyle to prevent health problems from developing. The final parts of the section describe how you can make the best use of the help that health professionals offer and how medical problems are investigated should they occur.

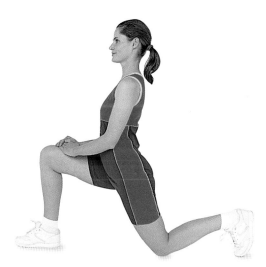

YOUR BODY

Skeleton

The skeleton provides form, support, and protection for the body. It consists of 206 bones, with further support from cartilage (a tough, fibrous material). The axial skeleton – the skull, spine, and ribcage – consists of 80 bones and protects the brain, spinal cord, heart, and lungs. The appendicular skeleton has 126 bones and consists of the limb bones, collarbones, shoulder blades, and bones of the pelvis. All bones are living tissue with cells that are constantly replacing old bone with new material. Bones contain a soft, fatty material called bone marrow; this is surrounded by spongy bone, which is in turn surrounded by denser compact bone. The marrow in the bones of the spine, skull, ribs, and pelvis manufactures blood cells.

Skull

Jawbone
(mandible)

Collarbone
(clavicle)

Shoulder blade
(scapula)

Breastbone (sternum)

Humerus

Rib

Spine

Ulna

Radius

Wrist bones
(carpals)

Hand bones
(metacarpals)

Finger bones
(phalanges)

Kneecap
(patella)

Pelvis

Femur

Fibula

Tibia

Ankle bones
(tarsals)

Foot bones
(metatarsals)

Toe bones
(phalanges)

Compact Spongy Bone
bone bone marrow

STRUCTURE OF BONE

Types of joint

Joints are formed where two or more bones meet. Different types of joint allow for differing degrees of movement. A few joints, such as those in the skull, are fixed. Semimovable joints, such as those in the spine, provide stability and some flexibility. The majority of joints, known as synovial joints, move freely. The main types of synovial joint, and their planes of movement, are illustrated below.

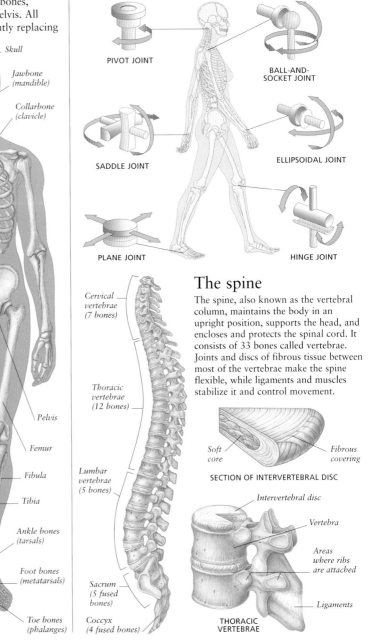

PIVOT JOINT

BALL-AND-SOCKET JOINT

SADDLE JOINT

ELLIPSOIDAL JOINT

PLANE JOINT

HINGE JOINT

The spine

The spine, also known as the vertebral column, maintains the body in an upright position, supports the head, and encloses and protects the spinal cord. It consists of 33 bones called vertebrae. Joints and discs of fibrous tissue between most of the vertebrae make the spine flexible, while ligaments and muscles stabilize it and control movement.

Cervical
vertebrae
(7 bones)

Thoracic
vertebrae
(12 bones)

Lumbar
vertebrae
(5 bones)

Sacrum
(5 fused
bones)

Coccyx
(4 fused bones)

Soft
core

Fibrous
covering

SECTION OF INTERVERTEBRAL DISC

Intervertebral disc

Vertebra

Areas
where ribs
are attached

Ligaments

**THORACIC
VERTEBRAE**

Muscles

Muscles are fibrous bundles of tissue that move the body, maintain its posture, and work internal organs such as the heart, intestines, and bladder. These functions are performed by three different types of muscle (right), of which skeletal muscle makes up the greatest bulk.

Muscles are controlled by signals from the nervous system. Skeletal muscle can be controlled consciously, while the other types work automatically. Most skeletal muscles connect two adjacent bones. One end of the muscle is attached by a flexible cord of fibrous tissue called a tendon; the other is attached by a tendon or by a sheet of connective tissue. The skeletal muscles not only move parts of the body but also help to maintain the posture when a person is standing, sitting, or lying down. The names of some muscles suggest their functions. Extensors straighten joints, flexors bend joints, adductors move limbs towards the body, abductors pull limbs outwards, and erectors raise or hold up parts of the body. Some of the main skeletal muscles are illustrated below. Deeper muscles are shown on the left of each image and the more superficial muscles are shown on the right.

Types of muscle

The three types of muscle are skeletal muscle, which covers and moves the skeleton; cardiac muscle, which forms the walls of the heart; and smooth muscle, found in the walls of the digestive tract, the blood vessels, and the genital and urinary tracts. Each type of muscle has a different function and consists of fibres of a particular shape. Skeletal muscle, which moves the limbs and body, is formed of long, strong, parallel fibres. This type of muscle is able to contract quickly and powerfully, but can work at maximum strength only for short periods of time. Heart muscle pumps blood around the body. It comprises short, branching, interlinked fibres that form a network within the walls of the heart. This type of muscle can work continually without tiring. Smooth muscle carries out functions such as moving food through the digestive tract. It is composed of short, spindle-shaped fibres that are connected to form sheets, and can work for prolonged periods.

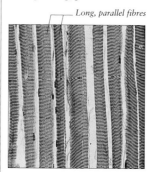

Long, parallel fibres

SKELETAL MUSCLE

How muscles work

Movement occurs when signals from the nervous system cause muscles to contract. Conscious movements of the body are produced by the interaction of skeletal muscles, bones, and joints. Most muscles connect one bone to another and cross a joint. When a muscle contracts, it pulls on the bones to move them. Many muscles are found in pairs, one on each side of a joint, and produce opposing movements. For example, in the upper arm the triceps contracts to pull the arm straight and the biceps contracts to bend the arm.

Triceps contracts

Biceps relaxes

STRAIGHTENING THE ARM

Triceps relaxes

Biceps contracts

BENDING THE ARM

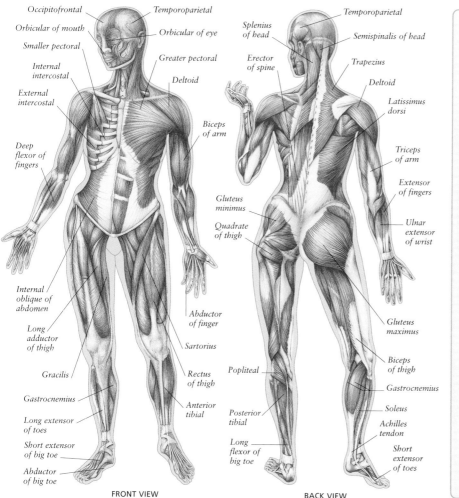

Occipitofrontal
Orbicular of mouth
Smaller pectoral
Internal intercostal
External intercostal
Deep flexor of fingers
Internal oblique of abdomen
Long adductor of thigh
Gracilis
Gastrocnemius
Long extensor of toes
Short extensor of big toe
Abductor of big toe

Temporoparietal
Orbicular of eye
Greater pectoral
Deltoid
Biceps of arm
Gluteus minimus
Quadrate of thigh
Abductor of finger
Sartorius
Rectus of thigh
Anterior tibial

FRONT VIEW

Splenius of head
Erector of spine
Temporoparietal
Semispinalis of head
Trapezius
Deltoid
Latissimus dorsi
Triceps of arm
Extensor of fingers
Ulnar extensor of wrist
Gluteus maximus
Biceps of thigh
Gastrocnemius
Soleus
Achilles tendon
Short extensor of toes
Popliteal
Posterior tibial
Long flexor of big toe

BACK VIEW

Cardiovascular system

The cardiovascular system transports blood around the body, taking oxygen and nutrients to body tissues and removing waste products. The heart is a hollow, muscular organ that pumps all the body's blood – roughly 5 litres (9 pints) – around the body about once a minute and faster during exercise. Blood flows through a network of vessels that reaches all parts of the body. Arteries carrying blood from the heart branch into smaller vessels and then into capillaries, which in turn join a network of veins that return blood to the heart.

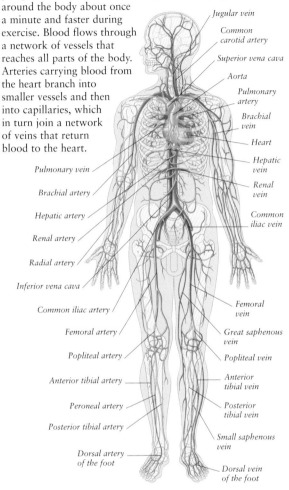

Jugular vein
Common carotid artery
Superior vena cava
Aorta
Pulmonary artery
Brachial vein
Heart
Hepatic vein
Renal vein
Common iliac vein
Pulmonary vein
Brachial artery
Hepatic artery
Renal artery
Radial artery
Inferior vena cava
Common iliac artery
Femoral vein
Femoral artery
Great saphenous vein
Popliteal artery
Popliteal vein
Anterior tibial artery
Anterior tibial vein
Peroneal artery
Posterior tibial vein
Posterior tibial artery
Small saphenous vein
Dorsal artery of the foot
Dorsal vein of the foot

Arteries and veins

Arteries have thick, muscular, elastic walls to withstand the high pressure of blood pumped out of the heart. Veins return blood to the heart. They have thinner walls that stretch easily, allowing them to expand and hold large volumes of blood when the body is at rest. The linings of many large veins have folds that act as one-way valves to stop blood from flowing the wrong way.

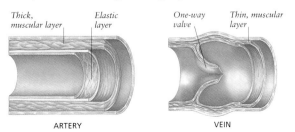

Thick, muscular layer
Elastic layer
One-way valve
Thin, muscular layer

ARTERY

VEIN

Structure of the heart

The heart is a double pump consisting mainly of muscle called myocardium. On each side, blood flows through veins into an upper chamber (atrium), then passes into a lower chamber (ventricle), which pumps the blood into the arteries. Blood flow through the chambers is controlled by one-way valves. The right side of the heart pumps blood into the pulmonary arteries and so to the lungs, and the left side pumps blood into the aorta and around the body.

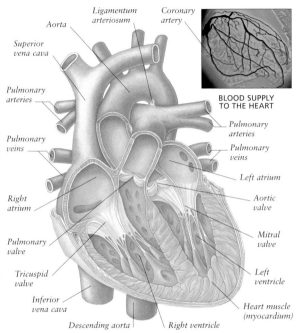

Ligamentum arteriosum
Coronary artery
Aorta
Superior vena cava
Pulmonary arteries
Pulmonary veins
Right atrium
Pulmonary valve
Tricuspid valve
Inferior vena cava
Descending aorta
Right ventricle

BLOOD SUPPLY TO THE HEART

Pulmonary arteries
Pulmonary veins
Left atrium
Aortic valve
Mitral valve
Left ventricle
Heart muscle (myocardium)

Blood circulation

The heart pumps blood into two linked circuits: the pulmonary and the systemic. The pulmonary circuit takes deoxygenated blood to the lungs, where it absorbs oxygen and releases carbon dioxide (a waste gas) through a network of capillaries; the oxygenated blood is then returned to the heart. The systemic circuit takes oxygenated blood to body tissues, where it releases oxygen and nutrients through capillary walls; carbon dioxide and other wastes pass from the tissues into the blood, and the deoxygenated blood is returned to the heart.

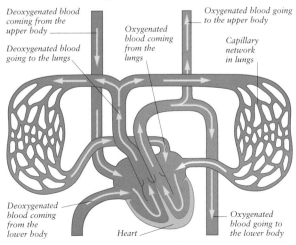

Deoxygenated blood coming from the upper body
Deoxygenated blood going to the lungs
Oxygenated blood coming from the lungs
Oxygenated blood going to the upper body
Capillary network in lungs
Deoxygenated blood coming from the lower body
Heart
Oxygenated blood going to the lower body

Respiratory system

Respiration is the process by which the body obtains oxygen, which it uses to produce energy, and expels carbon dioxide, the main waste product. Air breathed in through the nose or mouth passes down the trachea (windpipe) into the bronchi (lower airways), then into bronchioles (smaller airways) in the lungs. The bronchioles end in sacs called alveoli, which are surrounded by blood vessels. Here, oxygen passes into the blood and carbon dioxide enters the lungs to be breathed out. Breathing is powered by the diaphragm (a muscle) and the intercostal muscles. The respiratory system also includes the pharynx (throat), larynx (voicebox), and epiglottis. The tonsils and the adenoids in the pharynx help to fight infection. The larynx contains the vocal cords, which vibrate to produce sounds. The epiglottis seals the trachea during swallowing.

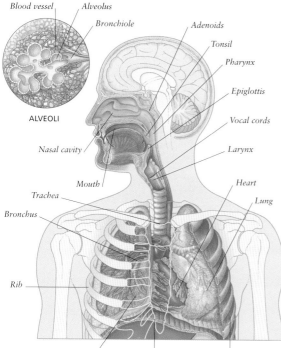

Blood vessel · Alveolus · Bronchiole · Adenoids · Tonsil · Pharynx · Epiglottis · Vocal cords · Larynx · Heart · Lung · Nasal cavity · Mouth · Trachea · Bronchus · Rib · Bronchiole · Diaphragm · Intercostal muscle

ALVEOLI

How breathing works

Breathing is the act by which the body takes in and expels air. The flow of air in and out of the body occurs because air moves from areas of high pressure to areas of low pressure. To breathe in (inhale), the diaphragm and the muscles between the ribs contract, causing the chest to enlarge. As a result the air pressure in the lungs decreases so that it is lower than the atmospheric pressure, and air is drawn into the lungs. To breathe out (exhale), the muscles relax, decreasing the volume of the lungs. The air pressure in the lungs becomes higher than that in the atmosphere, causing air to leave the body.

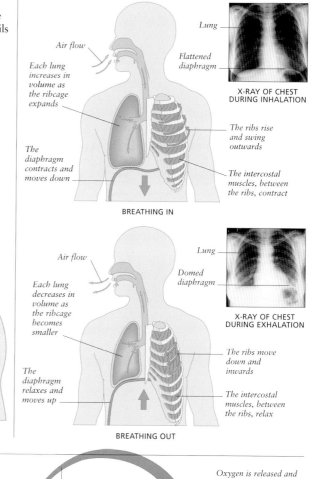

Lung · Air flow · Flattened diaphragm

X-RAY OF CHEST DURING INHALATION

Each lung increases in volume as the ribcage expands

The diaphragm contracts and moves down

The ribs rise and swing outwards

The intercostal muscles, between the ribs, contract

BREATHING IN

Air flow · Lung · Domed diaphragm

X-RAY OF CHEST DURING EXHALATION

Each lung decreases in volume as the ribcage becomes smaller

The diaphragm relaxes and moves up

The ribs move down and inwards

The intercostal muscles, between the ribs, relax

BREATHING OUT

Gas exchange in the body

The body's tissues constantly take up oxygen from the blood and release carbon dioxide back into the blood. Oxygen is breathed into the lungs, and passes from the alveoli (tiny sacs) into blood vessels called capillaries, where it binds to a substance called haemoglobin in the red blood cells. At the same time, carbon dioxide passes from the blood plasma (the fluid part of the blood) into the alveoli to be breathed out. In the capillaries in tissues, the red blood cells release oxygen, while carbon dioxide is absorbed into the plasma.

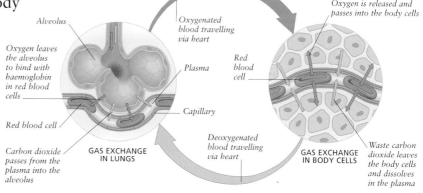

Alveolus · Oxygen leaves the alveolus to bind with haemoglobin in red blood cells · Red blood cell · Carbon dioxide passes from the plasma into the alveolus

Oxygenated blood travelling via heart · Plasma · Capillary · Deoxygenated blood travelling via heart

GAS EXCHANGE IN LUNGS

Oxygen is released and passes into the body cells · Red blood cell · Waste carbon dioxide leaves the body cells and dissolves in the plasma

GAS EXCHANGE IN BODY CELLS

Nervous system

The nervous system gathers, analyses, stores, and transmits information. It controls vital body functions and interacts with the outside world. There are two parts: the central nervous system, which comprises the brain and spinal cord, and the peripheral nervous system, which is made up of nerves that branch from the brain and spinal cord to all areas of the body. Signals, in the form of tiny electrical impulses, are transmitted through the nervous system from the brain to the rest of the body and vice versa. The brain controls almost all activities – both conscious activities, such as movement, and unconscious functions, such as maintaining body temperature. It also receives information from the nerves about the environment and the condition of other parts of the body. For example, the nerves leading from the eyes register visual information and nerves beneath the surface of the skin transmit sensations such as pain. In addition, the brain is capable of complex processes such as learning, memory, thought, and emotion, and can instruct the body to act on the basis of these processes.

Structure and function of the brain

The brain is the most complex organ in the body. It has more than 100 billion nerve cells and billions of pathways. The largest part of the brain is the cerebrum. It is divided into two halves (hemispheres), which are connected by a bundle of nerve fibres called the corpus callosum. The outer layer (cerebral cortex) consists of tissue called grey matter, which generates and processes nerve signals. The inner layer consists of white matter, which transmits the signals. The cerebrum controls conscious thought and movement and interprets sensory information; different parts govern specific activities such as speech and vision. A structure at the base of the brain called the cerebellum controls balance, coordination, and posture. The brain is connected to the spinal cord by the brainstem, which controls vital functions such as respiration. Just above the brainstem is the hypothalamus, which links the nervous system and the endocrine system and helps to regulate body temperature, sleep, and sexual behaviour. The brain is protected by the skull and by membranes called meninges. Clear cerebrospinal fluid cushions the brain and spinal cord from injury.

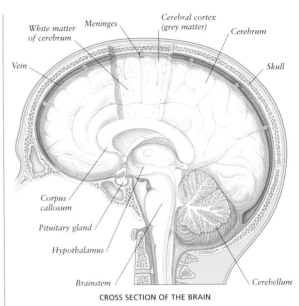

CROSS SECTION OF THE BRAIN

Organization of the nervous system

The central nervous system, comprising the brain and spinal cord, processes and coordinates nerve signals. The spinal cord forms the link between the brain and the rest of the body. Motor pathways, which carry messages from the brain, descend through the spinal cord, while sensory pathways from the skin and other sensory organs ascend through the spinal cord carrying messages to the brain. A network of peripheral nerves reaches all parts of the body. Each nerve is formed from hundreds of nerve fibres, which project from nerve cells, grouped in bundles. Thirty-one pairs of nerves branch off the spinal cord. These divide into smaller and smaller nerves throughout the torso and the limbs.

MAJOR SPINAL NERVES

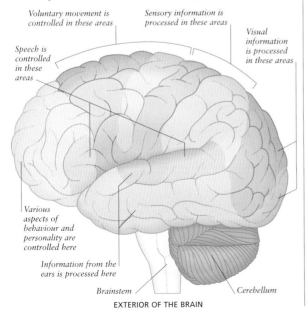

EXTERIOR OF THE BRAIN

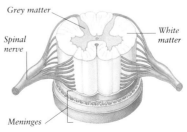

Structure of the spinal cord
The spinal cord is made up of grey matter, which contains nerve cells and supporting cells, and white matter, which contains nerve fibres. The cord is enclosed by protective membranes called meninges.

The senses

Our senses enable us to monitor all aspects of our environment. The eyes provide visual information; the ears detect sound and also aid balance; the nose and tongue respond to different smells and tastes respectively; and the sensory nerves in the skin allow us to feel physical contact (touch), changes in temperature, and pain. In each case, information about the environment detected by the sense organs is transmitted by nerves to the brain, where it is then analysed.

Vision

The organs of vision are the eyes. Light rays entering each eye are focused by the cornea and the lens so that they fall on the retina, producing an upside-down image on it. Cells in the retina convert this image into electrical impulses that pass along the optic nerve to the brain, where they are decoded to create vision. The iris alters the size of the pupil to control the amount of light reaching the retina. Blood vessels in the retina and a layer called the choroid supply the eye with nutrients.

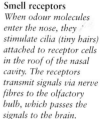

Sclera (white of eye)
Lens
Choroid
Cornea
Retina
Optic nerve
Pupil
Retinal blood vessel
Iris

CROSS SECTION OF AN EYE

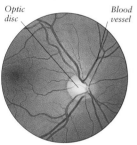

Optic disc
Blood vessel

View of the retina
The cells in the retina register colour and light intensity. At the back of the retina is the optic disc, where nerve fibres converge to form the optic nerve and where blood vessels enter the eye. The disc contains no light-sensitive cells and is called the "blind spot". This photograph was taken through an ophthalmoscope, which magnifies and illuminates the inside of the eye.

Hearing and balance

The ear is concerned not only with hearing but also with balance. It has outer, middle, and inner parts. The outer ear directs sound waves to the eardrum, causing it to vibrate. The bones of the middle ear transmit these vibrations to the inner ear, where they are converted into electrical signals. The signals pass along nerve cells to the brain, where they are analysed. The inner ear also contains structures that aid balance by detecting the position and movements of the head, allowing us to stay upright and move without falling over.

Structure of the ear
The outer ear comprises the pinna (the visible part) and the ear canal, which leads to the eardrum. The middle ear contains three tiny bones that connect the eardrum to a membrane separating the middle and inner ears. The inner ear houses the cochlea, which contains the sensory receptor for hearing, and structures that regulate balance.

Outer ear
Middle ear
Inner ear
Pinna
Ear canal
Eardrum
Nerve
Cochlea

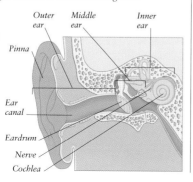

Smell

Smells are detected by specialized receptor cells in the roof of the nasal cavity. These receptor cells detect odour molecules in the air and convert the information into tiny electrical impulses. These impulses are transmitted along the olfactory nerve to the olfactory bulb (the end of the olfactory nerve) and then to the brain, where they are analysed. The human sense of smell is highly sensitive, allowing us to detect more than 10,000 different odours.

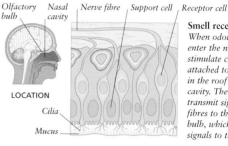

Olfactory bulb
Nasal cavity
Nerve fibre
Support cell
Receptor cell

LOCATION

Cilia
Mucus

Smell receptors
When odour molecules enter the nose, they stimulate cilia (tiny hairs) attached to receptor cells in the roof of the nasal cavity. The receptors transmit signals via nerve fibres to the olfactory bulb, which passes the signals to the brain.

Taste

Tastes are detected by the taste buds. These structures are located in the mouth and throat, with most of them – about 10,000 – on the upper surface of the tongue. The taste buds contain receptor cells, which respond to particular chemicals in food. The receptors can distinguish only five basic tastes: sweet, sour, salty, bitter, and "umami" (a savoury, meaty taste). It is actually our sense of smell, in combination with these five basic tastes, that allows us to differentiate a great range of more subtle flavours.

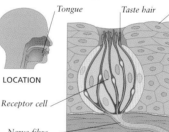

Tongue
Taste hair
Tongue surface

LOCATION

Receptor cell
Nerve fibre

Taste bud structure
Substances in the mouth come into contact with tiny hairs projecting from taste buds in the tongue. These hairs generate nerve impulses that travel along nerve fibres to a specialized area of the brain.

Touch

The sense of touch includes sensations such as pain, pressure, vibration, and temperature. These sensations are detected by two types of receptor under the surface of the skin: free (uncovered) nerve endings, and enclosed nerve endings called corpuscles. Different types of nerve ending or corpuscle monitor particular sensations. The number of receptors varies around the body: for example, the fingertips are highly sensitive and have many receptors, whereas the middle of the back has fewer receptors.

Touch receptors
Touch is detected by various receptors at different levels within the skin. Free (uncovered) nerve endings, near the surface of the skin, respond to touch, pain, pressure, and temperature. Merkel's and Meissner's corpuscles detect light touch, and Pacinian corpuscles detect deep pressure and vibration.

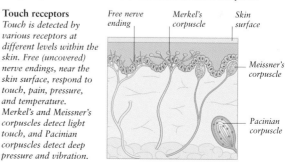

Free nerve ending
Merkel's corpuscle
Skin surface
Meissner's corpuscle
Pacinian corpuscle

Digestive system

The digestive system consists of the digestive tract and its associated organs. The digestive tract is a convoluted tube about 7 m (24 ft) long through which food passes while it is being broken down. The tract consists of the mouth, pharynx (throat), oesophagus, stomach, small and large intestines, rectum, and anus. The associated digestive organs include three pairs of salivary glands, the liver, the pancreas, and the gallbladder. The digestive system breaks down food into simpler components that can be used by the cells of the body and eliminates the remaining substances as waste.

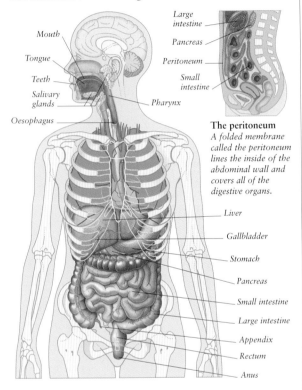

Mouth
Tongue
Teeth
Salivary glands
Oesophagus

Large intestine
Pancreas
Peritoneum
Small intestine
Pharynx

Liver
Gallbladder
Stomach
Pancreas
Small intestine
Large intestine
Appendix
Rectum
Anus

The peritoneum
A folded membrane called the peritoneum lines the inside of the abdominal wall and covers all of the digestive organs.

Mouth and oesophagus

The process of digestion begins in the mouth. The action of the teeth and tongue during chewing breaks food into small, soft pieces for swallowing, while substances in the saliva start to break down carbohydrates in the food. When you swallow, the tongue pushes the mixture of food and saliva, known as a bolus, down the throat into the oesophagus. At the same time, the soft palate closes off the nasal cavity, and the epiglottis, a flap of cartilage at the back of the tongue, moves to close off the larynx.

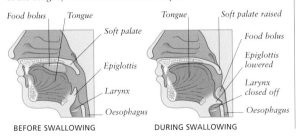

Food bolus
Tongue
Soft palate
Epiglottis
Larynx
Oesophagus

Tongue
Soft palate raised
Food bolus
Epiglottis lowered
Larynx closed off
Oesophagus

BEFORE SWALLOWING

DURING SWALLOWING

Stomach

Food moves down the oesophagus into the stomach. There, it may spend up to 5 hours being churned and partially broken down by digestive juices until it becomes a semi-liquid substance called chyme. Swallowed fluids, such as water and alcohol, pass straight through the stomach and into the intestine in a few minutes.

Small intestine

Chyme enters the duodenum (the first part of the small intestine) and is further broken down by digestive juices from the liver and pancreas. The final stage of digestion takes place in the rest of the small intestine. Here, digestive juices released from the intestinal walls split nutrients into chemical units small enough to pass through the wall of the intestine into the surrounding network of blood vessels.

Large intestine

After nutrients have been absorbed in the small intestine, the remaining material passes into the large intestine. Most of the water content is absorbed back into the body, and the semi-solid waste that remains is called faeces. It moves down into the rectum, where it is stored until it is released through the anus as a bowel motion.

Liver, gallbladder, and pancreas

The liver, gallbladder, and pancreas all help to break down food chemically. The liver uses the products of digestion to manufacture proteins such as antibodies (which help to fight infection) and blood clotting factors. It also breaks down worn-out blood cells and excretes the wastes as bile, which is stored in the gallbladder and plays a part in the digestion of fats. The entry of food into the duodenum (the first part of the small intestine) stimulates the gallbladder to release the bile into the duodenum via the bile duct. The pancreas secretes powerful digestive juices, which are released into the duodenum when food enters it. Together with digestive juices produced by the intestinal lining, they help to break down nutrients into substances that are absorbed into the blood and carried to the liver.

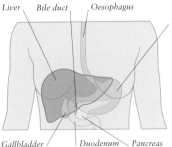

Liver
Bile duct
Oesophagus
Stomach
Gallbladder
Duodenum
Pancreas

The digestive organs
The liver, gallbladder, and pancreas, in the upper abdomen, secrete digestive juices into the duodenum. Bile from the liver and gallbladder passes down the bile duct, and pancreatic juices are released directly into the duodenum.

Peristalsis

Food is propelled along the digestive tract by a continuous sequence of muscular contractions known as peristalsis. The walls of the digestive tract are lined with smooth muscle. To move a piece of food (bolus) forwards, the muscle behind the food contracts while the muscle in front relaxes.

Peristaltic wave
To move pieces of food through the digestive tract, the muscles in the walls contract and relax in a sequence known as a peristaltic wave.

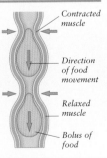

Contracted muscle
Direction of food movement
Relaxed muscle
Bolus of food

Endocrine system

The endocrine system produces hormones – chemicals that are carried in the bloodstream and control processes in other parts of the body. Such processes include metabolism (the chemical reactions constantly occurring in the body), responses to stress, growth, and sexual development.

The system comprises glands and other hormone-producing cells. Glands, such as the pituitary, adrenal, and thyroid glands, are organs whose only function is to produce specific hormones. Other organs and tissues, such as the ovaries, testes, heart, and kidneys, also contain hormone-producing cells.

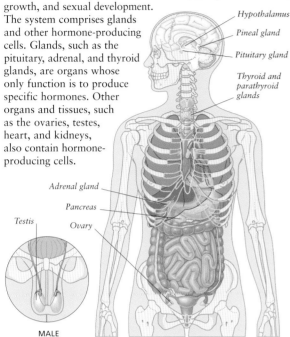

Hypothalamus
Pineal gland
Pituitary gland
Thyroid and parathyroid glands
Adrenal gland
Pancreas
Testis
Ovary

MALE

Pituitary gland and hypothalamus

The pituitary gland lies at the base of the brain. It is known as the "master gland" because it produces hormones that stimulate and control endocrine tissue in other glands and organs. It also secretes hormones that control growth, the volume of urine passed, and the contraction of the uterus during labour. The hypothalamus is a part of the brain that is linked to the pituitary gland. It secretes hormones called releasing factors that control the function of the pituitary, and also acts as a link between the nervous and endocrine systems.

Pineal gland

The pineal gland is situated deep inside the brain. Its precise function has yet to be clarified. However, the gland is known to produce a hormone called melatonin, which is thought to be associated with the daily cycle of sleep and waking.

Thyroid and parathyroid glands

The thyroid gland, in the neck, produces hormones that control metabolism. Some thyroid cells also secrete the hormone calcitonin, which lowers the blood level of calcium. The four parathyroid glands, behind the thyroid, produce a hormone that controls blood levels of calcium and phosphate. Calcium is vital for healthy bones and, with phosphate, plays an important part in nerve and muscle function.

Adrenal glands

The adrenal glands lie on top of the kidneys. Each gland has a cortex (outer layer) and a medulla (core). The cortex produces corticosteroid hormones, whose roles include helping to regulate blood levels of salt and glucose, and tiny amounts of male sex hormones, which promote the development of certain male sexual characteristics. The medulla secretes epinephrine (adrenaline) and norepinephrine (noradrenaline), which increase the heart rate and blood flow to the muscles in response to stress (a reaction called the "fight or flight response").

Pancreas

The pancreas lies behind the stomach. It produces digestive juices that help to break down food. It also releases the hormones insulin and glucagon, which play an important part in regulating the level of glucose, a sugar that forms the body's main energy source.

Ovaries

The ovaries lie on either side of the uterus. They release eggs and produce the female sex hormones progesterone and oestrogen, which regulate the menstrual cycle. Oestrogen also encourages the development of some female sexual characteristics, such as enlargement of the breasts.

Testes

The testes hang in a bag of skin and muscles called the scrotum. They produce sperm and secrete the male sex hormone testosterone. This hormone is responsible for the onset of puberty and the development of male secondary sexual characteristics, such as facial hair.

Lymphatic system

The lymphatic system consists of a network of lymph vessels that runs throughout the body, clumps of bean-shaped lymph nodes (commonly called lymph glands), the spleen, the thymus gland, and other areas of lymphatic tissue, such as Peyer's patches in the wall of the intestine. The lymphatic system helps to defend the body against infection and also to maintain the balance of body fluids.

Cervical lymph nodes
Lymph vessel
Axillary lymph nodes
Thoracic duct
Thymus gland
Spleen
Peyer's patch in intestine
Deep inguinal (groin) lymph nodes
Popliteal lymph nodes

Vessels and nodes

Lymph vessels carry a fluid called lymph around the body. Lymph helps to maintain the body's fluid balance by collecting excess fluid from the tissues and returning it to the bloodstream. It also carries white blood cells, which fight infection. Lymph nodes, situated at junctions between lymph vessels, filter infectious organisms from the lymph. They are packed with lymphocytes, a type of white blood cell. Clusters of nodes are found in many parts of the body, including the neck, armpits, and groin.

Spleen and thymus

The spleen and the thymus gland produce certain types of lymphocytes (white blood cells). These cells produce antibodies, which help to destroy infective organisms. The spleen also breaks down worn-out red blood cells.

Urinary system

The urinary system filters wastes from the blood, eliminating them together with excess water as urine. It also regulates body fluid levels and maintains the body's acid–alkali balance. The system consists of a pair of kidneys; the bladder; the ureters, which connect each kidney to the bladder; and the urethra, the tube through which urine leaves the body. The kidneys are red-brown, bean-shaped organs lying at the back of the abdomen, one on either side of the spine. They contain units called nephrons that filter the blood circulating through the kidneys and produce urine, which then passes down the ureters into the bladder. The bladder is kept closed by a ring of muscle (a sphincter) around its lower opening. This muscle can be relaxed voluntarily to allow urine to be expelled through the urethra. The male urethra is longer than the female urethra and also provides an outlet for semen (fluid that contains sperm and that is released during sexual activity). Because the female urethra is shorter and opens close to the vagina and anus, women are more prone to urinary infections than men.

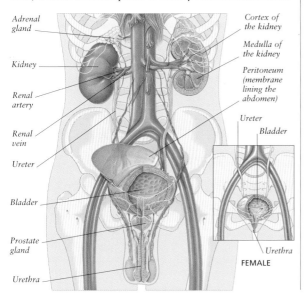

Adrenal gland

Kidney

Renal artery

Renal vein

Ureter

Bladder

Prostate gland

Urethra

Cortex of the kidney

Medulla of the kidney

Peritoneum (membrane lining the abdomen)

Ureter

Bladder

Urethra

FEMALE

Structure of the kidney

Inside the kidney, there are three regions: the cortex (outer layer), the medulla (middle layer), and the renal pelvis (inner region). The cortex contains functional units called nephrons. Each nephron consists of a glomerulus, a cluster of specialized capillaries in which the blood is filtered, and a renal tubule, through which the resulting waste fluids pass as they are turned into urine. The medulla consists of groups of urine-collecting ducts. Urine from these ducts passes into minor calyces and then into major calyces, which open into the renal pelvis. From here, the urine is funnelled into the ureter.

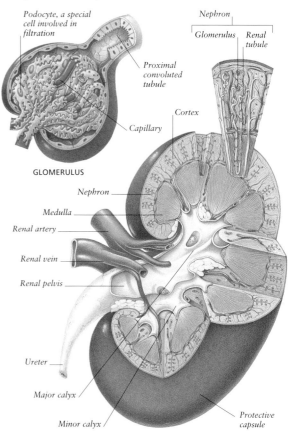

Podocyte, a special cell involved in filtration

Nephron

Glomerulus

Renal tubule

Proximal convoluted tubule

Cortex

Capillary

GLOMERULUS

Nephron

Medulla

Renal artery

Renal vein

Renal pelvis

Ureter

Major calyx

Minor calyx

Protective capsule

How urine is made

Urine is composed of substances that have been filtered from the blood in the nephrons. A kidney has about a million nephrons. Each consists of a cluster of tiny capillaries called a glomerulus and a tube called the renal tubule. This has three parts: the proximal convoluted tubule, the loop of Henle, and the distal convoluted tubule. Blood first passes through the glomerulus. The capillary walls have pores that allow water and small particles (such as salts) to pass through, while retaining larger particles, such as proteins and red blood cells. The fluid that has been removed from the blood, called filtrate, enters the renal tubule, where water, and other useful substances such as glucose and salts, are reabsorbed into the bloodstream as necessary.

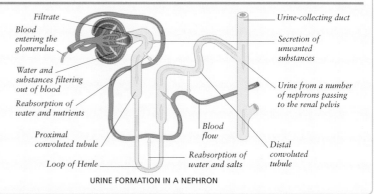

Filtrate

Blood entering the glomerulus

Water and substances filtering out of blood

Reabsorption of water and nutrients

Proximal convoluted tubule

Loop of Henle

Urine-collecting duct

Secretion of unwanted substances

Urine from a number of nephrons passing to the renal pelvis

Blood flow

Distal convoluted tubule

Reabsorption of water and salts

URINE FORMATION IN A NEPHRON

Male reproductive system

The male reproductive system produces sperm – cells that can fuse with eggs from a woman to form offspring. It also makes the male sex hormones needed for sperm production and for sexual development at puberty. The male genitals consist of the penis, the testes, and the scrotum, in which the testes are suspended. Each testis is packed with seminiferous tubules, which make sperm. The sperm are stored in the epididymis, a coiled tube that lies behind each testis. Another tube, the vas deferens, connects each epididymis to an ejaculatory duct, which in turn is connected to the urethra. Three glands – a pair of seminal vesicles and the prostate gland – secrete fluids to transport and nourish the sperm; the secretions and sperm form a fluid called semen. During sexual activity, the erectile tissue in the penis fills with blood, making the penis lengthen and stiffen in order to enter the woman's vagina. At orgasm, muscular contractions force semen along each vas deferens, down the urethra, and out of the penis.

Changes in boys during puberty

Puberty is the period during which sexual characteristics develop and sexual organs mature. In boys, puberty usually begins between the ages of about 12 and 15 and lasts for 3–4 years. The pituitary gland, at the base of the brain, starts to secrete hormones that stimulate the testes to produce the male sex hormone testosterone. This hormone stimulates changes such as enlargement of the genitals and the growth of body hair, and, later, sperm production and increased sex drive.

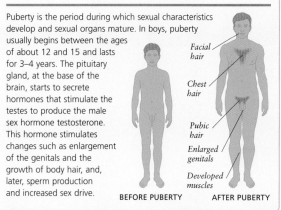

Facial hair

Chest hair

Pubic hair

Enlarged genitals

Developed muscles

BEFORE PUBERTY   AFTER PUBERTY

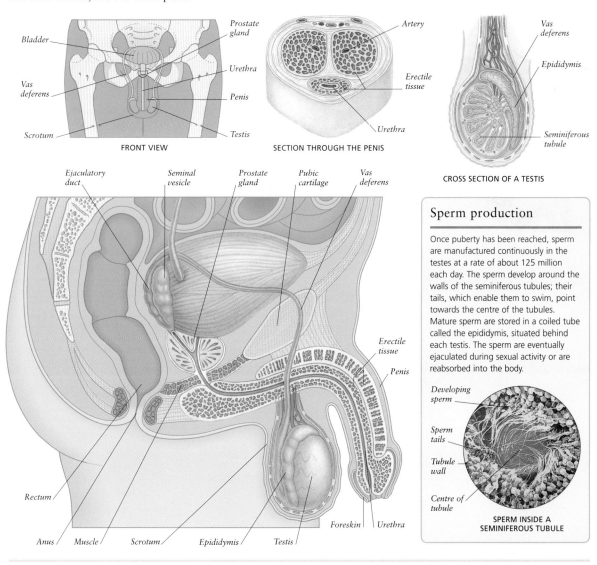

Bladder

Vas deferens

Scrotum

Prostate gland

Urethra

Penis

Testis

FRONT VIEW

Artery

Erectile tissue

Urethra

SECTION THROUGH THE PENIS

Vas deferens

Epididymis

Seminiferous tubule

CROSS SECTION OF A TESTIS

Ejaculatory duct

Seminal vesicle

Prostate gland

Pubic cartilage

Vas deferens

Erectile tissue

Penis

Rectum

Anus   Muscle   Scrotum   Epididymis   Testis

Foreskin   Urethra

Sperm production

Once puberty has been reached, sperm are manufactured continuously in the testes at a rate of about 125 million each day. The sperm develop around the walls of the seminiferous tubules; their tails, which enable them to swim, point towards the centre of the tubules. Mature sperm are stored in a coiled tube called the epididymis, situated behind each testis. The sperm are eventually ejaculated during sexual activity or are reabsorbed into the body.

Developing sperm

Sperm tails

Tubule wall

Centre of tubule

SPERM INSIDE A SEMINIFEROUS TUBULE

Female reproductive system

The internal structures of the female reproductive system – the ovaries, fallopian tubes, uterus, and vagina – lie in the lower third of the abdomen. The ovaries contain follicles that store eggs, cells that can fuse with sperm from a man to form offspring. Each month an egg matures and is released from an ovary; the fimbriae guide the egg into a fallopian tube, which propels it towards the uterus. The vagina, a passage with muscular walls, connects the uterus to the outside of the body. The external structures, collectively known as the vulva, include the sensitive clitoris and folds of skin called the labia, which protect the entrances to the vagina and the urethra. Just inside the vaginal entrance lie the Bartholin's glands, which secrete a fluid for lubrication during sexual intercourse.

Changes in girls during puberty

Puberty is the period during which sexual characteristics develop and sexual organs mature. In girls, puberty begins between the ages of about 10 and 14 and lasts for 3–4 years. The pituitary gland starts to secrete hormones that stimulate the ovaries to produce the female sex hormones oestrogen and progesterone. These hormones prompt physical changes such as enlargement of the breasts and hips and the growth of pubic and underarm hair. Later, they stimulate ovulation and menstruation.

Armpit hair
Enlarged breasts
Wider hips
Pubic hair
Thicker thighs

BEFORE PUBERTY   AFTER PUBERTY

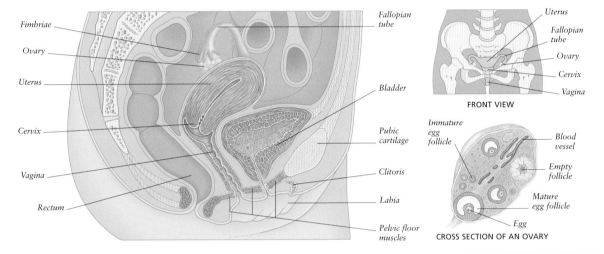

Fimbriae
Ovary
Uterus
Cervix
Vagina
Rectum

Fallopian tube
Bladder
Pubic cartilage
Clitoris
Labia
Pelvic floor muscles

Uterus
Fallopian tube
Ovary
Cervix
Vagina

FRONT VIEW

Immature egg follicle
Blood vessel
Empty follicle
Mature egg follicle
Egg

CROSS SECTION OF AN OVARY

The menstrual cycle

During the menstrual cycle, a woman's body is prepared for the possibility of pregnancy. The cycle is regulated by four sex hormones. Follicle-stimulating hormone and luteinizing hormone, which are secreted by the pituitary gland, cause an egg to mature in a follicle and be released. The egg and its follicle secrete oestrogen and progesterone, which make the uterus lining thicken. If an egg is fertilized, it embeds itself in the lining. If it is not fertilized it passes out of the body, together with blood and cells from the lining, during menstruation. The cycle lasts about 28 days but this can vary from month to month and from woman to woman.

A complete menstrual cycle
The chart shows changes that occur in the endometrium (uterus lining) and the ovary during a menstrual cycle. The egg can be fertilized by a sperm at ovulation, the time when it is released from its follicle.

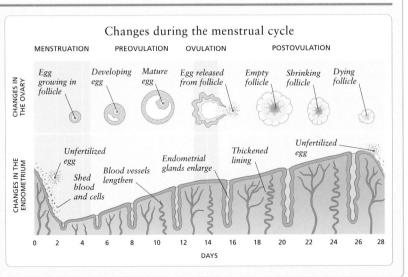

Changes during the menstrual cycle

MENSTRUATION   PREOVULATION   OVULATION   POSTOVULATION

CHANGES IN THE OVARY

Egg growing in follicle
Developing egg
Mature egg
Egg released from follicle
Empty follicle
Shrinking follicle
Dying follicle

CHANGES IN THE ENDOMETRIUM

Unfertilized egg
Shed blood and cells
Blood vessels lengthen
Endometrial glands enlarge
Thickened lining
Unfertilized egg

0   2   4   6   8   10   12   14   16   18   20   22   24   26   28
DAYS

Role of the breasts

Breasts play a part in sexual arousal, but their main role is to produce milk for babies. During puberty the hormone oestrogen causes the breasts to grow and develop. During pregnancy, hormonal changes make the breasts enlarge further and, in late pregnancy, stimulate milk production in glands called lobules. These glands are connected to ducts that lead to channels called ampullae, which open on to the surface of the nipple. The rest of the breast tissue is mostly fat, with a small amount of connective tissue, which helps to support the breasts.

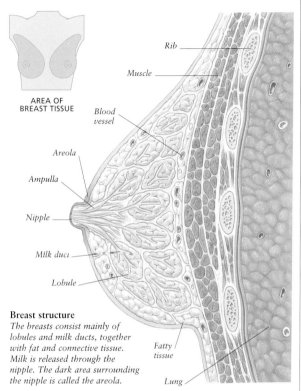

AREA OF
BREAST TISSUE

Rib

Muscle

Blood vessel

Areola

Ampulla

Nipple

Milk duct

Lobule

Fatty tissue

Lung

Breast structure
The breasts consist mainly of lobules and milk ducts, together with fat and connective tissue. Milk is released through the nipple. The dark area surrounding the nipple is called the areola.

The menopause

The menopause is the time when menstrual cycles cease. It usually occurs between the ages of 45 and 55. The ovaries stop responding to follicle-stimulating hormone and produce less of the female sex hormones oestrogen and progesterone. As a result ovulation and menstruation end, and once a woman has reached the menopause she is no longer fertile. In the years just before and after the menopause, hormone changes produce symptoms such as mood swings, hot flushes, vaginal dryness, and night sweats. The menopause may also result in long-term physical changes, such as osteoporosis.

Thin, brittle bone

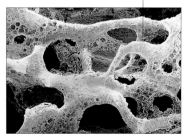

Osteoporotic bone
The sex hormone oestrogen is needed to give bones strength. Low oestrogen levels after the menopause can result in osteoporosis, a condition in which the bones lose density and may become thin and brittle, as shown in this microscopic image.

Conception and pregnancy

All organisms reproduce. In human beings, reproduction involves two types of cell: sperm, produced by the testes in men, and eggs, produced by the ovaries in women. These cells each contain half a set of DNA (genetic material). They are brought together by sexual intercourse; if a sperm penetrates and fertilizes an egg, the man's and woman's DNA combine to form new cells. Conception occurs when these cells embed themselves in the uterus. During pregnancy, which lasts for about 40 weeks (9 months), the cells develop into a baby.

Fertilization

During sexual intercourse, sperm are expelled into the woman's vagina, then swim up through the uterus and into the fallopian tubes. If the sperm meet an egg, they try to pierce its coating. If a sperm succeeds, it sheds its tail and fuses with the nucleus of the egg, while chemical changes in the egg stop any more sperm from entering. In this way a new cell is formed, combining DNA from the man and the woman.

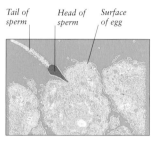

Tail of sperm   Head of sperm   Surface of egg

Sperm penetrating egg
The head of the sperm pushes through the egg's outer coating in order to reach the nucleus.

Beginning of pregnancy

The cell produced by the fusion of the egg and sperm is called a zygote. Within 2 days of fertilization, the zygote starts its journey along the fallopian tube towards the uterus, propelled by the muscular action of the tube's walls. At the same time, the zygote divides itself repeatedly to form a cluster of cells, which is called a morula. After 5–7 days, the cell cluster reaches the uterus. It embeds itself securely in the endometrium (the lining of the uterus) and continues to grow. From this moment onwards, the pregnancy is properly established. One part of the cell cluster grows into the endometrium and becomes the placenta, which will nourish the developing baby. The rest of the cells, from which the baby will grow, become an embryo.

LOCATION

A single cell called a zygote is formed if an egg fuses with a sperm

The zygote begins to divide soon after it has been formed

The cluster of dividing cells, called a morula, grows as it travels along the fallopian tube

An embryo starts to form once the cluster of cells has embedded itself in the lining of the uterus wall

Fallopian tube

An unfertilized egg is released from an ovary   Ovary

Lining of the uterus

From egg to embryo
As the cells passing along the fallopian tube divide, their number doubles every 12 hours. When the cell cluster reaches the uterus, it contains hundreds of cells. Once embedded in the uterus lining, the cells start developing into an embryo.

How the baby is nourished

An unborn baby depends on its mother to supply it with oxygen, nutrients, and antibodies against infection, and to remove its waste products. These substances pass between the mother's blood and the baby's blood inside the placenta, an organ that is attached to the uterus lining and is connected to the baby by the umbilical cord. In the placenta, the mother's and baby's blood supplies are brought close together, although they do not actually mix.

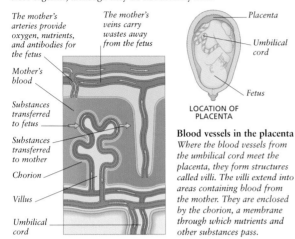

The mother's arteries provide oxygen, nutrients, and antibodies for the fetus

The mother's veins carry wastes away from the fetus

Mother's blood

Substances transferred to fetus

Substances transferred to mother

Chorion

Villus

Umbilical cord

Placenta

Umbilical cord

Fetus

LOCATION OF PLACENTA

Blood vessels in the placenta
Where the blood vessels from the umbilical cord meet the placenta, they form structures called villi. The villi extend into areas containing blood from the mother. They are enclosed by the chorion, a membrane through which nutrients and other substances pass.

The baby's development

The baby develops in a sac in the uterus. It is cushioned by amniotic fluid and nourished by blood from the umbilical cord. In the first 8 weeks, the baby is known as an embryo. During this time the limbs, head, and facial features appear, most of the organs form, and the heart begins to beat. From week 8, the baby is called a fetus. The body structures continue to develop throughout the pregnancy.

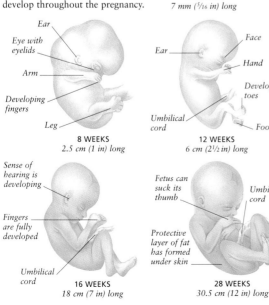

Developing head

Umbilical stalk

Developing arm

Developing leg

4 WEEKS
7 mm ($5/16$ in) long

Ear

Eye with eyelids

Arm

Developing fingers

Leg

8 WEEKS
2.5 cm (1 in) long

Ear

Face

Hand

Developing toes

Umbilical cord

Foot

12 WEEKS
6 cm ($2^{1}/_2$ in) long

Sense of hearing is developing

Fingers are fully developed

Umbilical cord

16 WEEKS
18 cm (7 in) long

Fetus can suck its thumb

Umbilical cord

Protective layer of fat has formed under skin

28 WEEKS
30.5 cm (12 in) long

Changes in the mother's body

Pregnancy is divided into three stages (trimesters), each about 3 months long. During pregnancy, the mother's body undergoes major changes. The most noticeable are the swelling of the abdomen as the baby grows and the enlargement of the breasts as they prepare to produce milk. In addition, specific changes occur in each trimester.

In the first trimester, there are few visible changes. However, the mother's heart rate increases by about 8 beats per minute in order to increase the blood circulation. Changes in hormone levels may cause symptoms such as nausea. During the second trimester, the mother may begin to experience backache due to the weight of the fetus. Her appetite may increase. By 18–20 weeks the fetus starts to make noticeable movements, producing fluttering feelings in the mother's abdomen. In the third trimester, the mother rapidly gains weight as the fetus undergoes a growth spurt. The uterus eventually becomes so large that the top reaches almost to the mother's breastbone. In the last weeks the fetus changes position so that it is lying with its head pointing downwards, ready for birth.

Mother at 12 weeks
The mother's breasts are tender and the areola (the area that surrounds the nipple) darkens. The enlarging uterus may press on the mother's bladder.

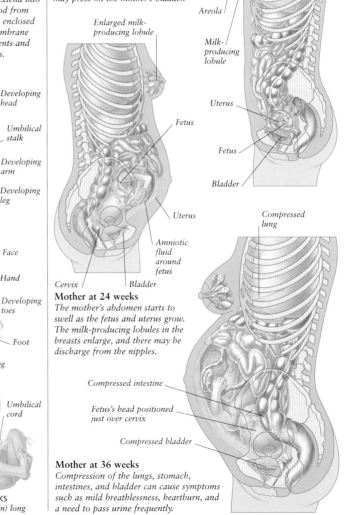

Enlarged milk-producing lobule

Areola

Milk-producing lobule

Uterus

Fetus

Fetus

Bladder

Fetus

Uterus

Amniotic fluid around fetus

Cervix

Bladder

Compressed lung

Mother at 24 weeks
The mother's abdomen starts to swell as the fetus and uterus grow. The milk-producing lobules in the breasts enlarge, and there may be discharge from the nipples.

Compressed intestine

Fetus's head positioned just over cervix

Compressed bladder

Mother at 36 weeks
Compression of the lungs, stomach, intestines, and bladder can cause symptoms such as mild breathlessness, heartburn, and a need to pass urine frequently.

The newborn baby

A newborn baby has to cope with dramatic physical changes as it leaves the total protection of the mother's uterus. In particular, the baby's body has to adapt in order to breathe air and function independently of the mother. The body systems can carry out the basic functions necessary for life, but they continue to develop and mature throughout childhood. A newborn baby also shows certain basic patterns of behaviour that aid his or her survival, such as finding the mother's breast, sucking, responding to stimuli such as noise, and crying to gain attention and care.

The skin may be blotchy. It may also be covered with a greasy substance called vernix, which protected the baby's skin in the uterus

The baby's hands may be clenched into fists

Many babies are born with hair. Premature babies may be covered with downy hair called lanugo hair, which disappears after about a month

The head may be temporarily misshapen due to pressure on the skull bones during birth. There are several soft areas called fontanelles, which are gaps between the bones

The nails may be long, and the ends may flake off by themselves

Babies born in hospital are fitted with an identification bracelet

The genitals are large in proportion to the rest of the body, and may also appear red and swollen

Right after delivery, the umbilical cord is clipped and cut to leave a small stump. The stump falls off within 10 days

The edges of the lips may develop white blisters due to vigorous sucking as the baby feeds

The eyelids are puffy. The baby can see, but only to a distance of 20–25 cm (8–10 in)

Reflex actions and movements

Babies are born with certain automatic patterns of behaviour. Some of these activities are involuntary actions, such as breathing and passing urine and faeces, and others are reflex actions, instinctive movements designed to protect and to aid survival. Some reflex actions, such as sucking and "rooting" (searching for the mother's breast), obviously aid survival. Others may be relics from a more primitive stage of human evolution; for example, the grasp reflex is thought to have originated with our ape ancestors, whose babies had to cling to their mothers as they were carried. The reflex actions, and involuntary actions such as passing urine, are eventually replaced by voluntary, controlled actions as the baby's nervous system and muscles mature. Two typical reflex responses are shown below.

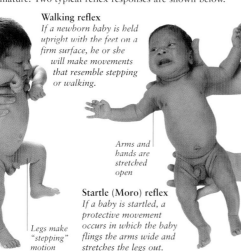

Walking reflex
If a newborn baby is held upright with the feet on a firm surface, he or she will make movements that resemble stepping or walking.

Legs make "stepping" motion

Arms and hands are stretched open

Startle (Moro) reflex
If a baby is startled, a protective movement occurs in which the baby flings the arms wide and stretches the legs out.

The heart before and after birth

In the fetus, the task of adding oxygen to the blood and filtering out waste gases is done by the placenta, but at birth the baby has to start breathing, obtaining oxygen from the lungs. Before birth, the fetus's heart pumps blood around the body and to the umbilical cord, but most of the blood bypasses the pulmonary arteries (the vessels leading to the lungs) by flowing through two special openings in the heart. With a baby's first breath the lungs expand and take in air; this triggers changes in the heart and circulation, causing the two openings in the heart to close so that all blood from the rest of the body then flows through the pulmonary arteries to the lungs to be oxygenated.

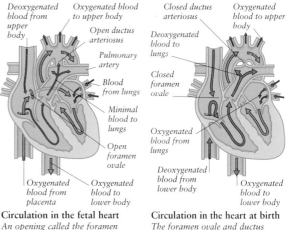

Deoxygenated blood from upper body

Oxygenated blood to upper body

Open ductus arteriosus

Pulmonary artery

Blood from lungs

Minimal blood to lungs

Open foramen ovale

Oxygenated blood from placenta

Oxygenated blood to lower body

Circulation in the fetal heart
An opening called the foramen ovale and a channel called the ductus arteriosus divert most blood away from the pulmonary arteries.

Closed ductus arteriosus

Oxygenated blood to upper body

Deoxygenated blood to lungs

Closed foramen ovale

Oxygenated blood from lungs

Deoxygenated blood from lower body

Oxygenated blood to lower body

Circulation in the heart at birth
The foramen ovale and ductus arteriosus close, so that all blood from the heart passes to the lungs to be oxygenated.

The growing child

Childhood is a time of dramatic physical, mental, and social development, during which a person grows from a dependent baby into a mature, self-sufficient individual. In addition, the child learns skills that allow him or her to interact with other people and with the environment. The rate of growth is fastest during the first year of life, and there is another period of rapid growth at puberty, the transition from childhood to adulthood. Children acquire many of the necessary physical, mental, and social skills during their first 5 years, but the learning process continues throughout life.

How bones grow and develop

At birth, much of the skeleton consists of tissue known as cartilage, with bone tissue only in the shafts of the largest bones. During childhood, the cartilage is gradually replaced by bone – a process called ossification. In the long bones of the limbs, areas called growth plates produce more cartilage to extend the bones, and this cartilage then turns to bone. By the beginning of adulthood, ossification is complete and the skeleton has reached its full size.

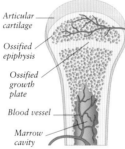

Epiphysis
Growth plate
Blood vessel
Marrow cavity
Diaphysis (shaft)

Long bone in a newborn baby
The diaphysis (shaft) is made of bone, while the epiphyses (ends) are made of cartilage.

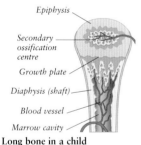

Epiphysis
Secondary ossification centre
Growth plate
Diaphysis (shaft)
Blood vessel
Marrow cavity

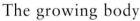

Long bone in a child
Growth and ossification (bone formation) take place in the ends of the long bone.

Articular cartilage
Ossified epiphysis
Ossified growth plate
Blood vessel
Marrow cavity

Long bone in an adult
All of the cartilage inside the bone has ossified. A layer of cartilage protects the ends of the bone.

How the skull and brain develop

A newborn baby has a full set of neurons (nerve cells), but the network of pathways between these cells is not yet mature. In the first 6 years, the brain grows and the neural (nerve) network rapidly becomes more complex, allowing a child to learn a wide range of skills and behaviour. To allow for this expansion, the cranium (the part of the skull covering the brain) grows at soft gaps called fontanelles and at seams called sutures; these areas gradually turn to bone. During the rest of childhood the brain, neural network, and skull develop at a slower rate.

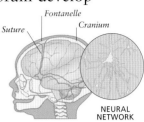

Fontanelle
Cranium
Suture

NEURAL NETWORK

Brain and skull at birth
The neural network is only partially developed. The skull bones are separated by sutures (seams) and fontanelles (soft gaps).

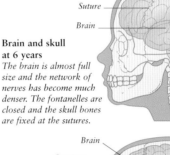

Suture
Brain

NEURAL NETWORK

Brain and skull at 6 years
The brain is almost full size and the network of nerves has become much denser. The fontanelles are closed and the skull bones are fixed at the sutures.

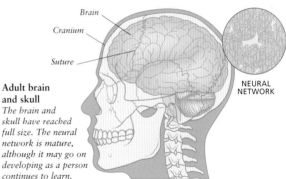

Brain
Cranium
Suture

NEURAL NETWORK

Adult brain and skull
The brain and skull have reached full size. The neural network is mature, although it may go on developing as a person continues to learn.

The growing body

Growth in childhood is controlled by hormones, and is also influenced by factors such as diet and general health. A child's body grows continuously, but the rate of growth varies depending on the stage of life: the most rapid overall growth occurs during infancy and puberty. In addition, some parts of the body develop faster than others, causing the body proportions to alter as the child grows. At birth, the head makes up about a quarter of the total body length, and until about age 6 it continues to grow quickly. The facial features change during childhood, as the face becomes larger in relation to the rest of the skull. The limbs, during infancy, are small in relation to the body and head, and lengthen as the child grows older, with especially rapid growth occurring during puberty. The body finally reaches its full size at around age 18. By this time, the head represents only about an eighth of the body length, while the legs comprise about a half.

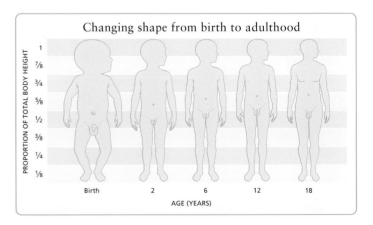

Changing shape from birth to adulthood

PROPORTION OF TOTAL BODY HEIGHT

1
7/8
3/4
5/8
1/2
3/8
1/4
1/8

Birth   2   6   12   18
AGE (YEARS)

Gaining skills during the first 5 years

Newborn babies can see, hear, perform reflex actions (such as sucking), and cry to gain their mother's attention. From birth to about age 5, young children learn a range of other essential skills. The four main areas of development are physical skills, manual dexterity, language, and social behaviour. Achievement of these skills occurs in well-recognized steps known as "developmental milestones"; these occur in a certain order and at roughly predictable times, although the exact age at which they are reached varies from one child to another. The ability to learn particular skills, such as bladder and bowel control, depends upon the maturity of the child's nervous system. In addition, before acquiring certain complex skills, children need to develop a lesser ability first; for example, babies must learn to stand before they can walk.

Physical skills
The most important skills are control of posture, balance, and movement. Babies first learn how to lift and turn their heads, then to sit up. They later learn how to crawl, stand, walk, and run.

Manual dexterity and vision
Children have to learn how to coordinate their hand movements and vision so that they can perform tasks such as picking up objects or drawing shapes.

Hearing and language
Early on, babies turn towards voices and respond to sounds by cooing. At about 1 year, children can speak their first word and begin to understand the meaning of words. They later learn to form sentences.

Social behaviour and play
The first social skill that babies master is smiling at people. They later learn to play with other children and tolerate separation from their parents. Children also acquire practical skills such as feeding and dressing themselves.

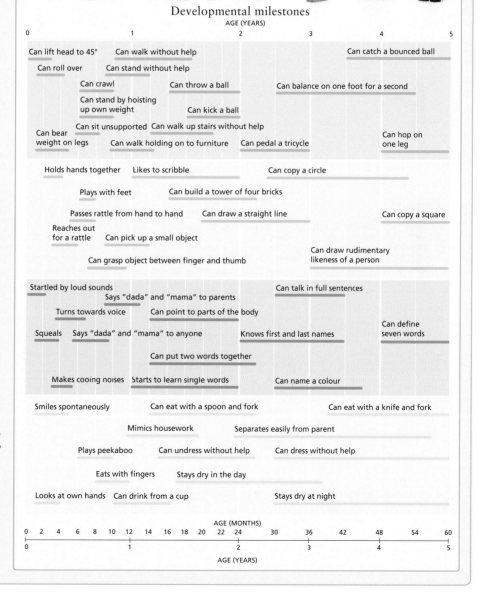

Developmental milestones

AGE (YEARS)

0 — 1 — 2 — 3 — 4 — 5

Physical skills
- Can lift head to 45°
- Can walk without help
- Can catch a bounced ball
- Can roll over
- Can stand without help
- Can crawl
- Can throw a ball
- Can balance on one foot for a second
- Can stand by hoisting up own weight
- Can kick a ball
- Can sit unsupported
- Can walk up stairs without help
- Can bear weight on legs
- Can walk holding on to furniture
- Can pedal a tricycle
- Can hop on one leg

Manual dexterity and vision
- Holds hands together
- Likes to scribble
- Can copy a circle
- Plays with feet
- Can build a tower of four bricks
- Passes rattle from hand to hand
- Can draw a straight line
- Can copy a square
- Reaches out for a rattle
- Can pick up a small object
- Can grasp object between finger and thumb
- Can draw rudimentary likeness of a person

Hearing and language
- Startled by loud sounds
- Can talk in full sentences
- Says "dada" and "mama" to parents
- Turns towards voice
- Can point to parts of the body
- Squeals
- Says "dada" and "mama" to anyone
- Knows first and last names
- Can define seven words
- Can put two words together
- Makes cooing noises
- Starts to learn single words
- Can name a colour

Social behaviour and play
- Smiles spontaneously
- Can eat with a spoon and fork
- Can eat with a knife and fork
- Mimics housework
- Separates easily from parent
- Plays peekaboo
- Can undress without help
- Can dress without help
- Eats with fingers
- Stays dry in the day
- Looks at own hands
- Can drink from a cup
- Stays dry at night

AGE (MONTHS)
0 2 4 6 8 10 12 14 16 18 20 22 24 30 36 42 48 54 60

AGE (YEARS)
0 — 1 — 2 — 3 — 4 — 5

Growth charts

Children have regular health checks during which their rate of growth is assessed. The weight and height (or, in a child under 2 years, length and head circumference), and the age, are plotted on charts with a shaded band to show the normal range of growth. There are different charts for boys and girls. Most children's measurements fall inside the band; if they fall outside, there may be a problem. You can also plot your child's growth yourself by measuring his or her height or, for babies, using measurements from the clinic.

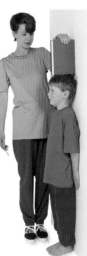

Measuring your child's height
To measure your child, ask him or her to take off his or her shoes and stand against a wall. Rest a flat object, such as a book, vertically on your child's head. Mark where the base meets the wall. Measure the distance from the mark to the floor.

Using the charts

Find your child's age on the bottom of the chart and follow a vertical line up, then find the height, head circumference, or weight on the left of the chart and follow a horizontal line across. Mark the point at which these lines cross. If you plot these points at regular intervals, the points will form a curve showing your child's growth.

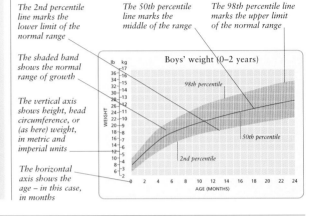

The 2nd percentile line marks the lower limit of the normal range

The 50th percentile line marks the middle of the range

The 98th percentile line marks the upper limit of the normal range

The shaded band shows the normal range of growth

The vertical axis shows height, head circumference, or (as here) weight, in metric and imperial units

The horizontal axis shows the age – in this case, in months

Children's head circumference 0–2 years

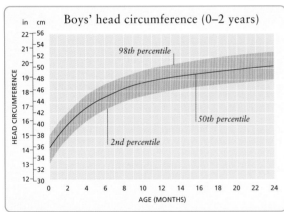

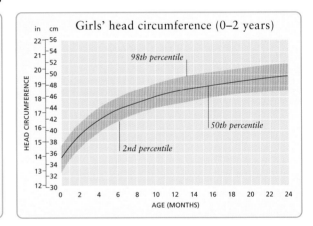

Children's weight 0–2 years

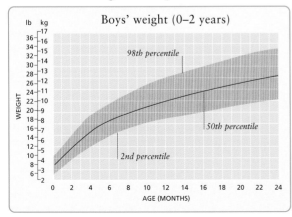

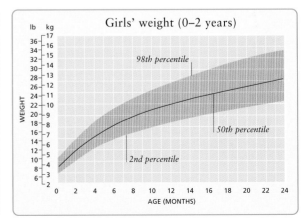

Children's length 0–2 years

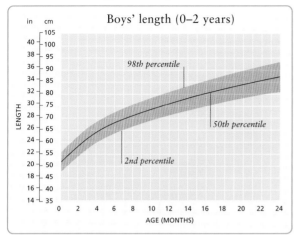

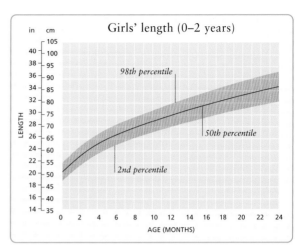

Children's weight 2–18 years

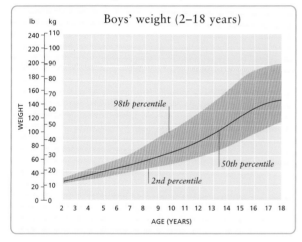

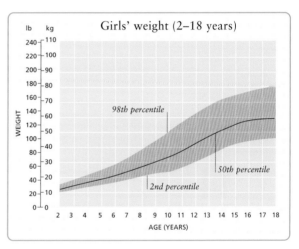

Children's height 2–18 years

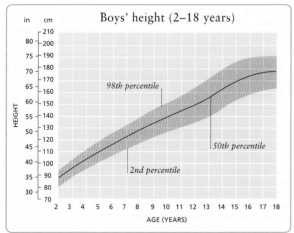

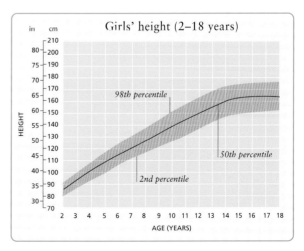

HEALTHY LIVING

A healthy diet

Diet has a major influence on health. It can affect your risk of developing many diseases; for example, a high-fat diet increases your risk of heart disease. It is also crucial in weight control. For a balanced diet you need the correct amounts of carbohydrates, fats, proteins, vitamins, and minerals. Eat plenty of high-fibre foods, limit foods with a high fat or sugar content, and avoid large amounts of salt, alcohol, and caffeine. In addition, water is vital for life, and you should aim to drink at least 8 glasses (2 litres) a day.

Meat, fish, and nuts are rich in protein, essential for building and repairing cells, and provide B vitamins and minerals such as iron. They can also be high in fat, so eat them only in moderation

Fruit and vegetables are high in fibre (which aids digestion), natural sugar, and water. Aim to eat at least five portions a day; examples of one portion include one medium-sized fruit, such as an apple, or one dessert bowl of salad

Milk and dairy foods provide protein, calcium, and certain vitamins, such as B_2, B_{12}, and D. They can form a fairly large part of your diet, but try to choose low-fat varieties so that you maintain a healthy weight

Food groups
This pie chart shows the five main food groups and their proportions in a healthy diet. Foods in the largest segments should form a greater part of your diet than those in the smaller segments.

Bread, potatoes, and pasta are high in fibre, starch, and some vitamins and minerals, so can form a large part of your diet

Limit your intake of fatty foods, which are high in energy, and sugary foods, which can cause tooth decay

Vitamins and minerals

The body requires a range of vitamins and minerals because these substances play vital roles in growth and metabolism (the chemical processes that occur in the body). Vitamins D and K can be made in the body, but the other vitamins, and all minerals, must be obtained from food. In affluent countries such as the UK, most people's diets supply the recommended daily allowances (RDAs) of vitamins and minerals, but certain people may need supplements. For example, pregnant women need extra folic acid for the health of the fetus, and vegans need extra vitamin B_{12} because they do not eat meat or other animal products (the usual source of this vitamin). You should not consume more than the recommended amounts of vitamins A, D, E, and K, because the body stores these substances and they can become toxic if excessive amounts build up in body tissues. In addition, pregnant women should avoid foods that contain high levels of vitamin A because the vitamin could have harmful effects on the developing fetus.

Good sources of vitamins and minerals

Vitamin/ mineral	Good sources	Uses in body
Vitamin A	Liver, eggs, whole milk, carrots	Important for healthy eyes, hair, skin, bones
Vitamin B_1	Meat, whole grains, peas, fortified cereals and breads	Aids release of energy from carbohydrates • Essential for proper nervous system function
Vitamin B_2	Eggs, meat, dairy products, leafy green vegetables	Involved in release of energy from food • Helps maintain nervous system and muscles
Vitamin B_3	Fish, whole grains, peanuts, peas	Aids release of energy from food • Helps maintain skin
Vitamin B_6	Meat, fish, whole grains, bananas	Needed to make blood • Aids function of nervous system
Vitamin B_{12}	Milk, fish, meat, eggs, yeast extract	Vital for blood cell growth and healthy nervous system
Vitamin C	Many fruits and vegetables	Strengthens tissues • Helps body absorb iron from food
Vitamin D	Dairy products, oily fish; also formed in skin by sunlight	Enhances calcium absorption for strong teeth and bones
Vitamin E	Vegetables, eggs, fish, margarine	Protects against degenerative disease
Vitamin K	Leafy green vegetables, pigs' liver; also formed by intestinal bacteria	Essential for proper blood clotting • Necessary for bone formation
Folic acid	Leafy green vegetables, organ meats, whole grains, fortified bread, nuts	Helps prevent neural tube defects (which can result in spina bifida) in fetuses • Helps maintain healthy cells and blood
Calcium	Tofu, fish with edible bones, dairy products, peas, beans	Needed for healthy bones, teeth, muscles • Aids conduction of nerve impulses
Iron	Eggs, meat, leafy green vegetables, pulses, fortified cereals	Aids formation of red blood cells and some proteins • Maintains healthy muscles

Assessing your weight

To avoid diseases associated with being overweight or underweight, you need to maintain your weight within the range considered normal for your height. To find out if you are within this range, you can use a height and weight chart such as the one shown below. You can also assess your weight by calculating your body mass index (BMI). To do this, divide your weight in kilograms by the square of your height in metres. A BMI figure under 20 indicates that you are underweight, while a figure over 25 shows that you are overweight.

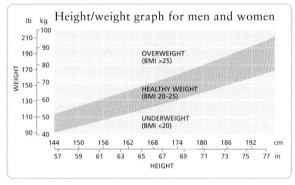

Height/weight graph for men and women

Exercise

Most people know that exercise is an important part of a healthy lifestyle. Regular exercise protects physical and mental health. It can also reduce your risk of developing long-term disease, increase your life expectancy, and improve your quality of life in later years. When you make exercise a part of your daily routine, you will probably find that you have a lot more energy for ordinary daily activities such as shopping, housework, child care, and gardening.

How exercise benefits health

Regular exercise benefits most of the body's systems, especially the cardiovascular, musculoskeletal, and respiratory systems. It can also benefit mental health by providing pleasure, reducing stress, and producing physical changes that improve mood.

The supply of blood to the brain is increased, thus promoting mental alertness, and chemical changes occur that improve mood

Blood pressure is reduced, and this decrease helps to lower the risk of cardiovascular disease

The heart becomes stronger and can pump more blood with every heartbeat

The lungs can take in more oxygen from each breath and supply more oxygen to the body

Muscles become stronger and more efficient so that they can work for longer periods of time

Joints become stronger and more flexible and mobile as a result of exercise

Bones maintain their strength and density so that they are less prone to damage and disease

Planning an exercise routine

For exercise to be beneficial, it has to be regular. The recommended amount is at least 30 minutes of moderate exercise, such as a brisk walk, on at least 5 days of the week. To become fitter or lose weight, you will have to exercise harder. You need to do activities that work the heart and lungs (build stamina), improve joint mobility (increase flexibility), and increase muscle strength. If you have never exercised regularly before, or if you have any health concerns, consult your doctor before starting an exercise routine.

Fitness benefits of different activities

Activity	Fitness benefits		
	Stamina	Flexibility	Strength
Aerobics	★★★★	★★★	★★
Basketball	★★★★	★★★	★★
Cycling (fast)	★★★★	★★	★★★
Climbing stairs	★★★	★	★★★
Dancing (aerobic)	★★★	★★★★	★
Golf	★	★★	★
Hiking	★★★	★	★★
Jogging	★★★★	★★	★★
Swimming	★★★★	★★★★	★★★★
Tennis	★★	★★★	★★
Walking (briskly)	★★	★	★
Yoga	★	★★★★	★

KEY

★ Small effect	★★ Good effect	★★★ Very good effect	★★★★ Excellent effect

Exercising safely

To avoid overexertion or injury, start by setting realistic goals. If you are not fit, begin exercising slowly and build up gradually. Take care not to overexert yourself so that you are in pain or feel ill. Make sure that you use the correct protective equipment, clothing, and footwear for your sport. Every time you exercise, start with a warming-up routine and finish with a cooling-down routine to prevent muscle cramps and stiffness and minimize the risk of injury. These types of routine involve gentle aerobic exercise, such as slow jogging, followed by a series of movements to stretch your muscles. Two typical stretches are shown here.

Keep your back straight while you move your hips

Rest your hands on your knee to steady yourself

Hip and thigh stretch
Kneel, then put one foot on the floor in front of you. Push your hips down and forwards to stretch the back thigh. Repeat for the other thigh.

Lower back stretch
Kneel, sitting on your heels. Stretch your arms above your head, bend forwards, and put your hands on the floor. Keep your arms, head, and body aligned.

Exercising at different ages

Most people, whatever their age, can derive physical and mental benefits from exercise. Apart from the overall improvements to your flexibility, strength, and stamina, exercise has different benefits for people at different stages of life. In children, it helps to build strong bones and muscles, improves coordination, and can also be fun. In adults, exercise helps to minimize the risk of heart disease. In older people, it helps to slow processes associated with aging, such as loss of bone density, and enables people to stay mobile for longer. Regular exercise can also enable pregnant women to cope better with the demands of pregnancy and childbirth.

Activities for children
Games such as football can improve physical aspects such as strength, balance, and coordination. Such games can also be fun and enable children to make new friends with the other players.

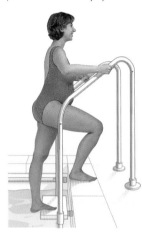

Pregnant women
During pregnancy, gentle swimming can allow you to stretch and exercise your muscles while the water supports your weight.

Older people
Activities such as walking can help to lessen the effects of aging by maintaining your bone and muscle strength and joint flexibility.

Alcohol

Alcohol is a drug that alters your mental and physical state. It can make you feel relaxed and happy; for this reason, it has been used socially for centuries. However, in excess, alcohol may cause physical, psychological, and social problems.

Harmful effects of alcohol

Although moderate alcohol consumption makes you feel relaxed and can have some health benefits, long-term, excessive drinking can cause serious health problems. Alcohol is absorbed into the blood through the stomach and small intestine, reaching its maximum concentration after 35–45 minutes. This level depends on various factors. One is weight: small, light people become intoxicated more easily than heavy people. Another is the drinker's sex. Women become intoxicated faster than men, and women's bodies are less efficient at breaking down alcohol. Another factor is whether or not you drink with food; if you drink alcohol with food, your body will absorb it at a slower rate.

Alcohol is broken down by the liver at an average rate of about 1 unit per hour (*see* SAFE ALCOHOL LIMITS, below). Your body cannot alter this rate, so the more you drink, the longer it takes for your body to break down the alcohol. If you drink heavily at night, you may still be intoxicated the next morning. This situation can be dangerous if you plan to drive a vehicle or operate machinery.

In the short term, excessive drinking can cause intoxication and hangovers. In the longer term, alcohol damages most body systems. Regular, excessive drinking can also lead to alcohol dependence and social problems such as domestic violence.

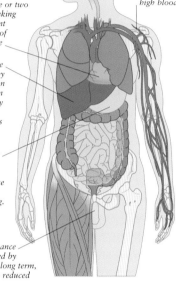

The brain's control of inhibitions and coordination is impaired by alcohol. Long-term drinking damages brain cells that control learning and memory

The heart may be protected against disease by one or two drinks a day, but drinking more than this amount will increase the risk of cardiovascular disease

The liver may become inflamed (hepatitis) by excessive consumption of alcohol. Long-term drinking can seriously damage the liver and cause diseases such as cirrhosis and cancer

The stomach and the duodenum (the first part of the small intestine) may become ulcerated as a result of long-term drinking. In addition, stomach cancer is a risk

Sexual performance may be impaired by alcohol. In the long term, fertility may be reduced

Drinking alcohol makes the blood vessels in the skin widen, causing the body to lose heat. Long-term drinking raises the risk of high blood pressure

Safe alcohol limits

To drink alcohol safely, you should limit your intake. Alcohol consumption is measured in units. Current UK government guidelines state that, in general, men should drink no more than 3–4 units a day, and women no more than 2–3 units. Try to keep within these limits and have at least one or two alcohol-free days a week. The volume of a drink containing 1 unit depends on the percentage of alcohol by volume (abv). The higher the abv, the smaller the volume equivalent to 1 unit. The box below shows a selection of alcoholic drinks, each equal to 1 unit. Measures served at home or in bars may be larger than those shown here.

Volume of drink equal to 1 unit of alcohol

HALF A PINT OF BEER
(250 ml/10fl oz; abv 3.5–4%)

SMALL GLASS OF WINE
(75 ml/3 fl oz; abv 13%)

SMALL GLASS OF SHERRY
(50 ml/2 fl oz; abv 20%)

SINGLE MEASURE OF A SPIRIT
(25ml/1 fl oz; abv 40%)

Tobacco

Tobacco is most commonly smoked in cigarettes but can also be smoked in cigars and pipes, inhaled as snuff, or chewed. However it is used, tobacco is harmful to health. In the UK, smoking is one of the main causes of death in people under the age of 65. Smoking also damages the health of "passive smokers", who inhale other people's smoke. The only way to avoid these health risks is to avoid smoking or coming into contact with other people's smoke.

Health hazards of smoking

Tobacco smoke contains many substances damaging to health, such as tar, carbon monoxide, and nicotine. Tar irritates the airways; carbon monoxide attaches itself to red blood cells, reducing their ability to carry oxygen; and nicotine is addictive. Tobacco smoke also contains cancer-causing substances that can harm the lungs and other organs.

Inhaling smoke from smokers' cigarettes and exhalations is known as passive smoking. The smoke can irritate the eyes, nose, and throat. In the long term, it may cause lung cancer and cardiovascular disease. In children, exposure to smoke increases the risk of infections, such as ear infections, and can trigger asthma and allergies. Babies born to mothers who smoke are likely to be smaller than average and at greater risk of sudden infant death syndrome (cot death).

Mouth and tongue cancers may be caused by irritants in smoke

The airways to the lungs are irritated by smoke. In the long term, smoke can cause disorders such as lung cancer and emphysema

The pharynx (throat) and larynx (voice box) may develop cancer due to smoking

The risk of cardiovascular disease is increased by smoking

Smoke can irritate the stomach lining, leading to ulcers. Long-term smoking may cause stomach cancer

Bladder cancer may result from smoking

Cancer of the cervix may develop as a result of smoking

FEMALE

Smoking and lung cancer

Smoking has been identified as the single most significant cause of preventable disease and early death in the UK. One of the main hazards associated with the habit is lung cancer; the vast majority of cases are caused by smoking, and the disease has a very low survival rate. Lung cancer is the leading cause of cancer-related death in men. It is also now the main cause of such deaths in women, resulting in more deaths than breast cancer. The more cigarettes a person smokes each day, the younger he or she starts, and the longer he or she is a smoker, the higher the risk of developing lung cancer. However, giving up can have significant health benefits, even for people who have been smoking for many years. Within 10–15 years of stopping, a former smoker's risk of developing lung cancer will be only slightly greater than the risk for a non-smoker.

Giving up smoking

You can help to prevent heart or lung disease by not smoking or by giving up before you begin to develop the diseases. No matter how long you have been smoking, you can prevent further damage to your health by giving up. If you need help in giving up, consult your doctor for advice. If you want to try on your own, list the reasons why you want to stop smoking, then work out the reasons why you smoke. Plan ways to cope with temptation and ask your family and friends for support. Telephone helplines staffed by ex-smokers can be helpful. Choose a fairly stress-free day on which to stop smoking completely and throw away cigarettes, lighters, and ashtrays. You may have withdrawal symptoms, such as irritability, and crave nicotine. Aids such as nicotine patches or gum can help to stop cravings. If you relapse, work out why it has happened, refer to your reasons for giving up, and try again.

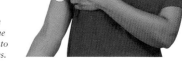

Nicotine patch in place

Using a nicotine patch
Nicotine patches deliver a constant supply of nicotine through the skin, helping to stop cravings for cigarettes.

Drugs

A drug is any chemical that alters the function of an organ or a biochemical process in the body. Drugs that are used to improve body functions or to treat diseases and disorders are known as medicines. Certain drugs, such as the sleeping drug temazepam, may be both used as medicines and abused for recreation. Other drugs, such as ecstasy, have no medicinal value and are used only for recreational purposes. Drug abuse can cause serious physical and mental problems, particularly if the abuser becomes dependent on a drug or takes an overdose, and may even cause death. In addition, the use of recreational drugs is illegal.

Effects of drug use on the body

People use recreational drugs to alter their mood. The main types of drug are classified according to the usual mood change that they cause, but often they have a mixture of effects. Stimulants, such as cocaine, increase mental and physical activity; relaxants, such as marijuana and heroin, produce a feeling of calm; intoxicants, such as glue, make users feel giggly and dreamy; and hallucinogens, such as lysergic acid diethylamine (LSD), alter perception and cause hallucinations (seeing or hearing things that do not exist).

Extreme reactions and risks of drugs

Drugs pose serious health risks. Overdoses of drugs such as heroin and cocaine can be fatal; other drugs, such as ecstasy, can also cause death. Some drugs affect vital functions; for example, heroin can slow breathing and heart rate. In addition, extreme reactions or adverse interactions with substances such as alcohol may occur. Another common effect is dependence, a condition in which users experience physical and mental cravings when they do not take a drug. Some problems may arise soon after taking a drug (even for the first time); others are associated with long-term abuse. Injected drugs carry additional risks associated with the use of nonsterile needles, such as HIV infection, hepatitis B or C, or blood poisoning. If you or someone close to you abuses drugs, ask your doctor for information on health risks and advice on counselling and treatment.

Sex and health

Puberty, when the body makes the change from childhood to adulthood, prepares you physically for sexual activity and reproduction. The development of emotional maturity often takes much longer, and involves both learning about yourself and gaining experience in dealing with other people.

Sex can be an intensely pleasurable experience that boosts the feeling of wellbeing. In addition, regular sex can improve cardiovascular fitness and help prolong life. However, you should be aware of the health risks of sex, such as unwanted pregnancy and diseases, called sexually transmitted infections (STIs), that are spread only or mainly by sexual intercourse.

Sexual relationships

Sexual fulfilment depends on a blend of physical and psychological factors, and what is right for one person or couple may not suit another. You and your partner should be happy with the frequency of sexual activity, and should be able to discuss which activities you enjoy or find unappealing. Anyone in a relationship should be aware of sexually transmitted infections (STIs) and understand how to minimize the risk of exposure to such conditions by practising safe sex (below). In addition, to avoid an unwanted pregnancy, you should be familiar with the options for contraception (see CONTRACEPTION CHOICES FOR MEN, p.250, and CONTRACEPTION CHOICES FOR WOMEN, p.272).

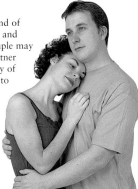

Physical and emotional benefits
Good sexual relationships fulfil both partners' needs for comfort and closeness as well as satisfying their physical desires.

It is common to experience a temporary lack of sexual desire or inability to perform sexually (see LOW SEX DRIVE IN MEN, p.246, and LOW SEX DRIVE IN WOMEN, p.268). Such problems are often due to stress or emotional difficulties, or to the use of alcohol, recreational drugs, or certain medications. Disorders such as diabetes mellitus can cause longer-term sexual problems. It is important to discuss concerns with your partner. Talk to your doctor if the problem is persistent.

Practising safe sex

Sexually transmitted infections (STIs) are usually spread by contact with infected skin or body fluids such as semen, blood, and vaginal secretions. Many STIs are uncomfortable but fairly minor problems, but some, such as HIV infection, are life-threatening. You can take simple steps to protect yourself. If you have sex with someone whom you do not know to be free of infection, use a condom, which gives protection against most STIs (apart from genital warts and pubic lice, which can affect body areas that are not covered by a condom). If you develop an STI, you should avoid sexual activity until you have been treated and are free of infection.

Stress

Stress is a physical or mental demand that provokes certain responses in us, allowing us to meet challenges or escape from danger. A moderate amount of stress can improve your performance in situations such as sports and work, but excessive stress can harm your health. You can minimize harmful stress by identifying situations that you find stressful and developing ways to cope with them.

Stress ratings of different life events

Very high	High
Death of a spouse	Retirement
Divorce or marital separation	Serious illness of family member
Personal injury or illness	Pregnancy
Loss of job	Change of job
Moving house	Death of close friend

Moderate	Low
Big mortgage	Change in work conditions
Legal action over debt	Change in schools
Trouble with in-laws	Small mortgage or loan
Spouse begins or stops work	Change in eating habits
Trouble with boss	Christmas or other holidays

Sources of stress

Stress may result from external events or circumstances, your personal reactions to pressure, or a combination of these factors. Major external sources of stress include long-term problems, such as an unhappy relationship, debilitating illness, or unemployment; major changes, even desirable ones, such as marriage or moving house; and a build-up of everyday stresses, such as being late for work or getting caught in a traffic jam. Behaviour patterns that cause or aggravate stress include impatience and aggression, lack of confidence, and suppressing feelings of tension or anxiety.

Recognizing signs of stress

If signs of stress are recognized early, action can be taken to prevent health problems. These signs may include having less energy than usual, a reduced appetite, or eating more than you do normally. You may have headaches, mouth ulcers, or be unusually susceptible to minor infections, such as colds. If you feel very stressed, you may be anxious, tearful, irritable, or low in spirits. Sleep may be disrupted, and relationships may suffer. To distract yourself, you may rely on alcohol, tobacco, or drugs. If stress is causing any of these problems, seek help from your family, friends, or doctor.

Making lifestyle changes

If your lifestyle is stressful, try to minimize the harmful effects that stress may cause. Find time to keep up with your family and friends, and take up leisure activities. Exercising regularly can help to relieve physical tension, as may learning to relax your body consciously (see RELAXATION EXERCISES, below). Break stressful tasks down into small, easy parts. Concentrate on important tasks and limit the number of less urgent ones to conserve your time and energy. If people make heavy demands on you, try to set limits on these demands.

Relaxation exercises

If you are under stress, your muscles tighten, the heart beats more rapidly, and breathing becomes fast and shallow. Relax both your mind and body by learning simple relaxation routines that slow down your body's stress responses. The breathing technique shown here may help to reduce stress. For more information, ask your doctor if he or she can recommend any relaxation classes.

Breathing to relax
Breathe slowly and deeply, using your diaphragm and abdominal muscles. Rest one hand on your chest and one on your abdomen: the lower hand should move more than the upper one.

PROFESSIONAL HEALTHCARE

Healthcare throughout life

Looking after your health involves not only following a healthy lifestyle but also making effective use of the healthcare system. Doctors and other professional healthcare workers provide treatment when you are ill and are also involved in some important elements of preventive healthcare. These include health education, checkups during childhood and later in life, screening tests to identify risk factors and early signs of disease, and immunizations to help prevent certain infectious diseases. To get the most from what professional healthcare has to offer, you need to be aware of the options for you and your family and to learn how to make the best use of the services that doctors and other healthcare professionals can provide.

Healthcare providers

Most disorders can be diagnosed and treated by general practitioners (GPs). GP practices provide a range of services, including antenatal care and clinics for immunizations and for minor surgery such as wart removal. Some large practices also have other healthcare providers including practice nurses, dentists, physiotherapists, and some practitioners of complementary therapy, such as osteopaths. In addition, the NHS helpline, NHS Direct, provides advice on health by telephone or on the internet (see USEFUL ADDRESSES, p.285).

The usual way to obtain hospital care is by referral from a GP. However, if you have a severe accident or a serious problem such as heavy bleeding, you should go straight to an accident and emergency department in a hospital for treatment. If your injury or symptoms are not severe, you should consider waiting to see your GP or contact NHS Direct. Hospital clinics for the treatment of sexually transmitted infections, called genito-urinary medicine (GUM) clinics, are also run on the basis of self-referral.

Choosing a doctor

If you are looking for a new GP, you can obtain a list of doctors in your area from your Patient & Public Involvement (PPI) forum or local library; you could also ask friends and neighbours for recommendations. When you find a likely practice, ask about their opening hours and how long, on average, you will have to wait for an appointment that is not urgent. In addition, ask whether the practice offers services provided by other healthcare professionals such as nurses, and special services, such as family planning clinics and clinics for people with diabetes or asthma. You may also wish to ask if you can choose a female doctor rather than a male doctor (or vice versa), if you have a strong preference in this matter.

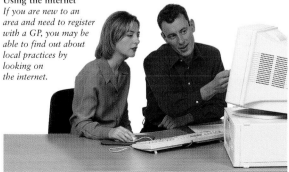

Using the internet
If you are new to an area and need to register with a GP, you may be able to find out about local practices by looking on the internet.

Visiting your doctor

Before your first appointment with a new doctor, you may be asked to fill in a questionnaire about your health and lifestyle. On your first visit, your doctor will ask further questions and check if you are up to date with immunizations and screening. During later visits, the doctor will add notes to your medical records, which are transferred if you change to another GP. You have the right to see your own or your child's records. During a visit, do not hesitate to ask questions about your health and treatments. Most appointments last 7–10 minutes.

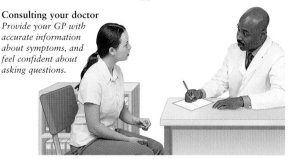

Consulting your doctor
Provide your GP with accurate information about symptoms, and feel confident about asking questions.

Your medical history

When you first visit a doctor, you will be questioned about your present and past health; treatments that you are having or have had; disorders that could run in your family; and aspects of your lifestyle, such as diet and exercise. The information gathered from these questions is known as a medical history. If you then visit your doctor with a disorder or unexplained symptoms, your medical history can help him or her to reach a diagnosis. In addition, if there is evidence that you are at risk of developing certain disorders, your doctor will suggest preventive measures or screening to detect early signs.

Having a physical examination

When you see your doctor, you may have a physical examination to assess your state of health, look for abnormalities, or confirm or rule out a diagnosis. The examination usually begins with a check of external areas, such as the eyes, ears, skin, and nails, and a test of nervous reflexes. In some cases, the doctor can gather information about other areas apart from the one being examined; for example, a pale-coloured tongue may be a sign of anaemia. He or she may also check for abnormalities by listening to organs with a stethoscope (auscultation), by feeling (palpation), or by tapping areas and listening to the sounds produced (percussion).

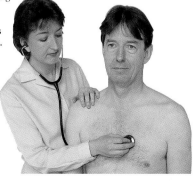

Listening to the chest
The doctor uses a stethoscope to listen to sounds within the chest, such as those made by the heart and lungs. A stethoscope is also used to listen to sounds made by the intestines or by blood flowing through vessels.

Health checks and screening

Health checks provide an opportunity to discuss with your doctor or health visitor your or your child's general health. In the UK, children are offered routine checks that focus on healthy growth and development. In adults, health checks usually are given after registering with a new doctor, for insurance purposes, or when starting a new job. In addition, pregnant women and those with a long-term illness, such as diabetes mellitus, are offered regular checks. Health checks for adults usually involve a physical examination (p.33) and basic screening, such as blood pressure measurement. Screening is important in preventing disease by looking for factors that increase the risk of disease and in detecting disease at an early stage when there is the greatest chance of treatment being successful. In some cases, screening may also be used to detect a rare inherited disease that may affect you or your children. Some tests may only be appropriate at certain ages: for example, newborn babies are screened for certain metabolic disorders; and women between the ages of 25 and 65 need regular cervical smear tests, which are used to screen for possible signs of cervical cancer.

Screening babies and children

In the uterus, babies may be tested for genetic disorders such as Down's syndrome. Immediately after birth, a baby's appearance and responses are checked for abnormalities, and a few days later, a blood sample is taken from the heel to look for hypothyroidism (underactivity of the thyroid gland) and phenylketonuria (a metabolic defect that can cause brain damage). In early childhood, the acquisition of certain skills, known as developmental milestones, is monitored (see GAINING SKILLS DURING THE FIRST 5 YEARS, p.25), and, throughout childhood, growth is checked (see GROWTH CHARTS, pp.26–27). Children should also have regular eye and ear tests (see VISION TESTING IN CHILDREN, p.97, and HEARING TESTS IN CHILDHOOD, p.101).

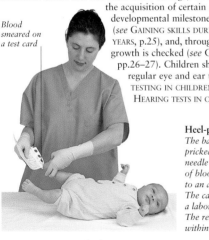

Blood smeared on a test card

Heel-prick test
The baby's heel is pricked with a small needle and a few drops of blood are smeared on to an absorbent card. The card is then sent to a laboratory for analysis. The results are available within a week or two.

Screening adults

Some screening tests are offered to adults at stages of life when the risk of certain diseases increases. For example, screening for early signs of breast cancer and cancer of the cervix is offered on the NHS to women in specific age groups (see COMMON SCREENING TESTS, right). Screening tests for other cancers, such as colorectal cancer and prostate cancer, are available, but these tests are not yet offered as part of national screening programmes in the UK. One of the most common screening tests is blood pressure measurement. Usually, high blood pressure, or hypertension, does not produce symptoms but is a major risk factor for heart disease and stroke. Other screening tests that are offered to adults include tests to check

blood cholesterol levels, which also affect your risk of heart disease and stroke, and eye pressure measurement, to check for glaucoma, a disorder that may cause blindness if left untreated. People with long-term disorders are usually offered regular screening to detect early signs of complications. For example, people with diabetes mellitus have regular screening for kidney disease, cardiovascular disorders, nerve damage, and problems in the blood vessels of the eye, which left untreated may lead to blindness.

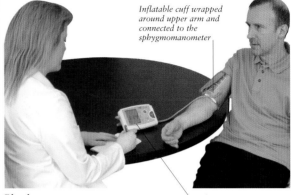

Inflatable cuff wrapped around upper arm and connected to the sphygmomanometer

Blood pressure measurement
To measure blood pressure, the doctor uses a sphygmomanometer. An inflatable cuff is wrapped around your upper arm. The cuff inflates and deflates automatically, then the device shows your blood pressure and pulse.

Sphygmomanometer has a digital display giving readings for both blood pressure and pulse rate

Common screening tests

Test	When recommended	What it screens for
Heel-prick test (left); a blood sample is taken from the baby's heel	Soon after birth	Hypothyroidism (an underactive thyroid gland) and phenylketonuria (a rare metabolic disorder)
Blood pressure measurement (above)	Every 5 years from about the age of 20	Hypertension (high blood pressure)
Blood cholesterol test; involves giving a blood sample for analysis	Recommended only for people who have risk factors for, or family history of, coronary artery disease	High blood cholesterol
Cervical smear test (p.260); a sample of cells is scraped from the cervix (neck of the womb)	Every 3–5 years for women between the ages of 25 and 65	Precancerous changes in cells of the cervix or cancer of the cervix
Faecal occult blood test; involves providing a sample of faeces for testing	Every year from age 50 for people at greater than normal risk of colorectal cancer; from 2006, will be available nationally for people aged 60–69	Colorectal cancer
Mammography (p.253); an X-ray of the breasts is taken	Every 3 years for women between the ages of 50 and 70	Breast cancer
Screening for glaucoma (p.184); the pressure inside the eye is measured	Every 2 years from the age of 40, or possibly more frequently if there is a family history of glaucoma	Glaucoma

Immunization

Immunization protects you from infectious disease for several months or years, or even for life. It can be conferred by using either vaccines or immunoglobulins. A vaccine contains a tiny amount of either a killed or modified infectious organism or a modified toxin (poison produced by bacteria). Once inside the body, the vaccine stimulates the immune system to make antibodies, proteins that help to destroy the organism or toxin if encountered in the body. Most vaccines involve several injections over a period of months or years to build up adequate protection. Immunoglobulins contain antibodies taken from the blood of a person or animal who is immune to a certain infection and give useful short-term protection. Immunizations may have side effects, such as mild fever. However, serious side effects are extremely rare.

Routine immunizations

Most routine immunizations are given during infancy and childhood according to an immunization schedule (below). The immunization schedule begins shortly after birth because it is important to protect babies against infectious diseases that may be life-threatening in infancy. You should keep records of all your immunizations and those of your children in case a doctor other than your GP needs to know about your immune status.

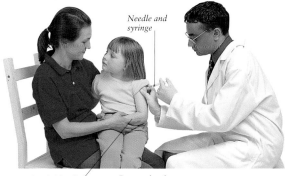

Needle and syringe

Arm held still during injection

Immunization
Immunizations are given by injection. Many are given in two or more doses over a period of several weeks or months.

Routine immunization schedule

Disease	Timing of immunization						
	Age (months)				Age (years)		
	2	3	4	12–15	3–5	10–14	13–18
Diphtheria*	✓	✓	✓		✓		✓
Tetanus*	✓	✓	✓		✓		✓
Pertussis*	✓	✓	✓		✓		
Poliomyelitis*	✓	✓	✓		✓		✓
Haemophilus influenzae type b (Hib)*	✓	✓	✓				
Meningitis C (Meningococcus C)	✓	✓	✓				
Measles, mumps, rubella (MMR)				✓	✓		
Tuberculosis (BCG)						✓	

*Given as one vaccine at indicated times

Immunizations for adults

Most immunizations give long-term protection from a disease, but in certain cases people may need a repeat dose known as a booster. For example, you need a booster immunization for tetanus if you sustain a dirty or deep wound; the bacterium responsible for this disease is very common in the environment and you are at risk of infection following this type of injury. In addition, make sure that you have been immunized for poliomyelitis if you missed out in childhood. Immunizations are often given to adults who are travelling to areas where certain diseases are common (*see* TRAVEL IMMUNIZATIONS, below) or if there is a high risk of an infectious disease for health or work reasons (*see* IMMUNIZATIONS FOR SPECIAL CASES, below).

Travel immunizations

The immunizations that you need before travelling depend on your destination, state of health, and current immune status, and the duration, type, and purpose of your travel. If you are planning to travel, make sure that you have been immunized against tetanus and poliomyelitis, and have booster doses if necessary. Most countries do not require visitors to have specific immunizations, but some may ask for a certificate showing that you have been immunized for yellow fever, a viral infection that can cause severe jaundice. Consult your doctor or local travel clinic about necessary immunizations at least 8 weeks before you travel because some immunizations require more than one dose to become effective. The table below shows the most common travel immunizations. Advice on immunizations for foreign travel changes frequently; always obtain current information.

Common travel immunizations

Disease	Dosage	Destination
Diphtheria	1 injection	Former USSR or developing countries
Hepatitis A	2 injections 6–12 months apart	Mediterranean countries (long stays) or developing countries
Hepatitis B	3 injections over 6 months, at least 4 weeks apart	Countries where hepatitis B is prevalent; necessary if you may need medical or dental treatment in such countries, or if you are likely to have unprotected sex
Japanese B encephalitis	2–3 injections 1–2 weeks apart	Rural areas of the Indian subcontinent, China, Southeast Asia, and the Far East; necessary if you plan an extended stay in any of these areas
Meningitis A and C	1 injection	Saudi Arabia (immunization certificate needed for Muslim pilgrims travelling to Mecca), remote areas of Sub-Saharan Africa, Nepal
Rabies	3 injections over 4 weeks	Areas where rabies is endemic; necessary if you will be working with animals or travelling in remote areas
Typhoid	1 injection	Areas with poor sanitation
Yellow fever	1 injection	Parts of Africa and South America

Immunizations for special cases

In some circumstances, specific groups of people may need to be given immunizations that are not normally offered to most people. These immunizations are usually offered because these groups are at increased risk of developing a serious illness if they become infected. For example, immunizations against influenza and pneumococcal pneumonia are commonly given to people over the age of 65; to those who have reduced immunity, such as people with diabetes mellitus, HIV infection, or AIDS; and to those with long-term heart or lung disease. In addition, some people may need immunization if their type of work puts them at increased risk of an infectious disease. For example, people who work with animals may need to be vaccinated against the virus that causes rabies.

MEDICAL TESTS

Testing samples

Tests that are carried out on samples of body fluids, such as blood or urine, are often the first investigations requested by a doctor before making or confirming a diagnosis. Samples of urine and faeces can usually be collected easily by the patient, and blood samples by the doctor in his or her surgery. Some samples, such as cell and tissue samples and certain body fluids, may need to be collected during a hospital procedure. The results of tests on body samples can provide information on the function of certain organs, such as the liver or kidneys, or reveal the presence of abnormal substances or abnormal levels of normal substances, such as hormones, in the body. In addition, some tests can reveal the presence of disease-causing microorganisms. Most tests on body samples are carried out in a laboratory, but some may be performed in a doctor's surgery or even at home.

Blood tests

Blood tests can be used to find information about the blood itself and to assess the function of other parts of the body, such as the liver. The samples are usually taken from a vein, but may also be taken from capillaries (tiny blood vessels) by a finger prick or occasionally from an artery. The most common blood tests performed are blood cell tests and blood chemistry tests. Blood cell tests include measuring the numbers of red and white blood cells and of platelets (cells that help blood to clot). Blood carries many substances apart from cells, and blood chemistry tests can measure the levels of these substances. These tests are used to detect kidney, liver, and muscle damage, certain bone disorders, and inflammation. One type is carried out to measure the level of cholesterol in the blood. In addition, blood chemistry tests are performed to see if a gland, such as the thyroid gland in the neck, is producing abnormal amounts of a hormone.

Urine tests

Urine is most commonly tested for evidence of urinary tract infections or diabetes, and can also be used to assess kidney function. Most urine tests are dipstick tests, which involve dipping a chemically treated stick into a sample of urine to show the presence or concentration of specific substances, such as glucose, protein, or blood. Dipstick tests are usually performed in a doctor's office. If the test suggests an infection, the sample may be sent to a laboratory to grow and identify the microorganism. A specific test for a hormone produced in pregnancy is the basis of the urine pregnancy test, which can be performed at home (see HOME PREGNANCY TEST, p.256).

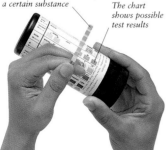

The intensity of each colour shows the concentration of a certain substance

The chart shows possible test results

Testing with a dipstick
A dipstick has squares along it, each of which reacts and changes colour on contact with a different chemical. The intensity of each colour shows the concentration of that substance in the urine. The dipstick is put into a urine sample and taken out again. The colours on the stick are then compared to reference colours on a chart.

Tests on body fluids

Tests may be performed on body fluids from wounds or abnormal areas of skin, from mucous membranes such as those of the nose and throat, or from internal areas such as the inside of a joint or around the brain and spinal cord. The tests may involve looking for infectious microorganisms, abnormal cells such as cancerous cells, or abnormal levels of certain chemicals. Other tests involve assessing cells or other substances that are normally found in the fluid, such as sperm in a sample of semen. Some samples, such as saliva, can be collected by the individual; others by a doctor. The samples are then usually sent to a laboratory for analysis.

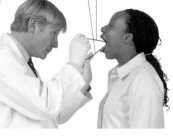

Tongue depressor
Swab

Having a swab taken
Fluids from wounds or from body cavities, such as the mouth, are usually collected with a swab – a sterile cotton bud on a plastic stick.

Tests on faeces

Samples of faeces may be tested for infectious microorganisms or for evidence of digestive disorders. One test is the faecal occult blood test, which can reveal tiny amounts of blood invisible to the naked eye. This test may be carried out if the doctor suspects that there may be bleeding in the digestive tract. The test may also be used to screen for colorectal cancer. Tests on samples of faeces are usually carried out in a laboratory.

Cell and tissue tests

Microscopic studies of individual cells, or of a larger sample of tissue containing a variety of cells, can give a definitive diagnosis for many disorders. Tests on cells are often used to diagnose cancer or screen for genetic disorders. Cells may be obtained from body fluids such as sputum (fluid coughed up from the lungs) or scraped from tissue surfaces such as the cervix (see CERVICAL SMEAR TEST, p.260). Cells may also be withdrawn from the body using a needle and syringe. This process, called aspiration, is often used to take cells from the lungs, thyroid gland, or breasts (see ASPIRATION OF A BREAST LUMP, p.252). Tissue tests are used to detect areas of abnormal tissue such as cirrhosis of the liver or tumours. Samples are taken by biopsy, in which a small piece of tissue is removed from parts of the body such as the skin (see SKIN BIOPSY, p.179) or the liver (below).

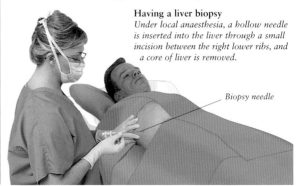

Having a liver biopsy
Under local anaesthesia, a hollow needle is inserted into the liver through a small incision between the right lower ribs, and a core of liver is removed.

Biopsy needle

Physiological tests

Certain investigations that do not involve testing samples (opposite) or imaging internal structures (*see* IMAGING TESTS, right) can be performed to assess the function of organs or systems. These physiological tests are commonly used to assess vision and hearing, the nervous system, and the heart and lungs.

Vision and hearing tests

The most common vision tests measure the ability to focus (*see* VISION TESTING, p.185, and VISION TESTING IN CHILDREN, p.97). Another test defines the visual field (the area that each eye can see independently). There is a range of tests for hearing. Some show how well sound is conducted through the ears; others measure how well sounds of varying pitch and volume can be heard or, in children, show the ability to hear speech (*see* HEARING TESTS, p.186, and HEARING TESTS IN CHILDHOOD, p.101).

Visual field test
This test is used to map the visual field. You are asked to look at a screen and press a button when you see flashes in different areas of the screen.

Nervous system tests

Some tests are used to establish whether nerves are able to conduct impulses normally. Abnormalities may be the result of something compressing a nerve or a disease such as diabetes mellitus. Another test, known as EEG, records the electrical activity produced in the brain and is useful for the diagnosis of disorders such as epilepsy.

Heart and lung tests

Heart rhythm and rate can be monitored by tests in which the electrical activity in the heart muscle is recorded: electrocardiography (p.199), ambulatory electrocardiography (p.201), and exercise ECG (below). Lung function can be tested in various ways. The simplest is measuring peak flow rate (p.193), which is the maximum rate at which you can breathe out. More complex tests show how quickly the lungs fill and empty (to detect narrowed airways), show lung capacity (to check for disorders that cause the lungs to shrink), and measure blood levels of oxygen (*see* MEASURING BLOOD OXYGEN, p.197).

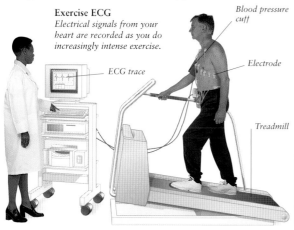

Exercise ECG
Electrical signals from your heart are recorded as you do increasingly intense exercise.

Blood pressure cuff

ECG trace

Electrode

Treadmill

Imaging tests

In imaging tests, energy is directed at or introduced into body tissues and detected by machines to produce images of internal structures. Many tests use X-rays; these tests range from conventional X-ray procedures to the computerized technique of CT scanning. X-rays carry the risk of exposure to harmful radiation, so some tests are available that use other forms of energy. For example, MRI uses magnetism and radio waves, and ultrasound scanning uses sound waves. Other imaging tests include radionuclide scanning, PET, and SPECT, which use radioactive substances introduced into certain tissues.

X-rays

X-rays are a form of radiation that can pass through body tissues to leave an image on photographic film. The ability of the rays to penetrate tissues depends on the density of those tissues. Solid, dense tissues such as bone let few rays through and appear white on the image. Muscular organs, such as the heart, appear grey. Tissues containing air, such as the lungs, and fluid-filled areas, such as the bladder, let most of the X-rays through and appear black on the film. X-ray images are often used to assess bone injuries such as fractures or disorders such as arthritis. The images can also show disorders in some soft tissues, such as infection in the lungs, and breast X-rays are used to screen women for breast cancer (*see* MAMMOGRAPHY, p.253). X-rays may also be used in other imaging techniques, such as bone densitometry (p.235).

Hollow or fluid-filled structures do not show clearly on plain X-rays but can be imaged by introducing a contrast medium into the area before taking the X-ray. The contrast medium blocks X-rays and makes the area appear white on the image. Types of contrast X-ray include barium contrast X-rays (p.38), used to image the digestive tract; angiography (p.38), which shows blood vessels; and intravenous urography (p.223), which shows the urinary tract.

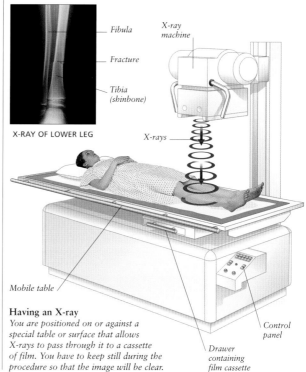

Fibula

Fracture

Tibia (shinbone)

X-RAY OF LOWER LEG

X-ray machine

X-rays

Mobile table

Having an X-ray
You are positioned on or against a special table or surface that allows X-rays to pass through it to a cassette of film. You have to keep still during the procedure so that the image will be clear.

Control panel

Drawer containing film cassette

Barium contrast X-rays

Parts of the digestive tract that are not visible on plain X-rays (p.37) can be imaged with barium contrast X-rays. Barium sulphate, which is a contrast medium (a substance that blocks X-rays), is introduced into the tract, then an X-ray is taken. If the oesophagus, stomach, or duodenum is to be investigated, the barium is swallowed in a drink, a procedure known as a barium swallow or meal. If the colon is to be viewed, the barium is given as an enema. These X-rays can reveal abnormalities such as tumours and narrowed or blocked areas.

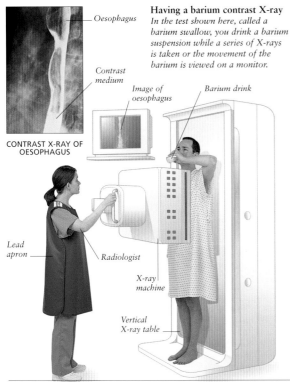

CONTRAST X-RAY OF OESOPHAGUS

Oesophagus

Contrast medium

Having a barium contrast X-ray
In the test shown here, called a barium swallow, you drink a barium suspension while a series of X-rays is taken or the movement of the barium is viewed on a monitor.

Image of oesophagus

Barium drink

Lead apron

Radiologist

X-ray machine

Vertical X-ray table

Angiography

In angiography, a dye is introduced into arteries to make them visible on X-rays (p.37) and reveal problems such as narrowed areas. First, a catheter is inserted into an artery some distance away and passed through the body, under X-ray control, until it reaches the artery to be imaged. The dye is injected through the catheter directly into the vessel, so that it is not diluted by the blood, and a series of X-rays is taken. Coronary angiography (below) shows the arteries supplying the heart muscle. Femoral angiography (p.228) shows arteries in the legs.

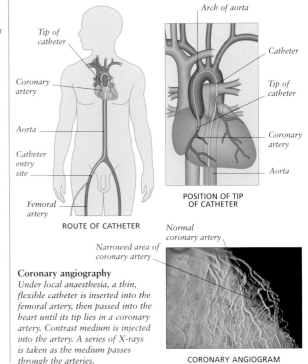

Tip of catheter

Coronary artery

Aorta

Catheter entry site

Femoral artery

ROUTE OF CATHETER

Arch of aorta

Catheter

Tip of catheter

Coronary artery

Aorta

POSITION OF TIP OF CATHETER

Coronary angiography
Under local anaesthesia, a thin, flexible catheter is inserted into the femoral artery, then passed into the heart until its tip lies in a coronary artery. Contrast medium is injected into the artery. A series of X-rays is taken as the medium passes through the arteries.

Normal coronary artery

Narrowed area of coronary artery

CORONARY ANGIOGRAM

CT scanning

Computerized tomography (CT) scanning is an X-ray-based technique that produces detailed cross-sectional images of the body. The images show a wide range of tissues of varying densities that do not show clearly on plain X-rays. CT scans reveal the anatomy of organs and other body structures, as well as abnormalities such as tumours or scar tissue inside organs. The scanner moves around the body; one section emits X-rays, which pass through the body to a detector on the other side of the machine. This X-ray detector transmits data to a computer, which creates an image that is shown on a monitor or reproduced on X-ray film. Hollow or fluid-filled areas usually appear black on the images but can be shown with a contrast medium, which blocks the passage of X-rays. In some cases, data from the scans can be used to create three-dimensional images. CT scans are most commonly used to investigate the brain or the solid abdominal organs but may also be carried out to view the lungs.

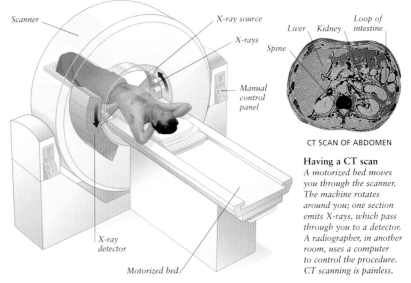

Scanner

X-ray source

X-rays

Manual control panel

X-ray detector

Motorized bed

Liver

Spine

Kidney

Loop of intestine

CT SCAN OF ABDOMEN

Having a CT scan
A motorized bed moves you through the scanner. The machine rotates around you; one section emits X-rays, which pass through you to a detector. A radiographer, in another room, uses a computer to control the procedure. CT scanning is painless.

MRI

Magnetic resonance imaging (MRI) uses magnetic force and radio waves. It can show fine details more clearly than other forms of imaging; in addition, unlike forms based on X-rays, it does not involve potentially harmful radiation. An MRI scanner contains two powerful magnets and a radiofrequency source. One magnet creates a strong magnetic field, which causes hydrogen atoms throughout the body to line up. The radiofrequency source emits radio waves that briefly knock the atoms out of alignment. As the atoms realign, they emit signals (resonance) that are picked up by the receiving magnet, which is placed around the area being scanned. Information about the signals is transmitted to a computer, which produces an image on a monitor. MRI is often used to examine the brain and spinal cord. It is also used to investigate sports injuries such as torn tendons.

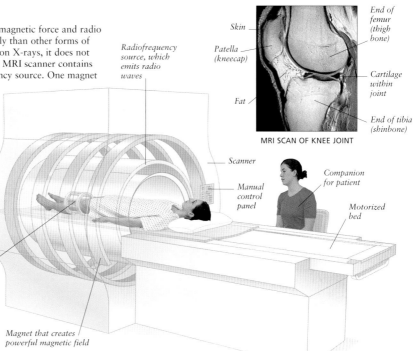

Radiofrequency source, which emits radio waves

Scanner

Manual control panel

Companion for patient

Motorized bed

Receiving magnet

Magnet that creates powerful magnetic field

Having an MRI scan
A motorized bed moves you into the scanner, and several scans are taken. If the machine makes you feel nervous, you may be allowed to have someone with you.

Skin

Patella (kneecap)

Fat

End of femur (thigh bone)

Cartilage within joint

End of tibia (shinbone)

MRI SCAN OF KNEE JOINT

Ultrasound scanning

In ultrasound scanning, images are created using ultrasound waves (high-frequency, inaudible sound waves). A device called a transducer is moved over the skin or, in some cases, inserted into a body opening such as the vagina or rectum, and sends ultrasound waves into the body. Where tissues of different densities meet, or where tissue meets fluid, the waves are reflected; the transducer picks up the echoes and passes them to a computer, which creates an image on a monitor. The images are updated continually so that movement can be seen. Doctors often use ultrasound to look at fetuses in the uterus (*see* ULTRASOUND SCANNING IN PREGNANCY, p.276) or the walls and valves of the heart, or to detect abnormalities such as cysts and kidney stones. A technique called Doppler ultrasound scanning (p.231), which shows the direction and speed of blood flow, is used to detect problems such as narrowed arteries or clots in veins.

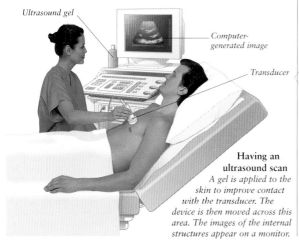

Ultrasound gel

Computer-generated image

Transducer

Having an ultrasound scan
A gel is applied to the skin to improve contact with the transducer. The device is then moved across this area. The images of the internal structures appear on a monitor.

Radionuclide scanning

Radionuclides are radioactive substances, and the radiation they emit can be used to create images. In radionuclide scanning, a tiny amount of the radionuclide is introduced into the body, usually by injection, then taken up by a specific type of tissue; for example, iodine is taken up by the thyroid gland. A device called a gamma camera detects the radiation and transmits data to a computer, which shows the tissue as areas of colour. The higher the level of cell activity in the tissue, the more radiation is emitted and the more intensely coloured the area appears. Radionuclide scans can show areas where cell activity is abnormally high, such as in tumours, or abnormally low, such as in damaged organs or cysts.

Having a radionuclide scan
Once your body has absorbed the radionuclide, you lie on a motorized bed that positions you over the gamma camera, which detects the radiation from the radionuclide. A computer interprets this as an image.

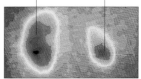

Normal kidney

Damaged kidney

SCAN OF KIDNEYS

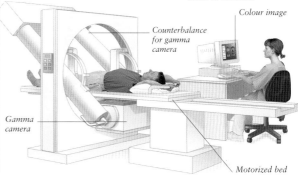

Counterbalance for gamma camera

Colour image

Gamma camera

Motorized bed

PET and SPECT scanning

Positron emission tomography (PET) and single-photon-emission computerized tomography (SPECT) are forms of radionuclide scanning (p.39). In both, a radionuclide (radioactive substance) is introduced into the body and taken up by tissues, and the radiation emitted is detected by a scanner. PET uses a radionuclide attached to glucose or other molecules essential to cell metabolism and can show the functioning of individual cells within tissues. It is mainly used to assess the heart and the brain. SPECT uses radionuclides that emit photons (a form of energy), whose movements can be traced by the scanner. The technique can show blood flow within organs and is used to assess if they are functioning normally. SPECT is chiefly used to assess the brain, heart, liver, and lungs.

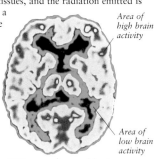

Area of high brain activity

Area of low brain activity

PET scan of normal brain
In this cross section of the brain, the yellow and red patches are highly active areas and the blue and black patches are less active areas.

Endoscopy

Endoscopy is a procedure in which a doctor views internal structures using a tube-like instrument called an endoscope, which includes a fibreoptic light source and magnifying lenses. The tip of the endoscope is passed through a natural body opening, such as the mouth, or a small incision in the skin. Most endoscopes are flexible, although rigid endoscopes are preferred in certain cases. The view may be seen directly through an eyepiece or shown on a monitor. Endoscopy may be used for diagnosis or for treatments.

Rigid endoscopes

A rigid endoscope is a short, straight metal viewing tube. It may be introduced through an incision in the skin and used to examine areas such as the abdominal cavity or the inside of joints, where the structures to be viewed are near the surface of the skin. Rigid endoscopes may also be inserted into natural orifices, such as the rectum. Procedures involving rigid endoscopes introduced through skin incisions are usually performed under general anaesthesia, but local anaesthesia may sometimes be used. Instruments may be passed down the endoscope or they may be introduced through separate incisions made in the skin.

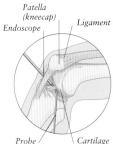

Patella (kneecap)
Endoscope
Ligament

Probe
Cartilage
POSITION OF INSTRUMENTS

Image of knee joint
Endoscope

Endoscopy of the knee
Small incisions are made on either side of the knee. The endoscope is inserted through one incision, and a probe is inserted through the other. The probe is used to move tissues so that certain structures can be viewed more clearly.

Probe

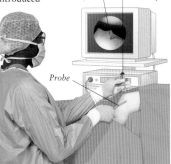

Flexible endoscopes

A flexible endoscope has a long, thin tube that can be steered round bends in internal passages and enter deep into the body. These endoscopes are often used for viewing inside the digestive, urinary, and respiratory tracts. The instrument is inserted through a natural opening such as the mouth, anus, or urethra; the person undergoing the procedure is first given a sedative or a local anaesthetic (for example, sprayed on to the back of the throat). The endoscope incorporates a system of lights, lenses, and optical fibres, and usually a video camera at the tip, allowing the doctor to view structures either directly through an eyepiece or on a monitor. If procedures, such as taking tissue samples, need to be carried out, very fine instruments can be passed down the tube, and the doctor can use the view from the tip as a guide during the procedure. The view may be recorded on videotape.

Endoscope
Oesophagus
Stomach
Tip of endoscope in duodenum

Upper digestive tract endoscopy
Before the procedure, you may be given a sedative. The endoscope is then passed into the body through the mouth. The view from the tip of the endoscope allows the doctor to detect abnormalities in the lining of the digestive tract.

ROUTE OF ENDOSCOPE

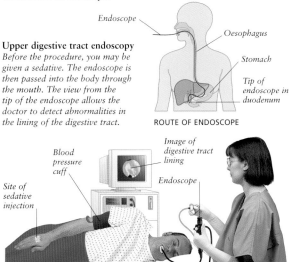

Blood pressure cuff
Site of sedative injection
Image of digestive tract lining
Endoscope

Endoscopic treatments

Endoscopy can be used for surgical treatments, often referred to as minimally invasive surgery. These treatments may even occur at the same time as the endoscopy is being used to make a diagnosis. The surgery is performed by using instruments passed down the endoscope. Endoscopic treatments include removal of intestinal polyps or diseased tissue (such as an inflamed gallbladder) and laser surgery to treat endometriosis. The doctor uses the endoscopic view as a guide during the procedure. Such operations are usually better for the patient than conventional surgery because the patient recovers faster and spends less time in hospital. In some procedures, such as laparoscopy (investigation of the abdomen), gas may be pumped into the abdomen to create more space and provide a better view.

Area of endometriosis
Probe
Uterus
Ovary

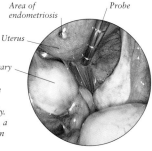

View of endometriosis
Endometriosis, in which tissue from the uterus lining grows outside the uterus, can be treated endoscopically. In this view through the endoscope, a probe holds tissues out of the way in preparation for laser surgery.

SYMPTOM

CHARTS

The charts help you identify the possible causes of a symptom, tell you when to seek medical help, and, if appropriate, suggest how you can treat the symptom or its cause yourself. The section consists of charts for children of different ages, charts for all adults, and charts specifically for men and for women. The information at the beginning of the section explains how to use the charts most effectively and how to identify the most appropriate chart for your symptom.

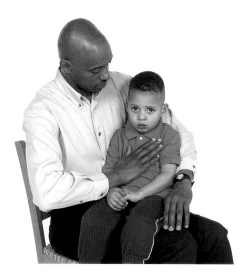

HOW TO USE THE CHARTS

Each of the 150 charts in this section covers a symptom or group of related symptoms and is similar to the example below. The chartfinder on page 44 will help you find the chart you need for your symptom. If you have more than one symptom, choose the chart that deals with the symptom that bothers you the most. To use a chart, follow the pathway of questions with yes/no answers until it leads to a possible cause or causes (there may be several possible diagnoses for a given set of symptoms) and action. The action tells you what your doctor may do or what might happen in hospital and, if self-help measures are appropriate, what you can do yourself. Many charts have boxes that give further self-help advice or provide information about disorders, tests, or treatments.

Warning box
This box highlights danger signs that need urgent medical attention or provides key information. Read the box first before working through the chart

Starting point
The starting point for each chart is always located in the top left corner of the page

Question boxes
These boxes ask for further information about your symptoms and can be answered YES or NO. Make sure that you read the questions carefully

Yes and No options
You can leave each question box by answering either YES or NO. YES is always to the right of a box, and NO is always at the bottom of a box

Pathway
The arrowed pathways lead you from one question to the next and eventually to a possible diagnosis

How the charts are organized

The charts are divided into four groups, each group indicated by a different colour bar down the edge of the page. The groups are:
- Charts for children: problems affecting children of all ages, as well as charts specifically for babies under one and adolescents
- General charts for adults: problems that can affect both men and women
- Charts for men: specific problems affecting men
- Charts for women: specific problems affecting women, including symptoms during pregnancy.

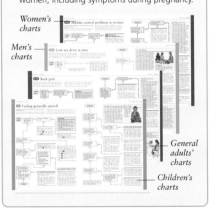

Women's charts

Men's charts

General adults' charts

Children's charts

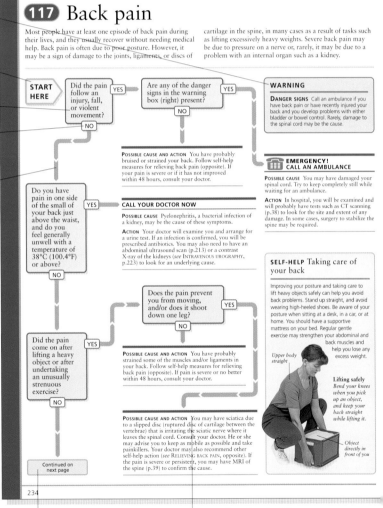

ADULTS: GENERAL

117 Back pain

Most people have at least one episode of back pain during their lives, and they usually recover without needing medical help. Back pain is often due to poor posture. However, it may be a sign of damage to the joints, ligaments, or discs of cartilage in the spine, in many cases as a result of tasks such as lifting excessively heavy weights. Severe back pain may be due to pressure on a nerve or, rarely, it may be due to a problem with an internal organ such as a kidney.

START HERE → **Did the pain follow an injury, fall, or violent movement?** — YES → **Are any of the danger signs in the warning box (right) present?** — YES →

NO

NO

WARNING
DANGER SIGNS Call an ambulance if you have back pain or have recently injured your back and you develop problems with either bladder or bowel control. Rarely, damage to the spinal cord may be the cause.

POSSIBLE CAUSE AND ACTION You have probably bruised or strained your back. Follow self-help measures for relieving back pain (opposite). If your pain is severe or if it has not improved within 48 hours, consult your doctor.

EMERGENCY!
CALL AN AMBULANCE
POSSIBLE CAUSE You may have damaged your spinal cord. Try to keep completely still while waiting for an ambulance.
ACTION In hospital, you will be examined and will probably have tests such as CT scanning (p.38) to look for the site and extent of any damage. In some cases, surgery to stabilize the spine may be required.

Do you have pain in one side of the small of your back just above the waist, and do you feel generally unwell with a temperature of 38°C (100.4°F) or above? — YES →

NO

CALL YOUR DOCTOR NOW
POSSIBLE CAUSE Pyelonephritis, a bacterial infection of a kidney, may be the cause of these symptoms.
ACTION Your doctor will examine you and arrange for a urine test. If an infection is confirmed, you will be prescribed antibiotics. You may also need to have an abdominal ultrasound scan (p.213) or a contrast X-ray of the kidneys (see INTRAVENOUS UROGRAPHY, p.223) to look for an underlying cause.

Does the pain prevent you from moving, and/or does it shoot down one leg? — YES →

NO

Did the pain come on after lifting a heavy object or after undertaking an unusually strenuous exercise? — YES →

NO

POSSIBLE CAUSE AND ACTION You have probably strained some of the muscles and/or ligaments in your back. Follow self-help measures for relieving back pain (opposite). If pain is severe or no better within 48 hours, consult your doctor.

SELF-HELP Taking care of your back

Improving your posture and taking care to lift heavy objects safely can help you avoid back problems. Stand up straight, and avoid wearing high-heeled shoes. Be aware of your posture when sitting at a desk, in a car, or at home. You should have a supportive mattress on your bed. Regular gentle exercise may strengthen your abdominal and back muscles and help you lose any excess weight.

Upper body straight

Lifting safely
Bend your knees when you pick up an object, and keep your back straight while lifting it.

Object directly in front of you

Continued on next page

POSSIBLE CAUSE AND ACTION You may have sciatica due to a slipped disc (ruptured disc of cartilage between the vertebrae) that is irritating the sciatic nerve where it leaves the spinal cord. Consult your doctor. He or she may advise you to keep as mobile as possible and take painkillers. Your doctor may also recommend other self-help action (see RELIEVING BACK PAIN, opposite). If the pain is severe or persistent, you may have MRI of the spine (p.39) to confirm the cause.

234

Continuation box
On two-page charts, these boxes show that the pathway continues on the second page. Another box appears on the second page in a matching colour to tell you where to pick up the pathway

Instructions for obtaining urgent medical help
These instructions tell you what to do when you need prompt medical help rather than a routine appointment with your doctor. They say whether to call an ambulance or how quickly to get in touch with your doctor

Possible cause or causes
This text tells you which condition or conditions are most likely to be responsible for your symptoms and whether you should consult your doctor

Action
This text tells you what can be done for your condition. If medical help is needed, it will tell you about tests you may have and likely treatments. If medical help is not necessary, information may be given on what you can do yourself

Self-help box
This type of box may outline practical measures that you can take to relieve symptoms or cope with your problem. Alternatively, there may be advice on how to assess the severity of a symptom; for example, by taking body temperature during a fever

Instructions for obtaining urgent medical help

If your symptoms suggest that you need urgent medical attention rather than just a routine appointment with your doctor, the instructions at the end of a pathway will tell you what to do. There are three different levels of urgency. In the most urgent cases, which are potentially life-threatening, you will be told to call an ambulance. For other urgent cases, you will be told to get help from your doctor either at once or within 24 hours. The instructions are fully explained below.

☎ EMERGENCY! CALL AN AMBULANCE

Your condition may be life-threatening unless given immediate medical attention in hospital. Usually, the best way to achieve this is by calling an ambulance so that you can be given medical care in transit. In some cases, going by car to the accident and emergency department of the nearest hospital may be a better option; for example, if an ambulance cannot reach you quickly.

CALL YOUR DOCTOR NOW

Your symptoms may indicate a serious problem that needs urgent medical assessment. Even if it is the middle of the night or the weekend, you should call your doctor immediately. He or she may visit you at home or want to see you at the surgery immediately. If you cannot get in touch with your doctor within 1 hour, call NHS Direct (*see* USEFUL ADDRESSES, p.285) or go to the accident and emergency department of your nearest hospital. If possible, go by car or taxi; failing that, phone for an ambulance.

SEE YOUR DOCTOR WITHIN 24 HOURS

You need prompt medical attention, but a short delay is unlikely to be damaging. Telephone your doctor and ask for an urgent appointment within the next 24 hours, or contact NHS Direct (*see* USEFUL ADDRESSES, p.285) for advice.

ADULTS: GENERAL

Continued from previous page

Are you over 50? YES / NO

Has your back gradually become stiff as well as painful over a period of months or years? YES / NO

POSSIBLE CAUSE You may have ankylosing spondylitis (inflammation of the joints between the vertebrae, resulting in the spinal column gradually becoming hard and inflexible). This is especially likely if you are between 20 and 40. Consult your doctor.

ACTION Your doctor will examine you and arrange for you to have a blood test and X-rays (p.37) of your back and pelvic areas. If you are found to have ankylosing spondylitis, you will probably be given nonsteroidal anti-inflammatory drugs. You will also be referred to a physiotherapist, who will teach you exercises to help keep your back mobile. These mobility exercises are an essential part of the treatment for this disorder and can be supplemented by other physical activities, such as swimming.

Did the pain come on suddenly after an extended stay in bed or confinement to a wheelchair, or are you over 60? YES / NO

SEE YOUR DOCTOR WITHIN 24 HOURS

POSSIBLE CAUSE You may have a crush fracture of a vertebra as a result of osteoporosis, in which bones throughout the body become thin and weak. Osteoporosis is symptomless unless a fracture occurs. The disorder is most common in women who have passed the menopause. However, a prolonged period of immobility will also lead to the development of osteoporosis.

ACTION Initial treatment for the pain is with painkillers. Your doctor may also request bone densitometry (below). Specific treatment for osteoporosis depends on the underlying cause. However, in all cases, it is important that you try to remain active and take weight-bearing exercise, such as walking.

Are you female and pregnant? YES / NO

CONSULT YOUR DOCTOR IF YOU ARE UNABLE TO MAKE A DIAGNOSIS FROM THIS CHART AND YOUR BACK PAIN IS SEVERE OR IF THE NATURE OF LONG-STANDING BACK PAIN SUDDENLY CHANGES.

Go to chart **147** BACK PAIN IN PREGNANCY (p.280)

SELF-HELP Relieving back pain

Most back pain is the result of minor sprains or strains that normally clear up on their own and can usually be helped by simple measures. Try the following:
- If possible, keep moving and carry out your normal daily activities.
- Rest in bed if the pain is severe, but do not stay in bed for more than 2 days.
- Take over-the-counter paracetamol or nonsteroidal anti-inflammatory drugs.
- Place a heating pad or wrapped hot-water bottle against the painful area.
- If heat does not provide relief, try using an ice pack (or a wrapped pack of frozen peas); place it over the painful area for 15 minutes every 2–3 hours.

If your backache is severe or is no better within 2 days, consult your doctor.

Once the pain has cleared up, follow the self-help advice for taking care of your back (opposite) to prevent a recurrence.

POSSIBLE CAUSE Osteoarthritis of the spine is probably the cause of your symptoms. In this condition, joints between the vertebrae in the spine are progressively damaged. This is particularly likely if you are over 50 and you are overweight. Consult your doctor.

ACTION Your doctor may arrange for blood tests and an X-ray (p.37) to confirm the diagnosis. Over-the-counter painkillers should help to relieve your symptoms. If you are overweight, it will help to lose weight (*see* HOW TO LOSE WEIGHT SAFELY, p.147). Your doctor may refer you for physiotherapy to help you strengthen the muscles that support the spine.

Bone densitometry

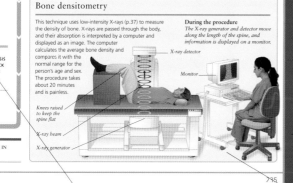

This technique uses low-intensity X-rays (p.37) to measure the density of bone. X-rays are passed through the body, and their absorption is interpreted by a computer and displayed as an image. The computer calculates the average bone density and compares it with the normal range for the person's age and sex. The procedure takes about 20 minutes and is painless.

During the procedure
The X-ray generator and detector move along the length of the spine, and information is displayed on a monitor.

X-ray detector
Monitor
Knees raised to keep the spine flat
X-ray beam
X-ray generator

Colour bar
Each group of charts is identified by a colour bar, helping you to find the chart you want more easily

---

Consult another chart
These instructions send you to another chart in the book that may be more appropriate for your symptoms or may give you additional information

Cause not identified
If you have not been able to find an explanation for your symptoms, you will usually be told to consult your doctor. In some cases, you will be given a suggested time, such as 48 hours, within which to consult your doctor if symptoms are no better

Information box
This type of box gives further information on what is involved in having a test or treatment mentioned elsewhere in the chart. In addition, some information boxes have key facts on a disease or extra detail of anatomy that is relevant to the chart

Symptom-by-symptom chartfinder

CHARTS FOR CHILDREN

1 Sleeping problems in babies

For children over 1 year, see chart 11, SLEEPING PROBLEMS
IN CHILDREN **(p.66).**
Most babies wake at regular intervals through the day and
night for feeds during the first few months of life. This is
perfectly normal, and there is no point in trying to force a

baby of this age into a routine that is more convenient for
you. Consult this chart only if you think your baby is waking
more frequently than is normal for him or her, if you have
difficulty settling your baby at night, or if a baby who has
previously slept well starts to wake during the night.

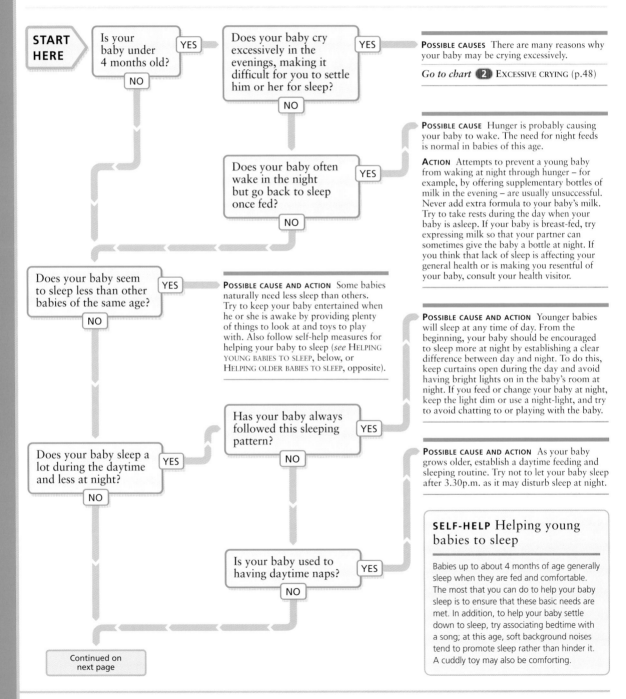

START HERE

Is your baby under 4 months old? — YES → **Does your baby cry excessively in the evenings, making it difficult for you to settle him or her for sleep?** — YES → **POSSIBLE CAUSES** There are many reasons why your baby may be crying excessively.

Go to chart **2** EXCESSIVE CRYING (p.48)

NO ↓ (from "under 4 months old")

NO ↓ (from "cry excessively")

Does your baby often wake in the night but go back to sleep once fed? — YES → **POSSIBLE CAUSE** Hunger is probably causing your baby to wake. The need for night feeds is normal in babies of this age.

ACTION Attempts to prevent a young baby from waking at night through hunger – for example, by offering supplementary bottles of milk in the evening – are usually unsuccessful. Never add extra formula to your baby's milk. Try to take rests during the day when your baby is asleep. If your baby is breast-fed, try expressing milk so that your partner can sometimes give the baby a bottle at night. If you think that lack of sleep is affecting your general health or is making you resentful of your baby, consult your health visitor.

NO ↓

Does your baby seem to sleep less than other babies of the same age? — YES → **POSSIBLE CAUSE AND ACTION** Some babies naturally need less sleep than others. Try to keep your baby entertained when he or she is awake by providing plenty of things to look at and toys to play with. Also follow self-help measures for helping your baby to sleep (*see* HELPING YOUNG BABIES TO SLEEP, below, or HELPING OLDER BABIES TO SLEEP, opposite).

NO ↓

Has your baby always followed this sleeping pattern? — YES → **POSSIBLE CAUSE AND ACTION** Younger babies will sleep at any time of day. From the beginning, your baby should be encouraged to sleep more at night by establishing a clear difference between day and night. To do this, keep curtains open during the day and avoid having bright lights on in the baby's room at night. If you feed or change your baby at night, keep the light dim or use a night-light, and try to avoid chatting to or playing with the baby.

NO ↓

Does your baby sleep a lot during the daytime and less at night? — YES → (up to "Has your baby always followed this sleeping pattern?")

NO ↓

Is your baby used to having daytime naps? — YES → **POSSIBLE CAUSE AND ACTION** As your baby grows older, establish a daytime feeding and sleeping routine. Try not to let your baby sleep after 3.30p.m. as it may disturb sleep at night.

NO ↓

Continued on next page

SELF-HELP Helping young babies to sleep

Babies up to about 4 months of age generally sleep when they are fed and comfortable. The most that you can do to help your baby sleep is to ensure that these basic needs are met. In addition, to help your baby settle down to sleep, try associating bedtime with a song; at this age, soft background noises tend to promote sleep rather than hinder it. A cuddly toy may also be comforting.

Continued from previous page

Does your baby seem unwell in any way? **YES**

NO

POSSIBLE CAUSES AND ACTION If your baby has specific symptoms, such as fever, diarrhoea, or vomiting, consult the relevant chart in this book. If there are no specific symptoms but your baby continues to seem unwell, you should contact your doctor.

Is your baby waking repeatedly at night after previously sleeping well? **YES**

NO

POSSIBLE CAUSE AND ACTION As your baby grows, he or she will need more food. Increasing feeds in the evening may stop him or her from waking at night. By the time your baby is 6 months old, he or she will be ready for weaning (p.59); consult your doctor or health visitor for advice.

CONSULT YOUR DOCTOR IF YOU ARE UNABLE TO MAKE A DIAGNOSIS FROM THIS CHART.

Could your baby be waking because he or she is hungry? **YES**

NO

POSSIBLE CAUSE Being too hot or cold may be causing your baby to wake in the night.

ACTION Try to keep the temperature in your baby's room at about 18°C (65°F). Your baby should need no more covers than you would in similar circumstances. Letting your baby get too hot may increase the risk of sudden infant death syndrome, or SIDS (left). If your baby kicks off the bedclothes and gets cold, try dressing him or her in a sleep suit at night.

SELF-HELP Reducing the risk of SIDS

To reduce the risk of sudden infant death syndrome (SIDS), also known as cot death, you can take the following measures:
- Both parents should avoid smoking during the pregnancy.
- If possible, let your baby sleep in a cot in your bedroom for the first 6 months.
- Always put your baby to sleep on his or her back near the foot of the cot. This position is the safest, since he or she cannot wriggle under the bedclothes.
- Use a firm mattress with no pillow.
- Keep your baby's head uncovered; pull bedclothes up just as far as the shoulders.
- Do not overwrap your baby in bedclothes. Use layers of sheets and thin blankets that can easily be added or taken off.
- Make sure your baby does not get too hot. Keep the room at a temperature that is comfortable for you. Do not place the cot close to a radiator or other type of heater.
- Do not let anyone smoke in the same room as your baby.

Could your baby be too cold or hot during the night? **YES**

NO

POSSIBLE CAUSE Babies sense anxiety or stress in their parents and can be disturbed by it.

ACTION It may take some time to reassure your baby. If you can, try to keep your baby's routine as stable as possible, even if your own life is unsettled. When your baby wakes at night, offer a drink and a cuddle, but make sure that your baby understands that he or she will be put back in the cot; otherwise, there is a danger that the baby will get into the habit of waking during the night and expecting to play (see HELPING OLDER BABIES TO SLEEP, below).

Has there been any recent domestic upheaval or possible cause of anxiety? **YES**

NO

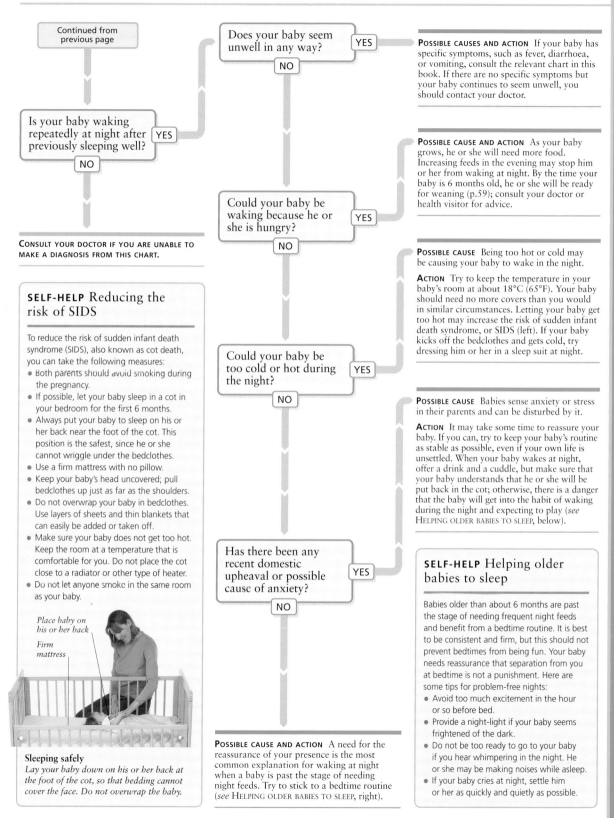

Place baby on his or her back
Firm mattress

Sleeping safely
Lay your baby down on his or her back at the foot of the cot, so that bedding cannot cover the face. Do not overwrap the baby.

POSSIBLE CAUSE AND ACTION A need for the reassurance of your presence is the most common explanation for waking at night when a baby is past the stage of needing night feeds. Try to stick to a bedtime routine (see HELPING OLDER BABIES TO SLEEP, right).

SELF-HELP Helping older babies to sleep

Babies older than about 6 months are past the stage of needing frequent night feeds and benefit from a bedtime routine. It is best to be consistent and firm, but this should not prevent bedtimes from being fun. Your baby needs reassurance that separation from you at bedtime is not a punishment. Here are some tips for problem-free nights:
- Avoid too much excitement in the hour or so before bed.
- Provide a night-light if your baby seems frightened of the dark.
- Do not be too ready to go to your baby if you hear whimpering in the night. He or she may be making noises while asleep.
- If your baby cries at night, settle him or her as quickly and quietly as possible.

2 Excessive crying

Crying is a young baby's only means of communicating physical discomfort or emotional distress. All babies sometimes cry when they are hungry, wet, upset, or in pain, and some babies occasionally cry for no obvious reason. Most parents soon learn to recognize the most common causes of their baby's crying and are usually able to deal with them according to need. You should consult this chart if your baby cries more often than you think is normal or if your baby suddenly starts to cry in an unusual way. In some cases, you may be advised to seek medical help.

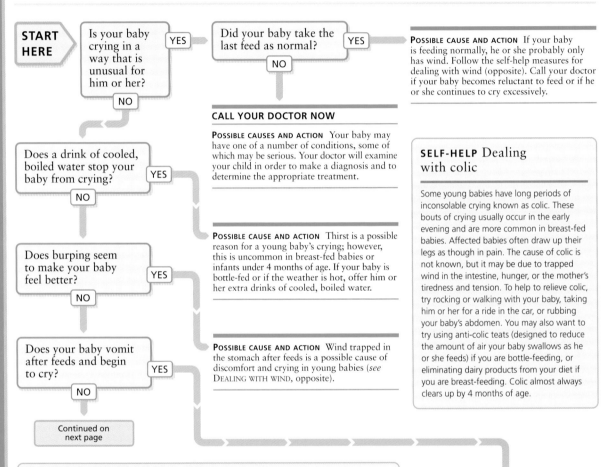

START HERE → **Is your baby crying in a way that is unusual for him or her?** — YES → **Did your baby take the last feed as normal?** — YES → **POSSIBLE CAUSE AND ACTION** If your baby is feeding normally, he or she probably only has wind. Follow the self-help measures for dealing with wind (opposite). Call your doctor if your baby becomes reluctant to feed or if he or she continues to cry excessively.

NO ↓ (from "Did your baby take the last feed as normal?")

CALL YOUR DOCTOR NOW

POSSIBLE CAUSES AND ACTION Your baby may have one of a number of conditions, some of which may be serious. Your doctor will examine your child in order to make a diagnosis and to determine the appropriate treatment.

NO ↓ (from "Is your baby crying")

Does a drink of cooled, boiled water stop your baby from crying? — YES →

POSSIBLE CAUSE AND ACTION Thirst is a possible reason for a young baby's crying; however, this is uncommon in breast-fed babies or infants under 4 months of age. If your baby is bottle-fed or if the weather is hot, offer him or her extra drinks of cooled, boiled water.

NO ↓

Does burping seem to make your baby feel better? — YES →

POSSIBLE CAUSE AND ACTION Wind trapped in the stomach after feeds is a possible cause of discomfort and crying in young babies (*see* DEALING WITH WIND, opposite).

NO ↓

Does your baby vomit after feeds and begin to cry? — YES →

NO ↓

Continued on next page

SELF-HELP Dealing with colic

Some young babies have long periods of inconsolable crying known as colic. These bouts of crying usually occur in the early evening and are more common in breast-fed babies. Affected babies often draw up their legs as though in pain. The cause of colic is not known, but it may be due to trapped wind in the intestine, hunger, or the mother's tiredness and tension. To help to relieve colic, try rocking or walking with your baby, taking him or her for a ride in the car, or rubbing your baby's abdomen. You may also want to try using anti-colic teats (designed to reduce the amount of air your baby swallows as he or she feeds) if you are bottle-feeding, or eliminating dairy products from your diet if you are breast-feeding. Colic almost always clears up by 4 months of age.

SELF-HELP Coping with crying

Many parents find it very stressful and feel unable to cope if their baby cries for hours on end. Such feelings are normal and do not mean that you are a bad parent. Ask neighbours or friends to look after your baby for an hour so that you can relax. If there is no one to ask, put your baby safely in his or her cot, close the door, and leave him or her for half an hour or so, until you feel better. Being left for a short while will not harm your baby. If the crying becomes unbearable and you are afraid that you might hit or shake your baby, put the baby in his or her cot and call your doctor, health visitor, or a self-help group (see USEFUL ADDRESSES, p.285).

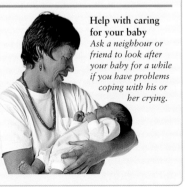

Help with caring for your baby
Ask a neighbour or friend to look after your baby for a while if you have problems coping with his or her crying.

SEE YOUR DOCTOR WITHIN 24 HOURS

POSSIBLE CAUSE Gastro-oesophageal reflux disease, in which the stomach contents leak back into the oesophagus, may be the cause.

ACTION Your doctor will examine your baby to exclude other causes. You may be advised to change your baby's nappy before a feed, burp the baby frequently during feeds, and keep him or her semi-upright during and after feeds. If you bottle-feed your baby, you may be advised to feed a pre-thickened formula. Your doctor may prescribe a medication to reduce reflux of acid from the stomach. If these measures do not help, your baby may be prescribed a drug to reduce stomach acid. Most babies grow out of the condition by the age of 12–18 months.

Continued from previous page

Is your baby under 4 months old? — **YES** →

Does your baby seem content for most of the day but cry a great deal during the late afternoon and evening? — **YES** →

POSSIBLE CAUSE Colic is the term often used to describe this common type of crying. It usually starts when a baby is about 6 weeks old and ceases by the age of 4 months. The precise cause of colic is not known.

ACTION There is no effective cure for colic. However, some self-help measures may give you and your baby temporary relief (*see* DEALING WITH COLIC, opposite). The main priority for parents is to find a way of coping with a constantly crying baby (*see* COPING WITH CRYING, opposite).

NO

NO

Does your baby usually stop crying when picked up and given your full attention? — **YES** →

POSSIBLE CAUSE The need for attention and physical comfort is a common cause of crying. Some babies are quite happy when left alone in their cot or playpen, but others need the constant reassurance of their parents' presence.

ACTION Cuddle your baby as much as he or she seems to want. At this age, there is no danger of "spoiling", and your baby will be happier as a result of an increased feeling of security. To enable you to get on with your everyday chores, you can try putting a young baby in a carrying sling while you go about the house. Once your baby seems content, you should avoid fussing over him or her.

NO

POSSIBLE CAUSE AND ACTION Teething can cause babies some discomfort. A hard, cooled object to chew on, such as a teething ring cooled in the refrigerator, may help. You can also give the recommended dose of painkillers to relieve the discomfort (*see* TEETHING, p.111).

Could your baby be teething? — **YES** →

NO

POSSIBLE CAUSE Some babies may feel uncomfortable or have a mild fever in the week after a routine immunization (p.35).

ACTION Take your baby's temperature (p.50). If he or she has a fever, follow the advice for dealing with fever after immunization (p.51). If your baby does not have a fever and his or her crying is still worrying you, consult your doctor.

POSSIBLE CAUSE Even young babies can be upset by increased tension in the home, particularly if the mother is affected.

ACTION Your baby will need more attention and reassurance than usual but should settle down within a week or so. Try to keep your baby's routine as stable as possible, even if other aspects of life are changing. If you think that your baby's crying could be a reaction to your own tension, try to find ways of reducing any strain you are under. Your doctor or health visitor may be able to suggest ways of helping.

Has your baby been immunized recently? — **YES** →

NO

Has there been a recent major domestic upheaval or other stressful event? — **YES** →

NO

SELF-HELP Dealing with wind

All babies swallow air when feeding. This air may then get trapped in the intestine, causing discomfort. Wind may be worse if your baby cries just before a feed or feeds greedily. Here are some tips that may prevent wind from occurring or may help to release the wind:

- If your baby is bottle-fed, make sure that the hole in the teat is the right size.
- Support your baby in a semi-upright position when feeding so that swallowed air rises to the top of the stomach.
- Burp your baby at intervals during each feed. Hold your baby upright against your shoulder or on your lap. Gently rub or pat his or her back to encourage the wind to come up.

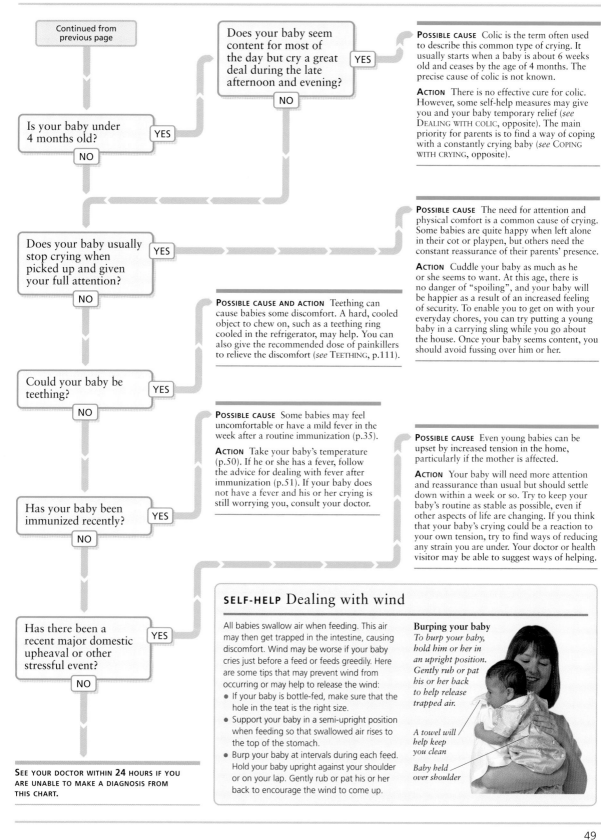

Burping your baby
To burp your baby, hold him or her in an upright position. Gently rub or pat his or her back to help release trapped air.

A towel will help keep you clean

Baby held over shoulder

SEE YOUR DOCTOR WITHIN **24** HOURS IF YOU ARE UNABLE TO MAKE A DIAGNOSIS FROM THIS CHART.

③ Fever in babies

For children over 1, see chart 14, FEVER IN CHILDREN **(p.72).**
A fever is an abnormally high body temperature, of 38°C (100.4°F) or above. A baby that has a fever will have a hot forehead and is likely to seem unhappy and fretful. If you think your baby may be unwell, take his or her temperature

(*see* TAKING YOUR BABY'S TEMPERATURE, below). A high fever may cause a baby to have a seizure, which is a medical emergency (*see* FEBRILE CONVULSIONS IN BABIES AND CHILDREN, opposite). If your baby has a fever, take steps to reduce it (*see* BRINGING DOWN A FEVER, p.73), and consult this chart.

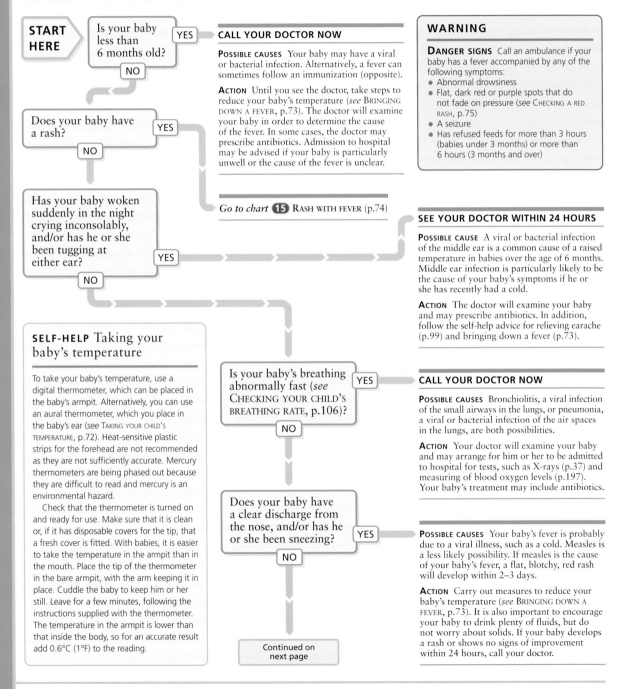

START HERE

Is your baby less than 6 months old? — YES →

CALL YOUR DOCTOR NOW

POSSIBLE CAUSES Your baby may have a viral or bacterial infection. Alternatively, a fever can sometimes follow an immunization (opposite).

ACTION Until you see the doctor, take steps to reduce your baby's temperature (*see* BRINGING DOWN A FEVER, p.73). The doctor will examine your baby in order to determine the cause of the fever. In some cases, the doctor may prescribe antibiotics. Admission to hospital may be advised if your baby is particularly unwell or the cause of the fever is unclear.

NO ↓

Does your baby have a rash? — YES → *Go to chart* **15** RASH WITH FEVER (p.74)

NO ↓

Has your baby woken suddenly in the night crying inconsolably, and/or has he or she been tugging at either ear? — YES →

SEE YOUR DOCTOR WITHIN 24 HOURS

POSSIBLE CAUSE A viral or bacterial infection of the middle ear is a common cause of a raised temperature in babies over the age of 6 months. Middle ear infection is particularly likely to be the cause of your baby's symptoms if he or she has recently had a cold.

ACTION The doctor will examine your baby and may prescribe antibiotics. In addition, follow the self-help advice for relieving earache (p.99) and bringing down a fever (p.73).

NO ↓

WARNING

DANGER SIGNS Call an ambulance if your baby has a fever accompanied by any of the following symptoms:
- Abnormal drowsiness
- Flat, dark red or purple spots that do not fade on pressure (*see* CHECKING A RED RASH, p.75)
- A seizure
- Has refused feeds for more than 3 hours (babies under 3 months) or more than 6 hours (3 months and over)

SELF-HELP Taking your baby's temperature

To take your baby's temperature, use a digital thermometer, which can be placed in the baby's armpit. Alternatively, you can use an aural thermometer, which you place in the baby's ear (*see* TAKING YOUR CHILD'S TEMPERATURE, p.72). Heat-sensitive plastic strips for the forehead are not recommended as they are not sufficiently accurate. Mercury thermometers are being phased out because they are difficult to read and mercury is an environmental hazard.

Check that the thermometer is turned on and ready for use. Make sure that it is clean or, if it has disposable covers for the tip, that a fresh cover is fitted. With babies, it is easier to take the temperature in the armpit than in the mouth. Place the tip of the thermometer in the bare armpit, with the arm keeping it in place. Cuddle the baby to keep him or her still. Leave for a few minutes, following the instructions supplied with the thermometer. The temperature in the armpit is lower than that inside the body, so for an accurate result add 0.6°C (1°F) to the reading.

Is your baby's breathing abnormally fast (*see* CHECKING YOUR CHILD'S BREATHING RATE, p.106)? — YES →

CALL YOUR DOCTOR NOW

POSSIBLE CAUSES Bronchiolitis, a viral infection of the small airways in the lungs, or pneumonia, a viral or bacterial infection of the air spaces in the lungs, are both possibilities.

ACTION Your doctor will examine your baby and may arrange for him or her to be admitted to hospital for tests, such as X-rays (p.37) and measuring of blood oxygen levels (p.197). Your baby's treatment may include antibiotics.

NO ↓

Does your baby have a clear discharge from the nose, and/or has he or she been sneezing? — YES →

POSSIBLE CAUSES Your baby's fever is probably due to a viral illness, such as a cold. Measles is a less likely possibility. If measles is the cause of your baby's fever, a flat, blotchy, red rash will develop within 2–3 days.

ACTION Carry out measures to reduce your baby's temperature (*see* BRINGING DOWN A FEVER, p.73). It is also important to encourage your baby to drink plenty of fluids, but do not worry about solids. If your baby develops a rash or shows no signs of improvement within 24 hours, call your doctor.

NO ↓

Continued on next page

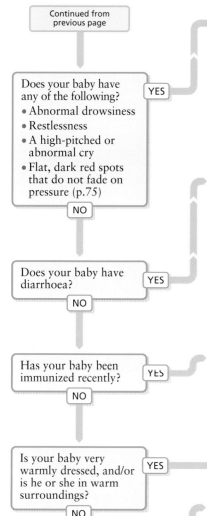

Continued from previous page

Does your baby have any of the following?
- Abnormal drowsiness
- Restlessness
- A high-pitched or abnormal cry
- Flat, dark red spots that do not fade on pressure (p.75)

YES →

NO ↓

Does your baby have diarrhoea?   **YES** →

NO ↓

Has your baby been immunized recently?   **YES** →

NO ↓

Is your baby very warmly dressed, and/or is he or she in warm surroundings?   **YES** →

NO ↓

☎ EMERGENCY! CALL AN AMBULANCE

POSSIBLE CAUSE Meningitis, inflammation of the membranes surrounding the brain due to infection, may be the cause of these symptoms.

ACTION If meningitis is suspected, your baby will be admitted to hospital immediately. He or she will be given urgent treatment with antibiotics and may need intensive care.

CALL YOUR DOCTOR NOW

POSSIBLE CAUSE Gastroenteritis, an infection of the digestive system, is the most likely cause of these symptoms, especially if your baby is also vomiting.

ACTION Your doctor will check whether your baby is dehydrated. He or she may also give you advice on preventing dehydration in babies (p.55) and self-help measures for treating gastroenteritis in babies (p.53).

POSSIBLE CAUSE Some babies may feel uncomfortable or have a mild fever in the week after a routine immunization (p.35).

ACTION Follow the advice for dealing with fever after immunization (right).

POSSIBLE CAUSE Overheating, caused by too much clothing or by being in excessively warm surroundings, can result in a fever.

ACTION A baby does not need to wear much more clothing than an adult would in similar conditions and will be comfortable in a room temperature of 15–20°C (60–68°F). A baby's cot should never be placed next to a radiator. Remove any excess clothing and move the baby to a slightly cooler (though not cold) place. If your baby's temperature is not down to normal within an hour, follow the advice for reducing a fever (p.73) and call your doctor.

SEE YOUR DOCTOR WITHIN 24 HOURS IF YOU ARE UNABLE TO MAKE A DIAGNOSIS FROM THIS CHART.

Fever after immunizations

Some babies and young children develop a mild fever after an immunization. Routine immunizations (p.35) are usually given at the ages of 2, 3, 4, and 12–15 months. If your child develops a fever after an immunization, you should follow the self-help advice for reducing his or her fever (see BRINGING DOWN A FEVER, p.73). Call your doctor immediately if your child's temperature rises above 39°C (102°F) or if he or she has other symptoms, such as an unusual or high-pitched cry. You should also call your doctor if self-help measures are not successful in reducing your child's temperature.

If your child has been unwell after having an immunization, mention it to your doctor or health visitor before the next immunization is due. He or she can advise you on how to deal with any symptoms that may develop.

If your child has a fever at the time when an immunization is due, it should be postponed until he or she is better.

Febrile convulsions in babies and children

A febrile convulsion is a type of seizure that affects some children aged 6 months to 5 years. It is triggered by an abrupt rise in body temperature, often at the onset of a feverish illness. During a convulsion, the child may:
- Lose consciousness
- Shake or jerk violently
- Stop breathing temporarily or breathe shallowly, which may result in a bluish tinge to the skin
- Pass urine and/or faeces
- Roll back his or her eyes

Febrile convulsions usually last for less than 5 minutes and, although frightening, are not often serious. About a third of children who have had a febrile convulsion have another one within 6 months. Most affected children stop having convulsions at about 5 years of age. Febrile convulsions are rarely an indication of epilepsy in later life.

To avoid convulsions, keep your child's temperature down (see BRINGING DOWN A FEVER, p.73). If he or she does have a febrile convulsion, remove excess clothes, and open a window or use an electric fan to ensure a flow of cool, fresh air. Surround him or her with soft objects, such as pillows, to prevent injury.

After the seizure has finished, place your child in the recovery position. He or she may fall asleep shortly afterwards. Call your doctor if your child has a convulsion. If it lasts more than 5 minutes, call an ambulance.

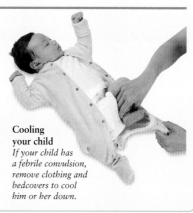

Cooling your child
If your child has a febrile convulsion, remove clothing and bedcovers to cool him or her down.

4 Vomiting in babies

For children over 1 year, see chart 38, VOMITING IN CHILDREN **(p.114).**

In young babies, it is easy for parents to confuse vomiting, which may indicate an illness, with regurgitation (posseting),

the effortless bringing up of small amounts of milk. Almost any minor upset can cause a baby to vomit once, and this is unlikely to be a cause for concern. However, persistent vomiting in babies can be a sign of an underlying problem.

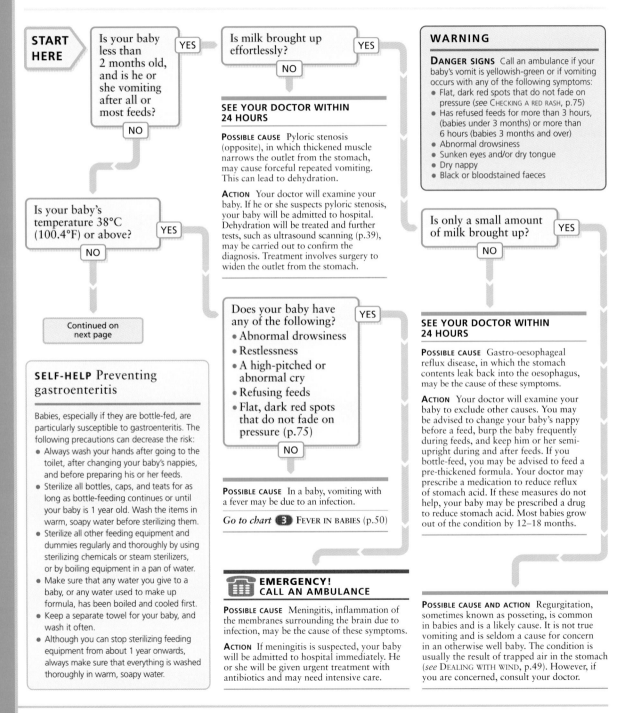

START HERE

Is your baby less than 2 months old, and is he or she vomiting after all or most feeds?

YES → Is milk brought up effortlessly?

YES →

NO

NO

SEE YOUR DOCTOR WITHIN 24 HOURS

POSSIBLE CAUSE Pyloric stenosis (opposite), in which thickened muscle narrows the outlet from the stomach, may cause forceful repeated vomiting. This can lead to dehydration.

ACTION Your doctor will examine your baby. If he or she suspects pyloric stenosis, your baby will be admitted to hospital. Dehydration will be treated and further tests, such as ultrasound scanning (p.39), may be carried out to confirm the diagnosis. Treatment involves surgery to widen the outlet from the stomach.

Is your baby's temperature 38°C (100.4°F) or above?

YES →

NO

Continued on next page

Does your baby have any of the following?
- Abnormal drowsiness
- Restlessness
- A high-pitched or abnormal cry
- Refusing feeds
- Flat, dark red spots that do not fade on pressure (p.75)

YES →

NO

POSSIBLE CAUSE In a baby, vomiting with a fever may be due to an infection.

Go to chart **3** FEVER IN BABIES (p.50)

WARNING

DANGER SIGNS Call an ambulance if your baby's vomit is yellowish-green or if vomiting occurs with any of the following symptoms:
- Flat, dark red spots that do not fade on pressure (see CHECKING A RED RASH, p.75)
- Has refused feeds for more than 3 hours, (babies under 3 months) or more than 6 hours (babies 3 months and over)
- Abnormal drowsiness
- Sunken eyes and/or dry tongue
- Dry nappy
- Black or bloodstained faeces

Is only a small amount of milk brought up?

YES →

NO

SEE YOUR DOCTOR WITHIN 24 HOURS

POSSIBLE CAUSE Gastro-oesophageal reflux disease, in which the stomach contents leak back into the oesophagus, may be the cause of these symptoms.

ACTION Your doctor will examine your baby to exclude other causes. You may be advised to change your baby's nappy before a feed, burp the baby frequently during feeds, and keep him or her semi-upright during and after feeds. If you bottle-feed, you may be advised to feed a pre-thickened formula. Your doctor may prescribe a medication to reduce reflux of stomach acid. If these measures do not help, your baby may be prescribed a drug to reduce stomach acid. Most babies grow out of the condition by 12–18 months.

SELF-HELP Preventing gastroenteritis

Babies, especially if they are bottle-fed, are particularly susceptible to gastroenteritis. The following precautions can decrease the risk:
- Always wash your hands after going to the toilet, after changing your baby's nappies, and before preparing his or her feeds.
- Sterilize all bottles, caps, and teats for as long as bottle-feeding continues or until your baby is 1 year old. Wash the items in warm, soapy water before sterilizing them.
- Sterilize all other feeding equipment and dummies regularly and thoroughly by using sterilizing chemicals or steam sterilizers, or by boiling equipment in a pan of water.
- Make sure that any water you give to a baby, or any water used to make up formula, has been boiled and cooled first.
- Keep a separate towel for your baby, and wash it often.
- Although you can stop sterilizing feeding equipment from about 1 year onwards, always make sure that everything is washed thoroughly in warm, soapy water.

EMERGENCY! CALL AN AMBULANCE

POSSIBLE CAUSE Meningitis, inflammation of the membranes surrounding the brain due to infection, may be the cause of these symptoms.

ACTION If meningitis is suspected, your baby will be admitted to hospital immediately. He or she will be given urgent treatment with antibiotics and may need intensive care.

POSSIBLE CAUSE AND ACTION Regurgitation, sometimes known as posseting, is common in babies and is a likely cause. It is not true vomiting and is seldom a cause for concern in an otherwise well baby. The condition is usually the result of trapped air in the stomach (see DEALING WITH WIND, p.49). However, if you are concerned, consult your doctor.

Continued from previous page

SELF-HELP Treating gastroenteritis in babies

Gastroenteritis does not usually need drug treatment; the priority is to replace fluids lost through vomiting and diarrhoea so your baby does not become dehydrated. If you are breast-feeding, give more frequent feeds. If you are bottle-feeding, give feeds at the normal strength but in smaller quantities and more frequently. If the baby becomes dehydrated, your doctor may advise giving oral rehydration solution as well. If your baby has started on solid food, keep to a normal diet if he or she feels like eating. If not, or if vomiting continues, give small, frequent drinks, then gradually return to a normal diet (see TREATING GASTROENTERITIS IN CHILDREN, p.114).

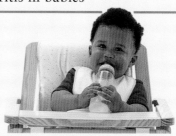

Giving rehydrating solutions
Rehydrating solutions should be prepared with cooled, boiled water and are available in different flavours to make them more palatable.

Does your baby have a cough? YES / NO

Does your baby have diarrhoea? YES / NO

Is your baby's vomit yellowish-green? YES / NO

Does the vomiting only occur during or after travel in a vehicle? YES / NO

Was your baby playing energetically just before vomiting, or were you playing boisterously with him or her? YES / NO

CALL YOUR DOCTOR NOW

POSSIBLE CAUSE Gastroenteritis, an infection of the digestive system, is the most likely cause of these symptoms. In some cases, a baby may also develop a fever.

ACTION Your doctor will check whether your baby is dehydrated and will give you advice on preventing dehydration in babies (p.55) and treating gastroenteritis in babies (above). To prevent future attacks, follow the advice for preventing gastroenteritis (opposite).

CALL YOUR DOCTOR NOW

POSSIBLE CAUSES Bronchiolitis, a viral infection affecting the small airways in the lungs, or whooping cough (pertussis), an infectious disease that causes bouts of severe coughing, may be the cause.

ACTION Your baby may be admitted to hospital, where his or her blood oxygen levels can be measured (p.197). If bronchiolitis is diagnosed, treatment may include bronchodilator drugs and oxygen. If whooping cough is diagnosed, he or she may need antibiotics to prevent the spread of the infection, although these do not always affect the severity of the symptoms.

EMERGENCY! CALL AN AMBULANCE

POSSIBLE CAUSE Intussusception, in which the intestine telescopes in on itself, causing an obstruction, is a possibility.

ACTION Your baby will probably be admitted to hospital, where he or she can be fully examined and an exact diagnosis made. Treatment for intussusception usually involves an enema to force the displaced intestinal tissue back into the right position. If the enema is not successful, surgery will be necessary.

POSSIBLE CAUSE AND ACTION Travel sickness is probably the cause. Although uncommon in children under the age of 1 year, some babies are particularly susceptible. The condition may run in families. For self-help measures, follow the advice on coping with travel sickness (p.115).

POSSIBLE CAUSE AND ACTION In babies, the muscles around the top of the stomach are relatively lax compared with those of older children, and enthusiastic playing may cause vomiting. This is no cause for concern and will be less of a problem as your baby grows older. In the meantime, try to avoid boisterous games, particularly after feeds.

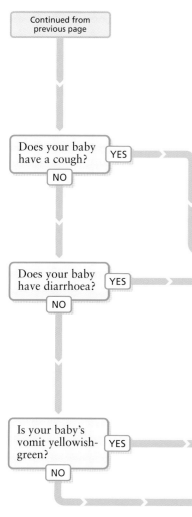

Pyloric stenosis

Pyloric stenosis is an uncommon disorder that occurs in babies under 2 months and is more common in boys. In this condition, the ring of muscle forming the outlet from the stomach into the small intestine becomes narrowed and thickened due to overgrowth of the muscle tissue. The cause is unknown. Because the stomach cannot empty into the intestine, the stomach contents build up until repeated, forceful vomiting occurs. Without treatment, the baby will lose weight and develop potentially life-threatening dehydration. Treatment involves surgery, in which the thickened muscle is cut to widen the stomach outlet. The baby should be able to resume normal feeding within 2–3 days and have no permanent ill effects.

AN ISOLATED ATTACK OF VOMITING IS UNLIKELY TO BE A SIGN OF A SERIOUS PROBLEM IN AN OTHERWISE WELL BABY. HOWEVER, IF YOUR BABY VOMITS MORE THAN ONCE IN A DAY OR SEEMS OTHERWISE UNWELL, CALL YOUR DOCTOR.

5 Diarrhoea in babies

For children over 1 year, see chart 40, Diarrhoea in children (p.118).
Diarrhoea is the frequent passing of abnormally loose or watery faeces. It is normal for a breast-fed baby to pass soft faeces up to 6 times a day, and this situation should not be mistaken for diarrhoea. If your baby does have diarrhoea, give him or her plenty of fluids to prevent dehydration (*see* Preventing dehydration in babies, opposite).

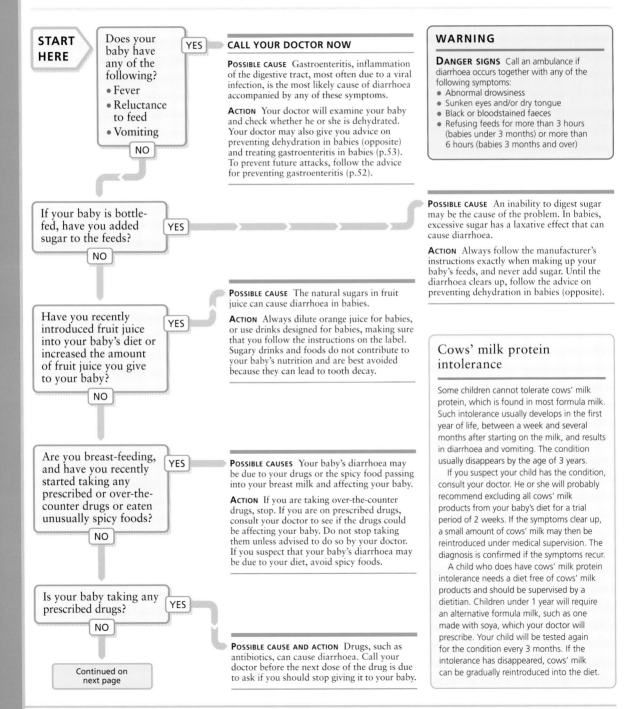

START HERE

Does your baby have any of the following?
- Fever
- Reluctance to feed
- Vomiting

YES →

CALL YOUR DOCTOR NOW

Possible cause Gastroenteritis, inflammation of the digestive tract, most often due to a viral infection, is the most likely cause of diarrhoea accompanied by any of these symptoms.

Action Your doctor will examine your baby and check whether he or she is dehydrated. Your doctor may also give you advice on preventing dehydration in babies (opposite) and treating gastroenteritis in babies (p.53). To prevent future attacks, follow the advice for preventing gastroenteritis (p.52).

NO

If your baby is bottle-fed, have you added sugar to the feeds?

YES ⇢

Possible cause An inability to digest sugar may be the cause of the problem. In babies, excessive sugar has a laxative effect that can cause diarrhoea.

Action Always follow the manufacturer's instructions exactly when making up your baby's feeds, and never add sugar. Until the diarrhoea clears up, follow the advice on preventing dehydration in babies (opposite).

NO

Have you recently introduced fruit juice into your baby's diet or increased the amount of fruit juice you give to your baby?

YES →

Possible cause The natural sugars in fruit juice can cause diarrhoea in babies.

Action Always dilute orange juice for babies, or use drinks designed for babies, making sure that you follow the instructions on the label. Sugary drinks and foods do not contribute to your baby's nutrition and are best avoided because they can lead to tooth decay.

NO

Are you breast-feeding, and have you recently started taking any prescribed or over-the-counter drugs or eaten unusually spicy foods?

YES →

Possible causes Your baby's diarrhoea may be due to your drugs or the spicy food passing into your breast milk and affecting your baby.

Action If you are taking over-the-counter drugs, stop. If you are on prescribed drugs, consult your doctor to see if the drugs could be affecting your baby. Do not stop taking them unless advised to do so by your doctor. If you suspect that your baby's diarrhoea may be due to your diet, avoid spicy foods.

NO

Is your baby taking any prescribed drugs?

YES →

Possible cause and action Drugs, such as antibiotics, can cause diarrhoea. Call your doctor before the next dose of the drug is due to ask if you should stop giving it to your baby.

NO

Continued on next page

WARNING

Danger signs Call an ambulance if diarrhoea occurs together with any of the following symptoms:
- Abnormal drowsiness
- Sunken eyes and/or dry tongue
- Black or bloodstained faeces
- Refusing feeds for more than 3 hours (babies under 3 months) or more than 6 hours (babies 3 months and over)

Cows' milk protein intolerance

Some children cannot tolerate cows' milk protein, which is found in most formula milk. Such intolerance usually develops in the first year of life, between a week and several months after starting on the milk, and results in diarrhoea and vomiting. The condition usually disappears by the age of 3 years.

If you suspect your child has the condition, consult your doctor. He or she will probably recommend excluding all cows' milk products from your baby's diet for a trial period of 2 weeks. If the symptoms clear up, a small amount of cows' milk may then be reintroduced under medical supervision. The diagnosis is confirmed if the symptoms recur.

A child who does have cows' milk protein intolerance needs a diet free of cows' milk products and should be supervised by a dietitian. Children under 1 year will require an alternative formula milk, such as one made with soya, which your doctor will prescribe. Your child will be tested again for the condition every 3 months. If the intolerance has disappeared, cows' milk can be gradually reintroduced into the diet.

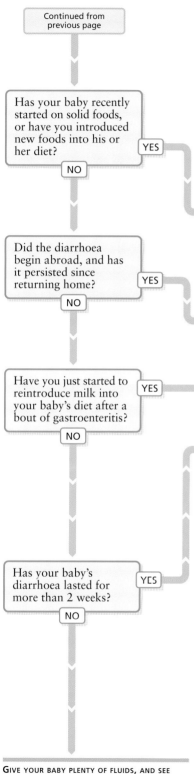

Continued from previous page

Has your baby recently started on solid foods, or have you introduced new foods into his or her diet?
YES
NO

Did the diarrhoea begin abroad, and has it persisted since returning home?
YES
NO

Have you just started to reintroduce milk into your baby's diet after a bout of gastroenteritis?
YES
NO

Has your baby's diarrhoea lasted for more than 2 weeks?
YES
NO

GIVE YOUR BABY PLENTY OF FLUIDS, AND SEE YOUR DOCTOR WITHIN 24 HOURS.

Babies' faeces

The first faeces that a baby passes are known as meconium, which is a sticky greenish-black substance consisting mainly of mucus and bile. Within a day or two, the faeces change to a greenish-brown colour, then settle to a regular colour. Most babies pass faeces several times a day, although some can go for a few days without passing any. As long as your baby seems well, there is probably nothing wrong.

Breast-fed babies can pass faeces very frequently. The faeces are very soft and usually orange-yellow, like mustard, and there may be visible mucus. They may smell of sour milk.

Bottle-fed babies pass bulkier and more substantial faeces than breast-fed babies. The faeces are usually light brown and smell strongly, rather like the faeces of an adult.

Green faeces are a sign that food has passed through the intestines very rapidly. For a breast-fed baby, green faeces may be normal, but in a bottle-fed baby, such faeces may result from a gastrointestinal infection.

POSSIBLE CAUSE AND ACTION A sudden change in your baby's diet can cause temporary diarrhoea. Introduce new foods slowly, with only one new food each week. Consult your doctor or health visitor if several foods appear to upset your baby's digestion.

POSSIBLE CAUSE AND ACTION Your baby may have acquired an infection abroad. Consult your doctor, and make sure that you mention your foreign travel.

POSSIBLE CAUSE Temporary intolerance to lactose (p.118), which is a natural sugar found in milk, is a possible cause of recurrent or persistent diarrhoea. If milk is reintroduced into your baby's diet too soon after an episode of gastroenteritis, the diarrhoea can recur.

ACTION Go back to giving your baby rehydrating solutions while he or she has diarrhoea. Then gradually reintroduce milk (see TREATING GASTROENTERITIS IN BABIES, p.53). If diarrhoea recurs again, see your doctor within 24 hours. Your doctor will advise a lactose-free diet until your baby recovers.

Are your baby's height and weight within the normal range for his or her age (see GROWTH CHARTS, p.26)?
YES
NO

POSSIBLE CAUSES Your baby may not be absorbing food normally. The cause may be either a food intolerance, such as cows' milk protein intolerance (opposite), or a disorder such as cystic fibrosis. Consult your doctor.

ACTION Your doctor will examine your baby and may arrange for his or her faeces to be tested for evidence of an infection. Your baby may be referred to a specialist to establish the underlying cause.

POSSIBLE CAUSE AND ACTION Some babies normally produce very soft faeces but do not have diarrhoea (see BABIES' FAECES, above). If you are not sure whether or not your baby's faeces are normal, you should consult your health visitor for advice.

SELF-HELP Preventing dehydration in babies

If your baby has diarrhoea or vomiting, it is essential to give plenty of fluids to help prevent dehydration, which is a potentially life-threatening condition. If you are breast-feeding, give your baby more frequent feeds. If you are bottle-feeding, make up the formula at the same strength but give smaller, more frequent feeds. If your baby has started on solid food, keep to a normal diet if he or she feels like eating. Do not worry, however, if your baby will not eat; it is more important to maintain fluid intake by giving small, frequent drinks such as water that has first been boiled and then cooled.

If the diarrhoea becomes worse, see your doctor. He or she may advise you to give your baby an oral rehydration preparation after each feed. This type of preparation, available from pharmacies, is designed to replace fluids, sugars, and salts lost from the body through diarrhoea and vomiting. Oral rehydration preparations are usually available as sachets of powder, which you mix with boiled, cooled water to form a drink for the baby. The powders are flavoured to make them more palatable.

55

6 Feeding problems

For children over 1, see chart 37, EATING PROBLEMS **(p.112).**
Feeding problems are a common source of irritability and
crying in young babies as well as concern in their parents.
Such problems may include a reluctance to feed, constant

hungry crying, and swallowing too much air, leading
to regurgitation. There may also be special problems for
mothers who are breast-feeding. This chart deals with most
of the common problems that may arise.

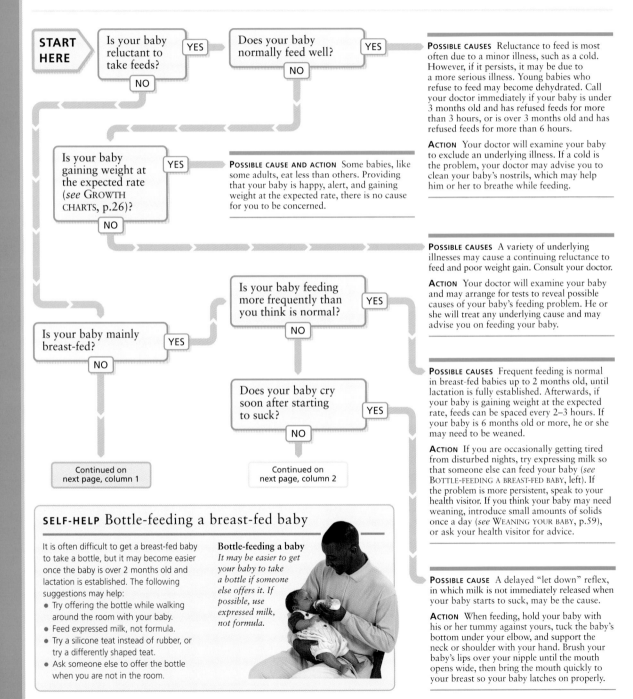

START HERE

Is your baby reluctant to take feeds?
— NO
— YES → **Does your baby normally feed well?**
— YES
— NO

POSSIBLE CAUSES Reluctance to feed is most
often due to a minor illness, such as a cold.
However, if it persists, it may be due to
a more serious illness. Young babies who
refuse to feed may become dehydrated. Call
your doctor immediately if your baby is under
3 months old and has refused feeds for more
than 3 hours, or is over 3 months old and has
refused feeds for more than 6 hours.

ACTION Your doctor will examine your baby
to exclude an underlying illness. If a cold is
the problem, your doctor may advise you to
clean your baby's nostrils, which may help
him or her to breathe while feeding.

Is your baby gaining weight at the expected rate *(see* GROWTH CHARTS, **p.26)?**
— NO
— YES → **POSSIBLE CAUSE AND ACTION** Some babies, like
some adults, eat less than others. Providing
that your baby is happy, alert, and gaining
weight at the expected rate, there is no cause
for you to be concerned.

POSSIBLE CAUSES A variety of underlying
illnesses may cause a continuing reluctance to
feed and poor weight gain. Consult your doctor.

ACTION Your doctor will examine your baby
and may arrange for tests to reveal possible
causes of your baby's feeding problem. He or
she will treat any underlying cause and may
advise you on feeding your baby.

Is your baby feeding more frequently than you think is normal?
— NO
— YES

Is your baby mainly breast-fed?
— NO
— YES

POSSIBLE CAUSES Frequent feeding is normal
in breast-fed babies up to 2 months old, until
lactation is fully established. Afterwards, if
your baby is gaining weight at the expected
rate, feeds can be spaced every 2–3 hours. If
your baby is 6 months old or more, he or she
may need to be weaned.

ACTION If you are occasionally getting tired
from disturbed nights, try expressing milk so
that someone else can feed your baby *(see*
BOTTLE-FEEDING A BREAST-FED BABY, left). If
the problem is more persistent, speak to your
health visitor. If you think your baby may need
weaning, introduce small amounts of solids
once a day *(see* WEANING YOUR BABY, **p.59),**
or ask your health visitor for advice.

Does your baby cry soon after starting to suck?
— NO
— YES

Continued on
next page, column 1

Continued on
next page, column 2

POSSIBLE CAUSE A delayed "let down" reflex,
in which milk is not immediately released when
your baby starts to suck, may be the cause.

ACTION When feeding, hold your baby with
his or her tummy against yours, tuck the baby's
bottom under your elbow, and support the
neck or shoulder with your hand. Brush your
baby's lips over your nipple until the mouth
opens wide, then bring the mouth quickly to
your breast so your baby latches on properly.

SELF-HELP Bottle-feeding a breast-fed baby

It is often difficult to get a breast-fed baby
to take a bottle, but it may become easier
once the baby is over 2 months old and
lactation is established. The following
suggestions may help:

- Try offering the bottle while walking
  around the room with your baby.
- Feed expressed milk, not formula.
- Try a silicone teat instead of rubber, or
  try a differently shaped teat.
- Ask someone else to offer the bottle
  when you are not in the room.

Bottle-feeding a baby
*It may be easier to get
your baby to take
a bottle if someone
else offers it. If
possible, use
expressed milk,
not formula.*

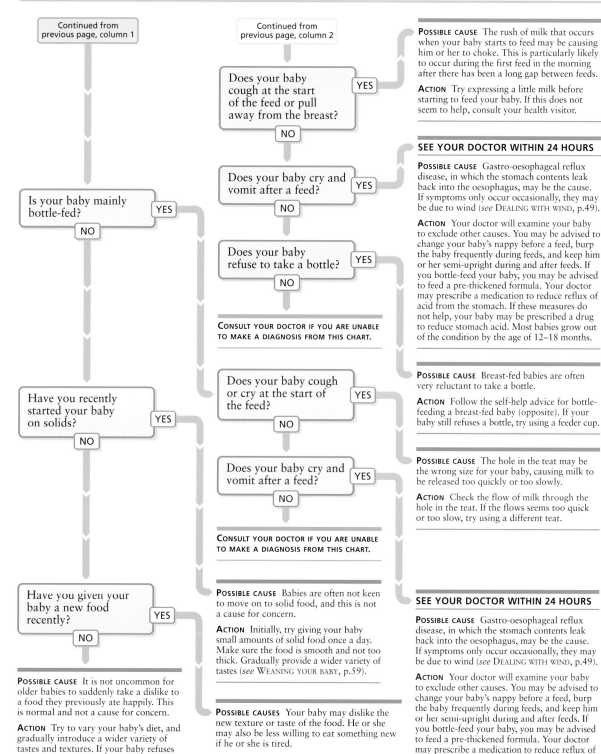

Continued from previous page, column 1

Continued from previous page, column 2

Does your baby cough at the start of the feed or pull away from the breast? YES / NO

POSSIBLE CAUSE The rush of milk that occurs when your baby starts to feed may be causing him or her to choke. This is particularly likely to occur during the first feed in the morning after there has been a long gap between feeds.

ACTION Try expressing a little milk before starting to feed your baby. If this does not seem to help, consult your health visitor.

Is your baby mainly bottle-fed? YES / NO

Does your baby cry and vomit after a feed? YES / NO

SEE YOUR DOCTOR WITHIN 24 HOURS

POSSIBLE CAUSE Gastro-oesophageal reflux disease, in which the stomach contents leak back into the oesophagus, may be the cause. If symptoms only occur occasionally, they may be due to wind (*see* DEALING WITH WIND, p.49).

ACTION Your doctor will examine your baby to exclude other causes. You may be advised to change your baby's nappy before a feed, burp the baby frequently during feeds, and keep him or her semi-upright during and after feeds. If you bottle-feed your baby, you may be advised to feed a pre-thickened formula. Your doctor may prescribe a medication to reduce reflux of acid from the stomach. If these measures do not help, your baby may be prescribed a drug to reduce stomach acid. Most babies grow out of the condition by the age of 12–18 months.

Does your baby refuse to take a bottle? YES / NO

CONSULT YOUR DOCTOR IF YOU ARE UNABLE TO MAKE A DIAGNOSIS FROM THIS CHART.

POSSIBLE CAUSE Breast-fed babies are often very reluctant to take a bottle.

ACTION Follow the self-help advice for bottle-feeding a breast-fed baby (opposite). If your baby still refuses a bottle, try using a feeder cup.

Have you recently started your baby on solids? YES / NO

Does your baby cough or cry at the start of the feed? YES / NO

POSSIBLE CAUSE The hole in the teat may be the wrong size for your baby, causing milk to be released too quickly or too slowly.

ACTION Check the flow of milk through the hole in the teat. If the flows seems too quick or too slow, try using a different teat.

Does your baby cry and vomit after a feed? YES / NO

CONSULT YOUR DOCTOR IF YOU ARE UNABLE TO MAKE A DIAGNOSIS FROM THIS CHART.

Have you given your baby a new food recently? YES / NO

POSSIBLE CAUSE Babies are often not keen to move on to solid food, and this is not a cause for concern.

ACTION Initially, try giving your baby small amounts of solid food once a day. Make sure the food is smooth and not too thick. Gradually provide a wider variety of tastes (*see* WEANING YOUR BABY, p.59).

SEE YOUR DOCTOR WITHIN 24 HOURS

POSSIBLE CAUSE Gastro-oesophageal reflux disease, in which the stomach contents leak back into the oesophagus, may be the cause. If symptoms only occur occasionally, they may be due to wind (*see* DEALING WITH WIND, p.49).

ACTION Your doctor will examine your baby to exclude other causes. You may be advised to change your baby's nappy before a feed, burp the baby frequently during feeds, and keep him or her semi-upright during and after feeds. If you bottle-feed your baby, you may be advised to feed a pre-thickened formula. Your doctor may prescribe a medication to reduce reflux of acid from the stomach. If these measures do not help, your baby may be prescribed a drug to reduce stomach acid. Most babies grow out of the condition by the age of 12–18 months.

POSSIBLE CAUSE It is not uncommon for older babies to suddenly take a dislike to a food they previously ate happily. This is normal and not a cause for concern.

ACTION Try to vary your baby's diet, and gradually introduce a wider variety of tastes and textures. If your baby refuses to eat one particular food, stop offering it to him or her, and reintroduce it at a later date. However, if you are concerned, consult your doctor or health visitor.

POSSIBLE CAUSES Your baby may dislike the new texture or taste of the food. He or she may also be less willing to eat something new if he or she is tired.

ACTION Stop giving your baby the new food for a while. Try it again at a later date, preferably at breakfast time when your baby is less likely to be tired.

7 Slow weight gain

For children over 1, see chart 12, GROWTH PROBLEMS (p.68). Consult this chart if you are worried that your baby is gaining weight too slowly. Most babies lose some weight in their first week of life (*see* WEIGHT LOSS IN THE NEWBORN, opposite), and this is not usually a cause for concern. After this, babies should put on weight at a steady rate. Your baby will be weighed and measured regularly at your local baby clinic, and his or her growth will be plotted on growth charts (*see* GROWTH CHARTS, p.26) so that any problems can be detected early. In the first year of life, growth is faster than at any other time and key body systems such as the nervous system are developing rapidly. For this reason, nutrition is particularly important at this time (*see* NUTRITIONAL REQUIREMENTS OF BABIES, below).

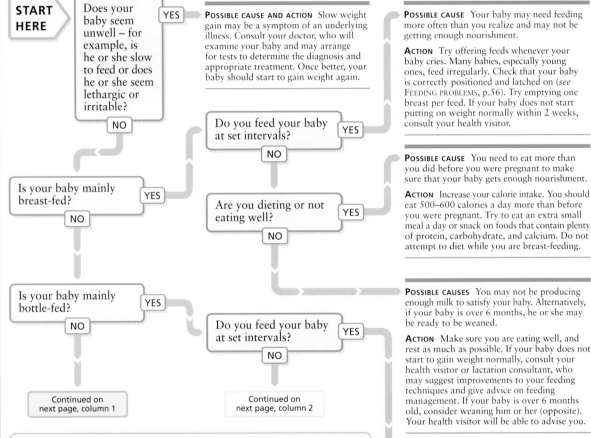

START HERE

Does your baby seem unwell – for example, is he or she slow to feed or does he or she seem lethargic or irritable?

YES → **POSSIBLE CAUSE AND ACTION** Slow weight gain may be a symptom of an underlying illness. Consult your doctor, who will examine your baby and may arrange for tests to determine the diagnosis and appropriate treatment. Once better, your baby should start to gain weight again.

NO

Is your baby mainly breast-fed? YES

NO

Do you feed your baby at set intervals? YES

NO

Are you dieting or not eating well? YES

NO

Is your baby mainly bottle-fed? YES

NO

Do you feed your baby at set intervals? YES

NO

POSSIBLE CAUSE Your baby may need feeding more often than you realize and may not be getting enough nourishment.

ACTION Try offering feeds whenever your baby cries. Many babies, especially young ones, feed irregularly. Check that your baby is correctly positioned and latched on (*see* FEEDING PROBLEMS, p.56). Try emptying one breast per feed. If your baby does not start putting on weight normally within 2 weeks, consult your health visitor.

POSSIBLE CAUSE You need to eat more than you did before you were pregnant to make sure that your baby gets enough nourishment.

ACTION Increase your calorie intake. You should eat 500–600 calories a day more than before you were pregnant. Try to eat an extra small meal a day or snack on foods that contain plenty of protein, carbohydrate, and calcium. Do not attempt to diet while you are breast-feeding.

POSSIBLE CAUSES You may not be producing enough milk to satisfy your baby. Alternatively, if your baby is over 6 months, he or she may be ready to be weaned.

ACTION Make sure you are eating well, and rest as much as possible. If your baby does not start to gain weight normally, consult your health visitor or lactation consultant, who may suggest improvements to your feeding techniques and give advice on feeding management. If your baby is over 6 months old, consider weaning him or her (opposite). Your health visitor will be able to advise you.

Continued on next page, column 1

Continued on next page, column 2

POSSIBLE CAUSE Your baby may need feeding more often than you realize and may not be getting enough nourishment.

ACTION Try feeding your baby whenever he or she cries, even if that means sometimes offering a feed when he or she is not hungry. Many babies, especially young ones, feed irregularly. If your baby is not putting on weight normally within 2 weeks, consult your health visitor.

Nutritional requirements of babies

Babies need a diet that is relatively high in energy (calories), high in fat, low in fibre, and low in salt. The foods should contain enough protein for growth and enough carbohydrates to provide energy. Liquid vitamin drops containing vitamins A, C, and D are generally recommended for babies over 6 months old who have breast milk as their main drink. These drops are available from mother and baby clinics or from your health visitor. Babies under 12 months who have mainly formula milk do not need supplements because the milk is already fortified with these vitamins. If you are vegetarian, you can bring up your baby on the same type of diet as yourself but be careful to include sufficient iron. Give your baby plenty of fruit and vegetables because these foods contain vitamin C, which helps the body absorb iron. Include pulses (such as beans, chickpeas, and lentils) and tofu to provide energy. A vegan diet is not nutritionally complete for a baby. If you are a vegan, consult your doctor or health visitor for advice on supplements.

SELF-HELP Weaning your baby

By the time your baby is 6 months old, he or she should be ready to be weaned. Weaning is the gradual transfer from a milk-only diet to solid foods. Start by introducing your baby to puréed fruit or vegetables and baby rice. Try giving him or her a taste after a milk feed. Gradually introduce other foods and textures. Your own food can be sieved or puréed, but do not add salt or sugar when preparing it. Do not give eggs, wheat-based foods, such as wheat cereals, citrus fruits, or fatty foods until your baby is at least 6 months old. Do not give cows' milk, honey, or foods containing nuts until he or she is at least 12 months.

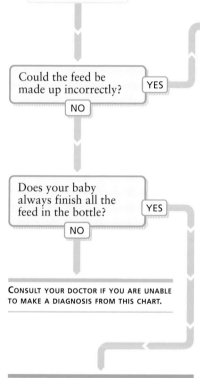

Eating from a spoon
As part of the weaning process, introduce your baby to the idea of taking food from a spoon.

Age (from)	Suggested weaning programme
6 months	Offer your baby puréed foods, including fruit, such as bananas, vegetables, pulses, and baby rice.
7–8 months	You can now give mashed or minced food, including eggs (as long as they are hard-boiled), fish, and chicken. You can also offer finger foods, such as toast, cubes of apple, or bits of hard cheese.
9–12 months	Introduce more variety into the diet, and provide food that contains small pieces, such as peas and chopped carrots.
Over 12 months	Your baby can now have the same diet as the rest of the family; but avoid salt and sugar, and give him or her full-cream, rather than semi-skimmed, milk.

Continued from previous page, column 1

Continued from previous page, column 2

POSSIBLE CAUSE If there is too little powder or too much water in the feed, your baby will not be receiving enough nourishment.

ACTION Always follow the manufacturer's instructions exactly when mixing feeds. Never add extra powder to your baby's feeds. If you think that your baby is thirsty, give him or her cooled, boiled water, and continue to offer feeds as normal. If your baby does not start putting on weight normally within 2 weeks, consult your health visitor.

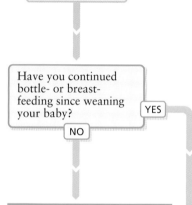

Have you continued bottle- or breast-feeding since weaning your baby?
NO — YES

Could the feed be made up incorrectly?
YES
NO

POSSIBLE CAUSE It is very difficult for newly weaned babies to get sufficient nourishment from solid food alone; milk feeds are still essential.

ACTION Offer your baby milk in addition to solid foods (*see* WEANING YOUR BABY, above). If your baby does not start putting on weight normally within 2 weeks or if you have trouble getting him or her to take solid food, consult your health visitor.

Does your baby always finish all the feed in the bottle?
YES
NO

CONSULT YOUR DOCTOR IF YOU ARE UNABLE TO MAKE A DIAGNOSIS FROM THIS CHART.

Weight loss in the newborn

Your baby may lose weight in the first week of life; however, this is unlikely to be a cause for concern. Most babies, particularly if they are breast-fed, may lose up to 200 g (7 oz) in the first few days after delivery. This weight loss is normal and is partly due to the relatively small amount of food they take in initially. In addition, newborn babies need to adjust to life outside the uterus and now have to take in, digest, and absorb their food, rather than have it supplied through the placenta. Most babies start to gain weight by the 5th day and are usually back to their birth weight by about 10 days after delivery.

Your baby will probably be weighed by the midwife or health visitor about three times a week for the first 2 weeks. Once your baby has regained his or her birth weight, he or she should continue to put on weight at a steady rate. For the first 3 months, your baby should gain approximately 170 g (6 oz) a week. By about 6 months, a baby should have roughly doubled his or her birth weight.

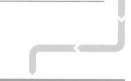

POSSIBLE CAUSE Check that you are giving your baby the right foods for his or her age. He or she may need more nourishment.

ACTION Follow the advice for weaning your baby (above), and offer food or milk whenever your baby seems hungry. If your baby does not start putting on weight normally within 2 weeks or if you are not sure what foods he or she should have, consult your health visitor.

POSSIBLE CAUSE As your baby grows, his or her appetite will increase, and he or she may need more food than you are now offering, even if you are giving the recommended amount for your baby's age.

ACTION Offer more milk than usual, and let your baby feed until he or she is satisfied. If your baby is over 6 months, he or she may be ready to start on solids (*see* WEANING YOUR BABY, above). If your baby does not start to gain weight normally or if you need further advice on weaning, consult your health visitor.

8 Skin problems in babies

If your baby has a rash with a temperature, see chart 15, RASH WITH FEVER (p.74).
The skin of newborn babies is very sensitive and can easily become irritated from rubbing on clothes or bedding. Such minor skin problems are usually no cause for concern. One of the most common skin problems in babies is nappy rash, which can be treated easily. Other rashes and skin abnormalities that occur for no apparent reason or that persist longer than a few days should be brought to your doctor's attention, especially if your baby seems unwell.

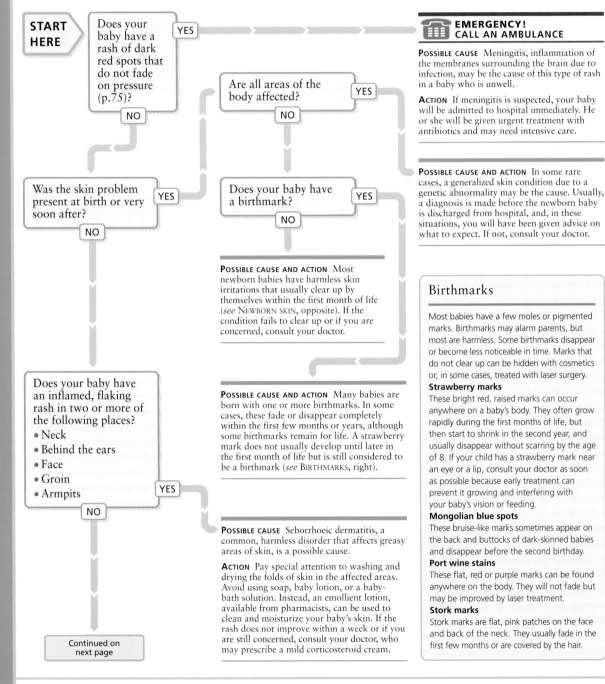

START HERE

Does your baby have a rash of dark red spots that do not fade on pressure (p.75)? — YES / NO

Are all areas of the body affected? — YES / NO

Was the skin problem present at birth or very soon after? — YES / NO

Does your baby have a birthmark? — YES / NO

Does your baby have an inflamed, flaking rash in two or more of the following places?
- Neck
- Behind the ears
- Face
- Groin
- Armpits
— YES / NO

☎ EMERGENCY! CALL AN AMBULANCE

POSSIBLE CAUSE Meningitis, inflammation of the membranes surrounding the brain due to infection, may be the cause of this type of rash in a baby who is unwell.

ACTION If meningitis is suspected, your baby will be admitted to hospital immediately. He or she will be given urgent treatment with antibiotics and may need intensive care.

POSSIBLE CAUSE AND ACTION In some rare cases, a generalized skin condition due to a genetic abnormality may be the cause. Usually, a diagnosis is made before the newborn baby is discharged from hospital, and, in these situations, you will have been given advice on what to expect. If not, consult your doctor.

POSSIBLE CAUSE AND ACTION Most newborn babies have harmless skin irritations that usually clear up by themselves within the first month of life (*see* NEWBORN SKIN, opposite). If the condition fails to clear up or if you are concerned, consult your doctor.

POSSIBLE CAUSE AND ACTION Many babies are born with one or more birthmarks. In some cases, these fade or disappear completely within the first few months or years, although some birthmarks remain for life. A strawberry mark does not usually develop until later in the first month of life but is still considered to be a birthmark (*see* BIRTHMARKS, right).

POSSIBLE CAUSE Seborrhoeic dermatitis, a common, harmless disorder that affects greasy areas of skin, is a possible cause.

ACTION Pay special attention to washing and drying the folds of skin in the affected areas. Avoid using soap, baby lotion, or a baby-bath solution. Instead, an emollient lotion, available from pharmacists, can be used to clean and moisturize your baby's skin. If the rash does not improve within a week or if you are still concerned, consult your doctor, who may prescribe a mild corticosteroid cream.

Birthmarks

Most babies have a few moles or pigmented marks. Birthmarks may alarm parents, but most are harmless. Some birthmarks disappear or become less noticeable in time. Marks that do not clear up can be hidden with cosmetics or, in some cases, treated with laser surgery.

Strawberry marks
These bright red, raised marks can occur anywhere on a baby's body. They often grow rapidly during the first months of life, but then start to shrink in the second year, and usually disappear without scarring by the age of 8. If your child has a strawberry mark near an eye or a lip, consult your doctor as soon as possible because early treatment can prevent it growing and interfering with your baby's vision or feeding.

Mongolian blue spots
These bruise-like marks sometimes appear on the back and buttocks of dark-skinned babies and disappear before the second birthday.

Port wine stains
These flat, red or purple marks can be found anywhere on the body. They will not fade but may be improved by laser treatment.

Stork marks
Stork marks are flat, pink patches on the face and back of the neck. They usually fade in the first few months or are covered by the hair.

Continued on next page

Continued from previous page

Does your baby have yellowish-brown crusts on the scalp?

YES

POSSIBLE CAUSE Your baby may have cradle cap, a form of seborrhoeic dermatitis. It is a common, harmless condition.

ACTION You can soften the crusts by rubbing your baby's scalp with baby or olive oil at night and then washing off the crusts the next morning. Alternatively, special shampoos to treat the condition are available over the counter. However, the condition usually clears up by itself within a few weeks. If it does not or if you are concerned, consult your doctor.

NO

Does your baby have a red, itchy rash on the face, inside the elbows, or behind the knees?

YES

POSSIBLE CAUSE Your child may have atopic eczema. This diagnosis is most likely if any other family members suffer from eczema or other allergic conditions. Consult your doctor.

ACTION If the diagnosis is confirmed, your doctor will advise you on dealing with atopic eczema (p.76). He or she may also prescribe a corticosteroid cream. If the rash is widespread or weepy, your child should see the doctor within 24 hours. Many children with atopic eczema grow out of it by the age of 8.

NO

Has your baby got an inflamed area of skin on his or her bottom with or without spots spreading from it?

YES

Is the skin broken or ulcerated?

YES

POSSIBLE CAUSE AND ACTION Your baby may have nappy rash that has become infected. Consult your doctor, who may prescribe a cream containing an antibiotic, possibly combined with a corticosteroid drug. In the meantime, follow the advice on treating nappy rash (below).

NO

NO

Are there several red spots outside the main area of the rash?

YES

NO

CONSULT YOUR DOCTOR IF YOU ARE UNABLE TO MAKE A DIAGNOSIS FROM THIS CHART.

Newborn skin

A newborn baby's skin is very delicate and easily irritated. Do not use soap or wipes to clean your baby until he or she is at least 6 weeks old because these can dry the skin. Water is usually sufficient for cleansing the nappy area, and a few drops of baby oil in the bath water will help avoid dry skin.

There are several harmless skin problems that commonly affect babies. These include:
- Blotchy skin partly due to blood vessels being visible because there is little fat below the skin and partly because circulation is not mature, resulting in uneven blood flow.
- Milia – white spots on the nose and cheeks caused by blocked sebaceous glands in the skin. The spots clear up without treatment within the first couple of weeks.
- Peeling or flaking skin on the hands and feet. Gently rub emollient lotion into the affected areas.
- Urticaria – a rash of spots with a white centre and red halo, which clears up quickly without treatment.
- Heat rash – small red spots, often on the face and chest. Make sure that your baby is not too warm. No treatment is needed.

SEE YOUR DOCTOR WITHIN 24 HOURS

POSSIBLE CAUSE A skin infection with the fungus that causes thrush is a possibility. It may accompany nappy rash and oral thrush.

ACTION Your doctor will probably prescribe an antifungal cream and will possibly also prescribe a corticosteroid cream.

SELF-HELP Nappy rash

Nappy rash affects most babies at some time. It is particularly common after diarrhoea but can also develop if the skin becomes irritated from wearing a wet or soiled nappy for a long time. You can help clear up your baby's nappy rash by following these steps:
- Leave your baby to play without wearing a nappy as often as possible – preferably at least once a day.
- Wash the baby's nappy area with water, dry it carefully, and avoid scented wipes.

- Change your baby's nappy often.
- Make sure that you dry the creases in your baby's skin thoroughly.
- Apply a water-repellent cream such as zinc and castor oil or petroleum jelly.
- If you use cloth nappies, make sure they are thoroughly rinsed, and avoid using biological detergents.

Consult your doctor if the rash becomes blistery, weepy, or ulcerated or if it does not clear up within a few days.

POSSIBLE CAUSE Your baby probably has nappy rash, which affects most babies at some time, particularly when they have diarrhoea. Some babies seem more susceptible than others.

ACTION Follow the advice on treating nappy rash (left). If the rash does not clear up within a few days or if it becomes worse, consult your doctor, who may prescribe a corticosteroid cream to reduce the inflammation.

9 Feeling generally unwell

For unusual or excessive tiredness in a child, see chart 10, TIREDNESS **(p.64).**

A child may sometimes complain of feeling unwell without giving you a clear idea of what exactly the matter is. At other times, you may suspect that your child is unwell if he or she seems quieter or more irritable than usual. Use this chart to look for specific signs of illness. Such signs may lead you to a more specific chart within this book or to consult a doctor.

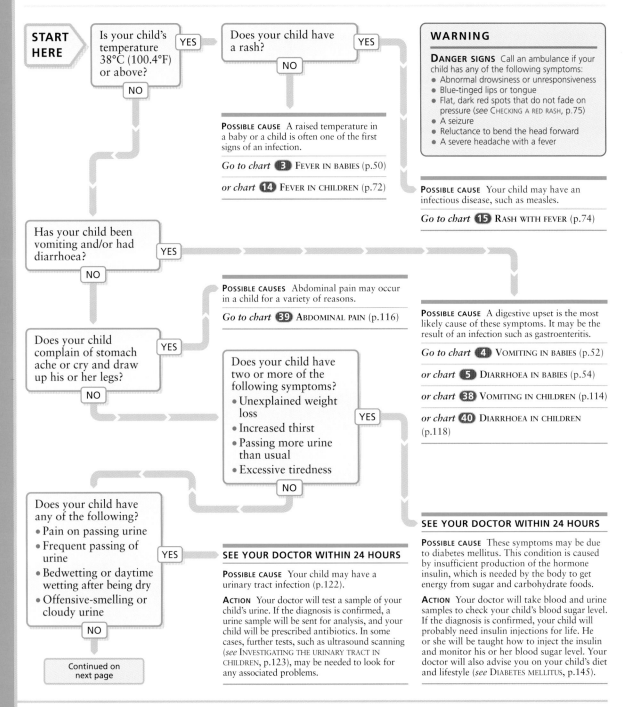

START HERE

Is your child's temperature 38°C (100.4°F) or above? — **NO**

YES → Does your child have a rash? — **NO**

YES →

WARNING

DANGER SIGNS Call an ambulance if your child has any of the following symptoms:
- Abnormal drowsiness or unresponsiveness
- Blue-tinged lips or tongue
- Flat, dark red spots that do not fade on pressure (*see* CHECKING A RED RASH, p.75)
- A seizure
- Reluctance to bend the head forward
- A severe headache with a fever

POSSIBLE CAUSE A raised temperature in a baby or a child is often one of the first signs of an infection.

Go to chart **3** FEVER IN BABIES (p.50)

or chart **14** FEVER IN CHILDREN (p.72)

POSSIBLE CAUSE Your child may have an infectious disease, such as measles.

Go to chart **15** RASH WITH FEVER (p.74)

Has your child been vomiting and/or had diarrhoea? — **NO** / **YES** →

POSSIBLE CAUSES Abdominal pain may occur in a child for a variety of reasons.

Go to chart **39** ABDOMINAL PAIN (p.116)

POSSIBLE CAUSE A digestive upset is the most likely cause of these symptoms. It may be the result of an infection such as gastroenteritis.

Go to chart **4** VOMITING IN BABIES (p.52)

or chart **5** DIARRHOEA IN BABIES (p.54)

or chart **38** VOMITING IN CHILDREN (p.114)

or chart **40** DIARRHOEA IN CHILDREN (p.118)

Does your child complain of stomach ache or cry and draw up his or her legs? — **NO** / **YES** →

Does your child have two or more of the following symptoms?
- Unexplained weight loss
- Increased thirst
- Passing more urine than usual
- Excessive tiredness

— **NO** / **YES** →

Does your child have any of the following?
- Pain on passing urine
- Frequent passing of urine
- Bedwetting or daytime wetting after being dry
- Offensive-smelling or cloudy urine

— **NO** / **YES** →

SEE YOUR DOCTOR WITHIN 24 HOURS

POSSIBLE CAUSE Your child may have a urinary tract infection (p.122).

ACTION Your doctor will test a sample of your child's urine. If the diagnosis is confirmed, a urine sample will be sent for analysis, and your child will be prescribed antibiotics. In some cases, further tests, such as ultrasound scanning (*see* INVESTIGATING THE URINARY TRACT IN CHILDREN, p.123), may be needed to look for any associated problems.

SEE YOUR DOCTOR WITHIN 24 HOURS

POSSIBLE CAUSE These symptoms may be due to diabetes mellitus. This condition is caused by insufficient production of the hormone insulin, which is needed by the body to get energy from sugar and carbohydrate foods.

ACTION Your doctor will take blood and urine samples to check your child's blood sugar level. If the diagnosis is confirmed, your child will probably need insulin injections for life. He or she will be taught how to inject the insulin and monitor his or her blood sugar level. Your doctor will also advise you on your child's diet and lifestyle (*see* DIABETES MELLITUS, p.145).

Continued on next page

Continued from previous page

Is your child refusing all food, including treats such as sweets that would normally be appealing?

NO **YES**

Has your child been in contact with an infectious illness within the past 2–3 weeks?

NO **YES**

Does your child seem to be better at weekends?

NO **YES**

Has there been a recent domestic upset, such as a house move, or is another child in the house ill?

NO **YES**

Has your child been feeling unwell for several weeks or more?

NO **YES**

CONSULT YOUR DOCTOR IF YOU ARE UNABLE TO MAKE A DIAGNOSIS FROM THIS CHART AND YOUR CHILD IS NO BETTER IN 48 HOURS.

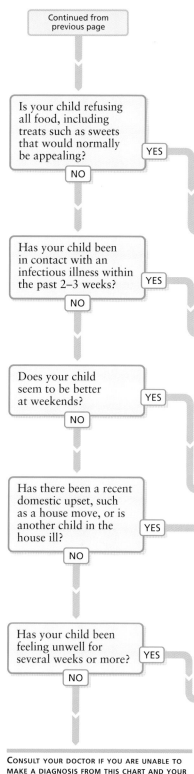

SELF-HELP Encouraging your child to drink

If your child is unwell, it is better to concentrate on encouraging him or her to drink rather than worrying about a poor appetite. The following measures may encourage your child to drink:

- Offer him or her interesting drinks, such as fruit-flavoured squashes, rather than plain water.
- Offer him or her ice lollies or ice cubes to suck.
- Offer small drinks frequently. Encourage your child to drink before an activity, such as a story.
- Use straws, bright or unusual cups, or "grown-up" cups to add interest.
- Let your child help prepare drinks or ice lollies.

Eating ice lollies
If your child is reluctant to drink, offer him or her an alternative such as a flavoured ice lolly instead.

Is your child also refusing to drink?

NO **YES**

POSSIBLE CAUSE Your child may be in the very early stages of a childhood infectious disease, such as chickenpox. It is common for children who are coming down with an infectious disease to feel unwell and listless for 2 or 3 days before any specific symptoms develop.

ACTION If your child develops any other symptoms, consult the relevant chart in this book. If your child is still feeling unwell after 48 hours and there is no obvious cause, consult your doctor.

POSSIBLE CAUSE Some children are easily unsettled by changes around them. They may express this by changes in behaviour or feeling unwell. An illness in another child in the family may cause conflicting feelings; your child may be anxious about the other child but also jealous of the extra attention given to him or her.

ACTION Talk to your child to find out what the problem is. Extra reassurance may help. If your child still feels unwell, consult your doctor.

Are your child's height and weight within the normal range for his or her age (*see* GROWTH CHARTS, p.26)?

NO **YES**

SEE YOUR DOCTOR WITHIN 24 HOURS

POSSIBLE CAUSE AND ACTION A sore mouth or throat is likely. However, refusing to drink can lead to dehydration. Your doctor will examine your child to establish the cause. Encourage your child to drink (above). If he or she is under 3 months and has refused feeds for 3 hours or is under 12 months and has refused to drink for 6 hours, contact your doctor immediately.

POSSIBLE CAUSE A refusal to eat is common in a child who is unwell for any reason.

ACTION Do not worry about your child's refusal to eat as long as he or she is drinking plenty (*see* ENCOURAGING YOUR CHILD TO DRINK, above). However, if your child is still not eating after 48 hours, and there is no obvious cause, consult your doctor.

POSSIBLE CAUSE Your child may be anxious about something at school, such as exams. Many children express anxiety by behaving in different ways than they normally do.

ACTION Talk to your child to find out what the problem is. You should also talk to his or her teachers to see if there is a problem you are not aware of, such as bullying. If your child continues to complain of feeling unwell, consult your doctor.

POSSIBLE CAUSE AND ACTION Your child may be unhappy or worried rather than physically ill. Some children find it hard to express feelings and may seem unwell instead. Take time to talk to your child, and, if necessary, consult your doctor, who may refer him or her to a specialist.

POSSIBLE CAUSE AND ACTION Your child may have an underlying disorder, such as a urinary tract infection. Consult your doctor, who may arrange for tests to look for an underlying cause and determine the appropriate treatment. Your child may be referred to a specialist.

10 Tiredness

For unusual drowsiness, see chart 22, CONFUSION AND/OR DROWSINESS (p.86).

It is normal for a child to be tired if he or she has slept badly the night before or had a particularly long or energetic day. It is also common for children to need more sleep than normal during growth spurts and at puberty. If your child seems tired most of time or tiredness is preventing him or her from taking part in social activities or keeping up at school, there may be an underlying medical problem. In many cases, such tiredness is short-lived and may be the result of a recent infection. However, you should consult your doctor to rule out a more serious problem.

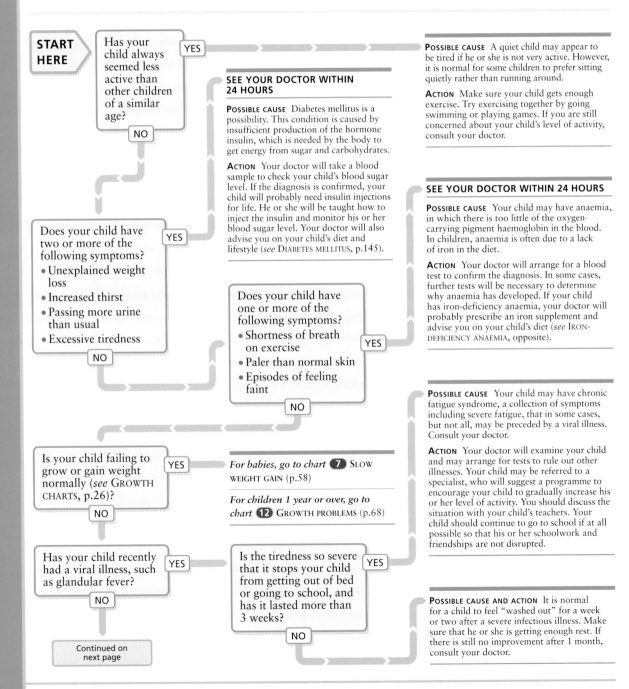

START HERE

Has your child always seemed less active than other children of a similar age?
YES / NO

Does your child have two or more of the following symptoms?
- Unexplained weight loss
- Increased thirst
- Passing more urine than usual
- Excessive tiredness

YES / NO

Does your child have one or more of the following symptoms?
- Shortness of breath on exercise
- Paler than normal skin
- Episodes of feeling faint

YES / NO

Is your child failing to grow or gain weight normally (*see* GROWTH CHARTS, p.26)?
YES / NO

Has your child recently had a viral illness, such as glandular fever?
YES / NO

Is the tiredness so severe that it stops your child from getting out of bed or going to school, and has it lasted more than 3 weeks?
YES / NO

Continued on next page

SEE YOUR DOCTOR WITHIN 24 HOURS

POSSIBLE CAUSE Diabetes mellitus is a possibility. This condition is caused by insufficient production of the hormone insulin, which is needed by the body to get energy from sugar and carbohydrates.

ACTION Your doctor will take a blood sample to check your child's blood sugar level. If the diagnosis is confirmed, your child will probably need insulin injections for life. He or she will be taught how to inject the insulin and monitor his or her blood sugar level. Your doctor will also advise you on your child's diet and lifestyle (*see* DIABETES MELLITUS, p.145).

For babies, go to chart **7** SLOW WEIGHT GAIN (p.58)

For children 1 year or over, go to chart **12** GROWTH PROBLEMS (p.68)

POSSIBLE CAUSE A quiet child may appear to be tired if he or she is not very active. However, it is normal for some children to prefer sitting quietly rather than running around.

ACTION Make sure your child gets enough exercise. Try exercising together by going swimming or playing games. If you are still concerned about your child's level of activity, consult your doctor.

SEE YOUR DOCTOR WITHIN 24 HOURS

POSSIBLE CAUSE Your child may have anaemia, in which there is too little of the oxygen-carrying pigment haemoglobin in the blood. In children, anaemia is often due to a lack of iron in the diet.

ACTION Your doctor will arrange for a blood test to confirm the diagnosis. In some cases, further tests will be necessary to determine why anaemia has developed. If your child has iron-deficiency anaemia, your doctor will probably prescribe an iron supplement and advise you on your child's diet (*see* IRON-DEFICIENCY ANAEMIA, opposite).

POSSIBLE CAUSE Your child may have chronic fatigue syndrome, a collection of symptoms including severe fatigue, that in some cases, but not all, may be preceded by a viral illness. Consult your doctor.

ACTION Your doctor will examine your child and may arrange for tests to rule out other illnesses. Your child may be referred to a specialist, who will suggest a programme to encourage your child to gradually increase his or her level of activity. You should discuss the situation with your child's teachers. Your child should continue to go to school if at all possible so that his or her schoolwork and friendships are not disrupted.

POSSIBLE CAUSE AND ACTION It is normal for a child to feel "washed out" for a week or two after a severe infectious illness. Make sure that he or she is getting enough rest. If there is still no improvement after 1 month, consult your doctor.

Continued from previous page

Is your child taking any prescribed drugs? — YES

POSSIBLE CAUSE AND ACTION Certain drugs, such as antihistamines and anticonvulsants, can cause tiredness as a side effect. Consult your doctor. Meanwhile, make sure your child does not stop taking his or her prescribed drugs.

NO

Does your child sleep badly? — YES

Does your child snore? — YES

POSSIBLE CAUSES Children often snore if they have a cold, and this is nothing to worry about. However, if your child snores all the time, he or she may have enlarged tonsils or adenoids (p.103), which may be blocking the airway during sleep. Consult your doctor.

ACTION Your doctor will examine your child's throat. In some cases, your doctor may refer your child to a specialist. Surgical removal of the tonsils and adenoids may improve the situation.

NO

Is your child's sleep disturbed by symptoms such as a cough or itchy skin? — YES

POSSIBLE CAUSE Symptoms of conditions such as asthma or eczema that do not bother a child during the day can disturb his or her sleep. Consult your doctor.

ACTION The doctor will examine your child and prescribe appropriate treatment. If your child is already receiving treatment for a condition such as asthma or eczema, it may need to be adjusted. Once the symptoms have been treated, your child should sleep better.

NO

NO

Go to chart **1** SLEEPING PROBLEMS IN BABIES (p.46)

or go to chart **11** SLEEPING PROBLEMS IN CHILDREN (p.66)

Could your child be getting too little sleep because of going to bed late or rising early? — YES

POSSIBLE CAUSE A lack of sleep is one of the most common causes of tiredness. Difficulty in getting your child to sleep is usually temporary and caused by lack of a fixed bedtime routine or anxiety. However, persistent problems may be the result of a behavioural problem.

ACTION Impose a regular bedtime routine, and be firm with your child (*see* GETTING YOUR CHILD TO SLEEP, p.66). If he or she is old enough, talk about any worries he or she may have. If your child is still not sleeping properly within a few weeks, consult your doctor.

NO

Has there been a recent upset at home or at school? — YES

POSSIBLE CAUSE Tiredness may be one sign of anxiety or depression as the result of a temporary upset.

ACTION Try to discover and deal with any underlying worries that your child has. Mild anxiety or depression can often be cleared up with extra reassurance and support. However, if your child's tiredness persists or becomes severe, consult your doctor.

NO

POSSIBLE CAUSE It is likely that your child is overdoing things due to long days or pressure to take part in various activities.

ACTION Talk to your child about dropping or rotating any optional activities. Encourage him or her to spend more time at home, playing quietly. Most children adjust to increased levels of activity at school within a term.

Do any of the following apply? — YES
- Your child is one of the youngest in his or her school year
- Your child has recently started going to a play group or school
- Your child has increased his or her after-school activities

NO

CONSULT YOUR DOCTOR IF YOU ARE UNABLE TO MAKE A DIAGNOSIS FROM THIS CHART AND YOUR CHILD'S TIREDNESS IS PERSISTENT OR SEVERE.

Iron-deficiency anaemia

In children, iron-deficiency anaemia is usually caused by a lack of iron in the diet. Try to get your child to eat foods that are rich in iron, such as dark green, leafy vegetables, eggs, and red meat. Certain foods, such as some breakfast cereals, are fortified with iron and are useful if your child will not eat other iron-rich foods. In addition, give your child plenty of fruit and vegetables, because they are rich in vitamin C, which helps the body absorb iron.

Providing an iron-rich diet
Offer your child plenty of iron-rich foods. Dark green vegetables such as broccoli are particularly high in iron.

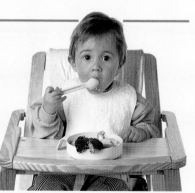

11 Sleeping problems in children

For children under 1 year, see chart 1, SLEEPING PROBLEMS IN BABIES (p.46).
The amount of sleep a child needs at night varies from about 9 to 12 hours according to age and individual requirements (*see* SLEEP REQUIREMENTS IN CHILDHOOD, right). Lack of sleep rarely affects health but may affect behaviour during the day

or performance at school. However, refusal to go to sleep at what you think is a reasonable time and/or waking in the middle of the night can be disruptive and distressing for the family if it occurs regularly. A number of factors, including physical illness, emotional upset, nightmares, and lack of a regular bedtime routine, may cause such sleeping problems.

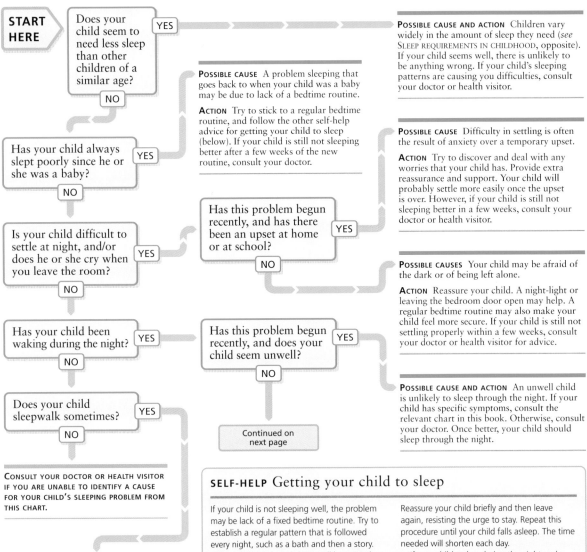

START HERE → Does your child seem to need less sleep than other children of a similar age?
YES → **POSSIBLE CAUSE AND ACTION** Children vary widely in the amount of sleep they need (*see* SLEEP REQUIREMENTS IN CHILDHOOD, opposite). If your child seems well, there is unlikely to be anything wrong. If your child's sleeping patterns are causing you difficulties, consult your doctor or health visitor.
NO ↓

Has your child always slept poorly since he or she was a baby?
YES → **POSSIBLE CAUSE** A problem sleeping that goes back to when your child was a baby may be due to lack of a bedtime routine.

ACTION Try to stick to a regular bedtime routine, and follow the other self-help advice for getting your child to sleep (below). If your child is still not sleeping better after a few weeks of the new routine, consult your doctor.
NO ↓

Is your child difficult to settle at night, and/or does he or she cry when you leave the room?
YES → Has this problem begun recently, and has there been an upset at home or at school?
YES → **POSSIBLE CAUSE** Difficulty in settling is often the result of anxiety over a temporary upset.

ACTION Try to discover and deal with any worries that your child has. Provide extra reassurance and support. Your child will probably settle more easily once the upset is over. However, if your child is still not sleeping better in a few weeks, consult your doctor or health visitor.
NO ↓

NO → **POSSIBLE CAUSES** Your child may be afraid of the dark or of being left alone.

ACTION Reassure your child. A night-light or leaving the bedroom door open may help. A regular bedtime routine may also make your child feel more secure. If your child is still not settling properly within a few weeks, consult your doctor or health visitor for advice.

Has your child been waking during the night?
YES → Has this problem begun recently, and does your child seem unwell?
YES → **POSSIBLE CAUSE AND ACTION** An unwell child is unlikely to sleep through the night. If your child has specific symptoms, consult the relevant chart in this book. Otherwise, consult your doctor. Once better, your child should sleep through the night.
NO ↓
NO ↓

Does your child sleepwalk sometimes?
YES
NO ↓

Continued on next page

CONSULT YOUR DOCTOR OR HEALTH VISITOR IF YOU ARE UNABLE TO IDENTIFY A CAUSE FOR YOUR CHILD'S SLEEPING PROBLEM FROM THIS CHART.

POSSIBLE CAUSE AND ACTION Sleepwalking is most common between the ages of 6 and 12. There is no need to worry as long as you ensure that your child is safe, for example by locking all outer doors. Do not try to wake your child, but guide him or her back to bed if necessary. Children usually grow out of it by age 12.

SELF-HELP Getting your child to sleep

If your child is not sleeping well, the problem may be lack of a fixed bedtime routine. Try to establish a regular pattern that is followed every night, such as a bath and then a story. Often, children do not sleep well because they are afraid of the dark. This problem can be solved by a night-light or leaving the bedroom door open. If you have difficulty in getting your child to sleep, settle him or her, say goodnight, and leave the room. If your child cries, leave him or her for a few minutes before returning.

Reassure your child briefly and then leave again, resisting the urge to stay. Repeat this procedure until your child falls asleep. The time needed will shorten each day.

If your child wakes during the night, only get up if he or she is truly crying. (A child who is only whimpering may drift back to sleep.) Go into the room to make sure nothing is wrong, reassure your child, and leave again. If your child still cries, try the method above. He or she will eventually settle back to sleep.

Continued from previous page

Is your child's sleep disturbed by symptoms such as a cough or itchy skin? — YES

POSSIBLE CAUSE Symptoms of conditions such as asthma or eczema that do not bother a child during the day can disturb his or her sleep. Consult your doctor.

ACTION Your doctor will examine your child and prescribe appropriate treatment. If your child is already receiving treatment for a condition such as asthma or eczema, it may need to be adjusted. Once the symptoms have been treated, your child should sleep better.

NO

Does your child wake several times a night to pass urine? — YES

POSSIBLE CAUSES Waking more than once or twice during the night to pass urine may be a sign of an underlying disorder – for example, a urinary tract infection. However, the most common cause is drinking too many fluids.

Go to chart **43** URINARY PROBLEMS (p.122)

NO

POSSIBLE CAUSE AND ACTION Certain drugs, such as some used to treat asthma, can cause disturbed sleep as a side effect. Consult your doctor. Meanwhile, do not stop giving your your child his or her prescribed drugs.

Is your child taking any prescribed drugs? — YES

NO

Is your child impossible to comfort at the time but has no memory of the event the following morning? — YES

Does your child seem to be having bad dreams? — YES

NO

NO

POSSIBLE CAUSE Your child is probably having nightmares. Bad dreams are common in children aged 5–6 and may be triggered by a frightening experience or events on television or in stories. Nightmares may be caused by anxiety.

ACTION Comfort your child until he or she manages to go back to sleep. In some cases, it may help to talk about the dream. If your child's nightmares are persistent or frequent, consult your doctor.

Does your child want to play on waking? — YES

NO

Does your child share a bedroom with you or another child? — YES

NO

POSSIBLE CAUSE Your child may be being disturbed by others in the room.

ACTION If possible, place your child in a separate room to sleep so that he or she is able to sleep through the night without being disturbed. After a few weeks, he or she may be able to share a room again without waking up at night.

CONSULT YOUR DOCTOR OR HEALTH VISITOR IF YOU ARE UNABLE TO IDENTIFY A CAUSE FOR YOUR CHILD'S SLEEPING PROBLEM FROM THIS CHART.

Sleep requirements in childhood

Children vary in the amount of sleep that they need, and it is normal for some children to sleep more than others of a similar age. In general, children sleep less as they grow up. The proportion of sleep spent dreaming also goes down, from about half in a newborn to about a fifth in a teenager. You should only worry about your child's sleeping if he or she seems unwell or if excessive sleepiness interferes with his or her activities.

Age	Average total sleep per 24 hours
Up to 3 months	16 hours
3–5 months	14 hours
5–24 months	13 hours
2–3 years	12 hours
3–5 years	11 hours
5–9 years	10½ hours
9–13 years	10 hours

Amount of sleep according to age
This table shows the average number of hours of sleep needed by babies and children at different ages.

POSSIBLE CAUSE Your child is probably having night terrors, a condition in which a child seems to be awake and terrified, although he or she is actually asleep and will not remember the incident in the morning. Night terrors are most common in 4–7 year olds.

ACTION You may be able to prevent a night terror by waking your child in the restless period that often precedes it. Night terrors usually occur about 2 hours after falling asleep. However, once one has started, there is little you can do except stay with your child. If he or she has frequent night terrors, consult your doctor. Night terrors will become less frequent as your child grows older.

POSSIBLE CAUSE AND ACTION Children are often ready to start their day earlier than their parents and may go through a phase of early waking. If you want your child to go back to sleep, follow the self-help advice for getting your child to sleep (opposite). If your child is old enough, you may wish to leave him or her to play quietly instead.

12 Growth problems

For children under 1, see chart 7, SLOW WEIGHT GAIN *(p.58). For weight problems in adolescents, see chart 51,* ADOLESCENT WEIGHT PROBLEMS *(p.135).*

Many parents worry that their child is too short or too thin; others worry that their child or is too tall or has put on too much weight. However, some children are naturally smaller or bigger than average, and serious disorders affecting growth

are rare. The best way to avoid unnecessary anxiety is to keep a regular record of your child's height and weight so that you can check that his or her growth rate is within the normal range (*see* GROWTH CHARTS, p.26). Consult this chart if your child is losing weight or is gaining weight at a much slower rate than you would expect, or if your child fails to grow in height as much as expected.

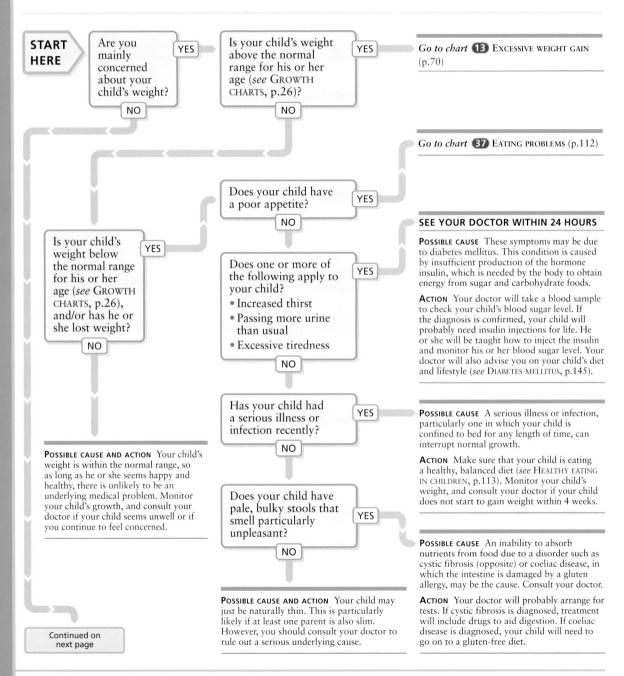

START HERE

Are you mainly concerned about your child's weight? — YES → **Is your child's weight above the normal range for his or her age (*see* GROWTH CHARTS, p.26)?** — YES → *Go to chart* **13** EXCESSIVE WEIGHT GAIN (p.70)

NO / NO

Go to chart **37** EATING PROBLEMS (p.112)

Does your child have a poor appetite? — YES →

SEE YOUR DOCTOR WITHIN 24 HOURS

POSSIBLE CAUSE These symptoms may be due to diabetes mellitus. This condition is caused by insufficient production of the hormone insulin, which is needed by the body to obtain energy from sugar and carbohydrate foods.

ACTION Your doctor will take a blood sample to check your child's blood sugar level. If the diagnosis is confirmed, your child will probably need insulin injections for life. He or she will be taught how to inject the insulin and monitor his or her blood sugar level. Your doctor will also advise you on your child's diet and lifestyle (*see* DIABETES MELLITUS, p.145).

NO

Is your child's weight below the normal range for his or her age (*see* GROWTH CHARTS, p.26), and/or has he or she lost weight? — YES →

Does one or more of the following apply to your child?
- Increased thirst
- Passing more urine than usual
- Excessive tiredness

— YES →

NO

Has your child had a serious illness or infection recently? — YES →

POSSIBLE CAUSE A serious illness or infection, particularly one in which your child is confined to bed for any length of time, can interrupt normal growth.

ACTION Make sure that your child is eating a healthy, balanced diet (*see* HEALTHY EATING IN CHILDREN, p.113). Monitor your child's weight, and consult your doctor if your child does not start to gain weight within 4 weeks.

NO

POSSIBLE CAUSE AND ACTION Your child's weight is within the normal range, so as long as he or she seems happy and healthy, there is unlikely to be an underlying medical problem. Monitor your child's growth, and consult your doctor if your child seems unwell or if you continue to feel concerned.

Does your child have pale, bulky stools that smell particularly unpleasant? — YES →

POSSIBLE CAUSE An inability to absorb nutrients from food due to a disorder such as cystic fibrosis (opposite) or coeliac disease, in which the intestine is damaged by a gluten allergy, may be the cause. Consult your doctor.

ACTION Your doctor will probably arrange for tests. If cystic fibrosis is diagnosed, treatment will include drugs to aid digestion. If coeliac disease is diagnosed, your child will need to go on to a gluten-free diet.

NO

POSSIBLE CAUSE AND ACTION Your child may just be naturally thin. This is particularly likely if at least one parent is also slim. However, you should consult your doctor to rule out a serious underlying cause.

Continued on next page

Continued from previous page

Are you mainly concerned about your child's height? — **YES**

NO

CONSULT YOUR DOCTOR IF YOU ARE UNABLE TO MAKE A DIAGNOSIS FROM THIS CHART.

Is your child's height above the normal range for his or her age (*see* GROWTH CHARTS, p.26)? — **YES**

NO

Is your child's height below the normal range for his or her age (*see* GROWTH CHARTS, p.26), and/or has he or she grown less than 2.5 cm (1 in) in the last 6 months? — **YES**

NO

IF YOU CANNOT MAKE A DIAGNOSIS FROM THIS CHART AND ARE STILL CONCERNED ABOUT ANY ASPECT OF YOUR CHILD'S GROWTH, CONSULT YOUR DOCTOR.

Cystic fibrosis

Cystic fibrosis is a genetic disorder in which secretions from the glands are abnormally thick. This results in a range of problems; in particular, thick mucus in the lungs causes a persistent cough and recurrent chest infections. Abnormal secretions from the pancreas interfere with the child's ability to digest food and cause him or her to pass pale, bulky, strong-smelling faeces. Children with cystic fibrosis frequently fail to grow normally and are often underweight. The condition is present from birth but is sometimes undetected for months or years, during which time the lungs may have become damaged. Regular chest physiotherapy performed by a parent, antibiotics, and drugs to aid digestion now enable most affected children to survive well into adulthood.

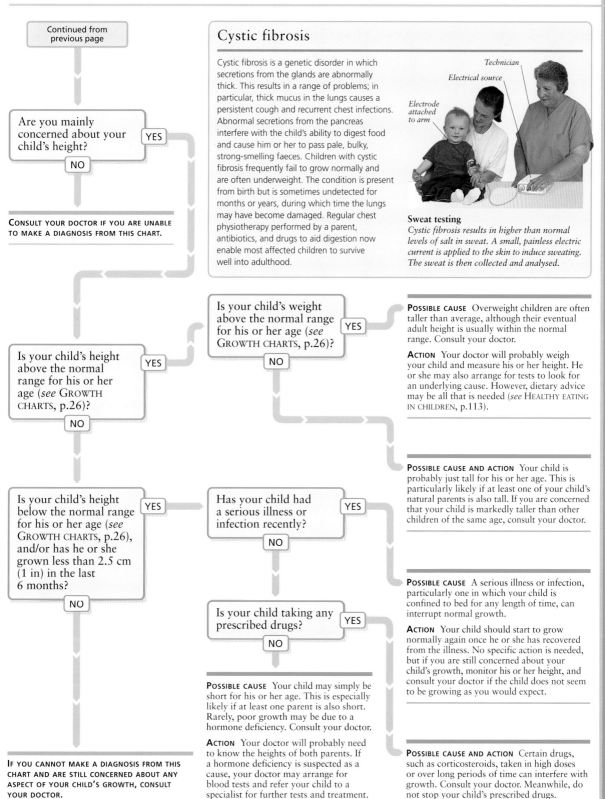

Technician
Electrical source
Electrode attached to arm

Sweat testing
Cystic fibrosis results in higher than normal levels of salt in sweat. A small, painless electric current is applied to the skin to induce sweating. The sweat is then collected and analysed.

Is your child's weight above the normal range for his or her age (*see* GROWTH CHARTS, p.26)? — **YES**

NO

POSSIBLE CAUSE Overweight children are often taller than average, although their eventual adult height is usually within the normal range. Consult your doctor.

ACTION Your doctor will probably weigh your child and measure his or her height. He or she may also arrange for tests to look for an underlying cause. However, dietary advice may be all that is needed (*see* HEALTHY EATING IN CHILDREN, p.113).

POSSIBLE CAUSE AND ACTION Your child is probably just tall for his or her age. This is particularly likely if at least one of your child's natural parents is also tall. If you are concerned that your child is markedly taller than other children of the same age, consult your doctor.

Has your child had a serious illness or infection recently? — **YES**

NO

POSSIBLE CAUSE A serious illness or infection, particularly one in which your child is confined to bed for any length of time, can interrupt normal growth.

ACTION Your child should start to grow normally again once he or she has recovered from the illness. No specific action is needed, but if you are still concerned about your child's growth, monitor his or her height, and consult your doctor if the child does not seem to be growing as you would expect.

Is your child taking any prescribed drugs? — **YES**

NO

POSSIBLE CAUSE Your child may simply be short for his or her age. This is especially likely if at least one parent is also short. Rarely, poor growth may be due to a hormone deficiency. Consult your doctor.

ACTION Your doctor will probably need to know the heights of both parents. If a hormone deficiency is suspected as a cause, your doctor may arrange for blood tests and refer your child to a specialist for further tests and treatment.

POSSIBLE CAUSE AND ACTION Certain drugs, such as corticosteroids, taken in high doses or over long periods of time can interfere with growth. Consult your doctor. Meanwhile, do not stop your child's prescribed drugs.

13 Excessive weight gain

Consult this chart if you think your child is overweight. Being overweight carries health risks and may contribute to emotional and social problems (*see* THE DANGERS OF CHILDHOOD OBESITY, opposite). It is therefore important to be alert to the possibility of excessive weight gain in your child. Appearance is not always a reliable sign of obesity because babies and toddlers are naturally chubby. The best way of ensuring that you notice any weight problem in your child is to keep a regular record of your child's growth (*see* GROWTH CHARTS, p.26). Increasing appreciation of the dangers of obesity in adults has led to a growing awareness that the problem often starts in childhood, when bad eating habits are established. It is extremely rare for excess weight to be due to a hormone problem.

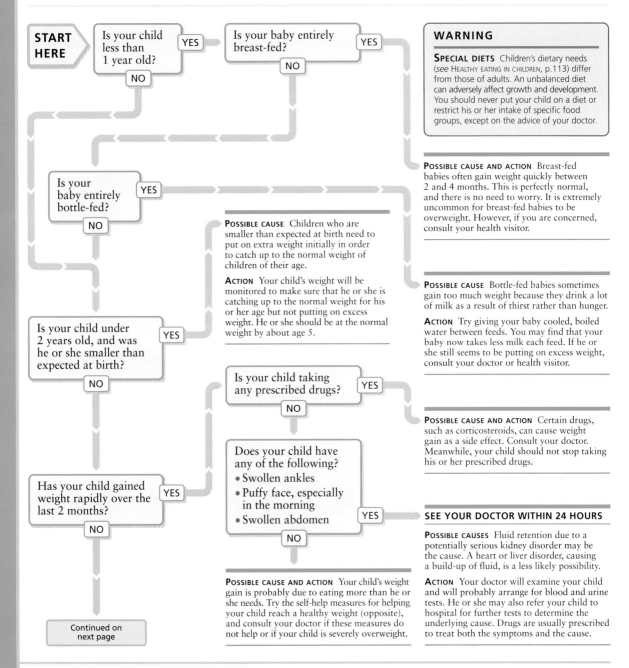

START HERE

Is your child less than 1 year old? — YES → **Is your baby entirely breast-fed?** — YES →
NO
NO

Is your baby entirely bottle-fed? — YES →
NO

POSSIBLE CAUSE Children who are smaller than expected at birth need to put on extra weight initially in order to catch up to the normal weight of children of their age.

ACTION Your child's weight will be monitored to make sure that he or she is catching up to the normal weight for his or her age but not putting on excess weight. He or she should be at the normal weight by about age 5.

Is your child under 2 years old, and was he or she smaller than expected at birth? — YES →
NO

Is your child taking any prescribed drugs? — YES →
NO

Does your child have any of the following?
• Swollen ankles
• Puffy face, especially in the morning
• Swollen abdomen — YES →
NO

Has your child gained weight rapidly over the last 2 months? — YES →
NO

Continued on next page

POSSIBLE CAUSE AND ACTION Your child's weight gain is probably due to eating more than he or she needs. Try the self-help measures for helping your child reach a healthy weight (opposite), and consult your doctor if these measures do not help or if your child is severely overweight.

WARNING

SPECIAL DIETS Children's dietary needs (*see* HEALTHY EATING IN CHILDREN, p.113) differ from those of adults. An unbalanced diet can adversely affect growth and development. You should never put your child on a diet or restrict his or her intake of specific food groups, except on the advice of your doctor.

POSSIBLE CAUSE AND ACTION Breast-fed babies often gain weight quickly between 2 and 4 months. This is perfectly normal, and there is no need to worry. It is extremely uncommon for breast-fed babies to be overweight. However, if you are concerned, consult your health visitor.

POSSIBLE CAUSE Bottle-fed babies sometimes gain too much weight because they drink a lot of milk as a result of thirst rather than hunger.

ACTION Try giving your baby cooled, boiled water between feeds. You may find that your baby now takes less milk each feed. If he or she still seems to be putting on excess weight, consult your doctor or health visitor.

POSSIBLE CAUSE AND ACTION Certain drugs, such as corticosteroids, can cause weight gain as a side effect. Consult your doctor. Meanwhile, your child should not stop taking his or her prescribed drugs.

SEE YOUR DOCTOR WITHIN 24 HOURS

POSSIBLE CAUSES Fluid retention due to a potentially serious kidney disorder may be the cause. A heart or liver disorder, causing a build-up of fluid, is a less likely possibility.

ACTION Your doctor will examine your child and will probably arrange for blood and urine tests. He or she may also refer your child to hospital for further tests to determine the underlying cause. Drugs are usually prescribed to treat both the symptoms and the cause.

Continued from previous page

Are other members of the family overweight? **YES**

NO

POSSIBLE CAUSE Overeating within the whole family is the most likely cause, although genetic factors may also play a part.

ACTION Look at the way the whole family eats. By changing your own eating patterns, you can encourage your child to lose weight. Follow the advice for helping your child achieve a healthy weight (below), and consult your doctor if these measures do not help or if your child is severely overweight.

Has your child been overweight since early childhood? **YES**

NO

Is your child always made to finish all the food on his or her plate? **YES**

NO

POSSIBLE CAUSE Your child is probably eating more than he or she needs.

ACTION Never force your child to eat. Allow him or her to stop eating, even if there is some food left, and serve smaller portions to avoid waste. Follow the advice for helping your child reach a healthy weight (below), and consult your doctor if these measures do not help or if your child is severely overweight.

Has your child been overweight for less than 6 months? **YES**

NO

POSSIBLE CAUSE AND ACTION Your child's weight gain is probably due to eating more than he or she needs. Try the self-help measures for helping your child reach a healthy weight (below), and consult your doctor if these measures do not help or if your child is severely overweight.

POSSIBLE CAUSE AND ACTION Your child's weight gain is probably due to eating more than he or she needs. Try the self-help measures for helping your child reach a healthy weight (right), and consult your doctor if these measures do not help or if your child is severely overweight.

Could your child be comfort eating, for example, because of stressful events at home or school? **YES**

NO

SELF-HELP Helping your child reach a healthy weight

Most overweight children eat more food than they need. To help your child lose weight, follow the advice for losing weight in adults (see HOW TO LOSE WEIGHT SAFELY, p.147) as well as the following measures:

- Make sure your child does not lose weight too quickly. He or she should lose a maximum of 0.5 kg (1 lb) per week.
- Involve your child, and let him or her take responsibility for losing weight.
- Stop buying high-fat and high-calorie foods, such as chocolate and fizzy drinks, so that the temptation is removed.
- Encourage your child to take up active leisure pursuits that he or she enjoys, such as football or dancing, instead of mostly watching TV or playing computer games.
- Encourage and reward your child for losing weight.

The dangers of childhood obesity

Being overweight can have a wide range of negative effects. Excess weight tends to reduce physical activity, which may compound the weight problem as well as contribute to poor fitness. Many overweight children also suffer from teasing or bullying from other children, making them insecure and unhappy. Low self-esteem, as a result of childhood teasing, often persists into adulthood.

Children who are overweight are likely to remain overweight as adults, putting them at increased risk of various disorders in later life, including life-threatening heart and circulatory disorders, such as a stroke or heart attack. Overweight adults are also more likely to suffer from joint problems, such as back or knee pain. Diabetes is more common in people who are overweight, as are some forms of cancer.

POSSIBLE CAUSE Erratic weight gain is common just before a growth spurt, especially in girls.

ACTION Monitor your child's weight. If he or she does not grow in height to balance the weight gain, follow the advice for helping your child reach a healthy weight (right). Consult your doctor if these measures do not help or if your child is severely overweight.

Eating healthily
High-fibre foods, such as wholemeal bread and muesli bars, are a healthy way to relieve hunger.

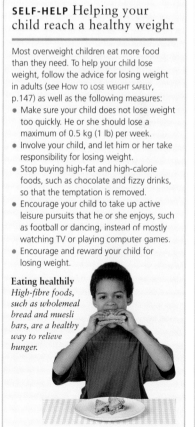

POSSIBLE CAUSE Overeating when under stress is common and can cause weight gain.

ACTION Try to discover and deal with any underlying worries that your child has. If necessary, talk to your child's teachers. Follow the advice for helping your child reach a healthy weight (right), and consult your doctor if these measures do not help or if your child is severely overweight.

14 Fever in children

For children under 1, see chart 3, FEVER IN BABIES (p.50). A fever is an abnormally high body temperature, of 38°C (100.4°F) or above. It is usually a sign that the body is fighting an infection. Heat exposure can also lead to a raised temperature. A child with a fever will feel generally unwell and be hot and sweaty. If your child does not feel well, you should take his or her temperature (*see* TAKING YOUR CHILD'S TEMPERATURE, below). If it is raised, take steps to reduce it (*see* BRINGING DOWN A FEVER, opposite). A high fever can cause seizures (febrile convulsions) in young children.

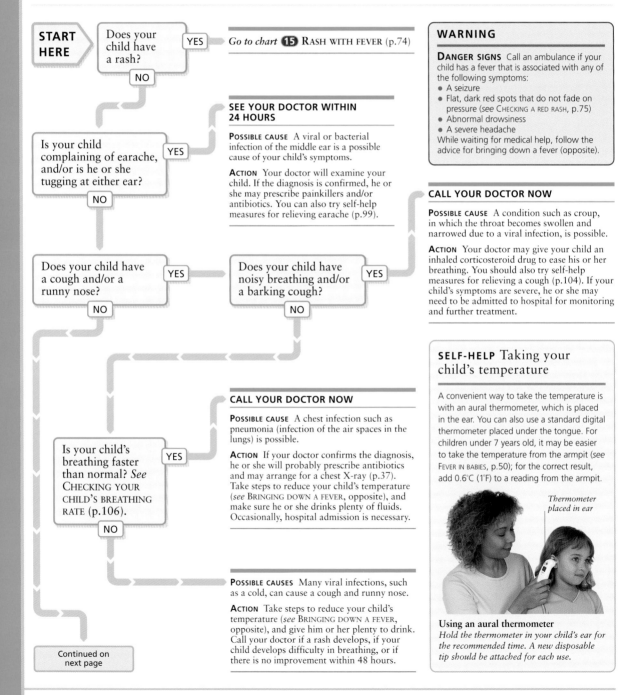

START HERE → **Does your child have a rash?** — YES → *Go to chart* **15** RASH WITH FEVER (p.74)

NO ↓

Is your child complaining of earache, and/or is he or she tugging at either ear? — YES →

NO ↓

Does your child have a cough and/or a runny nose? — YES → **Does your child have noisy breathing and/or a barking cough?** — YES →

NO ↓　　　　　　　　　　NO ↓

Is your child's breathing faster than normal? *See* CHECKING YOUR CHILD'S BREATHING RATE (p.106). — YES →

NO ↓

Continued on next page

SEE YOUR DOCTOR WITHIN 24 HOURS

POSSIBLE CAUSE A viral or bacterial infection of the middle ear is a possible cause of your child's symptoms.

ACTION Your doctor will examine your child. If the diagnosis is confirmed, he or she may prescribe painkillers and/or antibiotics. You can also try self-help measures for relieving earache (p.99).

CALL YOUR DOCTOR NOW

POSSIBLE CAUSE A chest infection such as pneumonia (infection of the air spaces in the lungs) is possible.

ACTION If your doctor confirms the diagnosis, he or she will probably prescribe antibiotics and may arrange for a chest X-ray (p.37). Take steps to reduce your child's temperature (*see* BRINGING DOWN A FEVER, opposite), and make sure he or she drinks plenty of fluids. Occasionally, hospital admission is necessary.

POSSIBLE CAUSES Many viral infections, such as a cold, can cause a cough and runny nose.

ACTION Take steps to reduce your child's temperature (*see* BRINGING DOWN A FEVER, opposite), and give him or her plenty to drink. Call your doctor if a rash develops, if your child develops difficulty in breathing, or if there is no improvement within 48 hours.

WARNING

DANGER SIGNS Call an ambulance if your child has a fever that is associated with any of the following symptoms:
- A seizure
- Flat, dark red spots that do not fade on pressure (*see* CHECKING A RED RASH, p.75)
- Abnormal drowsiness
- A severe headache

While waiting for medical help, follow the advice for bringing down a fever (opposite).

CALL YOUR DOCTOR NOW

POSSIBLE CAUSE A condition such as croup, in which the throat becomes swollen and narrowed due to a viral infection, is possible.

ACTION Your doctor may give your child an inhaled corticosteroid drug to ease his or her breathing. You should also try self-help measures for relieving a cough (p.104). If your child's symptoms are severe, he or she may need to be admitted to hospital for monitoring and further treatment.

SELF-HELP Taking your child's temperature

A convenient way to take the temperature is with an aural thermometer, which is placed in the ear. You can also use a standard digital thermometer placed under the tongue. For children under 7 years old, it may be easier to take the temperature from the armpit (*see* FEVER IN BABIES, p.50); for the correct result, add 0.6°C (1°F) to a reading from the armpit.

Thermometer placed in ear

Using an aural thermometer
Hold the thermometer in your child's ear for the recommended time. A new disposable tip should be attached for each use.

Continued from previous page

SELF-HELP Bringing down a fever

Lowering a temperature will make your child more comfortable and lessen the risk of a febrile convulsion (p.51). Remove your child's outer clothes and lay him or her in a cool room with a free flow of fresh air. Give plenty of cool drinks. If your child is over 3 months old, give the recommended dose of paracetamol. Alternatively, if your child is over 6 months old and weighs more than 7 kg (15½ lb), give the recommended dose of ibuprofen.

Flannel to wipe forehead

Cool drink

Fan

Cooling your child
Undress your child and open a door or window, or use an electric fan, to let cool air circulate over the skin.

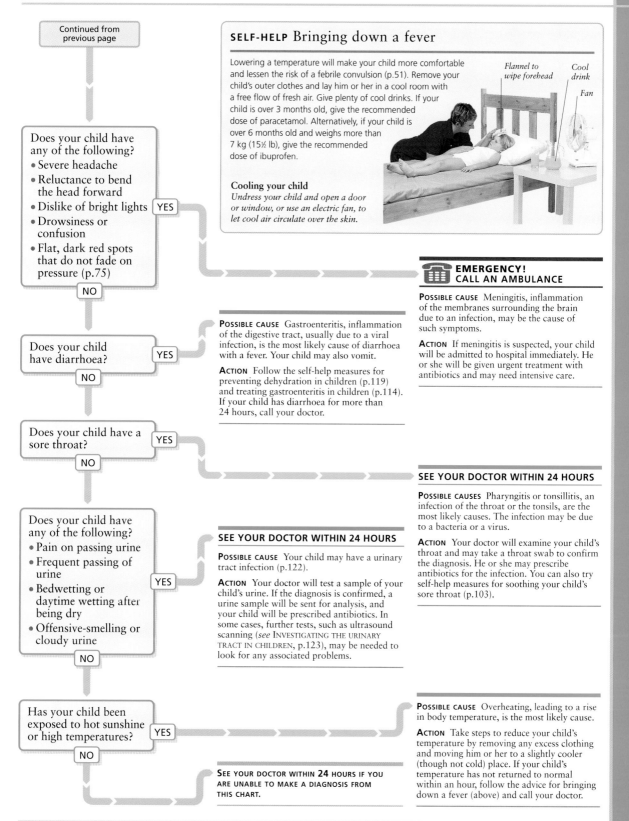

Does your child have any of the following?
- Severe headache
- Reluctance to bend the head forward
- Dislike of bright lights
- Drowsiness or confusion
- Flat, dark red spots that do not fade on pressure (p.75)

YES →

NO

📞 EMERGENCY! CALL AN AMBULANCE

POSSIBLE CAUSE Meningitis, inflammation of the membranes surrounding the brain due to an infection, may be the cause of such symptoms.

ACTION If meningitis is suspected, your child will be admitted to hospital immediately. He or she will be given urgent treatment with antibiotics and may need intensive care.

Does your child have diarrhoea?

YES →

NO

POSSIBLE CAUSE Gastroenteritis, inflammation of the digestive tract, usually due to a viral infection, is the most likely cause of diarrhoea with a fever. Your child may also vomit.

ACTION Follow the self-help measures for preventing dehydration in children (p.119) and treating gastroenteritis in children (p.114). If your child has diarrhoea for more than 24 hours, call your doctor.

Does your child have a sore throat?

YES →

NO

SEE YOUR DOCTOR WITHIN 24 HOURS

POSSIBLE CAUSES Pharyngitis or tonsillitis, an infection of the throat or the tonsils, are the most likely causes. The infection may be due to a bacteria or a virus.

ACTION Your doctor will examine your child's throat and may take a throat swab to confirm the diagnosis. He or she may prescribe antibiotics for the infection. You can also try self-help measures for soothing your child's sore throat (p.103).

Does your child have any of the following?
- Pain on passing urine
- Frequent passing of urine
- Bedwetting or daytime wetting after being dry
- Offensive-smelling or cloudy urine

YES →

NO

SEE YOUR DOCTOR WITHIN 24 HOURS

POSSIBLE CAUSE Your child may have a urinary tract infection (p.122).

ACTION Your doctor will test a sample of your child's urine. If the diagnosis is confirmed, a urine sample will be sent for analysis, and your child will be prescribed antibiotics. In some cases, further tests, such as ultrasound scanning (*see* INVESTIGATING THE URINARY TRACT IN CHILDREN, p.123), may be needed to look for any associated problems.

Has your child been exposed to hot sunshine or high temperatures?

YES →

NO

POSSIBLE CAUSE Overheating, leading to a rise in body temperature, is the most likely cause.

ACTION Take steps to reduce your child's temperature by removing any excess clothing and moving him or her to a slightly cooler (though not cold) place. If your child's temperature has not returned to normal within an hour, follow the advice for bringing down a fever (above) and call your doctor.

SEE YOUR DOCTOR WITHIN 24 HOURS IF YOU ARE UNABLE TO MAKE A DIAGNOSIS FROM THIS CHART.

15 Rash with fever

Consult this chart if your child develops a rash anywhere on the body associated with a temperature of 38°C (100.4°F) or higher. In children, this combination of symptoms is often caused by a viral infection, but, in some cases, it can be caused by a serious bacterial infection, such as meningitis, that needs urgent medical attention. Routine immunizations will protect your child against most serious infections. However, your child will still be at risk of developing a number of less serious infections and may even develop a mild form of diseases against which he or she has been immunized.

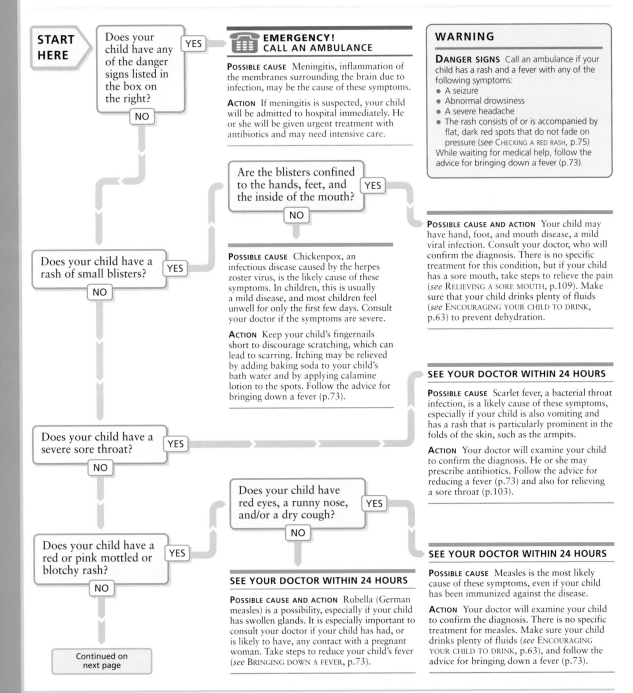

START HERE

Does your child have any of the danger signs listed in the box on the right? YES

NO

☎ **EMERGENCY! CALL AN AMBULANCE**

POSSIBLE CAUSE Meningitis, inflammation of the membranes surrounding the brain due to infection, may be the cause of these symptoms.

ACTION If meningitis is suspected, your child will be admitted to hospital immediately. He or she will be given urgent treatment with antibiotics and may need intensive care.

WARNING

DANGER SIGNS Call an ambulance if your child has a rash and a fever with any of the following symptoms:
- A seizure
- Abnormal drowsiness
- A severe headache
- The rash consists of or is accompanied by flat, dark red spots that do not fade on pressure (see CHECKING A RED RASH, p.75)

While waiting for medical help, follow the advice for bringing down a fever (p.73).

Are the blisters confined to the hands, feet, and the inside of the mouth? YES

NO

POSSIBLE CAUSE Chickenpox, an infectious disease caused by the herpes zoster virus, is the likely cause of these symptoms. In children, this is usually a mild disease, and most children feel unwell for only the first few days. Consult your doctor if the symptoms are severe.

ACTION Keep your child's fingernails short to discourage scratching, which can lead to scarring. Itching may be relieved by adding baking soda to your child's bath water and by applying calamine lotion to the spots. Follow the advice for bringing down a fever (p.73).

Does your child have a rash of small blisters? YES

NO

POSSIBLE CAUSE AND ACTION Your child may have hand, foot, and mouth disease, a mild viral infection. Consult your doctor, who will confirm the diagnosis. There is no specific treatment for this condition, but if your child has a sore mouth, take steps to relieve the pain (see RELIEVING A SORE MOUTH, p.109). Make sure that your child drinks plenty of fluids (see ENCOURAGING YOUR CHILD TO DRINK, p.63) to prevent dehydration.

Does your child have a severe sore throat? YES

NO

SEE YOUR DOCTOR WITHIN 24 HOURS

POSSIBLE CAUSE Scarlet fever, a bacterial throat infection, is a likely cause of these symptoms, especially if your child is also vomiting and has a rash that is particularly prominent in the folds of the skin, such as the armpits.

ACTION Your doctor will examine your child to confirm the diagnosis. He or she may prescribe antibiotics. Follow the advice for reducing a fever (p.73) and also for relieving a sore throat (p.103).

Does your child have red eyes, a runny nose, and/or a dry cough? YES

NO

Does your child have a red or pink mottled or blotchy rash? YES

NO

SEE YOUR DOCTOR WITHIN 24 HOURS

POSSIBLE CAUSE AND ACTION Rubella (German measles) is a possibility, especially if your child has swollen glands. It is especially important to consult your doctor if your child has had, or is likely to have, any contact with a pregnant woman. Take steps to reduce your child's fever (see BRINGING DOWN A FEVER, p.73).

SEE YOUR DOCTOR WITHIN 24 HOURS

POSSIBLE CAUSE Measles is the most likely cause of these symptoms, even if your child has been immunized against the disease.

ACTION Your doctor will examine your child to confirm the diagnosis. There is no specific treatment for measles. Make sure your child drinks plenty of fluids (see ENCOURAGING YOUR CHILD TO DRINK, p.63), and follow the advice for bringing down a fever (p.73).

Continued on next page

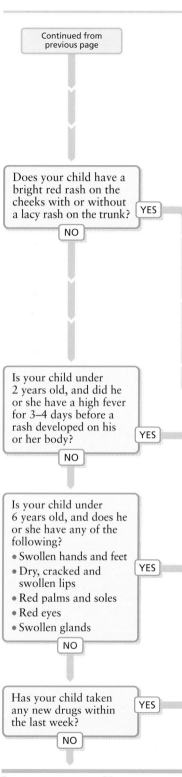

Continued from previous page

Does your child have a bright red rash on the cheeks with or without a lacy rash on the trunk? **YES** → **NO**

Is your child under 2 years old, and did he or she have a high fever for 3–4 days before a rash developed on his or her body? **YES** → **NO**

Is your child under 6 years old, and does he or she have any of the following?
- Swollen hands and feet
- Dry, cracked and swollen lips
- Red palms and soles
- Red eyes
- Swollen glands
YES → **NO**

Has your child taken any new drugs within the last week? **YES** → **NO**

SEE YOUR DOCTOR WITHIN 24 HOURS IF YOU ARE UNABLE TO MAKE A DIAGNOSIS FROM THIS CHART.

Viral infections that cause a rash

Many viral infections cause a fever and a rash. The more serious ones, such as measles, have become much less common as a result of routine immunizations. Many of these infections can also affect adults, whose symptoms can be more severe than children's. The incubation period is the time between acquiring an infection and first developing symptoms.

Disease (incubation period)	Symptoms	Period when infectious
Chickenpox: 10–21 days	Crops of raised, red, itchy spots that turn into blisters and then scabs, mainly on face and trunk	From 1–2 days before rash develops to 5–6 days after it has appeared, when all blisters have scabs
Erythema infectiosum (slapped cheek disease): 13–20 days	Bright red cheeks; lacy rash, mainly on trunk	Until rash has appeared
Hand, foot, and mouth disease: 3–5 days	Mild fever; rash of small blisters on hands, feet, and inside of mouth	For duration of blisters
Measles: 7–14 days	Cough; runny nose; red eyes; mottled or blotchy red rash, first on the face, then trunk and arms	Until 5 days after the rash develops
Roseola infantum: variable	High fever followed by flat, light-red rash on the trunk; swollen glands in neck	Until 5–15 days after onset of symptoms
Rubella: 14–19 days	Mild fever; swollen glands in neck; flat pink mottled or blotchy rash, mainly on face and trunk	From 1 week before rash develops until 4 days after rash has appeared
Scarlet fever: 2–5 days	High fever; severe sore throat; vomiting; red rash on body, most obvious in skin folds	Until prescribed course of antibiotics is completed

POSSIBLE CAUSE AND ACTION Your child may have roseola infantum, a common early childhood infection. This condition is difficult to diagnose before the rash appears as the fever is the only symptom. By the time the rash appears, the child is usually better. If you suspect your child has this condition and he or she still has a fever, consult your doctor. He or she will examine your child and may do tests to exclude more serious problems.

CALL YOUR DOCTOR NOW

POSSIBLE CAUSE Kawasaki disease, a rare condition of unknown cause, which can damage the heart and joints, is a possibility.

ACTION If your doctor suspects that your child has Kawasaki disease, your child will be admitted to hospital, where his or her condition can be monitored and treatment given to reduce the risk of heart complications.

CALL YOUR DOCTOR NOW

POSSIBLE CAUSES Your child may have an allergy to the prescribed medicine, or he or she may have a viral illness unrelated to the drug.

ACTION Your doctor will examine your child to determine the cause of the symptoms. If your child does have a drug allergy, your doctor will be able to tell you whether your child should avoid this drug in future.

POSSIBLE CAUSE AND ACTION Your child may have erythema infectiosum, also known as slapped-cheek disease or fifth disease. This viral condition is usually mild. Follow the advice on reducing a fever (p.73). The diagnosis should be confirmed by your doctor if your child has been in contact with a pregnant woman. If your are worried or if your child is no better in 48 hours, call your doctor.

Checking a red rash

If you or your child develops dark red or purple blotches, check whether they fade on pressure by pressing a clear glass against them. If the rash is visible through the glass, it may be a form of purpura, which is caused by bleeding under the skin and may occur in meningitis. If you or your child has a non-fading rash, call an ambulance.

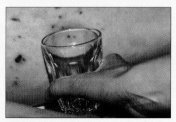

Checking a rash
Here, the rash is still visible when the glass is pressed against the skin – a sign that it may be caused by an illness such as meningitis.

16 Skin problems in children

For skin problems in children under 1, see chart 8, SKIN
PROBLEMS IN BABIES *(p.60).*
Childhood spots and rashes are usually due to irritation or
inflammation of the skin as a result of a local problem such as
an allergic reaction. However, a rash associated with a fever

may be due to a generalized infection (*see* VIRAL INFECTIONS
THAT CAUSE A RASH, p.75). A rash without a fever or a feeling
of being unwell is probably no cause for concern, but if it is
itchy or sore, consult your doctor. Call an ambulance if a rash
is accompanied by difficulty breathing and/or facial swelling.

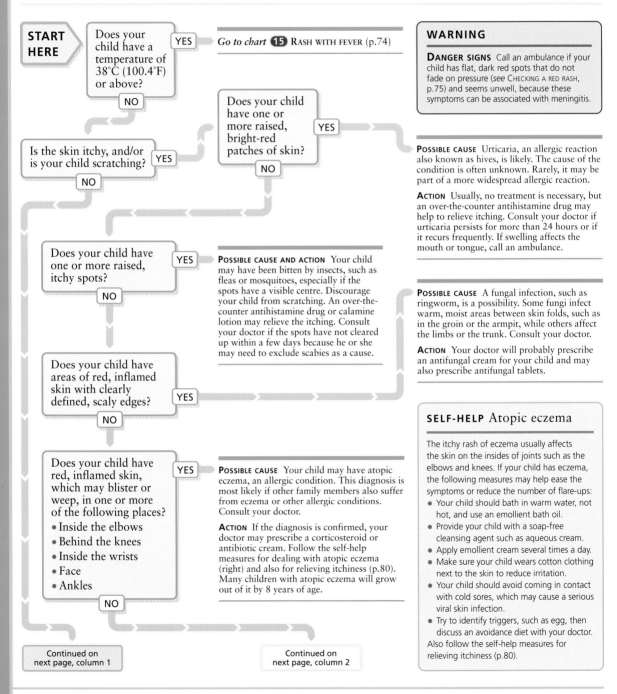

START HERE

Does your child have a temperature of 38°C (100.4°F) or above?
YES → *Go to chart* **15** RASH WITH FEVER (p.74)
NO

Is the skin itchy, and/or is your child scratching?
NO
YES

Does your child have one or more raised, bright-red patches of skin?
YES
NO

Does your child have one or more raised, itchy spots?
YES → **POSSIBLE CAUSE AND ACTION** Your child may have been bitten by insects, such as fleas or mosquitoes, especially if the spots have a visible centre. Discourage your child from scratching. An over-the-counter antihistamine drug or calamine lotion may relieve the itching. Consult your doctor if the spots have not cleared up within a few days because he or she may need to exclude scabies as a cause.
NO

Does your child have areas of red, inflamed skin with clearly defined, scaly edges?
YES
NO

Does your child have red, inflamed skin, which may blister or weep, in one or more of the following places?
- Inside the elbows
- Behind the knees
- Inside the wrists
- Face
- Ankles

YES → **POSSIBLE CAUSE** Your child may have atopic eczema, an allergic condition. This diagnosis is most likely if other family members also suffer from eczema or other allergic conditions. Consult your doctor.

ACTION If the diagnosis is confirmed, your doctor may prescribe a corticosteroid or antibiotic cream. Follow the self-help measures for dealing with atopic eczema (right) and also for relieving itchiness (p.80). Many children with atopic eczema will grow out of it by 8 years of age.

NO

Continued on next page, column 1

Continued on next page, column 2

WARNING

DANGER SIGNS Call an ambulance if your child has flat, dark red spots that do not fade on pressure (*see* CHECKING A RED RASH, p.75) and seems unwell, because these symptoms can be associated with meningitis.

POSSIBLE CAUSE Urticaria, an allergic reaction also known as hives, is likely. The cause of the condition is often unknown. Rarely, it may be part of a more widespread allergic reaction.

ACTION Usually, no treatment is necessary, but an over-the-counter antihistamine drug may help to relieve itching. Consult your doctor if urticaria persists for more than 24 hours or if it recurs frequently. If swelling affects the mouth or tongue, call an ambulance.

POSSIBLE CAUSE A fungal infection, such as ringworm, is a possibility. Some fungi infect warm, moist areas between skin folds, such as in the groin or the armpit, while others affect the limbs or the trunk. Consult your doctor.

ACTION Your doctor will probably prescribe an antifungal cream for your child and may also prescribe antifungal tablets.

SELF-HELP Atopic eczema

The itchy rash of eczema usually affects the skin on the insides of joints such as the elbows and knees. If your child has eczema, the following measures may help ease the symptoms or reduce the number of flare-ups:
- Your child should bath in warm water, not hot, and use an emollient bath oil.
- Provide your child with a soap-free cleansing agent such as aqueous cream.
- Apply emollient cream several times a day.
- Make sure your child wears cotton clothing next to the skin to reduce irritation.
- Your child should avoid coming in contact with cold sores, which may cause a serious viral skin infection.
- Try to identify triggers, such as egg, then discuss an avoidance diet with your doctor.
Also follow the self-help measures for relieving itchiness (p.80).

Continued from previous page, column 1

Continued from previous page, column 2

Is your child intensely itchy with or without grey lines between the fingers or on the wrists?
YES
NO

Does your child have inflamed or weeping skin that dries to form gold-coloured crusts?
YES
NO

Does your child have patches of red, inflamed skin that is also flaking?
YES
NO

Does your child have one or more small lumps of rough skin?
YES
NO

Does your child have several raised, pearly pimples up to 5 mm (¼ in) in diameter, each with a central dimple?
YES
NO

Is your child over 10 years old, and does he or she have any of the following?
• Blackheads
• Inflamed spots with white tops
• Painful red lumps under the skin
YES
NO

Is your child taking any prescribed or over-the-counter drugs?
YES
NO

SEE YOUR DOCTOR WITHIN 24 HOURS

POSSIBLE CAUSE Scabies, a parasitic infection, may be causing your child's symptoms. Scabies mites burrow under the skin between the fingers and at the wrists and can cause a widespread rash, which may affect the palms of the hands and soles of the feet in babies. Scabies is very contagious.

ACTION Your doctor will probably prescribe a treatment lotion, which you will need to apply to the whole of your child's body as directed. Everyone else in the household will need to be treated at the same time, and clothing and bedding also need to be washed. The mites should die within 3 days of treatment, but the itching may continue for up to 2 weeks.

POSSIBLE CAUSE Seborrhoeic dermatitis, a harmless skin disorder, is a possible cause of these symptoms. It often occurs in oily areas of skin, such as the hairline, eyebrows, and nose.

ACTION Avoid using soaps or other bath products on the affected areas. Instead, use an emollient, such as aqueous cream, to clean and moisturize the skin. The condition often improves if the scalp is treated with an over-the-counter dandruff shampoo or a shampoo containing ketocanazole. If the rash does not improve within a week or if you are concerned, consult your doctor, who may prescribe a corticosteroid cream.

SEE YOUR DOCTOR WITHIN 24 HOURS

POSSIBLE CAUSE Your child may have impetigo, a bacterial skin infection that commonly affects the face.

ACTION If your doctor confirms the diagnosis, you will probably be advised to wash the crusts away gently with warm water. Your doctor may also prescribe an antibiotic cream or, if the condition is widespread, oral antibiotics. Until the infection clears up, you should make sure that your child keeps a separate towel and other wash things to avoid infecting others. Keep your child away from other children while he or she is infected.

POSSIBLE CAUSE These may be warts, which are caused by a viral infection of the skin. A wart that grows into the sole of the foot is known as a verruca and may be painful.

ACTION Most warts disappear naturally, but this may take months or years. Over-the-counter wart treatments may speed the process. They should only be used on the hands and feet; never try self-treatment for a wart on the face. If a wart persists after you have treated it or if it is painful, consult your doctor. He or she may suggest other treatments, such as freezing.

POSSIBLE CAUSE AND ACTION Molluscum contagiosum, a harmless but contagious viral skin infection, is likely. The pimples clear up without treatment, but this may take up to 2 years. Meanwhile, they may catch on clothing and look unsightly. See your doctor. Individual pimples can be treated by your doctor, but because the treatment may be painful and may leave a scar, it is usually best not to treat the condition.

POSSIBLE CAUSE Your child may have acne, which is very common during adolescence.

Go to chart **55** ADOLESCENT SKIN PROBLEMS (p.140)

POSSIBLE CAUSE AND ACTION Certain drugs can cause skin problems as a side effect. Stop giving your child any over-the-counter drugs and consult your doctor. Meanwhile, do not stop giving your child any prescribed drugs.

CONSULT YOUR DOCTOR IF YOU ARE UNABLE TO MAKE A DIAGNOSIS FROM THIS CHART.

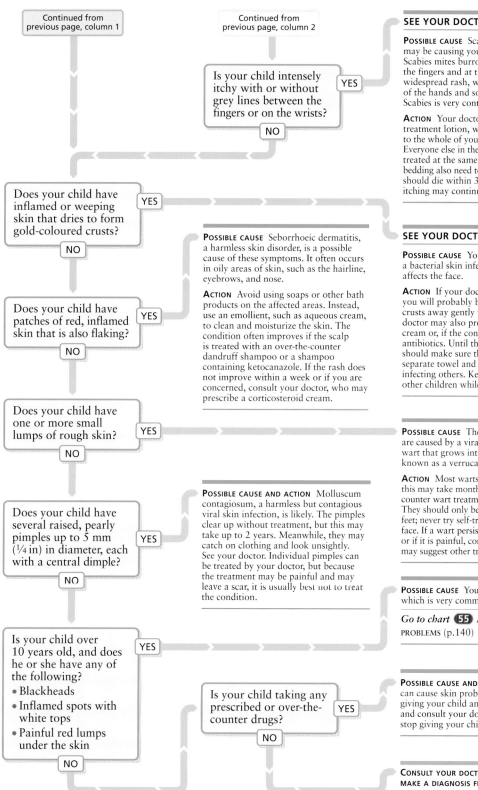

17 Hair, scalp, and nail problems

Consult this chart if your child has any problems affecting the hair, scalp, fingernails, or toenails. In general, eating a well-balanced diet will help keep your child's hair and nails strong and healthy. Use a soft hairbrush on a young child's hair because it can be easily damaged. If your child's hair is long, avoid braiding it tightly or using uncovered rubber bands to tie it back. In children, the most common hair problems needing treatment are fungal infections and head lice.

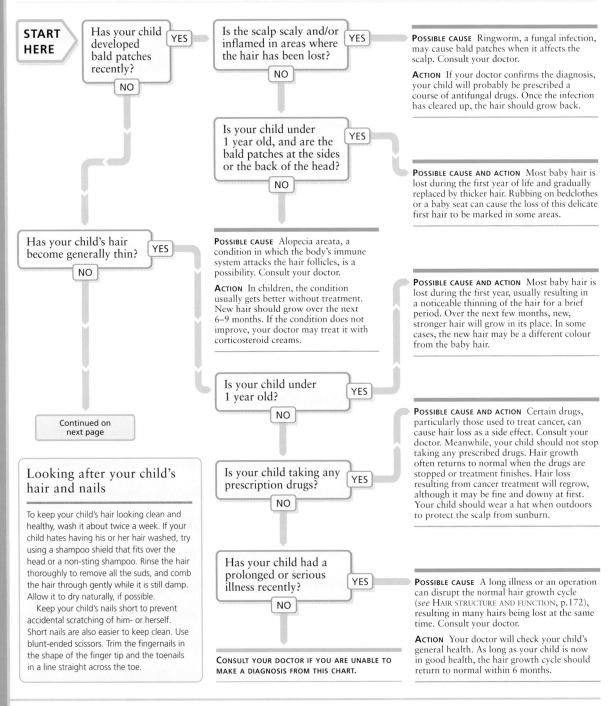

START HERE

Has your child developed bald patches recently?
— YES → **Is the scalp scaly and/or inflamed in areas where the hair has been lost?**
— YES → **POSSIBLE CAUSE** Ringworm, a fungal infection, may cause bald patches when it affects the scalp. Consult your doctor.
ACTION If your doctor confirms the diagnosis, your child will probably be prescribed a course of antifungal drugs. Once the infection has cleared up, the hair should grow back.

NO →
Is your child under 1 year old, and are the bald patches at the sides or the back of the head?
— YES → **POSSIBLE CAUSE AND ACTION** Most baby hair is lost during the first year of life and gradually replaced by thicker hair. Rubbing on bedclothes or a baby seat can cause the loss of this delicate first hair to be marked in some areas.

NO →
POSSIBLE CAUSE Alopecia areata, a condition in which the body's immune system attacks the hair follicles, is a possibility. Consult your doctor.
ACTION In children, the condition usually gets better without treatment. New hair should grow over the next 6–9 months. If the condition does not improve, your doctor may treat it with corticosteroid creams.

Has your child developed bald patches recently? NO →
Has your child's hair become generally thin?
— YES → **POSSIBLE CAUSE AND ACTION** Most baby hair is lost during the first year, usually resulting in a noticeable thinning of the hair for a brief period. Over the next few months, new, stronger hair will grow in its place. In some cases, the new hair may be a different colour from the baby hair.

Is your child under 1 year old?
— YES →

NO →
Is your child taking any prescription drugs?
— YES → **POSSIBLE CAUSE AND ACTION** Certain drugs, particularly those used to treat cancer, can cause hair loss as a side effect. Consult your doctor. Meanwhile, your child should not stop taking any prescribed drugs. Hair growth often returns to normal when the drugs are stopped or treatment finishes. Hair loss resulting from cancer treatment will regrow, although it may be fine and downy at first. Your child should wear a hat when outdoors to protect the scalp from sunburn.

NO →
Has your child had a prolonged or serious illness recently?
— YES → **POSSIBLE CAUSE** A long illness or an operation can disrupt the normal hair growth cycle (see HAIR STRUCTURE AND FUNCTION, p.172), resulting in many hairs being lost at the same time. Consult your doctor.
ACTION Your doctor will check your child's general health. As long as your child is now in good health, the hair growth cycle should return to normal within 6 months.

NO →

Has your child's hair become generally thin? NO →
Continued on next page

Looking after your child's hair and nails

To keep your child's hair looking clean and healthy, wash it about twice a week. If your child hates having his or her hair washed, try using a shampoo shield that fits over the head or a non-sting shampoo. Rinse the hair thoroughly to remove all the suds, and comb the hair through gently while it is still damp. Allow it to dry naturally, if possible.

Keep your child's nails short to prevent accidental scratching of him- or herself. Short nails are also easier to keep clean. Use blunt-ended scissors. Trim the fingernails in the shape of the finger tip and the toenails in a line straight across the toe.

CONSULT YOUR DOCTOR IF YOU ARE UNABLE TO MAKE A DIAGNOSIS FROM THIS CHART.

Continued from previous page

Does your child have an itchy scalp? — YES

NO

Does your child have a red, painful area around one or more nails? — YES

NO

Does your child bite his or her nails? — YES

NO

CONSULT YOUR DOCTOR IF YOU ARE UNABLE TO MAKE A DIAGNOSIS FROM THIS CHART.

SELF-HELP Treating head lice

Contrary to popular belief, head lice prefer clean, not dirty, hair. Head lice can be treated with an over-the-counter lotion or shampoo. Follow the directions on the packet, and then remove the dead lice and their eggs (known as nits) by combing through the hair with a fine-toothed nit comb. All family members, and anyone else who has come into contact with the child, also need to be treated, even if they have no symptoms, to eradicate the lice and prevent reinfestation. In addition, wash all combs, brushes, and towels in boiling water to kill any lice or nits attached to them.

Removing lice and eggs
Carefully combing through your child's hair with a fine-toothed nit comb will remove eggs and dead lice.

Fine-toothed nit comb

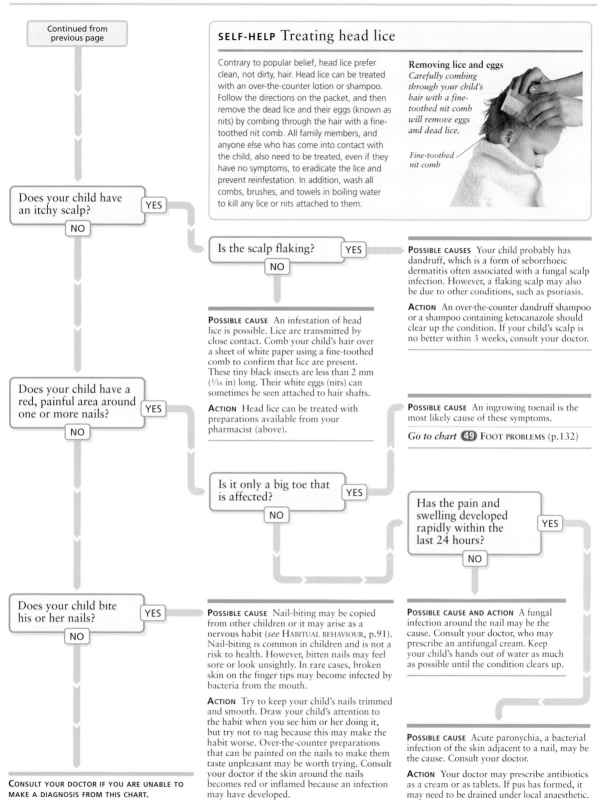

Is the scalp flaking? — YES

NO

POSSIBLE CAUSE An infestation of head lice is possible. Lice are transmitted by close contact. Comb your child's hair over a sheet of white paper using a fine-toothed comb to confirm that lice are present. These tiny black insects are less than 2 mm (1/16 in) long. Their white eggs (nits) can sometimes be seen attached to hair shafts.

ACTION Head lice can be treated with preparations available from your pharmacist (above).

Is it only a big toe that is affected? — YES

NO

POSSIBLE CAUSE Nail-biting may be copied from other children or it may arise as a nervous habit (*see* HABITUAL BEHAVIOUR, p.91). Nail-biting is common in children and is not a risk to health. However, bitten nails may feel sore or look unsightly. In rare cases, broken skin on the finger tips may become infected by bacteria from the mouth.

ACTION Try to keep your child's nails trimmed and smooth. Draw your child's attention to the habit when you see him or her doing it, but try not to nag because this may make the habit worse. Over-the-counter preparations that can be painted on the nails to make them taste unpleasant may be worth trying. Consult your doctor if the skin around the nails becomes red or inflamed because an infection may have developed.

POSSIBLE CAUSES Your child probably has dandruff, which is a form of seborrhoeic dermatitis often associated with a fungal scalp infection. However, a flaking scalp may also be due to other conditions, such as psoriasis.

ACTION An over-the-counter dandruff shampoo or a shampoo containing ketoconazole should clear up the condition. If your child's scalp is no better within 3 weeks, consult your doctor.

POSSIBLE CAUSE An ingrowing toenail is the most likely cause of these symptoms.

Go to chart **49** FOOT PROBLEMS (p.132)

Has the pain and swelling developed rapidly within the last 24 hours? — YES

NO

POSSIBLE CAUSE AND ACTION A fungal infection around the nail may be the cause. Consult your doctor, who may prescribe an antifungal cream. Keep your child's hands out of water as much as possible until the condition clears up.

POSSIBLE CAUSE Acute paronychia, a bacterial infection of the skin adjacent to a nail, may be the cause. Consult your doctor.

ACTION Your doctor may prescribe antibiotics as a cream or as tablets. If pus has formed, it may need to be drained under local anaesthetic.

18 Itching

Itching is a common and distressing symptom for a child and can have a variety of causes, including external irritants or infestation by parasites. It is important to deal promptly with any disorder that produces itching, because if it persists, scratching can lead to an infection or changes in the skin, which can, in turn, lead to further itching.

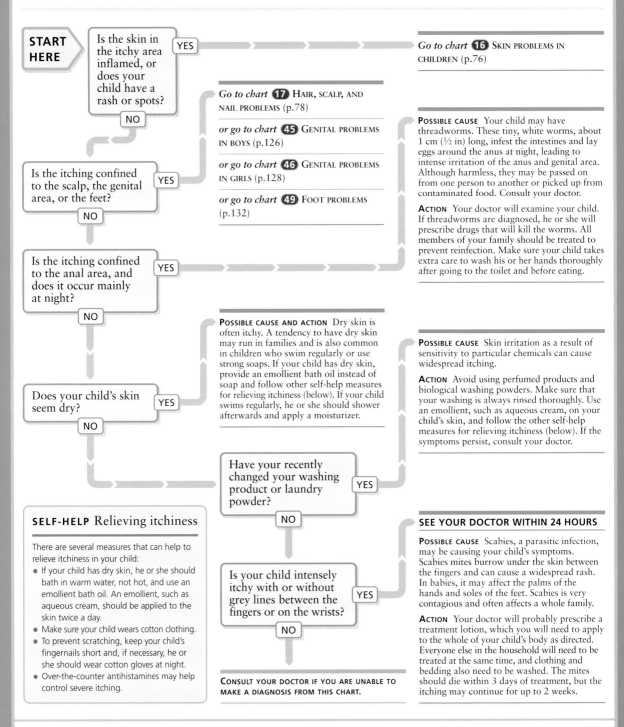

START HERE

Is the skin in the itchy area inflamed, or does your child have a rash or spots?

YES → *Go to chart* **16** SKIN PROBLEMS IN CHILDREN (p.76)

NO ↓

Is the itching confined to the scalp, the genital area, or the feet?

YES → *Go to chart* **17** HAIR, SCALP, AND NAIL PROBLEMS (p.78)

or go to chart **45** GENITAL PROBLEMS IN BOYS (p.126)

or go to chart **46** GENITAL PROBLEMS IN GIRLS (p.128)

or go to chart **49** FOOT PROBLEMS (p.132)

NO ↓

Is the itching confined to the anal area, and does it occur mainly at night?

YES → **POSSIBLE CAUSE** Your child may have threadworms. These tiny, white worms, about 1 cm (½ in) long, infest the intestines and lay eggs around the anus at night, leading to intense irritation of the anus and genital area. Although harmless, they may be passed on from one person to another or picked up from contaminated food. Consult your doctor.

ACTION Your doctor will examine your child. If threadworms are diagnosed, he or she will prescribe drugs that will kill the worms. All members of your family should be treated to prevent reinfection. Make sure your child takes extra care to wash his or her hands thoroughly after going to the toilet and before eating.

NO ↓

Does your child's skin seem dry?

YES → **POSSIBLE CAUSE AND ACTION** Dry skin is often itchy. A tendency to have dry skin may run in families and is also common in children who swim regularly or use strong soaps. If your child has dry skin, provide an emollient bath oil instead of soap and follow other self-help measures for relieving itchiness (below). If your child swims regularly, he or she should shower afterwards and apply a moisturizer.

NO ↓

Have your recently changed your washing product or laundry powder?

YES → **POSSIBLE CAUSE** Skin irritation as a result of sensitivity to particular chemicals can cause widespread itching.

ACTION Avoid using perfumed products and biological washing powders. Make sure that your washing is always rinsed thoroughly. Use an emollient, such as aqueous cream, on your child's skin, and follow the other self-help measures for relieving itchiness (below). If the symptoms persist, consult your doctor.

NO ↓

Is your child intensely itchy with or without grey lines between the fingers or on the wrists?

YES → **SEE YOUR DOCTOR WITHIN 24 HOURS**

POSSIBLE CAUSE Scabies, a parasitic infection, may be causing your child's symptoms. Scabies mites burrow under the skin between the fingers and can cause a widespread rash. In babies, it may affect the palms of the hands and soles of the feet. Scabies is very contagious and often affects a whole family.

ACTION Your doctor will probably prescribe a treatment lotion, which you will need to apply to the whole of your child's body as directed. Everyone else in the household will need to be treated at the same time, and clothing and bedding also need to be washed. The mites should die within 3 days of treatment, but the itching may continue for up to 2 weeks.

NO ↓

CONSULT YOUR DOCTOR IF YOU ARE UNABLE TO MAKE A DIAGNOSIS FROM THIS CHART.

SELF-HELP Relieving itchiness

There are several measures that can help to relieve itchiness in your child:

- If your child has dry skin, he or she should bath in warm water, not hot, and use an emollient bath oil. An emollient, such as aqueous cream, should be applied to the skin twice a day.
- Make sure your child wears cotton clothing.
- To prevent scratching, keep your child's fingernails short and, if necessary, he or she should wear cotton gloves at night.
- Over-the-counter antihistamines may help control severe itching.

19 Lumps and swellings

For lumps and swellings in the scrotum, see chart 45,
GENITAL PROBLEMS IN BOYS (p.126).
Consult this chart if your child has lumps or swellings on
any area of the body. Lumps and swellings under the surface
of the skin are often lymph nodes, commonly known as

glands, that have enlarged in response to an infection. Other
lumps and swellings may be due to injuries, bites, or stings.
A persistent lump or swelling should always be examined by
a doctor so that the cause can be established. However,
there is rarely cause for serious concern in a child.

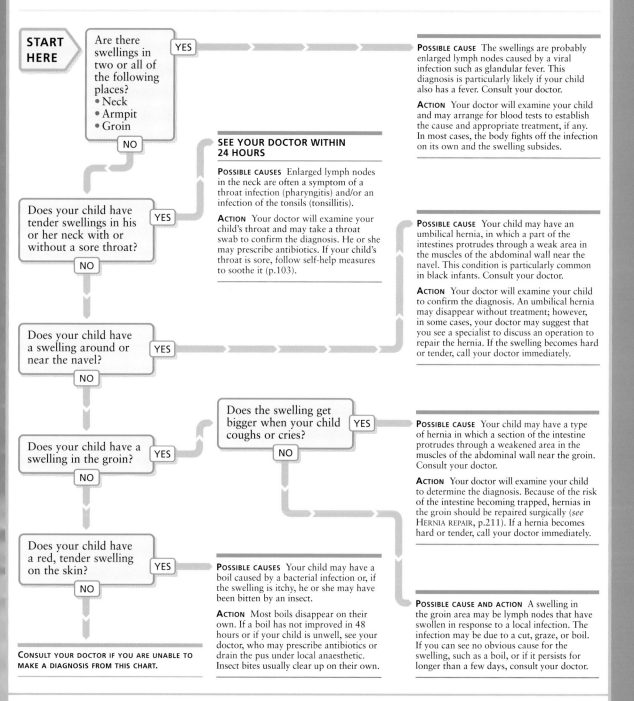

START HERE

Are there swellings in two or all of the following places?
• Neck
• Armpit
• Groin

YES → **POSSIBLE CAUSE** The swellings are probably enlarged lymph nodes caused by a viral infection such as glandular fever. This diagnosis is particularly likely if your child also has a fever. Consult your doctor.

ACTION Your doctor will examine your child and may arrange for blood tests to establish the cause and appropriate treatment, if any. In most cases, the body fights off the infection on its own and the swelling subsides.

NO ↓

Does your child have tender swellings in his or her neck with or without a sore throat?

YES → **SEE YOUR DOCTOR WITHIN 24 HOURS**

POSSIBLE CAUSES Enlarged lymph nodes in the neck are often a symptom of a throat infection (pharyngitis) and/or an infection of the tonsils (tonsillitis).

ACTION Your doctor will examine your child's throat and may take a throat swab to confirm the diagnosis. He or she may prescribe antibiotics. If your child's throat is sore, follow self-help measures to soothe it (p.103).

NO ↓

Does your child have a swelling around or near the navel?

YES → **POSSIBLE CAUSE** Your child may have an umbilical hernia, in which a part of the intestines protrudes through a weak area in the muscles of the abdominal wall near the navel. This condition is particularly common in black infants. Consult your doctor.

ACTION Your doctor will examine your child to confirm the diagnosis. An umbilical hernia may disappear without treatment; however, in some cases, your doctor may suggest that you see a specialist to discuss an operation to repair the hernia. If the swelling becomes hard or tender, call your doctor immediately.

NO ↓

Does your child have a swelling in the groin?

YES → **Does the swelling get bigger when your child coughs or cries?**

YES → **POSSIBLE CAUSE** Your child may have a type of hernia in which a section of the intestine protrudes through a weakened area in the muscles of the abdominal wall near the groin. Consult your doctor.

ACTION Your doctor will examine your child to determine the diagnosis. Because of the risk of the intestine becoming trapped, hernias in the groin should be repaired surgically (*see* HERNIA REPAIR, p.211). If a hernia becomes hard or tender, call your doctor immediately.

NO ↓

Does your child have a red, tender swelling on the skin?

YES → **POSSIBLE CAUSES** Your child may have a boil caused by a bacterial infection or, if the swelling is itchy, he or she may have been bitten by an insect.

ACTION Most boils disappear on their own. If a boil has not improved in 48 hours or if your child is unwell, see your doctor, who may prescribe antibiotics or drain the pus under local anaesthetic. Insect bites usually clear up on their own.

NO ↓

POSSIBLE CAUSE AND ACTION A swelling in the groin area may be lymph nodes that have swollen in response to a local infection. The infection may be due to a cut, graze, or boil. If you can see no obvious cause for the swelling, such as a boil, or if it persists for longer than a few days, consult your doctor.

CONSULT YOUR DOCTOR IF YOU ARE UNABLE TO
MAKE A DIAGNOSIS FROM THIS CHART.

20 Dizziness, fainting, and seizures

A brief loss of consciousness in a child is usually due to fainting and is seldom serious. However, if the loss of consciousness is accompanied by abnormal movements, such as jerking limbs, the child may be having a seizure. There are several possible causes for a seizure, some of which need urgent treatment. Children often become dizzy as a result of games that involve spinning or fairground rides, but dizziness for no obvious reason could be due to problems with the balance mechanism in the ear. If your child has regular episodes of dizziness or has a seizure, consult your doctor. Try to keep an accurate account of the episode and any related symptoms as this will help your doctor establish the cause.

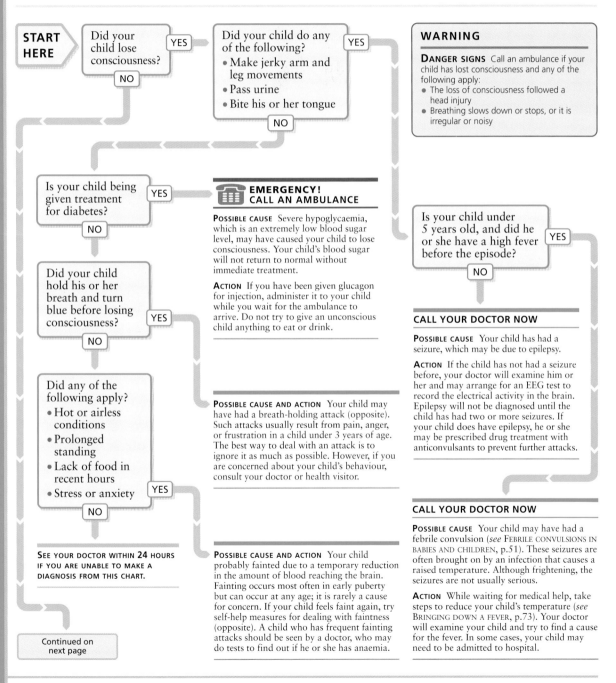

START HERE

Did your child lose consciousness? — YES →

NO ↓

Did your child do any of the following?
- Make jerky arm and leg movements
- Pass urine
- Bite his or her tongue

YES →

NO ↓

Is your child being given treatment for diabetes? — YES →

NO ↓

Did your child hold his or her breath and turn blue before losing consciousness? — YES →

NO ↓

Did any of the following apply?
- Hot or airless conditions
- Prolonged standing
- Lack of food in recent hours
- Stress or anxiety

YES →

NO ↓

SEE YOUR DOCTOR WITHIN **24** HOURS IF YOU ARE UNABLE TO MAKE A DIAGNOSIS FROM THIS CHART.

Continued on next page

WARNING

DANGER SIGNS Call an ambulance if your child has lost consciousness and any of the following apply:
- The loss of consciousness followed a head injury
- Breathing slows down or stops, or it is irregular or noisy

📞 EMERGENCY! CALL AN AMBULANCE

POSSIBLE CAUSE Severe hypoglycaemia, which is an extremely low blood sugar level, may have caused your child to lose consciousness. Your child's blood sugar will not return to normal without immediate treatment.

ACTION If you have been given glucagon for injection, administer it to your child while you wait for the ambulance to arrive. Do not try to give an unconscious child anything to eat or drink.

POSSIBLE CAUSE AND ACTION Your child may have had a breath-holding attack (opposite). Such attacks usually result from pain, anger, or frustration in a child under 3 years of age. The best way to deal with an attack is to ignore it as much as possible. However, if you are concerned about your child's behaviour, consult your doctor or health visitor.

POSSIBLE CAUSE AND ACTION Your child probably fainted due to a temporary reduction in the amount of blood reaching the brain. Fainting occurs most often in early puberty but can occur at any age; it is rarely a cause for concern. If your child feels faint again, try self-help measures for dealing with faintness (opposite). A child who has frequent fainting attacks should be seen by a doctor, who may do tests to find out if he or she has anaemia.

Is your child under 5 years old, and did he or she have a high fever before the episode? — YES →

NO ↓

CALL YOUR DOCTOR NOW

POSSIBLE CAUSE Your child has had a seizure, which may be due to epilepsy.

ACTION If the child has not had a seizure before, your doctor will examine him or her and may arrange for an EEG test to record the electrical activity in the brain. Epilepsy will not be diagnosed until the child has had two or more seizures. If your child does have epilepsy, he or she may be prescribed drug treatment with anticonvulsants to prevent further attacks.

CALL YOUR DOCTOR NOW

POSSIBLE CAUSE Your child may have had a febrile convulsion (see FEBRILE CONVULSIONS IN BABIES AND CHILDREN, p.51). These seizures are often brought on by an infection that causes a raised temperature. Although frightening, the seizures are not usually serious.

ACTION While waiting for medical help, take steps to reduce your child's temperature (see BRINGING DOWN A FEVER, p.73). Your doctor will examine your child and try to find a cause for the fever. In some cases, your child may need to be admitted to hospital.

Continued from previous page

Does your child have episodes in which he or she seems unaware of the surroundings for a few moments?
— **YES** →
— **NO** ↓

SELF-HELP Dealing with faintness

If your child suddenly turns pale, complains that his or her vision is closing in, and/or appears confused, he or she may be feeling faint. This state is more likely if the atmosphere is hot or stuffy; if your child has not eaten (and might therefore have a low blood sugar level); if he or she has been standing for a long time; or if the child is particularly stressed or anxious.

Your child should lie down with his or her feet raised to improve the blood flow to the brain. Make sure plenty of fresh air is available, and loosen the child's clothes, if necessary. If you are sure that your child is fully conscious, offer him or her a sweet drink to raise the blood sugar level. If your child loses consciousness and shows any of the danger signs listed opposite, call an ambulance.

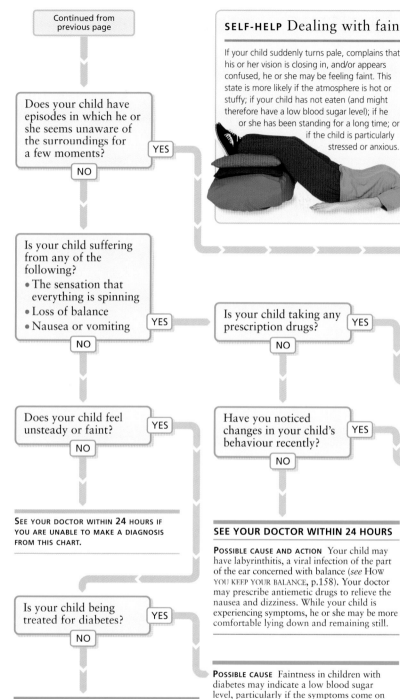

Relieving faintness
Lying down with the legs raised increases the flow of blood to the brain and usually quickly relieves feelings of faintness.

Is your child suffering from any of the following?
- The sensation that everything is spinning
- Loss of balance
- Nausea or vomiting
— **YES** →
— **NO** ↓

Is your child taking any prescription drugs?
— **YES** →
— **NO** ↓

CALL YOUR DOCTOR NOW

POSSIBLE CAUSE AND ACTION These may be generalized absence seizures, a type of epilepsy (formerly known as petit mal). Do not try to stop the seizures by shaking or slapping your child. Your doctor may refer your child for an EEG test to record the electrical activity in the brain. He or she may advise drug treatment with anticonvulsants to control the condition.

POSSIBLE CAUSE AND ACTION These symptoms may be the side effects of a drug. Call your doctor before the next dose of the drug is due to ask if it could be the cause and if you should stop giving it to your child.

Does your child feel unsteady or faint?
— **YES** →
— **NO** ↓

Have you noticed changes in your child's behaviour recently?
— **YES** →
— **NO** ↓

POSSIBLE CAUSE It is possible that your child is abusing drugs or solvents (*see* RECOGNIZING DRUG AND SOLVENT ABUSE, p.137). A nervous system problem is also a rare possibility. Consult your doctor.

ACTION Your doctor will examine your child and may refer him or her for tests such as MRI (p.39) to exclude a nervous system problem. If drug or substance abuse is the problem, your doctor may arrange counselling or suggest self-help groups (*see* USEFUL ADDRESSES, p.285).

SEE YOUR DOCTOR WITHIN 24 HOURS IF YOU ARE UNABLE TO MAKE A DIAGNOSIS FROM THIS CHART.

SEE YOUR DOCTOR WITHIN 24 HOURS

POSSIBLE CAUSE AND ACTION Your child may have labyrinthitis, a viral infection of the part of the ear concerned with balance (*see* HOW YOU KEEP YOUR BALANCE, p.158). Your doctor may prescribe antiemetic drugs to relieve the nausea and dizziness. While your child is experiencing symptoms, he or she may be more comfortable lying down and remaining still.

Breath-holding attacks

Young children sometimes hold their breath for up to 30 seconds. This can be in response to pain, but it can also be an attempt to manipulate parents. A child may hold his or her breath until he or she passes out. Once consciousness is lost, normal breathing will resume automatically.

If your child is attempting to get his or her way by breath-holding, try to ignore him or her as much as possible. Breath-holding is not harmful, and most children grow out of it by the age of 4 years. However, if you are worried, consult your doctor or health visitor.

Is your child being treated for diabetes?
— **YES** →
— **NO** ↓

POSSIBLE CAUSE Faintness in children with diabetes may indicate a low blood sugar level, particularly if the symptoms come on suddenly. Less commonly, these symptoms may be due to a high blood sugar level.

ACTION If your child is sufficiently alert, give him or her something very sweet to eat or drink. This should correct a low blood sugar level and will do no harm if the sugar level is too high. If your child cannot cooperate or is no better within 10 minutes, call a doctor at once.

POSSIBLE CAUSE AND ACTION Feeling faint is not uncommon in children, especially if they are in a stuffy atmosphere, hungry, or anxious, and is rarely a cause for concern. Follow self-help measures for dealing with faintness (above). Consult your doctor if your child has frequent fainting attacks; the doctor may need to determine whether your child has anaemia.

21 Headache

Headaches are a very common complaint. By the age of 7, 40 per cent of children have had a headache, and this figure rises to 75 per cent by the age of 15. Parents may worry that the pain is due to a serious condition, such as meningitis or a brain tumour. However, these conditions are extremely rare. Headaches often occur on their own but may accompany any infection that causes a fever. They can also be a symptom of a number of relatively minor disorders. Consult this chart if your child complains of a headache with or without other symptoms. Always consult your doctor if a headache is severe, persistent, or recurs frequently, or if this is the first time that your child has had a particular type of headache.

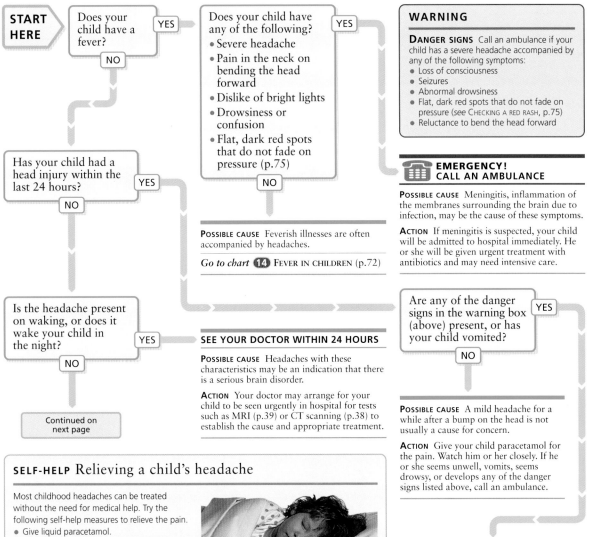

START HERE

Does your child have a fever? — YES → **Does your child have any of the following?** — YES →
- Severe headache
- Pain in the neck on bending the head forward
- Dislike of bright lights
- Drowsiness or confusion
- Flat, dark red spots that do not fade on pressure (p.75)

NO ↓ (fever)

NO ↓ (following)

Has your child had a head injury within the last 24 hours? — YES →

NO ↓

POSSIBLE CAUSE Feverish illnesses are often accompanied by headaches.

Go to chart **14** FEVER IN CHILDREN (p.72)

Is the headache present on waking, or does it wake your child in the night? — YES →

NO ↓

SEE YOUR DOCTOR WITHIN 24 HOURS

POSSIBLE CAUSE Headaches with these characteristics may be an indication that there is a serious brain disorder.

ACTION Your doctor may arrange for your child to be seen urgently in hospital for tests such as MRI (p.39) or CT scanning (p.38) to establish the cause and appropriate treatment.

Continued on next page

WARNING

DANGER SIGNS Call an ambulance if your child has a severe headache accompanied by any of the following symptoms:
- Loss of consciousness
- Seizures
- Abnormal drowsiness
- Flat, dark red spots that do not fade on pressure (*see* CHECKING A RED RASH, p.75)
- Reluctance to bend the head forward

📞 EMERGENCY! CALL AN AMBULANCE

POSSIBLE CAUSE Meningitis, inflammation of the membranes surrounding the brain due to infection, may be the cause of these symptoms.

ACTION If meningitis is suspected, your child will be admitted to hospital immediately. He or she will be given urgent treatment with antibiotics and may need intensive care.

Are any of the danger signs in the warning box (above) present, or has your child vomited? — YES →

NO ↓

POSSIBLE CAUSE A mild headache for a while after a bump on the head is not usually a cause for concern.

ACTION Give your child paracetamol for the pain. Watch him or her closely. If he or she seems unwell, vomits, seems drowsy, or develops any of the danger signs listed above, call an ambulance.

📞 EMERGENCY! CALL AN AMBULANCE

POSSIBLE CAUSE Your child's head injury may have resulted in damage to the brain.

ACTION Once in hospital, your child will be observed closely and may have tests such as CT scanning (p.38) to determine the treatment.

SELF-HELP Relieving a child's headache

Most childhood headaches can be treated without the need for medical help. Try the following self-help measures to relieve the pain.
- Give liquid paracetamol.
- Encourage your child to rest in a cool, quiet, dimly lit room. He or she may want to go to sleep for a while.
- If your child is hungry, offer him or her a snack, such as a biscuit and a drink of milk.

If the headache persists for more than 4 hours, if your child seems very unwell, or if other symptoms develop, call your doctor.

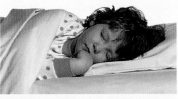

Headache relief
Encouraging a child to have a sleep or a rest, after first taking a painkiller, will often help to relieve his or her headache.

Continued from previous page

Does your child have recurrent headaches with or preceded by any of the following?
- Nausea or vomiting
- Abdominal pain
- Seeing flashing lights
- Pale appearance

YES →

Is your child completely well between attacks?

YES →

POSSIBLE CAUSE A severe headache associated with these symptoms may be a migraine, particularly if other members of the family also suffer from migraines. Consult your doctor.

ACTION Your doctor will probably examine your child to exclude other possible causes. Symptoms can often be eased by self-help measures, such as taking a painkiller and an antiemetic (drug that relieves nausea), drinking plenty of fluids, and resting in a darkened room. You should also try to discover whether there are any specific triggers, such as a food or an activity (*see* REDUCING THE FREQUENCY OF MIGRAINE, p.155).

NO

CALL YOUR DOCTOR NOW

POSSIBLE CAUSE If your child is not well between headaches or his or her performance at school has worsened recently, it may be an indication of a serious brain disorder that needs urgent investigation.

ACTION Your doctor will examine your child and may arrange for him or her to be seen urgently in hospital for tests such as MRI (p.39) or CT scanning (p.38) in order to establish the cause.

NO

Do headaches occur mainly after reading or using a computer?

YES →

POSSIBLE CAUSE Previously unrecognized eyesight problems may sometimes cause a child to develop a headache after activities such as these. Take your child to an optician for an eyesight test.

ACTION The optician will carry out a full sight test and, if a vision problem is found, will prescribe appropriate glasses for your child. If vision is normal, the optician will refer your child to the doctor, who will try to establish a cause for the headaches.

NO

Do either of the following describe your child's headache?
- Felt mainly in the forehead and face or teeth
- Worse when bending forward

YES →

SEE YOUR DOCTOR WITHIN 24 HOURS

POSSIBLE CAUSE Sinusitis (inflammation of the membranes lining the air spaces in the skull) may be the cause, especially if your child recently had a cold or a runny or blocked nose. Children under 8 are rarely affected because their sinuses have not yet developed.

ACTION Your doctor will examine your child. If sinusitis is suspected, he or she will prescribe antibiotics. In the meantime, give your child plenty of fluids, and give paracetamol to relieve pain. Steam inhalations (*see* TREATING A CHILD WITH A COLD, p.102) may ease congestion.

NO

Could your child be anxious or under stress at home or at school?

YES →

POSSIBLE CAUSE Anxiety is one of the most common causes of headaches in children.

ACTION Discuss your child's problems and worries with him or her, and see if you can identify a pattern to the headaches. Approach teachers for further information. Consult your doctor if you and your child cannot sort out the problem or if the headaches are frequent.

NO

POSSIBLE CAUSE AND ACTION Certain drugs can cause headaches as a side effect. Consult your doctor. Meanwhile, your child should not stop taking the prescribed drugs.

POSSIBLE CAUSE AND ACTION You should bring any frequent or unusual headaches to your doctor's attention. They are unlikely to be serious, but your doctor will want to rule out the possibility of an underlying disorder.

Is your child taking any prescription drugs?

YES →

NO

Are your child's headaches frequent, are they becoming more frequent, or has the nature of the headaches changed?

YES →

NO

CONSULT YOUR DOCTOR IF YOU ARE UNABLE TO MAKE A DIAGNOSIS FROM THIS CHART. IF THE HEADACHE IS SEVERE, CALL YOUR DOCTOR NOW.

22 Confusion and/or drowsiness

Children who are confused may talk nonsense, appear dazed or agitated, or see and hear things that are not real. This is a serious symptom that requires immediate medical attention. Drowsiness may be the result of a lack of sleep or a minor illness, or it may be a symptom of a serious disease, such as meningitis. Consult this chart if your child appears confused, or if he or she suddenly becomes unusually sleepy or unresponsive or is difficult to rouse from sleep.

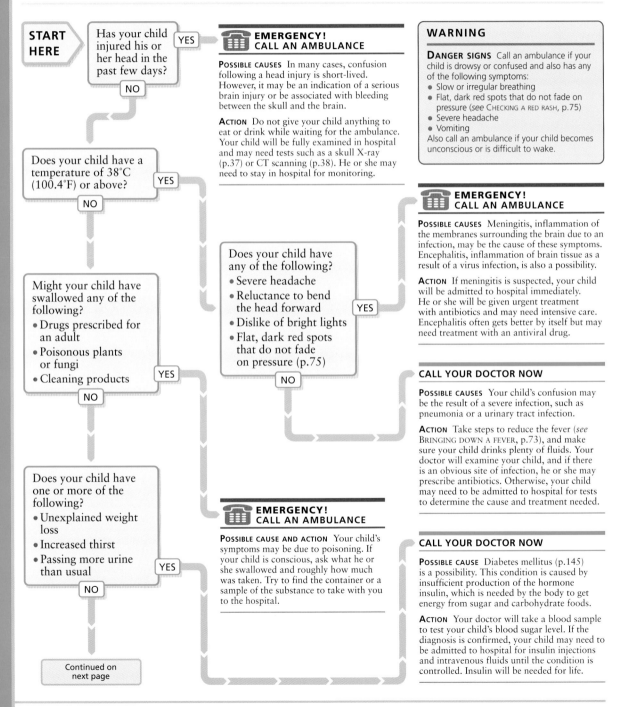

START HERE

Has your child injured his or her head in the past few days?
YES →

NO ↓

EMERGENCY! CALL AN AMBULANCE

POSSIBLE CAUSES In many cases, confusion following a head injury is short-lived. However, it may be an indication of a serious brain injury or be associated with bleeding between the skull and the brain.

ACTION Do not give your child anything to eat or drink while waiting for the ambulance. Your child will be fully examined in hospital and may need tests such as a skull X-ray (p.37) or CT scanning (p.38). He or she may need to stay in hospital for monitoring.

WARNING

DANGER SIGNS Call an ambulance if your child is drowsy or confused and also has any of the following symptoms:
- Slow or irregular breathing
- Flat, dark red spots that do not fade on pressure (see CHECKING A RED RASH, p.75)
- Severe headache
- Vomiting
Also call an ambulance if your child becomes unconscious or is difficult to wake.

Does your child have a temperature of 38°C (100.4°F) or above?
YES →

NO ↓

Might your child have swallowed any of the following?
- Drugs prescribed for an adult
- Poisonous plants or fungi
- Cleaning products

YES →

NO ↓

Does your child have any of the following?
- Severe headache
- Reluctance to bend the head forward
- Dislike of bright lights
- Flat, dark red spots that do not fade on pressure (p.75)

YES →

NO ↓

EMERGENCY! CALL AN AMBULANCE

POSSIBLE CAUSES Meningitis, inflammation of the membranes surrounding the brain due to an infection, may be the cause of these symptoms. Encephalitis, inflammation of brain tissue as a result of a virus infection, is also a possibility.

ACTION If meningitis is suspected, your child will be admitted to hospital immediately. He or she will be given urgent treatment with antibiotics and may need intensive care. Encephalitis often gets better by itself but may need treatment with an antiviral drug.

CALL YOUR DOCTOR NOW

POSSIBLE CAUSES Your child's confusion may be the result of a severe infection, such as pneumonia or a urinary tract infection.

ACTION Take steps to reduce the fever (see BRINGING DOWN A FEVER, p.73), and make sure your child drinks plenty of fluids. Your doctor will examine your child, and if there is an obvious site of infection, he or she may prescribe antibiotics. Otherwise, your child may need to be admitted to hospital for tests to determine the cause and treatment needed.

Does your child have one or more of the following?
- Unexplained weight loss
- Increased thirst
- Passing more urine than usual

YES →

NO ↓

EMERGENCY! CALL AN AMBULANCE

POSSIBLE CAUSE AND ACTION Your child's symptoms may be due to poisoning. If your child is conscious, ask what he or she swallowed and roughly how much was taken. Try to find the container or a sample of the substance to take with you to the hospital.

CALL YOUR DOCTOR NOW

POSSIBLE CAUSE Diabetes mellitus (p.145) is a possibility. This condition is caused by insufficient production of the hormone insulin, which is needed by the body to get energy from sugar and carbohydrate foods.

ACTION Your doctor will take a blood sample to test your child's blood sugar level. If the diagnosis is confirmed, your child may need to be admitted to hospital for insulin injections and intravenous fluids until the condition is controlled. Insulin will be needed for life.

Continued on next page

Continued from previous page

Is your child being treated for diabetes?

YES → **POSSIBLE CAUSES** Confusion or drowsiness in children with diabetes may indicate a low blood sugar level, particularly if the symptoms have come on suddenly. Less commonly, these symptoms may be the result of a high blood sugar level and may have developed gradually.

ACTION If your child is sufficiently alert, give him or her something very sweet to eat or drink. This should correct a low blood sugar level and will do no harm if the sugar level is too high. If your child cannot cooperate or is no better within 10 minutes, call your doctor at once. However, you should call an ambulance if your child becomes unconscious.

NO ↓

Is there evidence that your child has had a seizure; for example, has your child done either of the following?
- Bitten his or her tongue
- Wet him- or herself

YES → **POSSIBLE CAUSE AND ACTION** If your child has had an epileptic seizure, it may have left him or her drowsy or confused. If your child has been diagnosed as having epilepsy, consult your doctor because your child's treatment may need adjusting. However, you should call your doctor immediately if your child has not previously been diagnosed as having epilepsy: he or she needs to be assessed promptly.

NO ↓

Has your child had diarrhoea, with or without vomiting, in the past 24 hours?

YES → **CALL YOUR DOCTOR NOW**

POSSIBLE CAUSE Your child's symptoms may be due to dehydration.

ACTION Your doctor will examine your child to assess how severely dehydrated he or she is. In most cases, giving your child fluids at home will treat the dehydration and prevent it worsening (*see* PREVENTING DEHYDRATION IN CHILDREN, p.119). However, if your child is very unwell or unable to drink sufficient fluids to treat the dehydration, he or she may need to be admitted to hospital.

NO ↓

Has your child been exposed to hot sunshine or high temperatures recently?

YES → **EMERGENCY! CALL AN AMBULANCE**

POSSIBLE CAUSE Your child's symptoms may be due to heatstroke, in which a high temperature and dehydration can cause confusion and drowsiness.

ACTION While waiting for help, lay your child in a cool place and remove all his or her outer clothing. Open a window or use an electric fan to ensure a free flow of cool, fresh air over the skin. If your child is able to accept, offer cool drinks.

NO ↓

Is your child taking any prescription drugs or over-the-counter drugs?

YES → **CALL YOUR DOCTOR NOW**

POSSIBLE CAUSE AND ACTION Drowsiness or confusion may be a side effect of some drugs, including antihistamines and anticonvulsants. If your child is taking a prescribed drug, ask your doctor's advice before the next dose is due. Your child should stop taking any over-the-counter drugs.

NO ↓

Could your child have been drinking alcohol?

YES → **POSSIBLE CAUSE** Your child may be intoxicated or have alcohol poisoning.

ACTION Encourage your child to drink plenty of water, and wait for the effects to wear off. If your child becomes unconscious, call an ambulance.

NO ↓

Could your child be using recreational drugs or inhaling solvents?

YES → **POSSIBLE CAUSE** Drug or solvent abuse may cause drowsiness or confusion.

ACTION Watch your child carefully while he or she is confused or drowsy. If your child loses consciousness, call an ambulance. Delay discussing the problem with your child until he or she is well enough to understand. If you think your child is becoming dependent on drugs, consult your doctor. Many self-help groups also provide advice and support (*see* USEFUL ADDRESSES, p.285).

NO ↓

CALL YOUR DOCTOR NOW IF YOUR CHILD IS DROWSY OR CONFUSED AND YOU ARE UNABLE TO MAKE A DIAGNOSIS FROM THIS CHART.

23 Clumsiness

Children vary greatly in their levels of manual dexterity, physical coordination, and agility. Some children naturally acquire these skills later than others. They have difficulty in carrying out delicate tasks, such as tying shoelaces, and may often accidentally knock things over. Such clumsiness is unlikely to be a sign of an underlying disease, although poor vision can be an unrecognized cause. Severe clumsiness that has come on suddenly or that follows a head injury may result from a serious problem with the nervous system and needs urgent medical attention.

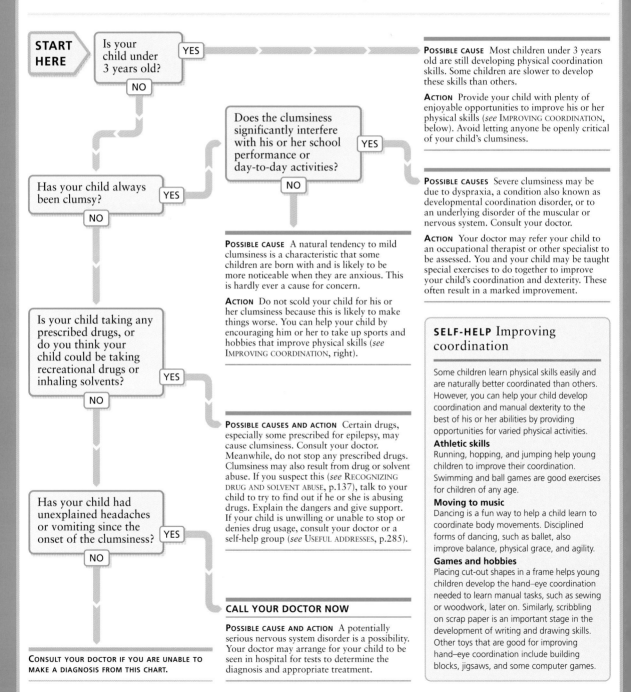

START HERE

Is your child under 3 years old?
YES →

NO ↓

POSSIBLE CAUSE Most children under 3 years old are still developing physical coordination skills. Some children are slower to develop these skills than others.

ACTION Provide your child with plenty of enjoyable opportunities to improve his or her physical skills (*see* IMPROVING COORDINATION, below). Avoid letting anyone be openly critical of your child's clumsiness.

Does the clumsiness significantly interfere with his or her school performance or day-to-day activities?
YES →

NO ↓

Has your child always been clumsy?
YES →

NO ↓

POSSIBLE CAUSES Severe clumsiness may be due to dyspraxia, a condition also known as developmental coordination disorder, or to an underlying disorder of the muscular or nervous system. Consult your doctor.

ACTION Your doctor may refer your child to an occupational therapist or other specialist to be assessed. You and your child may be taught special exercises to do together to improve your child's coordination and dexterity. These often result in a marked improvement.

POSSIBLE CAUSE A natural tendency to mild clumsiness is a characteristic that some children are born with and is likely to be more noticeable when they are anxious. This is hardly ever a cause for concern.

ACTION Do not scold your child for his or her clumsiness because this is likely to make things worse. You can help your child by encouraging him or her to take up sports and hobbies that improve physical skills (*see* IMPROVING COORDINATION, right).

Is your child taking any prescribed drugs, or do you think your child could be taking recreational drugs or inhaling solvents?
YES →

NO ↓

POSSIBLE CAUSES AND ACTION Certain drugs, especially some prescribed for epilepsy, may cause clumsiness. Consult your doctor. Meanwhile, do not stop any prescribed drugs. Clumsiness may also result from drug or solvent abuse. If you suspect this (*see* RECOGNIZING DRUG AND SOLVENT ABUSE, p.137), talk to your child to try to find out if he or she is abusing drugs. Explain the dangers and give support. If your child is unwilling or unable to stop or denies drug usage, consult your doctor or a self-help group (*see* USEFUL ADDRESSES, p.285).

Has your child had unexplained headaches or vomiting since the onset of the clumsiness?
YES →

NO ↓

CALL YOUR DOCTOR NOW

POSSIBLE CAUSE AND ACTION A potentially serious nervous system disorder is a possibility. Your doctor may arrange for your child to be seen in hospital for tests to determine the diagnosis and appropriate treatment.

CONSULT YOUR DOCTOR IF YOU ARE UNABLE TO MAKE A DIAGNOSIS FROM THIS CHART.

SELF-HELP Improving coordination

Some children learn physical skills easily and are naturally better coordinated than others. However, you can help your child develop coordination and manual dexterity to the best of his or her abilities by providing opportunities for varied physical activities.

Athletic skills
Running, hopping, and jumping help young children to improve their coordination. Swimming and ball games are good exercises for children of any age.

Moving to music
Dancing is a fun way to help a child learn to coordinate body movements. Disciplined forms of dancing, such as ballet, also improve balance, physical grace, and agility.

Games and hobbies
Placing cut-out shapes in a frame helps young children develop the hand–eye coordination needed to learn manual tasks, such as sewing or woodwork, later on. Similarly, scribbling on scrap paper is an important stage in the development of writing and drawing skills. Other toys that are good for improving hand–eye coordination include building blocks, jigsaws, and some computer games.

24 Speech difficulties

Consult this chart if your child has any problem with his or her speech, such as a delay in starting to talk, lack of clarity, defects in pronunciation, or stammering. Such difficulties often improve with time, but, in most cases, it is wise to seek the advice of your doctor or health visitor. If not addressed early, speech difficulties may cause behaviour and school problems. A speech therapist will usually be able to improve your child's ability to communicate effectively.

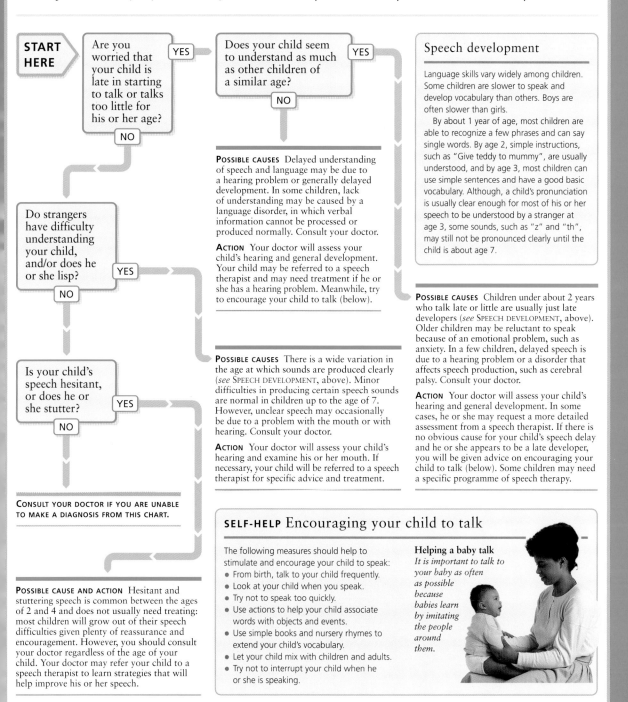

START HERE

Are you worried that your child is late in starting to talk or talks too little for his or her age? — YES →

NO ↓

Does your child seem to understand as much as other children of a similar age? — YES →

NO ↓

POSSIBLE CAUSES Delayed understanding of speech and language may be due to a hearing problem or generally delayed development. In some children, lack of understanding may be caused by a language disorder, in which verbal information cannot be processed or produced normally. Consult your doctor.

ACTION Your doctor will assess your child's hearing and general development. Your child may be referred to a speech therapist and may need treatment if he or she has a hearing problem. Meanwhile, try to encourage your child to talk (below).

Do strangers have difficulty understanding your child, and/or does he or she lisp? — YES →

NO ↓

POSSIBLE CAUSES There is a wide variation in the age at which sounds are produced clearly (*see* SPEECH DEVELOPMENT, above). Minor difficulties in producing certain speech sounds are normal in children up to the age of 7. However, unclear speech may occasionally be due to a problem with the mouth or with hearing. Consult your doctor.

ACTION Your doctor will assess your child's hearing and examine his or her mouth. If necessary, your child will be referred to a speech therapist for specific advice and treatment.

Is your child's speech hesitant, or does he or she stutter? — YES →

NO ↓

CONSULT YOUR DOCTOR IF YOU ARE UNABLE TO MAKE A DIAGNOSIS FROM THIS CHART.

POSSIBLE CAUSE AND ACTION Hesitant and stuttering speech is common between the ages of 2 and 4 and does not usually need treating: most children will grow out of their speech difficulties given plenty of reassurance and encouragement. However, you should consult your doctor regardless of the age of your child. Your doctor may refer your child to a speech therapist to learn strategies that will help improve his or her speech.

Speech development

Language skills vary widely among children. Some children are slower to speak and develop vocabulary than others. Boys are often slower than girls.

By about 1 year of age, most children are able to recognize a few phrases and can say single words. By age 2, simple instructions, such as "Give teddy to mummy", are usually understood, and by age 3, most children can use simple sentences and have a good basic vocabulary. Although, a child's pronunciation is usually clear enough for most of his or her speech to be understood by a stranger at age 3, some sounds, such as "z" and "th", may still not be pronounced clearly until the child is about age 7.

POSSIBLE CAUSES Children under about 2 years who talk late or little are usually just late developers (*see* SPEECH DEVELOPMENT, above). Older children may be reluctant to speak because of an emotional problem, such as anxiety. In a few children, delayed speech is due to a hearing problem or a disorder that affects speech production, such as cerebral palsy. Consult your doctor.

ACTION Your doctor will assess your child's hearing and general development. In some cases, he or she may request a more detailed assessment from a speech therapist. If there is no obvious cause for your child's speech delay and he or she appears to be a late developer, you will be given advice on encouraging your child to talk (below). Some children may need a specific programme of speech therapy.

SELF-HELP Encouraging your child to talk

The following measures should help to stimulate and encourage your child to speak:
- From birth, talk to your child frequently.
- Look at your child when you speak.
- Try not to speak too quickly.
- Use actions to help your child associate words with objects and events.
- Use simple books and nursery rhymes to extend your child's vocabulary.
- Let your child mix with children and adults.
- Try not to interrupt your child when he or she is speaking.

Helping a baby talk
It is important to talk to your baby as often as possible because babies learn by imitating the people around them.

25 Behaviour problems

Perception of what constitutes a behaviour problem varies widely between parents. At some stage, most children will behave in a way that causes their parents concern, even if it is by doing something as minor as nail-biting (see HABITUAL

BEHAVIOUR, opposite). However, most of these problems are outgrown. This chart covers some of the more common or serious behaviour problems that parents have to cope with. It will help you to decide if help from your doctor is advisable.

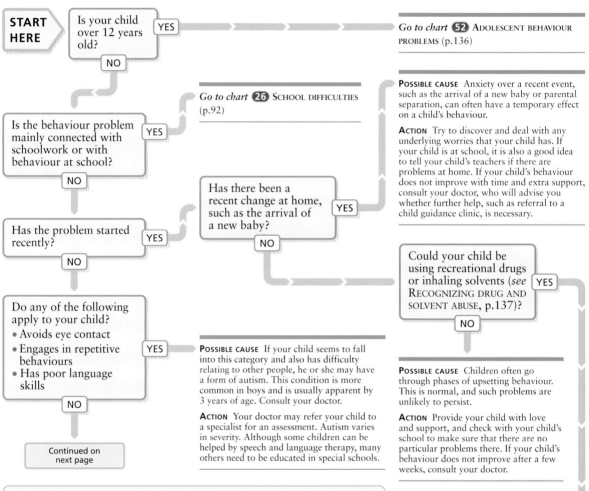

START HERE Is your child over 12 years old? — **YES** → *Go to chart* **52** ADOLESCENT BEHAVIOUR PROBLEMS (p.136)

NO

Is the behaviour problem mainly connected with schoolwork or with behaviour at school? — **YES** → *Go to chart* **26** SCHOOL DIFFICULTIES (p.92)

NO

Has the problem started recently? — **YES** → Has there been a recent change at home, such as the arrival of a new baby? — **YES**

NO (from Has there been a recent change)

POSSIBLE CAUSE Anxiety over a recent event, such as the arrival of a new baby or parental separation, can often have a temporary effect on a child's behaviour.

ACTION Try to discover and deal with any underlying worries that your child has. If your child is at school, it is also a good idea to tell your child's teachers if there are problems at home. If your child's behaviour does not improve with time and extra support, consult your doctor, who will advise you whether further help, such as referral to a child guidance clinic, is necessary.

NO (from Has the problem started recently?)

Do any of the following apply to your child?
- Avoids eye contact
- Engages in repetitive behaviours
- Has poor language skills

— **YES** → **POSSIBLE CAUSE** If your child seems to fall into this category and also has difficulty relating to other people, he or she may have a form of autism. This condition is more common in boys and is usually apparent by 3 years of age. Consult your doctor.

ACTION Your doctor may refer your child to a specialist for an assessment. Autism varies in severity. Although some children can be helped by speech and language therapy, many others need to be educated in special schools.

NO

Continued on next page

Could your child be using recreational drugs or inhaling solvents (see RECOGNIZING DRUG AND SOLVENT ABUSE, p.137)? — **YES**

NO

POSSIBLE CAUSE Children often go through phases of upsetting behaviour. This is normal, and such problems are unlikely to persist.

ACTION Provide your child with love and support, and check with your child's school to make sure that there are no particular problems there. If your child's behaviour does not improve after a few weeks, consult your doctor.

POSSIBLE CAUSE Drug or substance abuse often results in behaviour problems.

ACTION Talk to your child to try to find out whether there is an underlying problem. Try not to get aggressive or angry, but provide him or her with plenty of love. Giving your child support may provide him or her with the self-confidence to stop. If you think your child is becoming dependent on drugs, consult your doctor. Advice and support are also available from many self-help groups (see USEFUL ADDRESSES, p.285).

SELF-HELP Coping with the "terrible twos"

The period around the age of two years is a time during which children are beginning to appreciate that they have a separate identity and are able to influence their environment. It is often a time of alternating moods. Your child may have periods of self-assertion, during which he or she has violent temper tantrums if his or her wishes are frustrated. These may alternate with periods when he or she feels insecure and refuses to be separated from you. Such behaviour can make the "terrible twos" a very trying time for parents.

If your child has temper tantrums, try to keep calm and to ignore the behaviour, unless he or she could be injured. Also try to ignore other people who appear to be disapproving. If you are upset by the tantrums, it is better to leave the room than to show signs of distress yourself. Seek support from other parents of similar-aged children.

Your child will grow out of this phase, but, in the meantime, if you feel unable to cope with his or her behaviour, consult your doctor or health visitor for advice and support.

Continued from previous page

Has your child become unusually withdrawn and lost interest in activities that he or she previously enjoyed?

YES

NO

Is your child unruly, noisy, and disobedient?

YES

NO

CONSULT YOUR DOCTOR IF YOU ARE UNABLE TO FIND AN EXPLANATION FOR YOUR CHILD'S BEHAVIOUR ON THIS CHART AND YOUR CHILD CONTINUES TO BEHAVE IN A WAY THAT WORRIES YOU.

Habitual behaviour

Childhood habits, such as nail-biting, are common and rarely do any serious harm. They may provide comfort from stress or be a means of expressing emotion, such as anger. Rarely, habits such as breath-holding attacks (p.83) may be used to manipulate parents.

About a third of children bite their nails, a habit that may persist into adulthood. Thumb-sucking is common in children under 3. Some may continue up to the age of 6 or 7, when they should be persuaded to stop to prevent the adult teeth being pushed out of position.

Children are often unaware of habitual behaviour. To stop a habit, draw your child's attention to it when it occurs, but do not get angry. If you are worried, consult your doctor.

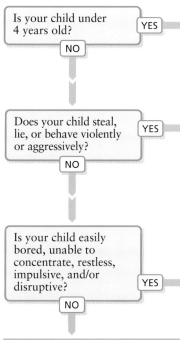

Twirling the hair
Children of all ages may play with their hair, often unaware that they are doing so. In some cases, this can lead to hair loss.

POSSIBLE CAUSES Both depression and anxiety can cause these symptoms.

ACTION Talk to your child to see if there is a reason for his or her behaviour. Offer support and encouragement, and try to remove or reduce any sources of stress that may be contributing. If your child's symptoms persist for more than 2 weeks or worsen, consult your doctor.

POSSIBLE CAUSE It is normal for small children to test the rules and disobey their parents. Many young children also go through a period of particularly difficult behaviour known as the "terrible twos".

ACTION All children grow out of this behaviour. Meanwhile, follow the advice for coping with the "terrible twos" (opposite). If, at any stage, you feel that you cannot cope, consult your doctor or health visitor.

Is your child under 4 years old?

YES

NO

Attention deficit hyperactivity disorder

Young children are normally very active. However, a child who is excessively restless, impulsive, and unable to concentrate may have attention deficit hyperactivity disorder (ADHD). Children with ADHD (usually boys) may be destructive, irritable, and aggressive and may also have difficulty making friends. Such behaviour is very hard to deal with and requires patience and understanding. Children with ADHD often have low self-esteem because of frequent scolding or criticism.

If you suspect that your child may have ADHD, consult your doctor, who will assess your child's behaviour and may refer him or her to a child psychologist, child psychiatrist, or paediatrician. You may be taught various techniques to improve your child's behaviour, and your child may be given drugs that will help calm him or her. Your child may also benefit from being taught in small groups. Although the disorder often continues through adolescence, behavioural problems may become less severe if the treatment is started early enough.

Does your child steal, lie, or behave violently or aggressively?

YES

NO

POSSIBLE CAUSE Children are often rebellious. However, if your child is persistently antisocial, disruptive, or violent, he or she may have a condition known as a conduct disorder. Consult your doctor.

ACTION Your doctor may refer your child to a specialist for assessment. Child guidance or family therapy will probably be needed. However, long-standing behaviour problems may be difficult to change.

Is your child easily bored, unable to concentrate, restless, impulsive, and/or disruptive?

YES

NO

CONSULT YOUR DOCTOR IF YOU ARE UNABLE TO FIND AN EXPLANATION FOR YOUR CHILD'S BEHAVIOUR ON THIS CHART AND YOUR CHILD CONTINUES TO BEHAVE IN A WAY THAT WORRIES YOU.

POSSIBLE CAUSE Although this type of behaviour is normal in small children, school-age children, particularly boys, who are constantly active and disruptive may have attention deficit hyperactivity disorder (left). Consult your doctor.

ACTION Your doctor will probably refer your child to a specialist to confirm the diagnosis. Children with this condition need extra support and help both at home and in school, and some also need drug treatment.

26 School difficulties

School difficulties fall into two main groups: those related mainly to learning, whether of a specific subject or of schoolwork in general; and those concerned with behaviour, including classroom behaviour and reluctance to go to school. Consult this chart if your child has any such difficulties. They may be the result of emotional problems, physical disorders, or social factors, or may arise from a general developmental problem. Discussion with school staff usually helps the situation. Your family doctor and the school medical services may also be able to help.

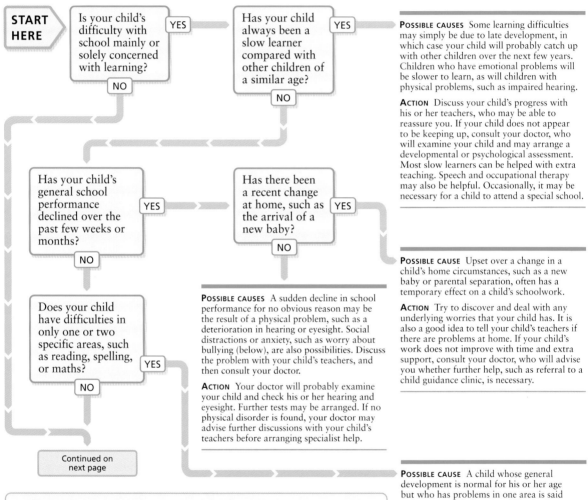

START HERE

Is your child's difficulty with school mainly or solely concerned with learning? — YES → **Has your child always been a slow learner compared with other children of a similar age?** — YES →

NO ↓

POSSIBLE CAUSES Some learning difficulties may simply be due to late development, in which case your child will probably catch up with other children over the next few years. Children who have emotional problems will be slower to learn, as will children with physical problems, such as impaired hearing.

ACTION Discuss your child's progress with his or her teachers, who may be able to reassure you. If your child does not appear to be keeping up, consult your doctor, who will examine your child and may arrange a developmental or psychological assessment. Most slow learners can be helped with extra teaching. Speech and occupational therapy may also be helpful. Occasionally, it may be necessary for a child to attend a special school.

Has your child's general school performance declined over the past few weeks or months? — YES → **Has there been a recent change at home, such as the arrival of a new baby?** — YES →

NO ↓

NO ↓

POSSIBLE CAUSE Upset over a change in a child's home circumstances, such as a new baby or parental separation, often has a temporary effect on a child's schoolwork.

ACTION Try to discover and deal with any underlying worries that your child has. It is also a good idea to tell your child's teachers if there are problems at home. If your child's work does not improve with time and extra support, consult your doctor, who will advise you whether further help, such as referral to a child guidance clinic, is necessary.

Does your child have difficulties in only one or two specific areas, such as reading, spelling, or maths? — YES →

NO ↓

POSSIBLE CAUSES A sudden decline in school performance for no obvious reason may be the result of a physical problem, such as a deterioration in hearing or eyesight. Social distractions or anxiety, such as worry about bullying (below), are also possibilities. Discuss the problem with your child's teachers, and then consult your doctor.

ACTION Your doctor will probably examine your child and check his or her hearing and eyesight. Further tests may be arranged. If no physical disorder is found, your doctor may advise further discussions with your child's teachers before arranging specialist help.

Continued on next page

POSSIBLE CAUSE A child whose general development is normal for his or her age but who has problems in one area is said to have a specific learning difficulty. For example, difficulty in reading and writing is known as dyslexia (opposite). Discuss the problem with your child's teachers initially, and consult your doctor.

ACTION Your doctor will probably examine your child to make sure that a physical problem, such as poor eyesight or an unrecognized illness, is not contributing to your child's difficulties. Your doctor may liaise with the school medical services. Work with your child's school to encourage your child as much as possible. In some cases, extra support in school may be necessary.

Bullying

Bullying can take many forms. As well as physical violence, it includes teasing, name-calling, spreading unpleasant stories, and excluding children from groups. Bullying is especially common in primary school.

A child who is being bullied is singled out for attention by the bully and may become very unhappy and insecure. He or she may not want to go to school, and his or her schoolwork may suffer. If your child is being bullied, it is vitally important that you reassure him or her that the bullying is not his or her fault. Build up your child's self-esteem, and talk to his or her school. Schools should have a policy on bullying.

The bully needs help, too. In many cases, bullying is an expression of an underlying problem such as a need for attention. If your child is a bully, it is important that you make it clear that this behaviour is harmful and unacceptable while trying to find the cause.

Continued from previous page

Has your child been playing truant? — **YES**

NO

Has your child become reluctant to go to school? — **YES**

NO

Have teachers complained about your child's behaviour at school? — **YES**

NO

SCHOOL DIFFICULTIES THAT HAVE NOT BEEN DESCRIBED ON THIS CHART SHOULD BE DISCUSSED WITH YOUR CHILD'S TEACHERS. YOUR DOCTOR'S ADVICE MAY ALSO BE HELPFUL IN SOME CASES.

Do any of the following apply to your child?
- He or she often comes home with unexplained bruises or cuts.
- Money or belongings are frequently "lost" at school.
- He or she comes home with broken belongings.

YES

NO

Does your child resist all attempts to get him or her into school? — **YES**

NO

POSSIBLE CAUSES Dislike of school may be caused by a variety of factors. For example, children starting a new school may be anxious. Your child may be having difficulties with work at school or be afraid of certain teachers or pupils. If not tackled, a dislike of school may progress into a refusal to attend school.

ACTION Try to find out the cause of the problem, and discuss your child's feelings with his or her teachers so that they can watch out for signs of bullying (opposite). Do not keep your child at home. Depending on the cause of the problem, it may be necessary for your child to receive extra teaching or help through a child guidance clinic.

Is your child easily bored, unable to concentrate, restless, impulsive, and/or disruptive? — **YES**

NO

Is your child's behaviour at home acceptable? — **YES**

NO

POSSIBLE CAUSE Truancy combined with other antisocial behaviours, such as stealing, is more common in adolescents. In some cases, it is due to bullying (opposite) or the influence of friends. Talk to your child's teachers and your doctor.

ACTION If problems persist despite intervention at school, it may be necessary to refer your child to a child guidance clinic. Long-standing behaviour problems may be difficult to change.

POSSIBLE CAUSE This type of problem may be due to bullying, even if your child is initially reluctant to admit it (*see* BULLYING, opposite).

ACTION Talk to your child about the situation, and speak to his or her teachers. Bullying or other violence at school should be taken very seriously. Your child's school should have a policy for dealing with bullying, and you can help by building up your child's confidence.

POSSIBLE CAUSES School refusal may be a sign that something is seriously wrong. There may be a problem at school, such as bullying (opposite), or a failure of the school to meet the child's needs. Occasionally, refusal to go to school is caused by anxiety at home or, in a young child, by anxiety over separation from his or her parents.

ACTION Try to discover the underlying cause of your child's refusal to go to school so that it can be dealt with, and make every effort to ensure that your child attends school. In the meantime, discuss the problem with your child's teachers. If the situation does not improve, consult your doctor. He or she may recommend you seek help for your child through a child guidance clinic.

POSSIBLE CAUSE Although this type of behaviour is normal in small children, school-age children who are constantly active and disruptive may have attention deficit hyperactivity disorder (p.91). Consult your doctor.

ACTION Your doctor will probably refer your child to a specialist to confirm the diagnosis. Children with this condition need extra support at home and in school, and some need drug treatment.

POSSIBLE CAUSES Bad behaviour that is confined to school can be due to a number of problems. Schoolwork may be too easy, leading to boredom, or it may be too difficult, possibly because of an unrecognized learning difficulty, resulting in loss of interest. Bad behaviour may also be the result of rejecting authority. In some cases, poor behaviour at school may be due to bullying (opposite).

ACTION Talk to your child to try to uncover the cause of the problem. It is also wise to discuss the problem with your child's teachers. Adjustments may need to be made to your child's schoolwork so that it meets his or her needs more closely. In some cases, help through a child guidance clinic may be arranged by your doctor.

Dyslexia

Dyslexia means difficulty with words. Early signs include difficulty in learning to read, write, and spell. Dyslexia is not linked to low intelligence. If you think your child may be dyslexic, talk to your doctor and your child's teachers. They should be able to arrange for a formal assessment of your child and subsequent support (*see also* USEFUL ADDRESSES, p.285).

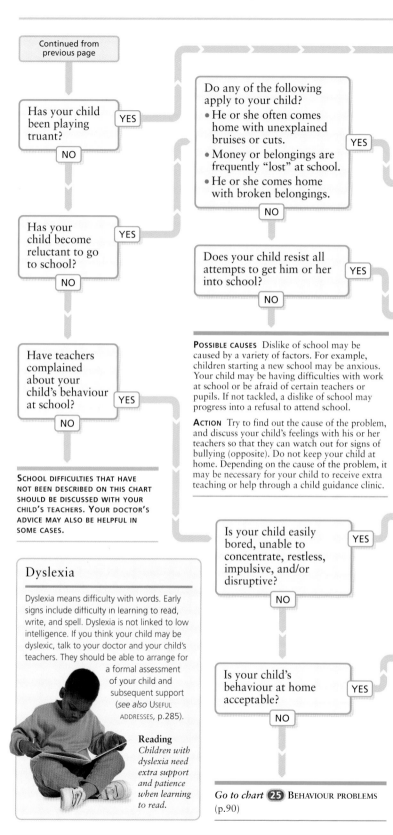

Reading
Children with dyslexia need extra support and patience when learning to read.

Go to chart **25** BEHAVIOUR PROBLEMS (p.90)

27 Eye problems

For blurred vision in children, see chart 28, DISTURBED OR IMPAIRED VISION (p.96).

This chart deals with pain, itching, redness, and/or discharge from one or both eyes. In children, such symptoms are most commonly the result of infection or local irritation. In most cases, it is reasonable to treat these problems at home initially. Always seek immediate medical advice about injury to the eye or for any foreign body in the eye that cannot be removed by simple self-help measures. You should also seek medical help if home treatment is not effective.

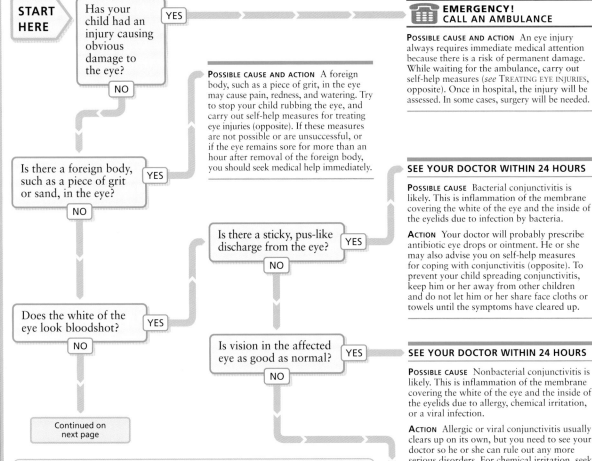

START HERE → Has your child had an injury causing obvious damage to the eye? — **YES** →

NO ↓

Is there a foreign body, such as a piece of grit or sand, in the eye? — **YES** →

POSSIBLE CAUSE AND ACTION A foreign body, such as a piece of grit, in the eye may cause pain, redness, and watering. Try to stop your child rubbing the eye, and carry out self-help measures for treating eye injuries (opposite). If these measures are not possible or are unsuccessful, or if the eye remains sore for more than an hour after removal of the foreign body, you should seek medical help immediately.

NO ↓

Is there a sticky, pus-like discharge from the eye? — **YES** →

NO ↓

Does the white of the eye look bloodshot? — **YES** →

NO ↓

Is vision in the affected eye as good as normal? — **YES** →

NO ↓

Continued on next page

EMERGENCY! CALL AN AMBULANCE

POSSIBLE CAUSE AND ACTION An eye injury always requires immediate medical attention because there is a risk of permanent damage. While waiting for the ambulance, carry out self-help measures (see TREATING EYE INJURIES, opposite). Once in hospital, the injury will be assessed. In some cases, surgery will be needed.

SEE YOUR DOCTOR WITHIN 24 HOURS

POSSIBLE CAUSE Bacterial conjunctivitis is likely. This is inflammation of the membrane covering the white of the eye and the inside of the eyelids due to infection by bacteria.

ACTION Your doctor will probably prescribe antibiotic eye drops or ointment. He or she may also advise you on self-help measures for coping with conjunctivitis (opposite). To prevent your child spreading conjunctivitis, keep him or her away from other children and do not let him or her share face cloths or towels until the symptoms have cleared up.

SEE YOUR DOCTOR WITHIN 24 HOURS

POSSIBLE CAUSE Nonbacterial conjunctivitis is likely. This is inflammation of the membrane covering the white of the eye and the inside of the eyelids due to allergy, chemical irritation, or a viral infection.

ACTION Allergic or viral conjunctivitis usually clears up on its own, but you need to see your doctor so he or she can rule out any more serious disorders. For chemical irritation, seek immediate medical help, and carry out self-help measures for treating eye injuries (opposite).

CALL YOUR DOCTOR NOW

POSSIBLE CAUSE Iritis, inflammation of the coloured part of the eye, is a possibility.

ACTION Your doctor will refer your child to a specialist for a detailed eye examination and for other tests to look for disorders that sometimes occur with iritis, such as arthritis. Iritis needs immediate treatment with corticosteroid eye drops or tablets to prevent permanent damage to vision.

Blocked tear duct

Tears are produced continuously to clean and moisturize the front of the eye. Excess tears drain away through the tear ducts. These are narrow passages that lead from the inner corner of the lower eyelid to the inside of the nose. If a tear duct becomes blocked, tears cannot drain away normally and the eye waters.

Blocked tear ducts are common in babies. One or both tear ducts may be blocked at birth. This is not a cause for concern, as in most cases the ducts open naturally by the time a child is 1 year old. Massage may help unblock a tear duct. Wash your hands thoroughly, and use a forefinger to massage the skin just below the inner corner of the eye in a gentle circular motion. Repeat the massage three or four times a day for 1 or 2 weeks. This technique may help the tear duct to open. If a blocked tear duct has not opened by the age of 1 year, the doctor may refer your child to a specialist for treatment. The duct may have to be opened with a thin probe under a general anaesthetic.

Continued from previous page

Are the eyelids red and itchy? — YES

NO

POSSIBLE CAUSE Blepharitis, inflammation of the lid margins, is the most likely cause of itchy, scaly eyelids. This condition is often associated with dandruff. Consult your doctor.

ACTION Your doctor will probably prescribe an ointment to apply to the eyelids. Treating the scalp with an over-the-counter anti-dandruff shampoo may also result in an improvement in the eyelids.

Is there a tender red lump on one eyelid? — YES

NO

POSSIBLE CAUSE A stye, a boil-like infection at the root of an eyelash, is likely.

ACTION A stye will usually clear up within a week without special treatment. It will either burst, releasing pus, or gradually disappear. If pus is released, use a clean piece of cotton wool moistened with warm water to clear away the discharge, wiping towards the outer side of the eye. To prevent infection spreading, try to discourage your child from touching the affected eye. Consult your doctor if a stye fails to heal within a week or if styes recur often.

Do one or both eyes water continuously? — YES

NO

Is your child less than 1 year old? — YES

NO

CONSULT YOUR DOCTOR IF YOU ARE UNABLE TO MAKE A DIAGNOSIS FROM THIS CHART.

CONSULT YOUR DOCTOR IF YOU ARE UNABLE TO MAKE A DIAGNOSIS FROM THIS CHART.

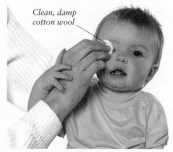

SELF-HELP Coping with conjunctivitis

A common cause of conjunctivitis in children is a bacterial infection, which is easily spread. If your child has conjunctivitis, you should try to stop him or her from touching the affected eye. Remove the discharge from your child's eye with warm water and cotton wool as often as necessary. Keep your child away from other children until his or her symptoms have cleared up. You can help prevent other family members from catching conjunctivitis by having a separate towel and face cloth for your child.

Clean, damp cotton wool

Cleaning your child's eye
Gently wipe from the inside to the outer edge of the eye. Use a clean piece of damp cotton wool each time.

POSSIBLE CAUSE A blocked tear duct may be causing your baby's symptoms. This condition is common in babies and usually corrects itself without treatment by the end of the first year.

ACTION You may be able to help a blocked duct to open by gentle massage (see BLOCKED TEAR DUCT, opposite). In rare cases, the duct does not open and an operation is needed.

SELF-HELP Treating eye injuries

You should seek prompt medical attention for a blow to the eye or an eye wound. If there is a visible wound, lay the victim down with his or her head elevated and place a pad of clean, non-fluffy material gently over the eye. Do not press down on it. Keep the victim as still as possible while you are waiting for medical help to arrive.

A foreign body floating on the white of the eye is usually easily removed (right). However, if it is embedded in the eye or rests on the coloured part of the eye, do not attempt to remove it. Take the person to hospital.

If chemicals have splashed into someone's eye, seek immediate medical help. In the meantime, self-help treatment (far right) can help minimize damage to the eye.

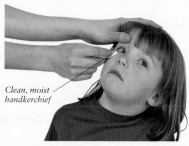

Clean, moist handkerchief

Foreign bodies in the eye
Gently ease the eyelid away from the eye. Lift the foreign body off the surface of the eye using the corner of a clean, moist handkerchief.

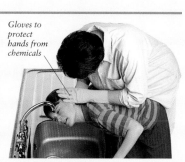

Gloves to protect hands from chemicals

Chemicals in the eye
Gently run cold water over the eye for 10 minutes. Keep the unaffected eye uppermost to prevent chemicals being washed into it.

28 Disturbed or impaired vision

Serious defects in a child's vision are usually picked up during a routine eye test. However, you may suspect that your child has an undetected problem with his or her eyesight if he or she squints or always holds books very close to the face. When your child begins school, a teacher may notice that he or she performs less well sitting at the back of the classroom, where it may be difficult to see the board. Consult your optician if you suspect a problem with your child's eyesight. If your child develops a sudden problem with his or her vision, he or she should receive urgent medical assessment. Fortunately, disorders causing a sudden disturbance of vision are rare in childhood.

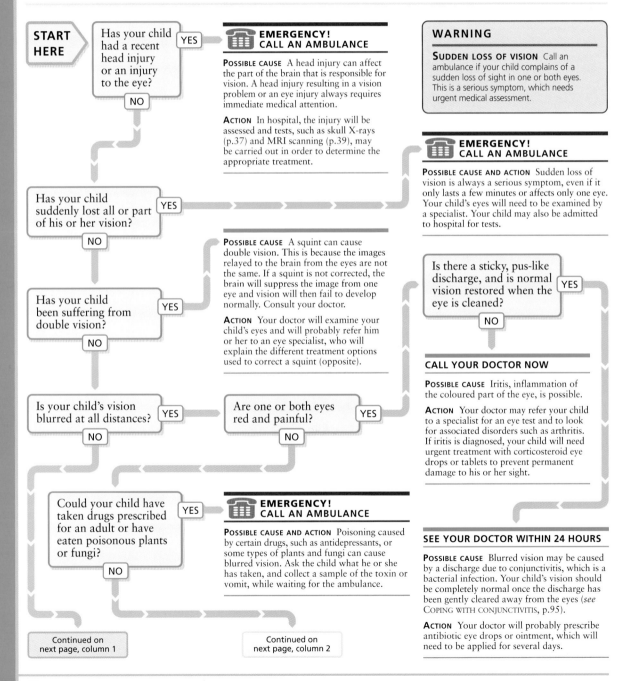

START HERE

Has your child had a recent head injury or an injury to the eye? — YES / NO

EMERGENCY! CALL AN AMBULANCE

POSSIBLE CAUSE A head injury can affect the part of the brain that is responsible for vision. A head injury resulting in a vision problem or an eye injury always requires immediate medical attention.

ACTION In hospital, the injury will be assessed and tests, such as skull X-rays (p.37) and MRI scanning (p.39), may be carried out in order to determine the appropriate treatment.

Has your child suddenly lost all or part of his or her vision? — YES / NO

Has your child been suffering from double vision? — YES / NO

POSSIBLE CAUSE A squint can cause double vision. This is because the images relayed to the brain from the eyes are not the same. If a squint is not corrected, the brain will suppress the image from one eye and vision will then fail to develop normally. Consult your doctor.

ACTION Your doctor will examine your child's eyes and will probably refer him or her to an eye specialist, who will explain the different treatment options used to correct a squint (opposite).

Is your child's vision blurred at all distances? — YES / NO

Are one or both eyes red and painful? — YES / NO

Could your child have taken drugs prescribed for an adult or have eaten poisonous plants or fungi? — YES / NO

EMERGENCY! CALL AN AMBULANCE

POSSIBLE CAUSE AND ACTION Poisoning caused by certain drugs, such as antidepressants, or some types of plants and fungi can cause blurred vision. Ask the child what he or she has taken, and collect a sample of the toxin or vomit, while waiting for the ambulance.

WARNING

SUDDEN LOSS OF VISION Call an ambulance if your child complains of a sudden loss of sight in one or both eyes. This is a serious symptom, which needs urgent medical assessment.

EMERGENCY! CALL AN AMBULANCE

POSSIBLE CAUSE AND ACTION Sudden loss of vision is always a serious symptom, even if it only lasts a few minutes or affects only one eye. Your child's eyes will need to be examined by a specialist. Your child may also be admitted to hospital for tests.

Is there a sticky, pus-like discharge, and is normal vision restored when the eye is cleaned? — YES / NO

CALL YOUR DOCTOR NOW

POSSIBLE CAUSE Iritis, inflammation of the coloured part of the eye, is possible.

ACTION Your doctor may refer your child to a specialist for an eye test and to look for associated disorders such as arthritis. If iritis is diagnosed, your child will need urgent treatment with corticosteroid eye drops or tablets to prevent permanent damage to his or her sight.

SEE YOUR DOCTOR WITHIN 24 HOURS

POSSIBLE CAUSE Blurred vision may be caused by a discharge due to conjunctivitis, which is a bacterial infection. Your child's vision should be completely normal once the discharge has been gently cleared away from the eyes (*see* COPING WITH CONJUNCTIVITIS, p.95).

ACTION Your doctor will probably prescribe antibiotic eye drops or ointment, which will need to be applied for several days.

Continued on next page, column 1

Continued on next page, column 2

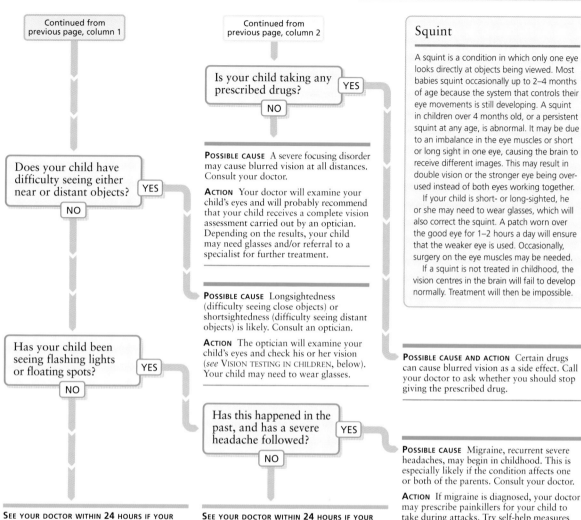

Continued from previous page, column 1

Continued from previous page, column 2

Is your child taking any prescribed drugs? — **YES**

NO

POSSIBLE CAUSE A severe focusing disorder may cause blurred vision at all distances. Consult your doctor.

ACTION Your doctor will examine your child's eyes and will probably recommend that your child receives a complete vision assessment carried out by an optician. Depending on the results, your child may need glasses and/or referral to a specialist for further treatment.

Does your child have difficulty seeing either near or distant objects? — **YES**

NO

POSSIBLE CAUSE Longsightedness (difficulty seeing close objects) or shortsightedness (difficulty seeing distant objects) is likely. Consult an optician.

ACTION The optician will examine your child's eyes and check his or her vision (*see* VISION TESTING IN CHILDREN, below). Your child may need to wear glasses.

Has your child been seeing flashing lights or floating spots? — **YES**

NO

Has this happened in the past, and has a severe headache followed? — **YES**

NO

Squint

A squint is a condition in which only one eye looks directly at objects being viewed. Most babies squint occasionally up to 2–4 months of age because the system that controls their eye movements is still developing. A squint in children over 4 months old, or a persistent squint at any age, is abnormal. It may be due to an imbalance in the eye muscles or short or long sight in one eye, causing the brain to receive different images. This may result in double vision or the stronger eye being over-used instead of both eyes working together.

If your child is short- or long-sighted, he or she may need to wear glasses, which will also correct the squint. A patch worn over the good eye for 1–2 hours a day will ensure that the weaker eye is used. Occasionally, surgery on the eye muscles may be needed.

If a squint is not treated in childhood, the vision centres in the brain will fail to develop normally. Treatment will then be impossible.

POSSIBLE CAUSE AND ACTION Certain drugs can cause blurred vision as a side effect. Call your doctor to ask whether you should stop giving the prescribed drug.

POSSIBLE CAUSE Migraine, recurrent severe headaches, may begin in childhood. This is especially likely if the condition affects one or both of the parents. Consult your doctor.

ACTION If migraine is diagnosed, your doctor may prescribe painkillers for your child to take during attacks. Try self-help measures for relieving a child's headache (p.84) and for reducing the frequency of migraine (p.155).

SEE YOUR DOCTOR WITHIN **24** HOURS IF YOUR CHILD HAS A VISION PROBLEM AND YOU ARE UNABLE TO MAKE A DIAGNOSIS FROM THIS CHART.

SEE YOUR DOCTOR WITHIN **24** HOURS IF YOUR CHILD HAS A VISION PROBLEM AND YOU ARE UNABLE TO MAKE A DIAGNOSIS FROM THIS CHART.

Vision testing in children

Simple vision tests are routinely carried out in babies as part of their developmental checks. Further tests may be recommended if a problem is suspected. Vision tests for babies and children vary depending on their age. In infants, eye drops are given to dilate the pupil. A beam of light is then shone into each eye in turn using an instrument called a retinoscope. The effect of different lenses on the beam of light determines whether vision is normal. Older children are often tested by being asked to identify letters on cards held at a distance. Each eye is tested separately.

At all ages, a vision test also includes careful examination of the retina, which is the light-sensitive membrane at the back of the eye.

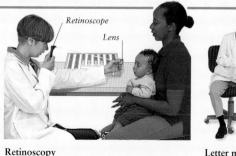

Retinoscope

Lens

Letter card held at a set distance

Patch worn over one eye

Retinoscopy
The test is performed in a darkened room. An instrument called a retinoscope is used to shine a beam of light through a lens into each of the child's eyes in turn.

Letter matching test
The tester points to a letter and asks the child to identify a matching letter.

29 Painful or irritated ear

For hearing problems in children, see chart 30, HEARING PROBLEMS (p.100).

Earache is common in children and can be very distressing. In most cases, earache is caused by an infection spreading from the back of the throat to the ear (*see* STRUCTURE OF THE EAR IN CHILDREN, opposite). Fortunately, such ear infections become less common as children grow up. A child who is not old enough to tell you that he or she has an earache may wake unexpectedly in the night and may cry inconsolably, shriek loudly, or pull at the affected ear.

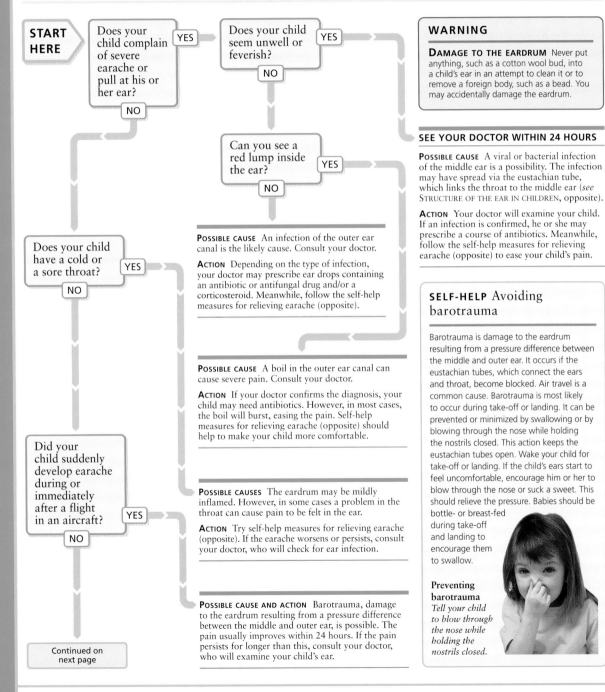

START HERE

Does your child complain of severe earache or pull at his or her ear? — YES → **Does your child seem unwell or feverish?** — YES →

NO → **Can you see a red lump inside the ear?** — YES →

NO

NO ↓

Does your child have a cold or a sore throat? — YES →

NO ↓

Did your child suddenly develop earache during or immediately after a flight in an aircraft? — YES →

NO ↓

Continued on next page

POSSIBLE CAUSE An infection of the outer ear canal is the likely cause. Consult your doctor.

ACTION Depending on the type of infection, your doctor may prescribe ear drops containing an antibiotic or antifungal drug and/or a corticosteroid. Meanwhile, follow the self-help measures for relieving earache (opposite).

POSSIBLE CAUSE A boil in the outer ear canal can cause severe pain. Consult your doctor.

ACTION If your doctor confirms the diagnosis, your child may need antibiotics. However, in most cases, the boil will burst, easing the pain. Self-help measures for relieving earache (opposite) should help to make your child more comfortable.

POSSIBLE CAUSES The eardrum may be mildly inflamed. However, in some cases a problem in the throat can cause pain to be felt in the ear.

ACTION Try self-help measures for relieving earache (opposite). If the earache worsens or persists, consult your doctor, who will check for ear infection.

POSSIBLE CAUSE AND ACTION Barotrauma, damage to the eardrum resulting from a pressure difference between the middle and outer ear, is possible. The pain usually improves within 24 hours. If the pain persists for longer than this, consult your doctor, who will examine your child's ear.

WARNING

DAMAGE TO THE EARDRUM Never put anything, such as a cotton wool bud, into a child's ear in an attempt to clean it or to remove a foreign body, such as a bead. You may accidentally damage the eardrum.

SEE YOUR DOCTOR WITHIN 24 HOURS

POSSIBLE CAUSE A viral or bacterial infection of the middle ear is a possibility. The infection may have spread via the eustachian tube, which links the throat to the middle ear (*see* STRUCTURE OF THE EAR IN CHILDREN, opposite).

ACTION Your doctor will examine your child. If an infection is confirmed, he or she may prescribe a course of antibiotics. Meanwhile, follow the self-help measures for relieving earache (opposite) to ease your child's pain.

SELF-HELP Avoiding barotrauma

Barotrauma is damage to the eardrum resulting from a pressure difference between the middle and outer ear. It occurs if the eustachian tubes, which connect the ears and throat, become blocked. Air travel is a common cause. Barotrauma is most likely to occur during take-off or landing. It can be prevented or minimized by swallowing or by blowing through the nose while holding the nostrils closed. This action keeps the eustachian tubes open. Wake your child for take-off or landing. If the child's ears start to feel uncomfortable, encourage him or her to blow through the nose or suck a sweet. This should relieve the pressure. Babies should be bottle- or breast-fed during take-off and landing to encourage them to swallow.

Preventing barotrauma
Tell your child to blow through the nose while holding the nostrils closed.

Continued from
previous page

Is there a
discharge from
the affected ear? **YES**

NO

Does your child
have itching
or irritation
inside the ear? **YES**

NO

**CONSULT YOUR DOCTOR IF YOU ARE UNABLE
TO MAKE A DIAGNOSIS FROM THIS CHART.**

Is the skin
around the
child's ear red
and inflamed? **YES**

NO

Structure of the ear in children

From the outside, children's ears look similar to those of adults. However, the eustachian tube, which connects the middle ear to the back of the throat, is shorter and more horizontal than in adults, allowing infections to reach the middle ear more easily. In addition, the adenoids (*see* TONSILS AND ADENOIDS, p.103), areas of lymphatic tissue that lie close to the back of the throat, tend to be larger in children; they can readily block the eustachian tubes, preventing drainage and increasing the risk of infection.

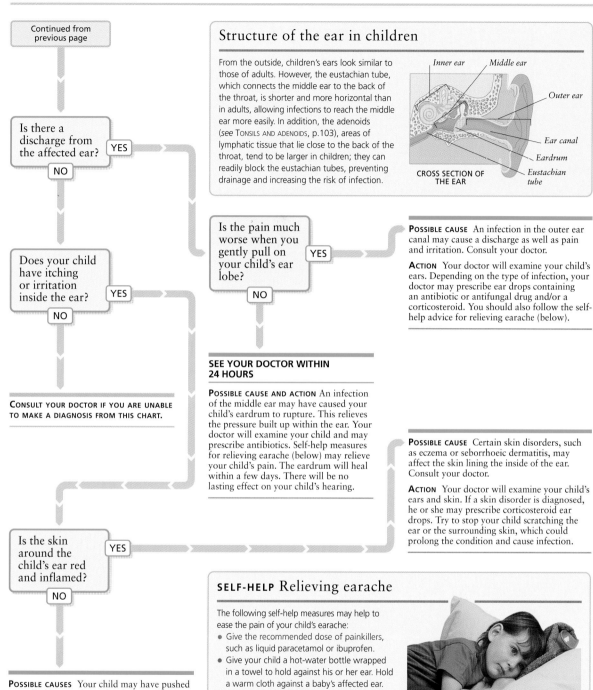

Inner ear   *Middle ear*

Outer ear

Ear canal

Eardrum

**CROSS SECTION OF
THE EAR**   *Eustachian
tube*

Is the pain much
worse when you
gently pull on
your child's ear
lobe? **YES**

NO

POSSIBLE CAUSE An infection in the outer ear canal may cause a discharge as well as pain and irritation. Consult your doctor.

ACTION Your doctor will examine your child's ears. Depending on the type of infection, your doctor may prescribe ear drops containing an antibiotic or antifungal drug and/or a corticosteroid. You should also follow the self-help advice for relieving earache (below).

**SEE YOUR DOCTOR WITHIN
24 HOURS**

POSSIBLE CAUSE AND ACTION An infection of the middle ear may have caused your child's eardrum to rupture. This relieves the pressure built up within the ear. Your doctor will examine your child and may prescribe antibiotics. Self-help measures for relieving earache (below) may relieve your child's pain. The eardrum will heal within a few days. There will be no lasting effect on your child's hearing.

POSSIBLE CAUSE Certain skin disorders, such as eczema or seborrhoeic dermatitis, may affect the skin lining the inside of the ear. Consult your doctor.

ACTION Your doctor will examine your child's ears and skin. If a skin disorder is diagnosed, he or she may prescribe corticosteroid ear drops. Try to stop your child scratching the ear or the surrounding skin, which could prolong the condition and cause infection.

SELF-HELP Relieving earache

The following self-help measures may help to ease the pain of your child's earache:
- Give the recommended dose of painkillers, such as liquid paracetamol or ibuprofen.
- Give your child a hot-water bottle wrapped in a towel to hold against his or her ear. Hold a warm cloth against a baby's affected ear.
- Encourage your child to sit or lie with his or her head raised on pillows (lying flat may worsen the pain). Resting with the affected ear facing downwards will allow any discharge to drain out.

Do not put ear drops or olive oil into your child's ear unless advised otherwise by your doctor. Do not put cotton wool in the ear – it could prevent a discharge from draining out.

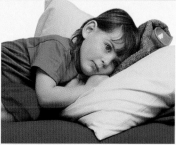

Easing earache
Resting the ear against a covered hot-water bottle with the head slightly raised may help to ease the pain of earache.

POSSIBLE CAUSES Your child may have pushed a small object, such as a bead or small piece of food, into his or her ear. Alternatively, an insect may have flown or crawled into the ear. Consult your doctor.

ACTION Your doctor will examine your child's ear. If there is an insect or any other foreign body in the ear canal, it may be possible for your doctor to wash it out. If the doctor cannot remove it, he or she will refer your child to hospital to have it removed.

30 Hearing problems

Hearing problems are often not noticed in a child. If your child always needs to have the television or radio on louder than you think necessary or there is a sudden deterioration in your child's school performance, a hearing problem may be the cause. Hearing problems in babies are often detected at routine developmental checks by your health visitor or doctor, but you may be the first to notice that your baby is not responding to sounds or learning to speak as quickly as you think he or she should. This should always be brought to your doctor's attention.

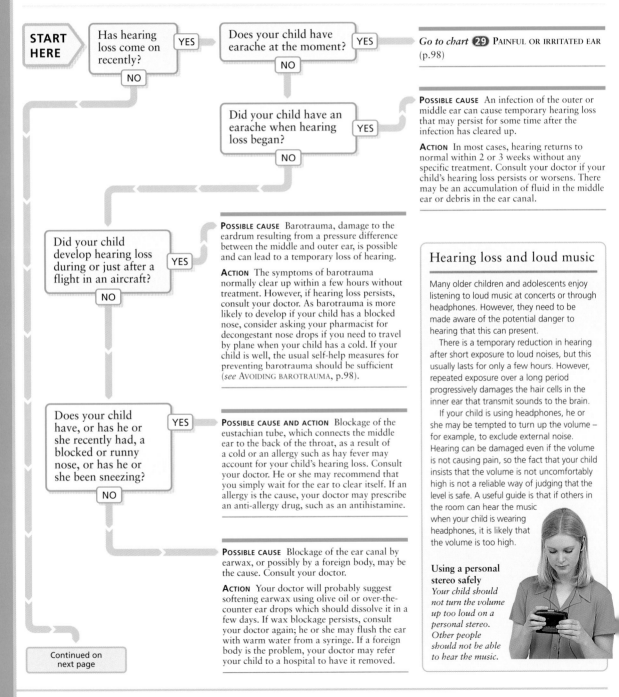

START HERE

Has hearing loss come on recently? — YES → **Does your child have earache at the moment?** — YES → *Go to chart* **29** **PAINFUL OR IRRITATED EAR** (p.98)

NO

NO

Did your child have an earache when hearing loss began? — YES →

POSSIBLE CAUSE An infection of the outer or middle ear can cause temporary hearing loss that may persist for some time after the infection has cleared up.

ACTION In most cases, hearing returns to normal within 2 or 3 weeks without any specific treatment. Consult your doctor if your child's hearing loss persists or worsens. There may be an accumulation of fluid in the middle ear or debris in the ear canal.

NO

Did your child develop hearing loss during or just after a flight in an aircraft? — YES →

POSSIBLE CAUSE Barotrauma, damage to the eardrum resulting from a pressure difference between the middle and outer ear, is possible and can lead to a temporary loss of hearing.

ACTION The symptoms of barotrauma normally clear up within a few hours without treatment. However, if hearing loss persists, consult your doctor. As barotrauma is more likely to develop if your child has a blocked nose, consider asking your pharmacist for decongestant nose drops if you need to travel by plane when your child has a cold. If your child is well, the usual self-help measures for preventing barotrauma should be sufficient (*see* AVOIDING BAROTRAUMA, p.98).

NO

Does your child have, or has he or she recently had, a blocked or runny nose, or has he or she been sneezing? — YES →

POSSIBLE CAUSE AND ACTION Blockage of the eustachian tube, which connects the middle ear to the back of the throat, as a result of a cold or an allergy such as hay fever may account for your child's hearing loss. Consult your doctor. He or she may recommend that you simply wait for the ear to clear itself. If an allergy is the cause, your doctor may prescribe an anti-allergy drug, such as an antihistamine.

NO

POSSIBLE CAUSE Blockage of the ear canal by earwax, or possibly by a foreign body, may be the cause. Consult your doctor.

ACTION Your doctor will probably suggest softening earwax using olive oil or over-the-counter ear drops which should dissolve it in a few days. If wax blockage persists, consult your doctor again; he or she may flush the ear with warm water from a syringe. If a foreign body is the problem, your doctor may refer your child to a hospital to have it removed.

Continued on next page

Hearing loss and loud music

Many older children and adolescents enjoy listening to loud music at concerts or through headphones. However, they need to be made aware of the potential danger to hearing that this can present.

There is a temporary reduction in hearing after short exposure to loud noises, but this usually lasts for only a few hours. However, repeated exposure over a long period progressively damages the hair cells in the inner ear that transmit sounds to the brain.

If your child is using headphones, he or she may be tempted to turn up the volume – for example, to exclude external noise. Hearing can be damaged even if the volume is not causing pain, so the fact that your child insists that the volume is not uncomfortably high is not a reliable way of judging that the level is safe. A useful guide is that if others in the room can hear the music when your child is wearing headphones, it is likely that the volume is too high.

Using a personal stereo safely
Your child should not turn the volume up too loud on a personal stereo. Other people should not be able to hear the music.

Continued from previous page

Do any of the following apply to your child?
- Suffers from recurrent ear infections
- Has a persistently runny or blocked nose
- Snores

YES →

POSSIBLE CAUSES Your child may have glue ear (chronic secretory otitis media), in which fluid builds up in the middle ear, causing hearing problems. This condition may be due to an allergy or to persistently enlarged adenoids blocking the eustachian tube, which connects the middle ear and the back of the throat (see STRUCTURE OF THE EAR IN CHILDREN, p.99).

ACTION Your doctor will probably arrange for hearing tests, including tympanometry (see HEARING TESTS IN CHILDHOOD, below), to confirm the diagnosis. He or she may suggest anti allergy drugs such as antihistamines. If the fluid persists, your doctor may recommend surgical removal of the adenoids and/or the insertion of a tiny tube through the eardrum to drain the fluid (see TREATING GLUE EAR, right). In most cases, normal hearing is restored.

NO ↓

During pregnancy, did you come into contact with someone who had rubella or did you have a fever with a rash?

YES →

NO ↓

Are you worried that your child has never been able to hear properly?

YES →

POSSIBLE CAUSE Your child may have an inherited hearing problem, possibly due to abnormal development of the inner ear or the nerve that transmits sounds to the brain. This type of hearing problem is most likely if there is a family history of such abnormalities. Consult your doctor.

ACTION Your doctor will probably arrange for your child to have hearing tests (below). If your child is found to have a problem with hearing, he or she will need additional help with language development at school and at home.

NO ↓

CONSULT YOUR DOCTOR IF YOU ARE UNABLE TO MAKE A DIAGNOSIS FROM THIS CHART.

Treating glue ear

In the disorder glue ear (chronic secretory otitis media), fluid builds up in the middle ear, resulting in reduced hearing. The condition may be treated surgically by inserting a tiny plastic tube, called a grommet, through the eardrum. The grommet allows air into the middle ear and lets fluid drain away. The grommet is left in place and usually falls out after 6–12 months. The eardrum then heals. Although grommets relieve hearing problems caused by fluid build-up, they do not prevent future ear infections. The operation to insert a grommet is usually performed under general anaesthesia as day surgery and rarely needs to be repeated.

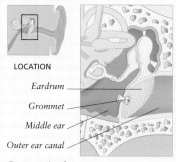

LOCATION

Eardrum
Grommet
Middle ear
Outer ear canal

Grommet in place
The grommet inserted into the eardrum provides a channel between the middle and outer ear, allowing air to circulate normally in the ear, which improves hearing.

POSSIBLE CAUSE Exposure of the unborn child to rubella and certain other infections can damage hearing. Consult your doctor.

ACTION Your doctor will arrange for your child to have hearing tests (below) and may refer him or her to a specialist for assessment.

Hearing tests in childhood

Tests to assess hearing are performed throughout childhood as part of routine developmental screening; the type of test depends on the age of the child. Newborn babies can be assessed using tests such as otoacoustic emission, in which a sound is played into the ear and an ear piece measures the resulting echo from the inner ear. Speech discrimination tests can be used to detect hearing loss in young children who have a simple vocabulary. For example, in the McCormick toy discrimination test, the child is shown various toys and is asked to identify pairs of toys that have similar sounding names, such as tree and key. Tympanometry (p.186) is a test that is also used for adults. It measures movement of the eardrum in response to sound and is useful in detecting a build-up of fluid in the middle ear. By age 4, most children are able to cooperate with a simple form of audiometry (p.186), which measures how loud sounds of various frequencies need to be for the child to hear them.

The McCormick test
The doctor prevents the child from lip-reading by covering his or her mouth and then asks the child to identify various toys.

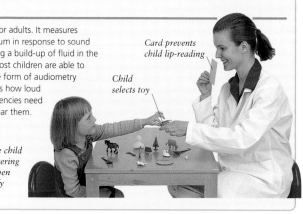

Card prevents child lip-reading

Child selects toy

31 Runny or blocked nose

A runny nose can be irritating for a child, and a blocked nose can be distressing for a baby because it makes feeding difficult, but neither symptom on its own is likely to be a sign of serious disease. All children have a runny or blocked nose from time to time (often accompanied by sneezing), and, in most cases, a common cold is responsible. If your child gets a nosebleed from picking or blowing a blocked nose, follow the treatment advice for nosebleeds (p.190).

START HERE

Has your child had a runny or blocked nose for more than 1 month?
YES →

POSSIBLE CAUSE Your child may have enlarged adenoids (*see* TONSILS AND ADENOIDS, p.103). This is common in children and is often the result of an infection or allergies. Consult your doctor.

ACTION Your doctor will examine your child and may arrange for hearing tests as enlarged adenoids can cause hearing difficulties. The adenoids shrink as a child grows and are rarely a problem after the age of 8. In some cases, anti-allergy drugs may help. If the symptoms are severe, your doctor may refer your child to a specialist to see whether it is necessary to remove the adenoids.

POSSIBLE CAUSE Seasonal allergic rhinitis (hay fever) is a possibility. This condition is caused by an allergy to pollen and usually occurs in the spring or the summer.

ACTION If possible, keep your child inside when the pollen count is high, and keep him or her away from areas of long grass. Oral antihistamine drugs may help and are available over the counter. If these measures do not help, consult your doctor.

NO

Does your child have a clear, watery discharge from both nostrils?
YES →

Are your child's eyes itchy?
YES →

NO

Does your child have a green or yellow discharge from the nose?
YES →

NO

POSSIBLE CAUSE A common cold or other viral infection is probably the cause.

ACTION Follow the self-help measures for treating a child with a cold (right). If your child has a fever, take steps to reduce it (*see* BRINGING DOWN A FEVER, p.73). Your child's symptoms should begin to improve after a few days. If they do not or if your child develops other symptoms, consult your doctor.

CONSULT YOUR DOCTOR IF YOU ARE UNABLE TO MAKE A DIAGNOSIS FROM THIS CHART.

Is the discharge from one nostril only?
YES →

NO

POSSIBLE CAUSE A foreign body, such as a bead or a peanut, may be lodged in your child's nose and may have caused an infection. Consult your doctor.

ACTION Never try to remove a foreign body from your child's nose yourself, because you may only force it further into the nose. Your doctor may be able to remove the obstruction. However, if the foreign body is difficult to reach, your child may need to be admitted to hospital for a minor operation under general anaesthetic to remove it. The infection should then clear up by itself, but in some cases antibiotics are needed to treat it.

POSSIBLE CAUSE A common cold or other viral infection is probably the cause.

ACTION Follow the self-help measures for treating a child with a cold (right). If your child has a fever, take steps to reduce it (*see* BRINGING DOWN A FEVER, p.73). Your child's symptoms should begin to improve after a few days. If they do not or if your child develops other symptoms, consult your doctor.

SELF-HELP Treating a child with a cold

Children often have 4–6 colds a year until their bodies start to build up immunity to the numerous viruses that can cause a cold. Infections are particularly common after a child joins a playgroup or school. The following measures may help:
- Encourage your child to drink fluids.
- Give liquid paracetamol.
- Keep the air in your child's room moist by placing wet towels near a radiator or by using a humidifier.
- Try to teach your child to blow his or her nose one nostril at a time.
- Apply a barrier cream, such as petroleum jelly, around your child's nose and upper lip to prevent soreness.
- If your baby has difficulty feeding because of a blocked nose, try giving him or her the recommended dose of children's nose drops before a feed.

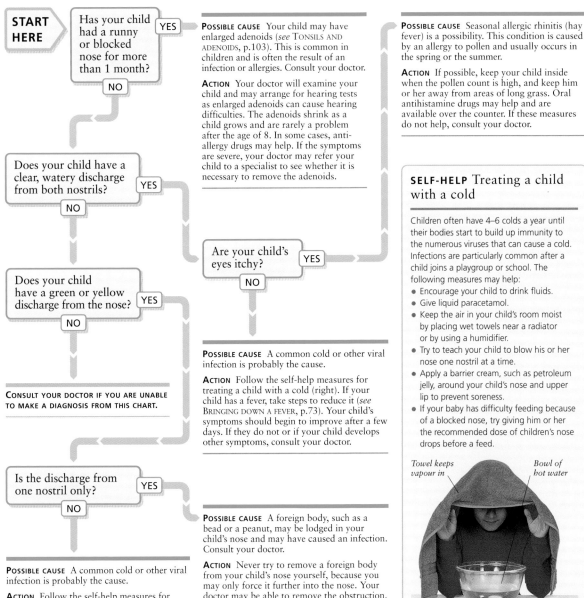

Towel keeps vapour in *Bowl of hot water*

Relieving congestion
Inhaling steam from a bowl of hot, but not boiling, water can help clear a blocked nose. Children should always be supervised.

32 Sore throat

Sore throats are common in childhood. An older child will usually tell you if his or her throat hurts. In a baby or a young child, the first sign you may have that something is wrong may be a reluctance to eat because of the pain caused by swallowing. Most sore throats are the result of minor viral infections that clear up within 2–3 days without the need for medical treatment. In a few cases, however, antibiotics may be needed to treat a bacterial infection.

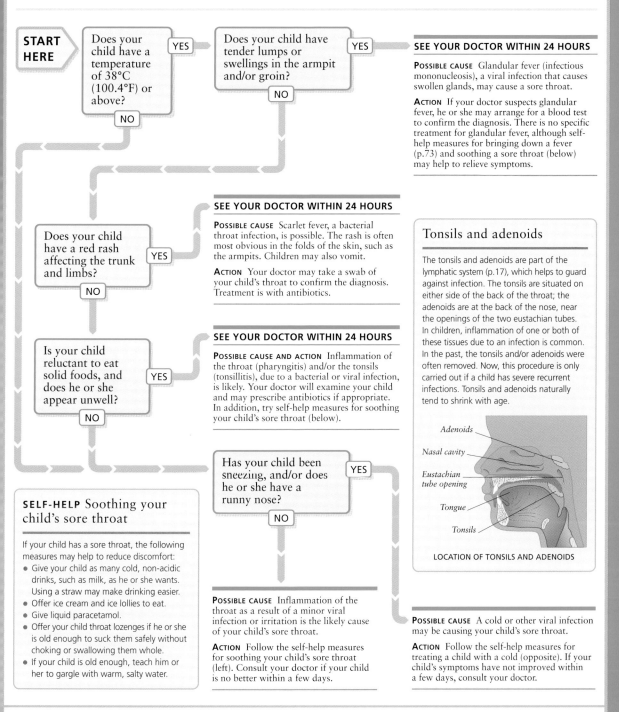

START HERE

Does your child have a temperature of 38°C (100.4°F) or above? → **YES**

NO

Does your child have tender lumps or swellings in the armpit and/or groin? → **YES**

NO

SEE YOUR DOCTOR WITHIN 24 HOURS

POSSIBLE CAUSE Glandular fever (infectious mononucleosis), a viral infection that causes swollen glands, may cause a sore throat.

ACTION If your doctor suspects glandular fever, he or she may arrange for a blood test to confirm the diagnosis. There is no specific treatment for glandular fever, although self-help measures for bringing down a fever (p.73) and soothing a sore throat (below) may help to relieve symptoms.

Does your child have a red rash affecting the trunk and limbs? → **YES**

NO

SEE YOUR DOCTOR WITHIN 24 HOURS

POSSIBLE CAUSE Scarlet fever, a bacterial throat infection, is possible. The rash is often most obvious in the folds of the skin, such as the armpits. Children may also vomit.

ACTION Your doctor may take a swab of your child's throat to confirm the diagnosis. Treatment is with antibiotics.

Is your child reluctant to eat solid foods, and does he or she appear unwell? → **YES**

NO

SEE YOUR DOCTOR WITHIN 24 HOURS

POSSIBLE CAUSE AND ACTION Inflammation of the throat (pharyngitis) and/or the tonsils (tonsillitis), due to a bacterial or viral infection, is likely. Your doctor will examine your child and may prescribe antibiotics if appropriate. In addition, try self-help measures for soothing your child's sore throat (below).

Has your child been sneezing, and/or does he or she have a runny nose? → **YES**

NO

Tonsils and adenoids

The tonsils and adenoids are part of the lymphatic system (p.17), which helps to guard against infection. The tonsils are situated on either side of the back of the throat; the adenoids are at the back of the nose, near the openings of the two eustachian tubes. In children, inflammation of one or both of these tissues due to an infection is common. In the past, the tonsils and/or adenoids were often removed. Now, this procedure is only carried out if a child has severe recurrent infections. Tonsils and adenoids naturally tend to shrink with age.

Adenoids

Nasal cavity

Eustachian tube opening

Tongue

Tonsils

LOCATION OF TONSILS AND ADENOIDS

SELF-HELP Soothing your child's sore throat

If your child has a sore throat, the following measures may help to reduce discomfort:
- Give your child as many cold, non-acidic drinks, such as milk, as he or she wants. Using a straw may make drinking easier.
- Offer ice cream and ice lollies to eat.
- Give liquid paracetamol.
- Offer your child throat lozenges if he or she is old enough to suck them safely without choking or swallowing them whole.
- If your child is old enough, teach him or her to gargle with warm, salty water.

POSSIBLE CAUSE Inflammation of the throat as a result of a minor viral infection or irritation is the likely cause of your child's sore throat.

ACTION Follow the self-help measures for soothing your child's sore throat (left). Consult your doctor if your child is no better within a few days.

POSSIBLE CAUSE A cold or other viral infection may be causing your child's sore throat.

ACTION Follow the self-help measures for treating a child with a cold (opposite). If your child's symptoms have not improved within a few days, consult your doctor.

33 Coughing

Coughing is a normal protective reaction to irritation of the throat or lungs. In babies under 6 months, coughs are unusual and can be a sign of a serious lung infection if the child is also unwell. In older children, the vast majority of coughs are due to minor infections of the throat or upper airways, such as colds. A runny nose can cause a cough, particularly at night as fluid drips down the back of the throat and causes irritation. A cough at night, even if it is not accompanied by wheezing, can be a symptom of asthma, and you should consult your doctor if you are concerned.

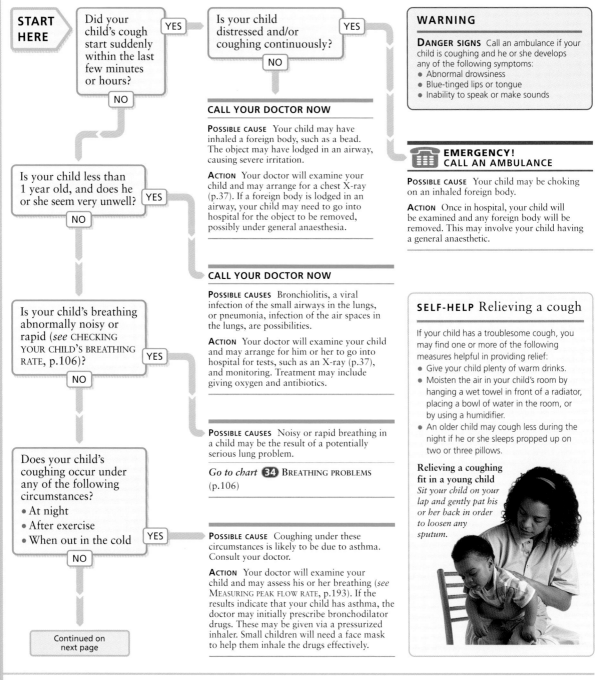

START HERE

Did your child's cough start suddenly within the last few minutes or hours? **YES** → Is your child distressed and/or coughing continuously? **YES** →

NO ↓ / **NO** ↓

CALL YOUR DOCTOR NOW

POSSIBLE CAUSE Your child may have inhaled a foreign body, such as a bead. The object may have lodged in an airway, causing severe irritation.

ACTION Your doctor will examine your child and may arrange for a chest X-ray (p.37). If a foreign body is lodged in an airway, your child may need to go into hospital for the object to be removed, possibly under general anaesthesia.

Is your child less than 1 year old, and does he or she seem very unwell? **YES** →

NO ↓

CALL YOUR DOCTOR NOW

POSSIBLE CAUSES Bronchiolitis, a viral infection of the small airways in the lungs, or pneumonia, infection of the air spaces in the lungs, are possibilities.

ACTION Your doctor will examine your child and may arrange for him or her to go into hospital for tests, such as an X-ray (p.37), and monitoring. Treatment may include giving oxygen and antibiotics.

Is your child's breathing abnormally noisy or rapid (*see* CHECKING YOUR CHILD'S BREATHING RATE, p.106)? **YES** →

NO ↓

POSSIBLE CAUSES Noisy or rapid breathing in a child may be the result of a potentially serious lung problem.

***Go to chart* 34** BREATHING PROBLEMS (p.106)

Does your child's coughing occur under any of the following circumstances?
- At night
- After exercise
- When out in the cold

YES →

NO ↓

POSSIBLE CAUSE Coughing under these circumstances is likely to be due to asthma. Consult your doctor.

ACTION Your doctor will examine your child and may assess his or her breathing (*see* MEASURING PEAK FLOW RATE, p.193). If the results indicate that your child has asthma, the doctor may initially prescribe bronchodilator drugs. These may be given via a pressurized inhaler. Small children will need a face mask to help them inhale the drugs effectively.

Continued on next page

WARNING

DANGER SIGNS Call an ambulance if your child is coughing and he or she develops any of the following symptoms:
- Abnormal drowsiness
- Blue-tinged lips or tongue
- Inability to speak or make sounds

EMERGENCY! CALL AN AMBULANCE

POSSIBLE CAUSE Your child may be choking on an inhaled foreign body.

ACTION Once in hospital, your child will be examined and any foreign body will be removed. This may involve your child having a general anaesthetic.

SELF-HELP Relieving a cough

If your child has a troublesome cough, you may find one or more of the following measures helpful in providing relief:
- Give your child plenty of warm drinks.
- Moisten the air in your child's room by hanging a wet towel in front of a radiator, placing a bowl of water in the room, or by using a humidifier.
- An older child may cough less during the night if he or she sleeps propped up on two or three pillows.

Relieving a coughing fit in a young child
Sit your child on your lap and gently pat his or her back in order to loosen any sputum.

Continued from previous page

Has your child been immunized against whooping cough? **YES**

NO

POSSIBLE CAUSE Even though your child has been immunized, a mild attack of whooping cough (pertussis), an infectious disease that causes bouts of coughing, may be the cause. The infection is much less serious in children who have been immunized than in those who have not. Consult your doctor.

ACTION Your doctor will probably prescribe antibiotics for your child to reduce the chance of him or her passing the infection on to others. Coughing may persist for several weeks, but symptoms are rarely severe enough for the child to need hospital admission.

Does your child have bouts of uncontrollable coughing followed by a noisy intake of breath, and/or is coughing often accompanied by vomiting? **YES**

NO

SEE YOUR DOCTOR WITHIN 24 HOURS

POSSIBLE CAUSE Your child may have whooping cough (pertussis), an infectious disease that causes bouts of severe, uncontrollable coughing.

ACTION Your doctor will probably prescribe antibiotics to reduce the chance of your child passing the infection on to others. If the condition is severe, your doctor may send your child to hospital for treatment. Episodes of coughing may persist for several months. Severe cases of whooping cough, which are more likely in children aged under 1 year, may result in permanent damage to the lungs.

POSSIBLE CAUSES Your child may have enlarged tonsils or adenoids (p.103), which can block the airway. Consult your doctor.

ACTION Your doctor will examine your child and may arrange for hearing tests (p.101) or refer your child to a specialist. In some cases, removal of the tonsils and/or adenoids is advised, although symptoms often improve as the child grows up. Adenoids rarely cause a problem in children over 8 years.

Does your child always have a runny nose? **YES**

NO

Does your child have any of the following? **YES**
- Frequent ear infections
- Nasal speech
- Snoring
- Poor hearing

NO

POSSIBLE CAUSE Perennial allergic rhinitis may be the cause. In this condition, an allergic reaction to substances such as house dust, animal fur, or mould spores causes symptoms all year round.

ACTION If you think you know the trigger for your child's allergy, try to limit his or her contact with it. Antihistamines, which are available over the counter, may provide relief. If these do not help, consult your doctor, who may prescribe alternative drug treatment.

Does your child have a temperature of 38°C (100.4°F) or above and/or a runny nose? **YES**

NO

POSSIBLE CAUSES A common cold or other viral infection is a possibility. However, if a rash also develops, your child may have measles. This is especially likely if he or she has not been vaccinated against measles.

ACTION Take steps to lower your child's temperature (see BRINGING DOWN A FEVER, p.73), and follow the self-help measures for treating a child with a cold (p.102) and relieving a cough (opposite). If your child develops a rash or is no better within 2 days, consult your doctor.

Does anyone in the home smoke, or could your child have been smoking? **YES**

NO

POSSIBLE CAUSE AND ACTION A smoky atmosphere and smoking itself will irritate a child's throat and lungs, causing a persistent cough. If your child has begun to smoke, you should persuade him or her to stop. The longer he or she smokes, the more difficult it will be to give up. If family members continue to smoke, they should avoid smoking in the home.

CONSULT YOUR DOCTOR IF YOU ARE UNABLE TO MAKE A DIAGNOSIS FROM THIS CHART.

34 Breathing problems

Breathing problems in children include excessively noisy or fast breathing and shortness of breath. Although rapid or noisy breathing is usually obvious, shortness of breath may be less noticeable because a child may simply avoid activities that make him or her breathless. Any child who starts to wheeze needs to be seen by a doctor, and a child with severe difficulty in breathing needs urgent attention. Breathing problems that occur suddenly also need immediate attention.

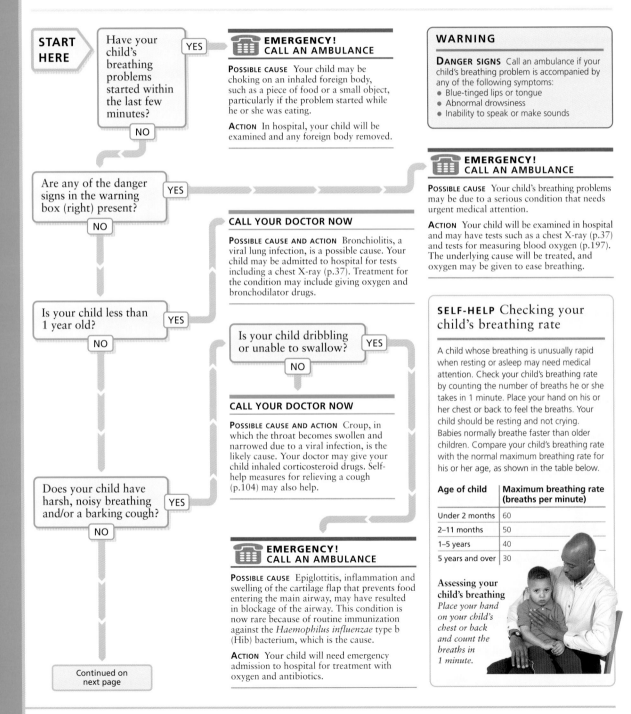

START HERE

Have your child's breathing problems started within the last few minutes?

YES →

📞 **EMERGENCY! CALL AN AMBULANCE**

POSSIBLE CAUSE Your child may be choking on an inhaled foreign body, such as a piece of food or a small object, particularly if the problem started while he or she was eating.

ACTION In hospital, your child will be examined and any foreign body removed.

NO

WARNING

DANGER SIGNS Call an ambulance if your child's breathing problem is accompanied by any of the following symptoms:
● Blue-tinged lips or tongue
● Abnormal drowsiness
● Inability to speak or make sounds

Are any of the danger signs in the warning box (right) present?

YES →

📞 **EMERGENCY! CALL AN AMBULANCE**

POSSIBLE CAUSE Your child's breathing problems may be due to a serious condition that needs urgent medical attention.

ACTION Your child will be examined in hospital and may have tests such as a chest X-ray (p.37) and tests for measuring blood oxygen (p.197). The underlying cause will be treated, and oxygen may be given to ease breathing.

NO

CALL YOUR DOCTOR NOW

POSSIBLE CAUSE AND ACTION Bronchiolitis, a viral lung infection, is a possible cause. Your child may be admitted to hospital for tests including a chest X-ray (p.37). Treatment for the condition may include giving oxygen and bronchodilator drugs.

Is your child less than 1 year old?

YES →

Is your child dribbling or unable to swallow?

YES →

NO

NO

CALL YOUR DOCTOR NOW

POSSIBLE CAUSE AND ACTION Croup, in which the throat becomes swollen and narrowed due to a viral infection, is the likely cause. Your doctor may give your child inhaled corticosteroid drugs. Self-help measures for relieving a cough (p.104) may also help.

Does your child have harsh, noisy breathing and/or a barking cough?

YES →

NO

📞 **EMERGENCY! CALL AN AMBULANCE**

POSSIBLE CAUSE Epiglottitis, inflammation and swelling of the cartilage flap that prevents food entering the main airway, may have resulted in blockage of the airway. This condition is now rare because of routine immunization against the *Haemophilus influenzae* type b (Hib) bacterium, which is the cause.

ACTION Your child will need emergency admission to hospital for treatment with oxygen and antibiotics.

SELF-HELP Checking your child's breathing rate

A child whose breathing is unusually rapid when resting or asleep may need medical attention. Check your child's breathing rate by counting the number of breaths he or she takes in 1 minute. Place your hand on his or her chest or back to feel the breaths. Your child should be resting and not crying. Babies normally breathe faster than older children. Compare your child's breathing rate with the normal maximum breathing rate for his or her age, as shown in the table below.

Age of child	Maximum breathing rate (breaths per minute)
Under 2 months	60
2–11 months	50
1–5 years	40
5 years and over	30

Assessing your child's breathing
Place your hand on your child's chest or back and count the breaths in 1 minute.

Continued on next page

SELF-HELP Easing breathing in an asthma attack

If your child is having severe difficulty in breathing, call an ambulance. While waiting for help to arrive, you should:
- Help your child to sit upright, leaning forwards slightly, with his or her forearms supported on a table or the back of a chair.
- Make sure any prescribed reliever drugs for asthma have been taken according to the treatment plan.
- Try to stay calm and keep your child calm. Do not leave him or her alone. Try to keep other people from crowding around your child, to prevent him or her from becoming more anxious.

Easing breathing
Sit your child upright with his or her arms supported. Do not leave your child alone.

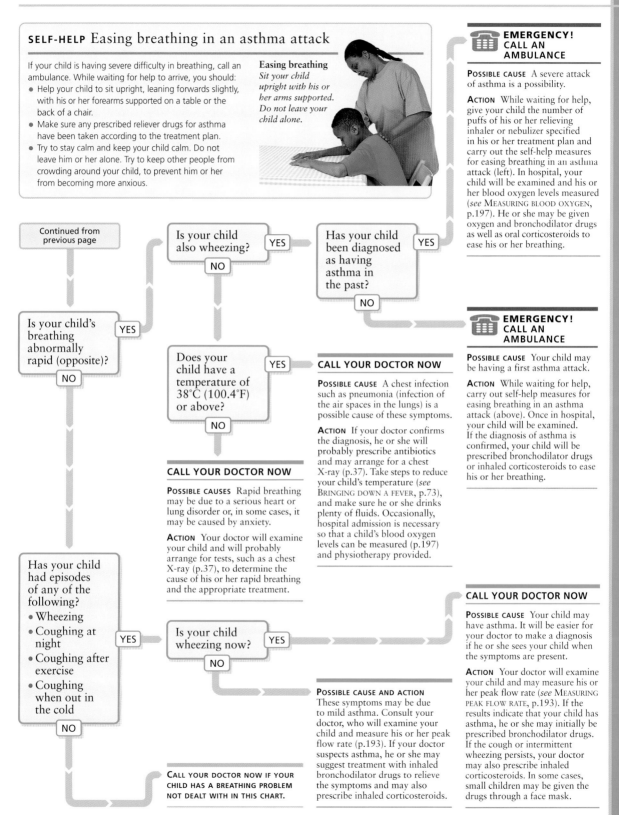

EMERGENCY! CALL AN AMBULANCE

POSSIBLE CAUSE A severe attack of asthma is a possibility.

ACTION While waiting for help, give your child the number of puffs of his or her relieving inhaler or nebulizer specified in his or her treatment plan and carry out the self-help measures for easing breathing in an asthma attack (left). In hospital, your child will be examined and his or her blood oxygen levels measured (*see* MEASURING BLOOD OXYGEN, p.197). He or she may be given oxygen and bronchodilator drugs as well as oral corticosteroids to ease his or her breathing.

Continued from previous page

Is your child also wheezing? — YES → **Has your child been diagnosed as having asthma in the past?** — YES →

NO

Is your child's breathing abnormally rapid (opposite)? — YES →

NO

Does your child have a temperature of 38°C (100.4°F) or above? — YES →

NO

NO

EMERGENCY! CALL AN AMBULANCE

POSSIBLE CAUSE Your child may be having a first asthma attack.

ACTION While waiting for help, carry out self-help measures for easing breathing in an asthma attack (above). Once in hospital, your child will be examined. If the diagnosis of asthma is confirmed, your child will be prescribed bronchodilator drugs or inhaled corticosteroids to ease his or her breathing.

CALL YOUR DOCTOR NOW

POSSIBLE CAUSE A chest infection such as pneumonia (infection of the air spaces in the lungs) is a possible cause of these symptoms.

ACTION If your doctor confirms the diagnosis, he or she will probably prescribe antibiotics and may arrange for a chest X-ray (p.37). Take steps to reduce your child's temperature (*see* BRINGING DOWN A FEVER, p.73), and make sure he or she drinks plenty of fluids. Occasionally, hospital admission is necessary so that a child's blood oxygen levels can be measured (p.197) and physiotherapy provided.

CALL YOUR DOCTOR NOW

POSSIBLE CAUSES Rapid breathing may be due to a serious heart or lung disorder or, in some cases, it may be caused by anxiety.

ACTION Your doctor will examine your child and will probably arrange for tests, such as a chest X-ray (p.37), to determine the cause of his or her rapid breathing and the appropriate treatment.

Has your child had episodes of any of the following?
- Wheezing
- Coughing at night
- Coughing after exercise
- Coughing when out in the cold

YES → **Is your child wheezing now?** — YES →

NO

NO

CALL YOUR DOCTOR NOW

POSSIBLE CAUSE Your child may have asthma. It will be easier for your doctor to make a diagnosis if he or she sees your child when the symptoms are present.

ACTION Your doctor will examine your child and may measure his or her peak flow rate (*see* MEASURING PEAK FLOW RATE, p.193). If the results indicate that your child has asthma, he or she may initially be prescribed bronchodilator drugs. If the cough or intermittent wheezing persists, your doctor may also prescribe inhaled corticosteroids. In some cases, small children may be given the drugs through a face mask.

POSSIBLE CAUSE AND ACTION These symptoms may be due to mild asthma. Consult your doctor, who will examine your child and measure his or her peak flow rate (p.193). If your doctor suspects asthma, he or she may suggest treatment with inhaled bronchodilator drugs to relieve the symptoms and may also prescribe inhaled corticosteroids.

CALL YOUR DOCTOR NOW IF YOUR CHILD HAS A BREATHING PROBLEM NOT DEALT WITH IN THIS CHART.

35 Mouth problems

For problems specifically relating to the teeth, see chart 36,
TEETH PROBLEMS (p.110).
Consult this chart if your child complains of a painful mouth
or has sores in the mouth or on the tongue or lips. Because
the lining of the mouth and the skin of the lips are thin
and delicate, these areas are susceptible to minor injuries
and infections. Younger children often pick up infections
affecting the mouth and lips because they tend to put objects
into their mouths. Allergies can cause swelling of the mouth
or tongue, which can be serious (*see* WARNING, below).

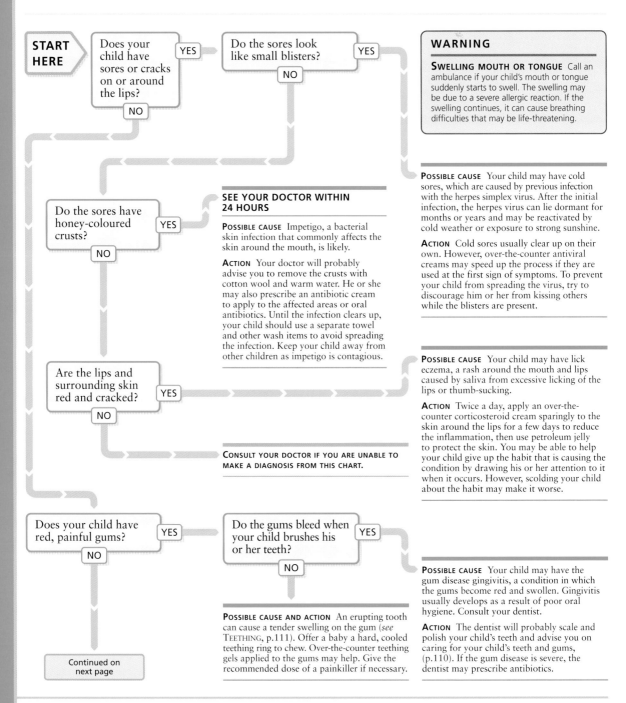

START HERE

Does your child have sores or cracks on or around the lips? — YES → **Do the sores look like small blisters?** — YES →

NO

NO

WARNING

SWELLING MOUTH OR TONGUE Call an ambulance if your child's mouth or tongue suddenly starts to swell. The swelling may be due to a severe allergic reaction. If the swelling continues, it can cause breathing difficulties that may be life-threatening.

POSSIBLE CAUSE Your child may have cold sores, which are caused by previous infection with the herpes simplex virus. After the initial infection, the herpes virus can lie dormant for months or years and may be reactivated by cold weather or exposure to strong sunshine.

ACTION Cold sores usually clear up on their own. However, over-the-counter antiviral creams may speed up the process if they are used at the first sign of symptoms. To prevent your child from spreading the virus, try to discourage him or her from kissing others while the blisters are present.

Do the sores have honey-coloured crusts? — YES →

NO

SEE YOUR DOCTOR WITHIN 24 HOURS

POSSIBLE CAUSE Impetigo, a bacterial skin infection that commonly affects the skin around the mouth, is likely.

ACTION Your doctor will probably advise you to remove the crusts with cotton wool and warm water. He or she may also prescribe an antibiotic cream to apply to the affected areas or oral antibiotics. Until the infection clears up, your child should use a separate towel and other wash items to avoid spreading the infection. Keep your child away from other children as impetigo is contagious.

Are the lips and surrounding skin red and cracked? — YES →

NO

POSSIBLE CAUSE Your child may have lick eczema, a rash around the mouth and lips caused by saliva from excessive licking of the lips or thumb-sucking.

ACTION Twice a day, apply an over-the-counter corticosteroid cream sparingly to the skin around the lips for a few days to reduce the inflammation, then use petroleum jelly to protect the skin. You may be able to help your child give up the habit that is causing the condition by drawing his or her attention to it when it occurs. However, scolding your child about the habit may make it worse.

CONSULT YOUR DOCTOR IF YOU ARE UNABLE TO MAKE A DIAGNOSIS FROM THIS CHART.

Does your child have red, painful gums? — YES → **Do the gums bleed when your child brushes his or her teeth?** — YES →

NO

NO

POSSIBLE CAUSE AND ACTION An erupting tooth can cause a tender swelling on the gum (*see* TEETHING, p.111). Offer a baby a hard, cooled teething ring to chew. Over-the-counter teething gels applied to the gums may help. Give the recommended dose of a painkiller if necessary.

POSSIBLE CAUSE Your child may have the gum disease gingivitis, a condition in which the gums become red and swollen. Gingivitis usually develops as a result of poor oral hygiene. Consult your dentist.

ACTION The dentist will probably scale and polish your child's teeth and advise you on caring for your child's teeth and gums, (p.110). If the gum disease is severe, the dentist may prescribe antibiotics.

Continued on next page

Continued from previous page

Does your child have creamy yellow or white patches inside the mouth and/or on the tongue? — **YES** →

Does your child also have blisters on the palms of the hands and the soles of the feet? — **YES** →

NO

SEE YOUR DOCTOR WITHIN 24 HOURS

POSSIBLE CAUSE Oral thrush, a fungal infection, is a possibility. This condition is most common in young babies or in older children whose immunity has been lowered by certain diseases or drug treatments.

ACTION Your doctor will probably prescribe antifungal gel or lozenges to clear up the infection. To prevent reinfection, sterilize any dummies, bottle teats, and teething rings that your child uses.

NO

POSSIBLE CAUSE Your child may have hand, foot, and mouth disease, a mild infection caused by a virus. The blisters on the hands and feet often appear about 48 hours after the ones in the mouth. Consult your doctor.

ACTION There is no specific treatment for this condition. If the blisters burst and form ulcers, encourage your child to rinse his or her mouth with a solution of bicarbonate of soda. Give your child the recommended dose of a painkiller if necessary (*see* RELIEVING A SORE MOUTH, below). Make sure your child drinks plenty of fluids (*see* ENCOURAGING YOUR CHILD TO DRINK, p.63).

Does your child have one or more shallow, grey, ulcerated patches or blisters in the mouth? — **YES** →

Does your child have a fever and/or seem generally unwell? — **YES** →

NO

NO

POSSIBLE CAUSE Your child may have mouth ulcers. These often develop for no apparent reason but tend to recur in times of stress or at the site of a minor injury, such as damage from a toothbrush. Mouth ulcers can be painful but are not serious.

ACTION Rinsing the mouth with a solution of bicarbonate of soda may help relieve the pain (*see* RELIEVING A SORE MOUTH, below). Over-the-counter treatments can also relieve pain and may help the ulcers to heal. If an ulcer does not heal within 10 days or your child has several ulcers at the same time, consult your doctor.

SEE YOUR DOCTOR WITHIN 24 HOURS

POSSIBLE CAUSES The most likely cause is infection with the herpes simplex virus, the virus that causes cold sores. When babies or young children have a first infection with this virus they may be unwell and have a very sore mouth. Similar symptoms can be due to other viruses or, in some cases, to prescription drugs.

ACTION If the child's mouth is so sore that he or she is unable to drink, your doctor may recommend hospital admission. In less severe cases, your doctor will recommend self-help measures (*see* RELIEVING A SORE MOUTH, below). If prescription drugs are thought to be the cause they will be stopped.

Does your child have a sore area inside a cheek or on the side of the tongue? — **YES** →

NO

CONSULT YOUR DOCTOR IF YOU ARE UNABLE TO MAKE A DIAGNOSIS FROM THIS CHART.

POSSIBLE CAUSE AND ACTION A new or jagged tooth may cause enough friction to make your child's cheek or tongue sore. Take steps to relieve the pain (*see* RELIEVING A SORE MOUTH, right). If the sore persists or appears to be cause by a jagged tooth, consult your dentist, who may be able to smooth a rough edge.

SELF-HELP Relieving a sore mouth

The following self-help measures may help to relieve the pain of a sore mouth:
- If necessary, give your child the appropriate dose of a painkiller, such as paracetamol.
- If your child is old enough to cooperate, he or she should rinse the mouth hourly with ¼ teaspoon of bicarbonate of soda dissolved in 100 ml (3½ fl.oz) of warm water.
- Offer soft foods, such as ice cream.
- Serve drinks with drinking straws to keep liquids away from sores on the lips.
- Avoid giving acidic foods and drinks, such as oranges or fruit juices.
- Try to continue brushing your child's teeth twice daily, but take care near the sore areas.

Easy-to-eat foods
Soft foods are easy for a child with a sore mouth to eat. Ice cream is ideal because the coldness helps to numb the mouth, relieving pain.

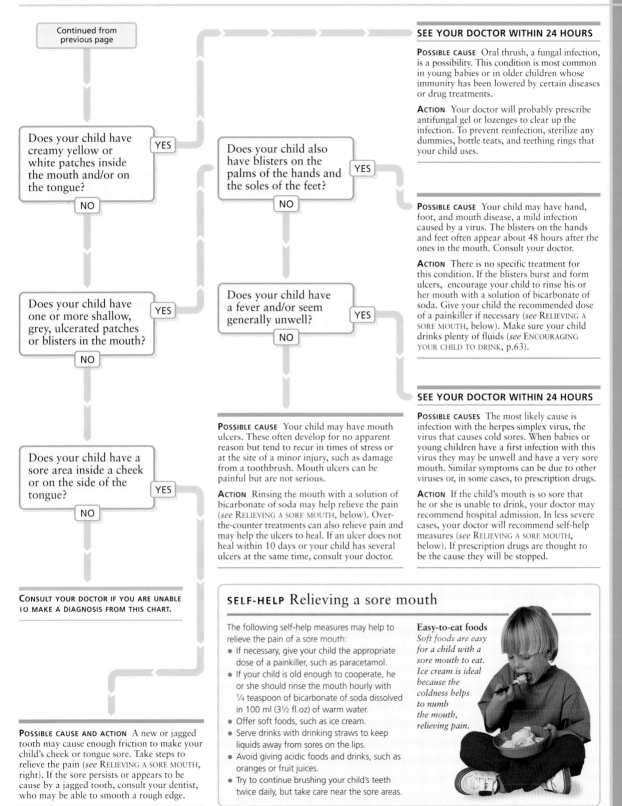

36 Teeth problems

Your child's teeth are constantly at risk of decay, which, if untreated, could spread to central parts of the tooth, causing serious damage. Regular brushing (*see* CARING FOR YOUR CHILD'S TEETH AND GUMS, below) can help prevent decay. Your child should also have regular dental checkups from about 3 years of age. If symptoms of decay, such as toothache, develop between checkups, make an appointment with your dentist. In young children, pain associated with the teeth may be due to teething (opposite), which is usually no cause for concern. If your child has toothache or an accident needing urgent dental treatment and your dentist is unavailable, call the casualty department of a local hospital for details of an on-call dentist.

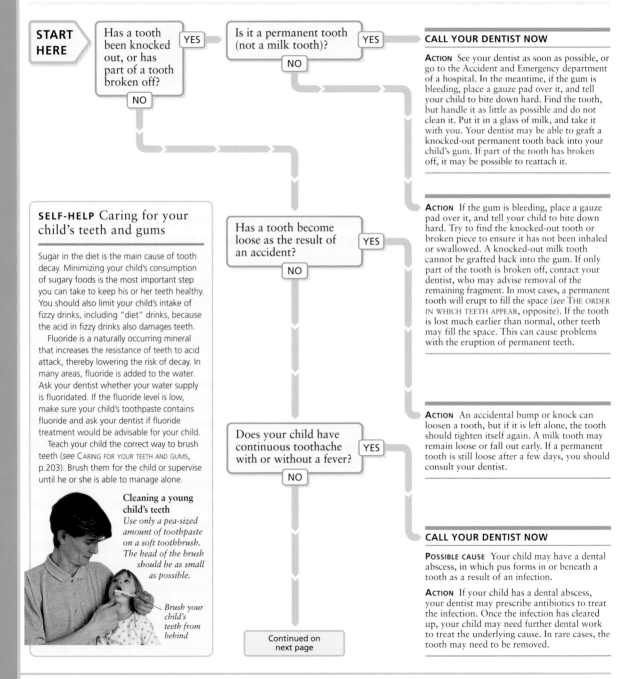

START HERE

Has a tooth been knocked out, or has part of a tooth broken off?
YES → **Is it a permanent tooth (not a milk tooth)?** YES →

CALL YOUR DENTIST NOW

ACTION See your dentist as soon as possible, or go to the Accident and Emergency department of a hospital. In the meantime, if the gum is bleeding, place a gauze pad over it, and tell your child to bite down hard. Find the tooth, but handle it as little as possible and do not clean it. Put it in a glass of milk, and take it with you. Your dentist may be able to graft a knocked-out permanent tooth back into your child's gum. If part of the tooth has broken off, it may be possible to reattach it.

NO (permanent tooth question)

NO (knocked out question)

ACTION If the gum is bleeding, place a gauze pad over it, and tell your child to bite down hard. Try to find the knocked-out tooth or broken piece to ensure it has not been inhaled or swallowed. A knocked-out milk tooth cannot be grafted back into the gum. If only part of the tooth is broken off, contact your dentist, who may advise removal of the remaining fragment. In most cases, a permanent tooth will erupt to fill the space (*see* THE ORDER IN WHICH TEETH APPEAR, opposite). If the tooth is lost much earlier than normal, other teeth may fill the space. This can cause problems with the eruption of permanent teeth.

Has a tooth become loose as the result of an accident?
YES →

NO

SELF-HELP Caring for your child's teeth and gums

Sugar in the diet is the main cause of tooth decay. Minimizing your child's consumption of sugary foods is the most important step you can take to keep his or her teeth healthy. You should also limit your child's intake of fizzy drinks, including "diet" drinks, because the acid in fizzy drinks also damages teeth.

Fluoride is a naturally occurring mineral that increases the resistance of teeth to acid attack, thereby lowering the risk of decay. In many areas, fluoride is added to the water. Ask your dentist whether your water supply is fluoridated. If the fluoride level is low, make sure your child's toothpaste contains fluoride and ask your dentist if fluoride treatment would be advisable for your child.

Teach your child the correct way to brush teeth (*see* CARING FOR YOUR TEETH AND GUMS, p.203). Brush them for the child or supervise until he or she is able to manage alone.

ACTION An accidental bump or knock can loosen a tooth, but if it is left alone, the tooth should tighten itself again. A milk tooth may remain loose or fall out early. If a permanent tooth is still loose after a few days, you should consult your dentist.

Does your child have continuous toothache with or without a fever?
YES →

NO

Cleaning a young child's teeth
Use only a pea-sized amount of toothpaste on a soft toothbrush. The head of the brush should be as small as possible.

Brush your child's teeth from behind

Continued on next page

CALL YOUR DENTIST NOW

POSSIBLE CAUSE Your child may have a dental abscess, in which pus forms in or beneath a tooth as a result of an infection.

ACTION If your child has a dental abscess, your dentist may prescribe antibiotics to treat the infection. Once the infection has cleared up, your child may need further dental work to treat the underlying cause. In rare cases, the tooth may need to be removed.

Continued from previous page

Does your child feel pain in his or her teeth when they are exposed to hot or cold foods? — YES / NO

Does the pain last only a few seconds? — YES / NO

Teething

The eruption of a tooth, particularly a molar, can be uncomfortable and may make your child irritable and restless. You may be able to feel the emerging tooth if you run your finger over the gum. A baby may have flushed cheeks, be less willing to feed, and may sleep poorly when teething. However, you should not attribute other symptoms, such as a fever or diarrhoea, to teething.

Babies who are teething often seem to like chewing on a cold, hard object, such as a chilled teething ring or a raw carrot. Over-the-counter local anaesthetic gels can be soothing if gently applied to the affected gums. The recommended dose of a painkiller can also be given if necessary.

Does your child feel pain when he or she bites on a tooth that has been filled recently? — YES / NO

SEE YOUR DENTIST WITHIN 24 HOURS

POSSIBLE CAUSE Your child may have decay deep within a tooth or in a crack in a tooth. This is especially likely if your child also has bouts of throbbing tooth pain not brought on by food or drink.

ACTION Your dentist will examine your child's teeth and may need to remove and fill any decayed areas.

POSSIBLE CAUSE AND ACTION It is quite common for a tooth to feel uncomfortable for a while after a filling has been put in, especially if the filling is large. If the pain gets worse or if your child is no better within 48 hours, consult your dentist, who will check the filling and adjust it if necessary.

SEE YOUR DOCTOR WITHIN 24 HOURS

POSSIBLE CAUSE Aching in several teeth can be a symptom of sinusitis (inflammation of the membranes lining the air spaces in the skull), especially if your child has recently had a cold or a runny or blocked nose. Children under the age of 8 are rarely affected because their sinuses have not yet developed.

ACTION If sinusitis is confirmed, your doctor may prescribe antibiotics. To ease symptoms, carry out self-help action for treating a child with a cold (p.102).

POSSIBLE CAUSE Teeth can become sensitive to extremes of temperature if their protective surfaces become thin or damaged. This may be due to tooth decay. Consult your dentist.

ACTION Your dentist will examine your child's teeth and treat any decay. If no abnormality is found, he or she may advise that your child brushes with a toothpaste for sensitive teeth and rubs a small amount over the teeth afterwards.

Does your child have pain in several of the teeth in the upper jaw? — YES / NO

Does your child have tender gums behind the back teeth? — YES / NO

CONSULT YOUR DENTIST IF YOU ARE UNABLE TO MAKE A DIAGNOSIS FROM THIS CHART.

POSSIBLE CAUSE Your child's second molars may be beginning to emerge (see THE ORDER IN WHICH TEETH APPEAR, right). The gums may become inflamed as the teeth erupt, but this is usually short-lived.

ACTION If necessary, give your child the recommended does of a painkiller, such as paracetamol. Consult your dentist if the pain is severe or if it is no better within 48 hours.

The order in which teeth appear

The ages at which teeth appear vary from child to child. A few children have one or more teeth at birth, while others still have none at a year old. There are 20 teeth in the first, or primary, set. The sequence in which they erupt is more important than the age of eruption. By the age of 13, the primary teeth have usually fallen out and most of the 32 permanent, or adult, teeth have erupted. In some people, the third molars, known as the wisdom teeth, never appear.

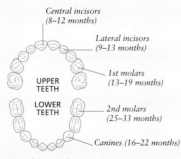

Central incisors
(8–12 months)

Lateral incisors
(9–13 months)

1st molars
(13–19 months)

2nd molars
(25–33 months)

Canines (16–22 months)

UPPER TEETH

LOWER TEETH

MILK (PRIMARY) TEETH

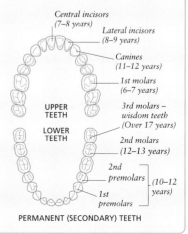

Central incisors
(7–8 years)

Lateral incisors
(8–9 years)

Canines
(11–12 years)

1st molars
(6–7 years)

3rd molars – wisdom teeth
(Over 17 years)

2nd molars
(12–13 years)

2nd premolars (10–12 years)

1st premolars

UPPER TEETH

LOWER TEETH

PERMANENT (SECONDARY) TEETH

The ages at which teeth appear
The figures in brackets indicate the average ages at which the teeth erupt. However, neither early nor late eruption is a cause for concern.

37 Eating problems

For children under 1 year, see chart 6, FEEDING PROBLEMS (p.56). The appetites of children are more closely governed by their body's energy requirements than are the appetites of adults. Most children alternate between active periods, during which they have large appetites, and inactive periods, when they eat much less. In addition, when children are growing rapidly, their appetites will be larger than usual. Some children naturally burn up less energy than others and have smaller appetites. Such variations in appetite are normal and are not a problem as long as your child seems well and is growing normally. Some children may refuse to eat to gain their parents' attention or control. This is relatively common in young children, but they usually grow out of it. In older children and adolescents, however, a refusal to eat may be a symptom of the potentially life-threatening disorder anorexia nervosa (*see* EATING DISORDERS, p.135).

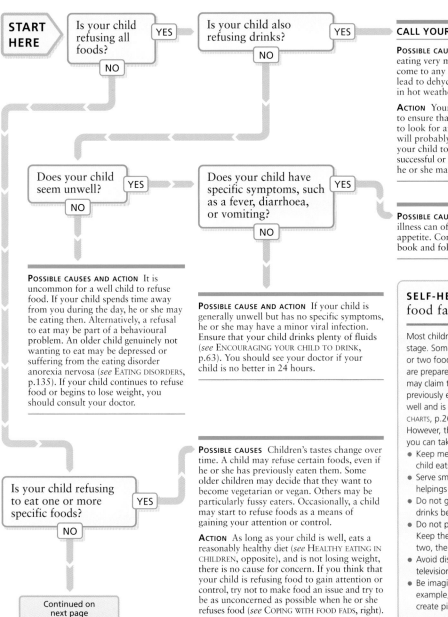

START HERE

Is your child refusing all foods? — YES → **Is your child also refusing drinks?** — YES →

NO

NO

CALL YOUR DOCTOR NOW

POSSIBLE CAUSES A child can go without eating very much for several days and not come to any harm, but refusal to drink can lead to dehydration within hours, particularly in hot weather or if the child has a fever.

ACTION Your doctor will examine your child to ensure that he or she is not dehydrated and to look for an underlying cause. Your doctor will probably give you advice on encouraging your child to drink (p.63). If this is not successful or if your child is already dehydrated, he or she may need to be admitted to hospital.

Does your child seem unwell? — YES →

NO

Does your child have specific symptoms, such as a fever, diarrhoea, or vomiting? — YES →

NO

POSSIBLE CAUSE AND ACTION An underlying illness can often cause a temporary loss of appetite. Consult the relevant chart in this book and follow the advice given.

POSSIBLE CAUSES AND ACTION It is uncommon for a well child to refuse food. If your child spends time away from you during the day, he or she may be eating then. Alternatively, a refusal to eat may be part of a behavioural problem. An older child genuinely not wanting to eat may be depressed or suffering from the eating disorder anorexia nervosa (*see* EATING DISORDERS, p.135). If your child continues to refuse food or begins to lose weight, you should consult your doctor.

POSSIBLE CAUSE AND ACTION If your child is generally unwell but has no specific symptoms, he or she may have a minor viral infection. Ensure that your child drinks plenty of fluids (*see* ENCOURAGING YOUR CHILD TO DRINK, p.63). You should see your doctor if your child is no better in 24 hours.

SELF-HELP Coping with food fads

Most children become faddy eaters at some stage. Sometimes a child will refuse only one or two foods or will accept foods only if they are prepared in a particular way. The child may claim to dislike foods that he or she previously enjoyed. As long as your child is well and is growing normally (*see* GROWTH CHARTS, p.26), there is no need for concern. However, there are some self-help measures you can take to encourage your child to eat:

- Keep mealtimes relaxed. Do not insist your child eats everything on his or her plate.
- Serve small portions, giving second helpings if requested.
- Do not give your child snacks and lots of drinks between meals.
- Do not persist in offering rejected foods. Keep them off the menu for a week or two, then try again.
- Avoid distractions, such as toys or television, during mealtimes.
- Be imaginative when preparing food; for example, cut it into decorative shapes or create pictures on the plate.

Is your child refusing to eat one or more specific foods? — YES →

NO

POSSIBLE CAUSES Children's tastes change over time. A child may refuse certain foods, even if he or she has previously eaten them. Some older children may decide that they want to become vegetarian or vegan. Others may be particularly fussy eaters. Occasionally, a child may start to refuse foods as a means of gaining your attention or control.

ACTION As long as your child is well, eats a reasonably healthy diet (*see* HEALTHY EATING IN CHILDREN, opposite), and is not losing weight, there is no cause for concern. If you think that your child is refusing food to gain attention or control, try not to make food an issue and try to be as unconcerned as possible when he or she refuses food (*see* COPING WITH FOOD FADS, right).

Continued on next page

Continued from previous page

Has your child been eating less than you think is appropriate for longer than 3 months? **NO**

YES → Are your child's height and weight within the normal range for his or her age (*see* GROWTH CHARTS, p.26)?

YES →

POSSIBLE CAUSE Your child's appetite may be reduced if he or she is in a phase of slow growth or is taking less exercise then previously.

ACTION As long as your child seems well and happy and is not losing weight, there is no cause for concern. However, if your child begins to lose weight or fails to grow normally, you should consult your doctor.

NO → Is your child over 12 years old? **NO**

YES →

POSSIBLE CAUSES Your child may have an underlying illness such as an intestinal disorder that is causing a loss of appetite and poor growth. However, dieting or the eating disorder anorexia nervosa (*see* EATING DISORDERS, p.135) need to be considered. Consult your doctor.

ACTION Your doctor will examine your child and may arrange for tests to exclude an underlying disorder. If it is appropriate, an assessment by a psychiatrist may be suggested.

Does your child refuse to eat when at home but eat well at school or other people's homes? **NO**

YES →

POSSIBLE CAUSES AND ACTION When away from home, it is quite common for peer pressure to lead a child to eat foods he or she would not normally eat. Alternatively, a child may refuse to eat at home as a means of gaining your attention. Try not to make food an issue, and show as little concern as possible when your child refuses food. Follow self-help measures for coping with food fads (opposite).

POSSIBLE CAUSES Your child may have an underlying illness such as an intestinal disorder that is causing a loss of appetite and poor growth. The eating disorder anorexia nervosa (*see* EATING DISORDERS, p.135) may develop in children under 12 years of age but is not common. Consult your doctor.

ACTION Your doctor will examine your child and may arrange for tests to look for an underlying illness and determine the appropriate treatment. If it is appropriate, an assessment by a psychiatrist may be suggested.

Is your child taking any prescribed drugs? **NO**

YES →

POSSIBLE CAUSE AND ACTION Certain drugs can interfere with appetite, in some cases by causing mild nausea as a side effect. Consult your doctor. Meanwhile, do not stop your child's prescribed drugs.

Has there been a recent change or upset at home or at school? **NO**

YES →

CONSULT YOUR DOCTOR IF YOU ARE UNABLE TO MAKE A DIAGNOSIS FROM THIS CHART.

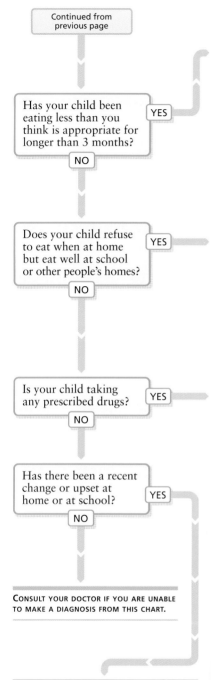

POSSIBLE CAUSE Your child may be anxious or upset about a recent event. This can often lead to a loss of appetite.

ACTION Try to discover and deal with any underlying worries your child has. It may help to talk to your child's teachers in case there are problems at school that you are unaware of. If your child's appetite does not improve or if he or she seems unwell, consult your doctor.

Healthy eating in children

Relative to their size, children need to eat more food than adults because they need fuel for growth and are more active. Over the age of 5, children should eat carbohydrates, proteins, and fats in the same proportions as adults: carbohydrates should make up roughly half of the diet; fats, just over a third; and proteins, the remainder. Children under 5 need more fats, as fats are high in calories and are important for the development of nerves. Children under 2 should have full-cream milk, rather than semi-skimmed. A varied diet that includes fruit, vegetables, meats, dairy products, and carbohydrates such as bread will provide your child with the nutrients he or she needs (*see* A HEALTHY DIET, p.28).

On the whole, fresh foods are better than processed. If the pressures of time mean that you often buy convenience foods, provide a balance with plenty of fresh fruit and vegetables. Give your child healthy snacks, such as muesli bars, yoghurts, and dried fruit, but introduce healthier foods into your child's diet gradually. Keep fried and sugary foods to a minimum. Do not give your child tea or coffee or put salt on his or her meals. If you establish sensible eating habits now, your child will be less likely to become overweight or suffer from diet-related health problems in later life.

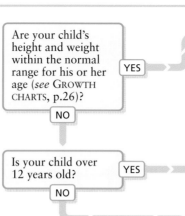

Healthy meals
Encourage your child to enjoy healthy eating by providing a range of tasty, nutritious meals.

38 Vomiting in children

For children under 1 year, see chart 4, VOMITING IN BABIES (p.52).

When a child vomits only once, this is usually caused by overeating or an emotional upset and is rarely due to a serious disorder. Repeated vomiting is most likely to be due to an infection of the digestive tract. Infections elsewhere in the body, such as in the urinary tract, can also cause vomiting in children, but there will usually be other symptoms as well. Rarely, vomiting can be a symptom of a serious condition needing urgent treatment. If your child is vomiting, make sure he or she drinks plenty of fluids to avoid dehydration (*see* PREVENTING DEHYDRATION IN CHILDREN, p.119).

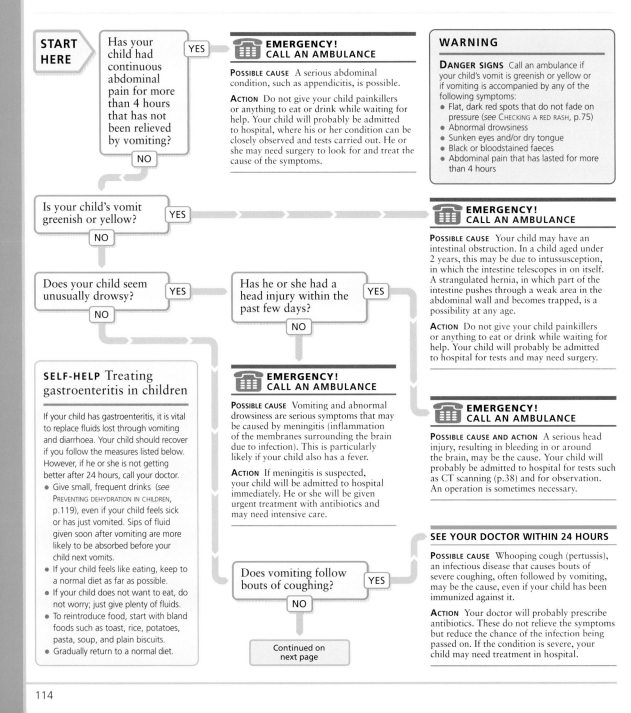

START HERE → Has your child had continuous abdominal pain for more than 4 hours that has not been relieved by vomiting?

YES →

EMERGENCY! CALL AN AMBULANCE

POSSIBLE CAUSE A serious abdominal condition, such as appendicitis, is possible.

ACTION Do not give your child painkillers or anything to eat or drink while waiting for help. Your child will probably be admitted to hospital, where his or her condition can be closely observed and tests carried out. He or she may need surgery to look for and treat the cause of the symptoms.

NO ↓

Is your child's vomit greenish or yellow?

YES →

NO ↓

Does your child seem unusually drowsy?

YES → Has he or she had a head injury within the past few days?

YES →

NO ↓

NO ↓

SELF-HELP Treating gastroenteritis in children

If your child has gastroenteritis, it is vital to replace fluids lost through vomiting and diarrhoea. Your child should recover if you follow the measures listed below. However, if he or she is not getting better after 24 hours, call your doctor.

- Give small, frequent drinks (*see* PREVENTING DEHYDRATION IN CHILDREN, p.119), even if your child feels sick or has just vomited. Sips of fluid given soon after vomiting are more likely to be absorbed before your child next vomits.
- If your child feels like eating, keep to a normal diet as far as possible.
- If your child does not want to eat, do not worry; just give plenty of fluids.
- To reintroduce food, start with bland foods such as toast, rice, potatoes, pasta, soup, and plain biscuits.
- Gradually return to a normal diet.

EMERGENCY! CALL AN AMBULANCE

POSSIBLE CAUSE Vomiting and abnormal drowsiness are serious symptoms that may be caused by meningitis (inflammation of the membranes surrounding the brain due to infection). This is particularly likely if your child also has a fever.

ACTION If meningitis is suspected, your child will be admitted to hospital immediately. He or she will be given urgent treatment with antibiotics and may need intensive care.

Does vomiting follow bouts of coughing?

YES →

NO ↓

Continued on next page

WARNING

DANGER SIGNS Call an ambulance if your child's vomit is greenish or yellow or if vomiting is accompanied by any of the following symptoms:
- Flat, dark red spots that do not fade on pressure (*see* CHECKING A RED RASH, p.75)
- Abnormal drowsiness
- Sunken eyes and/or dry tongue
- Black or bloodstained faeces
- Abdominal pain that has lasted for more than 4 hours

EMERGENCY! CALL AN AMBULANCE

POSSIBLE CAUSE Your child may have an intestinal obstruction. In a child aged under 2 years, this may be due to intussusception, in which the intestine telescopes in on itself. A strangulated hernia, in which part of the intestine pushes through a weak area in the abdominal wall and becomes trapped, is a possibility at any age.

ACTION Do not give your child painkillers or anything to eat or drink while waiting for help. Your child will probably be admitted to hospital for tests and may need surgery.

EMERGENCY! CALL AN AMBULANCE

POSSIBLE CAUSE AND ACTION A serious head injury, in which bleeding in or around the brain, may be the cause. Your child will probably be admitted to hospital for tests such as CT scanning (p.38) and for observation. An operation is sometimes necessary.

SEE YOUR DOCTOR WITHIN 24 HOURS

POSSIBLE CAUSE Whooping cough (pertussis), an infectious disease that causes bouts of severe coughing, often followed by vomiting, may be the cause, even if your child has been immunized against it.

ACTION Your doctor will probably prescribe antibiotics. These do not relieve the symptoms but reduce the chance of the infection being passed on. If the condition is severe, your child may need treatment in hospital.

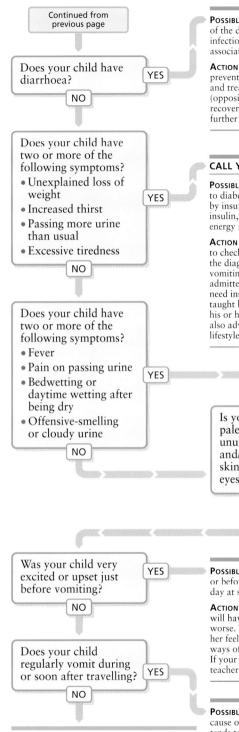

Continued from previous page

Does your child have diarrhoea? YES

NO

POSSIBLE CAUSE Gastroenteritis, inflammation of the digestive tract, usually due to a viral infection, is the most likely cause and may be associated with abdominal pain.

ACTION Follow the self-help measures for preventing dehydration in children (p.119) and treating gastroenteritis in children (opposite). If your child has not started to recover after 24 hours or if he or she develops further symptoms, call your doctor.

Does your child have two or more of the following symptoms?
- Unexplained loss of weight
- Increased thirst
- Passing more urine than usual
- Excessive tiredness

YES

NO

CALL YOUR DOCTOR NOW

POSSIBLE CAUSE These symptoms may be due to diabetes mellitus. This condition is caused by insufficient production of the hormone insulin, which is needed by the body to get energy from sugar and carbohydrate foods.

ACTION Your doctor will take a blood sample to check your child's blood sugar level. If the diagnosis is confirmed and your child is vomiting, he or she will probably need to be admitted to hospital. Your child will probably need insulin injections for life and will be taught how to inject the insulin and monitor his or her blood sugar level. Your doctor will also advise you on your child's diet and lifestyle (see DIABETES MELLITUS, p.145).

Does your child have two or more of the following symptoms?
- Fever
- Pain on passing urine
- Bedwetting or daytime wetting after being dry
- Offensive-smelling or cloudy urine

YES

NO

Is your child passing pale faeces and unusually dark urine, and/or are your child's skin and whites of the eyes yellow? YES

NO

Was your child very excited or upset just before vomiting? YES

NO

POSSIBLE CAUSE Vomiting when excited or before stressful events, such as the first day at school, is common in children.

ACTION Be sympathetic: the vomiting will have made your child feel even worse. Talk to your child about his or her feelings, and help him or her to find ways of coping with stressful situations. If your child is at school, his or her teachers may also be able to help.

Does your child regularly vomit during or soon after travelling? YES

NO

POSSIBLE CAUSE Travel sickness is the probable cause of your child's vomiting. The condition tends to run in families.

ACTION When your child travels, follow self-help measures for coping with travel sickness (above). Most children become less susceptible to travel sickness as they grow older.

AN OCCASIONAL BOUT OF VOMITING IS COMMON DURING CHILDHOOD AND MAY OFTEN HAVE NO OBVIOUS PHYSICAL CAUSE. HOWEVER, IF YOU ARE CONCERNED OR THE VOMITING IS RECURRENT, CONSULT YOUR DOCTOR.

SELF-HELP Coping with travel sickness

If your child suffers from travel sickness, some of the following suggestions may help:
- Give only light meals or snacks before and during your journey.
- Try to travel at night to encourage your child to sleep through the journey.
- Keep a car window open.
- Discourage your child from reading during your journey.
- Provide plenty of distractions, such as tapes of stories and songs.
- Try giving your child an over-the-counter travel sickness remedy before the journey. Your pharmacist can advise you.
- Be prepared. For example, bring a change of clothes for your child.

Looking out of the window
If your child suffers from travel sickness, games that encourage him or her to look out of the window may help.

SEE YOUR DOCTOR WITHIN 24 HOURS

POSSIBLE CAUSE Your child's symptoms may be due to a urinary tract infection (p.122).

ACTION Your doctor will test a sample of your child's urine. If the diagnosis is confirmed, a urine sample will be sent to a laboratory for analysis, and your child will be prescribed antibiotics. In some cases, further tests, such as ultrasound scanning (see INVESTIGATING THE URINARY TRACT IN CHILDREN, p.123), may be needed to look for any associated problems.

SEE YOUR DOCTOR WITHIN 24 HOURS

POSSIBLE CAUSE Your child may have a liver problem such as hepatitis, in which a viral infection causes inflammation of liver cells.

ACTION Your doctor will arrange for a blood test to confirm the diagnosis. He or she may also refer your child to hospital for further tests. To prevent the infection from spreading within the family, keep your child's eating utensils and towels separate. Your doctor may recommend that other members of the family are immunized against the disease.

39 Abdominal pain

In, most cases, abdominal pain is short-lived and disappears on its own without treatment. However, in some cases, there may be a serious physical cause, such as appendicitis, that needs urgent medical attention. It can be difficult to decide whether abdominal pain in a child, particularly a young child, needs medical attention or whether to wait and see. If your child has stomach ache or if his or her behaviour causes you to suspect abdominal pain, consult this chart for advice.

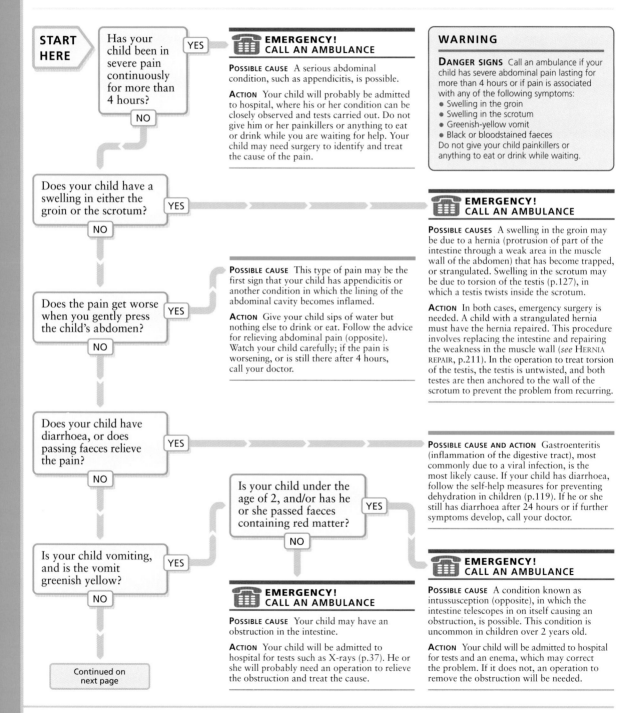

START HERE

Has your child been in severe pain continuously for more than 4 hours?

YES → **EMERGENCY! CALL AN AMBULANCE**

POSSIBLE CAUSE A serious abdominal condition, such as appendicitis, is possible.

ACTION Your child will probably be admitted to hospital, where his or her condition can be closely observed and tests carried out. Do not give him or her painkillers or anything to eat or drink while you are waiting for help. Your child may need surgery to identify and treat the cause of the pain.

NO ↓

WARNING

DANGER SIGNS Call an ambulance if your child has severe abdominal pain lasting for more than 4 hours or if pain is associated with any of the following symptoms:
- Swelling in the groin
- Swelling in the scrotum
- Greenish-yellow vomit
- Black or bloodstained faeces

Do not give your child painkillers or anything to eat or drink while waiting.

Does your child have a swelling in either the groin or the scrotum?

YES → **EMERGENCY! CALL AN AMBULANCE**

POSSIBLE CAUSES A swelling in the groin may be due to a hernia (protrusion of part of the intestine through a weak area in the muscle wall of the abdomen) that has become trapped, or strangulated. Swelling in the scrotum may be due to torsion of the testis (p.127), in which a testis twists inside the scrotum.

ACTION In both cases, emergency surgery is needed. A child with a strangulated hernia must have the hernia repaired. This procedure involves replacing the intestine and repairing the weakness in the muscle wall (see HERNIA REPAIR, p.211). In the operation to treat torsion of the testis, the testis is untwisted, and both testes are then anchored to the wall of the scrotum to prevent the problem from recurring.

NO ↓

Does the pain get worse when you gently press the child's abdomen?

YES → **POSSIBLE CAUSE** This type of pain may be the first sign that your child has appendicitis or another condition in which the lining of the abdominal cavity becomes inflamed.

ACTION Give your child sips of water but nothing else to drink or eat. Follow the advice for relieving abdominal pain (opposite). Watch your child carefully; if the pain is worsening, or is still there after 4 hours, call your doctor.

NO ↓

Does your child have diarrhoea, or does passing faeces relieve the pain?

YES → **POSSIBLE CAUSE AND ACTION** Gastroenteritis (inflammation of the digestive tract), most commonly due to a viral infection, is the most likely cause. If your child has diarrhoea, follow the self-help measures for preventing dehydration in children (p.119). If he or she still has diarrhoea after 24 hours or if further symptoms develop, call your doctor.

NO ↓

Is your child under the age of 2, and/or has he or she passed faeces containing red matter?

YES → **EMERGENCY! CALL AN AMBULANCE**

POSSIBLE CAUSE A condition known as intussusception (opposite), in which the intestine telescopes in on itself causing an obstruction, is possible. This condition is uncommon in children over 2 years old.

ACTION Your child will be admitted to hospital for tests and an enema, which may correct the problem. If it does not, an operation to remove the obstruction will be needed.

NO ↓

Is your child vomiting, and is the vomit greenish yellow?

YES → **EMERGENCY! CALL AN AMBULANCE**

POSSIBLE CAUSE Your child may have an obstruction in the intestine.

ACTION Your child will be admitted to hospital for tests such as X-rays (p.37). He or she will probably need an operation to relieve the obstruction and treat the cause.

NO ↓

Continued on next page

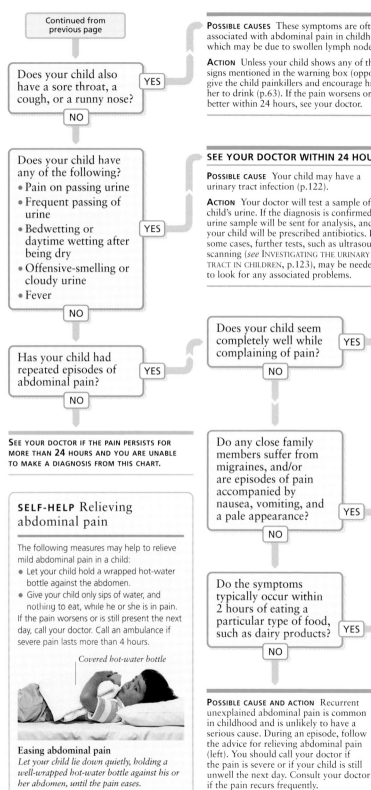

Continued from previous page

Does your child also have a sore throat, a cough, or a runny nose? **YES** → **NO**

Does your child have any of the following?
- Pain on passing urine
- Frequent passing of urine
- Bedwetting or daytime wetting after being dry
- Offensive-smelling or cloudy urine
- Fever

YES → **NO**

Has your child had repeated episodes of abdominal pain? **YES** → **NO**

SEE YOUR DOCTOR IF THE PAIN PERSISTS FOR MORE THAN 24 HOURS AND YOU ARE UNABLE TO MAKE A DIAGNOSIS FROM THIS CHART.

Does your child seem completely well while complaining of pain? **YES** → **NO**

Do any close family members suffer from migraines, and/or are episodes of pain accompanied by nausea, vomiting, and a pale appearance? **YES** → **NO**

Do the symptoms typically occur within 2 hours of eating a particular type of food, such as dairy products? **YES** → **NO**

POSSIBLE CAUSES These symptoms are often associated with abdominal pain in childhood, which may be due to swollen lymph nodes.

ACTION Unless your child shows any of the signs mentioned in the warning box (opposite), give the child painkillers and encourage him or her to drink (p.63). If the pain worsens or is no better within 24 hours, see your doctor.

SEE YOUR DOCTOR WITHIN 24 HOURS

POSSIBLE CAUSE Your child may have a urinary tract infection (p.122).

ACTION Your doctor will test a sample of your child's urine. If the diagnosis is confirmed, a urine sample will be sent for analysis, and your child will be prescribed antibiotics. In some cases, further tests, such as ultrasound scanning (*see* INVESTIGATING THE URINARY TRACT IN CHILDREN, p.123), may be needed to look for any associated problems.

POSSIBLE CAUSE AND ACTION Recurrent unexplained abdominal pain is common in childhood and is unlikely to have a serious cause. During an episode, follow the advice for relieving abdominal pain (left). You should call your doctor if the pain is severe or if your child is still unwell the next day. Consult your doctor if the pain recurs frequently.

Intussusception

In intussusception, part of the intestine telescopes into itself, causing an obstruction. The cause is unknown, but the problem may occur during viral infections. If your doctor suspects that your child has intussusception, your child will be admitted to hospital and may be given intravenous fluids. An enema will probably be given to confirm the diagnosis. This may also correct the problem by forcing the intestine back into position. If the enema does not help, emergency surgery may be needed to relieve the obstruction and remove any damaged intestine.

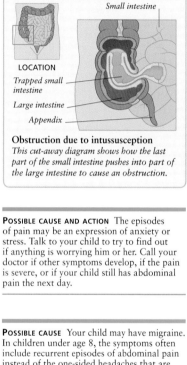

Small intestine

LOCATION
Trapped small intestine
Large intestine
Appendix

Obstruction due to intussusception
This cut-away diagram shows how the last part of the small intestine pushes into part of the large intestine to cause an obstruction.

POSSIBLE CAUSE AND ACTION The episodes of pain may be an expression of anxiety or stress. Talk to your child to try to find out if anything is worrying him or her. Call your doctor if other symptoms develop, if the pain is severe, or if your child still has abdominal pain the next day.

POSSIBLE CAUSE Your child may have migraine. In children under age 8, the symptoms often include recurrent episodes of abdominal pain instead of the one-sided headaches that are typical of migraine in older children and adults. Consult your doctor.

ACTION Your doctor will examine your child and may arrange for tests such as a urine test (p.36) to exclude other disorders. Taking painkillers should help to relieve the symptoms.

POSSIBLE CAUSE Your child may have a food intolerance, such as lactose intolerance (p.118), in which symptoms such as abdominal pain, vomiting, and/or diarrhoea occur whenever a certain food is eaten. Consult your doctor.

ACTION Your doctor may suggest excluding possible problem foods or food groups from your child's diet for a trial period. If you need to exclude a food permanently from the diet, you may be referred to a dietician for advice.

SELF-HELP Relieving abdominal pain

The following measures may help to relieve mild abdominal pain in a child:
- Let your child hold a wrapped hot-water bottle against the abdomen.
- Give your child only sips of water, and nothing to eat, while he or she is in pain.

If the pain worsens or is still present the next day, call your doctor. Call an ambulance if severe pain lasts more than 4 hours.

Covered hot-water bottle

Easing abdominal pain
Let your child lie down quietly, holding a well-wrapped hot-water bottle against his or her abdomen, until the pain eases.

40 Diarrhoea in children

For children under 1 year, see chart 5, DIARRHOEA IN
BABIES *(p.54).*
Diarrhoea is the frequent passing of abnormally loose or
watery faeces. While diarrhoea can be serious in babies, in
older children it is unlikely to be a cause for concern.

The most common cause of diarrhoea in children is a viral
infection of the digestive tract. In most cases, drug treatment is
inappropriate; avoiding food, so that the intestines are rested,
and drinking plenty of fluids (*see* PREVENTING DEHYDRATION
IN CHILDREN, opposite) is the best course of action.

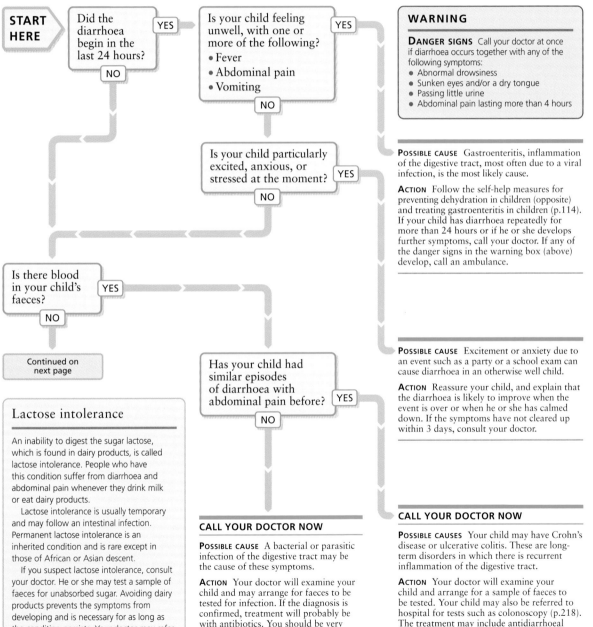

START HERE

Did the diarrhoea begin in the last 24 hours?
— **YES** →
— **NO** ↓

Is your child feeling unwell, with one or more of the following?
- Fever
- Abdominal pain
- Vomiting
— **YES** →
— **NO** ↓

Is your child particularly excited, anxious, or stressed at the moment?
— **YES** →
— **NO** ↓

Is there blood in your child's faeces?
— **YES** →
— **NO** ↓

Continued on next page

Has your child had similar episodes of diarrhoea with abdominal pain before?
— **YES** →
— **NO** ↓

WARNING

DANGER SIGNS Call your doctor at once
if diarrhoea occurs together with any of the
following symptoms:
- Abnormal drowsiness
- Sunken eyes and/or a dry tongue
- Passing little urine
- Abdominal pain lasting more than 4 hours

POSSIBLE CAUSE Gastroenteritis, inflammation
of the digestive tract, most often due to a viral
infection, is the most likely cause.

ACTION Follow the self-help measures for
preventing dehydration in children (opposite)
and treating gastroenteritis in children (p.114).
If your child has diarrhoea repeatedly for
more than 24 hours or if he or she develops
further symptoms, call your doctor. If any of
the danger signs in the warning box (above)
develop, call an ambulance.

POSSIBLE CAUSE Excitement or anxiety due to
an event such as a party or a school exam can
cause diarrhoea in an otherwise well child.

ACTION Reassure your child, and explain that
the diarrhoea is likely to improve when the
event is over or when he or she has calmed
down. If the symptoms have not cleared up
within 3 days, consult your doctor.

Lactose intolerance

An inability to digest the sugar lactose,
which is found in dairy products, is called
lactose intolerance. People who have
this condition suffer from diarrhoea and
abdominal pain whenever they drink milk
or eat dairy products.

Lactose intolerance is usually temporary
and may follow an intestinal infection.
Permanent lactose intolerance is an
inherited condition and is rare except in
those of African or Asian descent.

If you suspect lactose intolerance, consult
your doctor. He or she may test a sample of
faeces for unabsorbed sugar. Avoiding dairy
products prevents the symptoms from
developing and is necessary for as long as
the condition persists. Your doctor may refer
you to a dietician for advice.

CALL YOUR DOCTOR NOW

POSSIBLE CAUSE A bacterial or parasitic
infection of the digestive tract may be
the cause of these symptoms.

ACTION Your doctor will examine your
child and may arrange for faeces to be
tested for infection. If the diagnosis is
confirmed, treatment will probably be
with antibiotics. You should be very
careful about hygiene so that other
family members do not become infected.

CALL YOUR DOCTOR NOW

POSSIBLE CAUSES Your child may have Crohn's
disease or ulcerative colitis. These are long-
term disorders in which there is recurrent
inflammation of the digestive tract.

ACTION Your doctor will examine your
child and arrange for a sample of faeces to
be tested. Your child may also be referred to
hospital for tests such as colonoscopy (p.218).
The treatment may include antidiarrhoeal
drugs, and, in some cases, corticosteroid drugs
may also be needed.

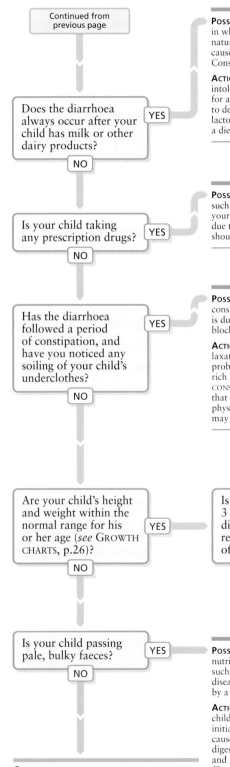

Continued from previous page

Does the diarrhoea always occur after your child has milk or other dairy products? — YES

NO

POSSIBLE CAUSE Lactose intolerance (opposite), in which the body cannot digest lactose, the natural sugar found in milk, may be the cause. This condition is usually temporary. Consult your doctor.

ACTION If your doctor suspects lactose intolerance, he or she will probably arrange for a sample of your child's faeces to be tested to detect undigested sugars. If your child is lactose-intolerant, you will need advice from a dietitian on a lactose-free diet.

Is your child taking any prescription drugs? — YES

NO

POSSIBLE CAUSE AND ACTION Certain drugs, such as antibiotics, can cause diarrhoea. Call your doctor before the next dose of the drug is due to ask if it could be the cause and if you should stop giving it to your child.

Has the diarrhoea followed a period of constipation, and have you noticed any soiling of your child's underclothes? — YES

NO

POSSIBLE CAUSE Your child may have chronic constipation blocking the rectum. The soiling is due to the overflow of liquid faeces past the blockage. Consult your doctor.

ACTION Your doctor may initially prescribe a laxative to clear the blockage. He or she will probably also recommend adding extra fibre-rich foods to your child's diet (see AVOIDING CONSTIPATION, p.120). If your doctor suspects that the condition is caused by an underlying physical or behavioural problem, he or she may refer your child to a specialist.

Are your child's height and weight within the normal range for his or her age (see GROWTH CHARTS, p.26)? — YES

NO

Is your child under 3 years, and does the diarrhoea contain any recognizable pieces of food? — YES

NO

Is your child passing pale, bulky faeces? — YES

NO

POSSIBLE CAUSE An inability to absorb nutrients from food due to a disorder such as cystic fibrosis (p.69) or coeliac disease, in which the intestine is damaged by a gluten allergy, may be the cause.

ACTION Your doctor will examine your child and will probably arrange for initial tests. Treatment depends on the cause but may include drugs to aid digestion or a special diet with vitamin and mineral supplements. If cystic fibrosis is suspected, your child may be referred to hospital for further tests.

GIVE YOUR CHILD PLENTY OF FLUIDS, AND SEE YOUR DOCTOR WITHIN 24 HOURS.

SELF-HELP Preventing dehydration in children

If your child has diarrhoea, vomiting, and/or a fever, it is important to give him or her plenty of fluids to prevent or treat dehydration, a potentially life-threatening condition.

The most suitable fluid to give your child is water. In addition, give diluted, unsweetened fruit juice because this contains some sugar. If your child is at risk of dehydration, your doctor may advise oral rehydration solution, available over the counter from chemists. It is usually supplied as powder, to be mixed with water as directed. Give the solution in addition to, or instead of, normal drinks.

While symptoms last, offer small drinks at frequent intervals. Even if your child vomits, give him or her sips of fluid soon afterwards to replace the fluid lost from the body.

If your child still has diarrhoea after 24 hours, call your doctor.

Oral rehydration fluids are usually flavoured to make them palatable

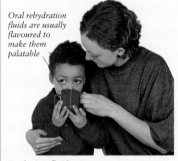

Replacing fluids
Encourage your child to sip rehydrating solution or diluted fruit juice at least once an hour while symptoms last. He or she should also drink soon after vomiting.

POSSIBLE CAUSE AND ACTION Toddler diarrhoea, a common condition in which a young child fails to digest food properly, is likely. This may be due partly to your child not being able to chew his or her food enough. It is not a danger to health; however, you should consult your doctor so that he or she can make sure an infection is not the cause.

POSSIBLE CAUSE AND ACTION Some children routinely produce soft faeces that can be mistaken for diarrhoea. If you are not sure whether or not your child's faeces are normal, consult your doctor or health visitor for advice.

41 Constipation

Consult this chart if your child is not having regular bowel movements or if he or she is passing very hard or pellet-like faeces. There is a wide variation in the normal frequency with which children empty their bowels. Some children have a bowel movement several times a day; others have one every 2 or 3 days. Both of these extremes are normal so long as the child is otherwise well and that the faeces are not hard or painful to pass. It is also normal for babies and toddlers to strain and go bright red in the face when passing normal, soft faeces, although parents sometimes mistake this as a sign that their child is constipated. Minor changes to a child's usual bowel habit are often caused by a change in diet or in the daily routine, an illness, dehydration (especially in hot weather), or emotional stress.

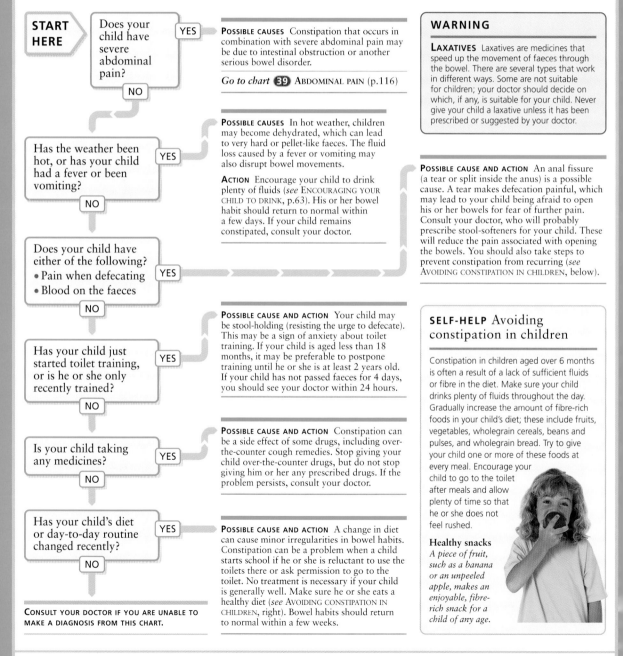

START HERE → **Does your child have severe abdominal pain?** → **YES**

POSSIBLE CAUSES Constipation that occurs in combination with severe abdominal pain may be due to intestinal obstruction or another serious bowel disorder.

Go to chart **39** ABDOMINAL PAIN (p.116)

NO ↓

Has the weather been hot, or has your child had a fever or been vomiting? → **YES**

POSSIBLE CAUSES In hot weather, children may become dehydrated, which can lead to very hard or pellet-like faeces. The fluid loss caused by a fever or vomiting may also disrupt bowel movements.

ACTION Encourage your child to drink plenty of fluids (*see* ENCOURAGING YOUR CHILD TO DRINK, p.63). His or her bowel habit should return to normal within a few days. If your child remains constipated, consult your doctor.

NO ↓

Does your child have either of the following?
● **Pain when defecating**
● **Blood on the faeces** → **YES**

POSSIBLE CAUSE AND ACTION An anal fissure (a tear or split inside the anus) is a possible cause. A tear makes defecation painful, which may lead to your child being afraid to open his or her bowels for fear of further pain. Consult your doctor, who will probably prescribe stool-softeners for your child. These will reduce the pain associated with opening the bowels. You should also take steps to prevent constipation from recurring (*see* AVOIDING CONSTIPATION IN CHILDREN, below).

NO ↓

Has your child just started toilet training, or is he or she only recently trained? → **YES**

POSSIBLE CAUSE AND ACTION Your child may be stool-holding (resisting the urge to defecate). This may be a sign of anxiety about toilet training. If your child is aged less than 18 months, it may be preferable to postpone training until he or she is at least 2 years old. If your child has not passed faeces for 4 days, you should see your doctor within 24 hours.

NO ↓

Is your child taking any medicines? → **YES**

POSSIBLE CAUSE AND ACTION Constipation can be a side effect of some drugs, including over-the-counter cough remedies. Stop giving your child over-the-counter drugs, but do not stop giving him or her any prescribed drugs. If the problem persists, consult your doctor.

NO ↓

Has your child's diet or day-to-day routine changed recently? → **YES**

POSSIBLE CAUSE AND ACTION A change in diet can cause minor irregularities in bowel habits. Constipation can be a problem when a child starts school if he or she is reluctant to use the toilets there or ask permission to go to the toilet. No treatment is necessary if your child is generally well. Make sure he or she eats a healthy diet (*see* AVOIDING CONSTIPATION IN CHILDREN, right). Bowel habits should return to normal within a few weeks.

NO ↓

CONSULT YOUR DOCTOR IF YOU ARE UNABLE TO MAKE A DIAGNOSIS FROM THIS CHART.

WARNING

LAXATIVES Laxatives are medicines that speed up the movement of faeces through the bowel. There are several types that work in different ways. Some are not suitable for children; your doctor should decide on which, if any, is suitable for your child. Never give your child a laxative unless it has been prescribed or suggested by your doctor.

SELF-HELP Avoiding constipation in children

Constipation in children aged over 6 months is often a result of a lack of sufficient fluids or fibre in the diet. Make sure your child drinks plenty of fluids throughout the day. Gradually increase the amount of fibre-rich foods in your child's diet; these include fruits, vegetables, wholegrain cereals, beans and pulses, and wholegrain bread. Try to give your child one or more of these foods at every meal. Encourage your child to go to the toilet after meals and allow plenty of time so that he or she does not feel rushed.

Healthy snacks
A piece of fruit, such as a banana or an unpeeled apple, makes an enjoyable, fibre-rich snack for a child of any age.

42 Abnormal-looking faeces

For hard or pellet-like faeces, see chart 41, CONSTIPATION (p.120). For runny faeces in a child under 1 year, see chart 5, DIARRHOEA IN BABIES (p.54); for a child over 1 year, see chart 40, DIARRHOEA IN CHILDREN (p.118).
It is normal for faeces to vary slightly in their colour, smell, or consistency. Consult this chart only if there is a marked change in the appearance of your child's faeces. Sudden

differences are almost always caused by something your child has eaten, and the change should only last a few days. However, there may be an underlying disorder causing the problem. If the faeces still look abnormal in 48 hours or if they are accompanied by other symptoms such as abdominal pain, you should consult your doctor, taking a sample of the faeces in a clean container for him or her to examine.

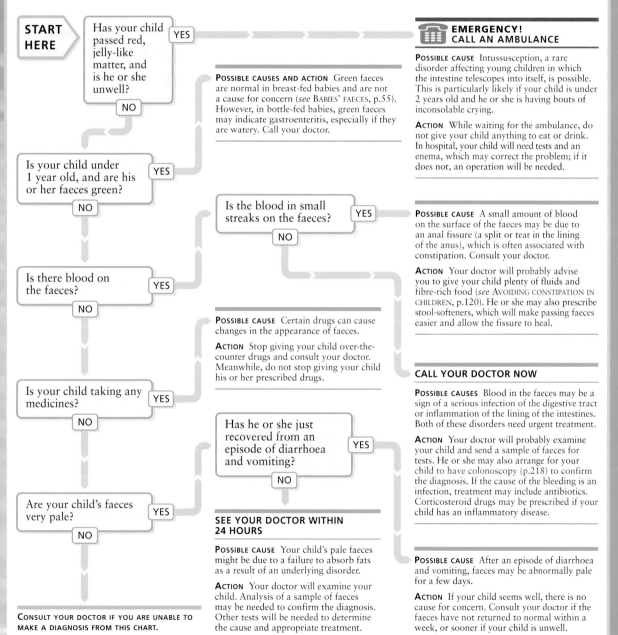

START HERE

Has your child passed red, jelly-like matter, and is he or she unwell? — YES →

EMERGENCY! CALL AN AMBULANCE

POSSIBLE CAUSE Intussusception, a rare disorder affecting young children in which the intestine telescopes into itself, is possible. This is particularly likely if your child is under 2 years old and he or she is having bouts of inconsolable crying.

ACTION While waiting for the ambulance, do not give your child anything to eat or drink. In hospital, your child will need tests and an enema, which may correct the problem; if it does not, an operation will be needed.

NO ↓

Is your child under 1 year old, and are his or her faeces green? — YES →

POSSIBLE CAUSES AND ACTION Green faeces are normal in breast-fed babies and are not a cause for concern (see BABIES' FAECES, p.55). However, in bottle-fed babies, green faeces may indicate gastroenteritis, especially if they are watery. Call your doctor.

NO ↓

Is there blood on the faeces? — YES →

Is the blood in small streaks on the faeces? — YES →

POSSIBLE CAUSE A small amount of blood on the surface of the faeces may be due to an anal fissure (a split or tear in the lining of the anus), which is often associated with constipation. Consult your doctor.

ACTION Your doctor will probably advise you to give your child plenty of fluids and fibre-rich food (see AVOIDING CONSTIPATION IN CHILDREN, p.120). He or she may also prescribe stool-softeners, which will make passing faeces easier and allow the fissure to heal.

NO (blood in streaks) ↓

CALL YOUR DOCTOR NOW

POSSIBLE CAUSES Blood in the faeces may be a sign of a serious infection of the digestive tract or inflammation of the lining of the intestines. Both of these disorders need urgent treatment.

ACTION Your doctor will probably examine your child and send a sample of faeces for tests. He or she may also arrange for your child to have colonoscopy (p.218) to confirm the diagnosis. If the cause of the bleeding is an infection, treatment may include antibiotics. Corticosteroid drugs may be prescribed if your child has an inflammatory disease.

NO ↓

Is your child taking any medicines? — YES →

POSSIBLE CAUSE Certain drugs can cause changes in the appearance of faeces.

ACTION Stop giving your child over-the-counter drugs and consult your doctor. Meanwhile, do not stop giving your child his or her prescribed drugs.

NO ↓

Are your child's faeces very pale? — YES →

Has he or she just recovered from an episode of diarrhoea and vomiting? — YES →

POSSIBLE CAUSE After an episode of diarrhoea and vomiting, faeces may be abnormally pale for a few days.

ACTION If your child seems well, there is no cause for concern. Consult your doctor if the faeces have not returned to normal within a week, or sooner if your child is unwell.

NO ↓

SEE YOUR DOCTOR WITHIN 24 HOURS

POSSIBLE CAUSE Your child's pale faeces might be due to a failure to absorb fats as a result of an underlying disorder.

ACTION Your doctor will examine your child. Analysis of a sample of faeces may be needed to confirm the diagnosis. Other tests will be needed to determine the cause and appropriate treatment.

NO ↓

CONSULT YOUR DOCTOR IF YOU ARE UNABLE TO MAKE A DIAGNOSIS FROM THIS CHART.

43 Urinary problems

For problems with bladder control, see chart 44, TOILET-TRAINING PROBLEMS (p.124).

Most children pass urine more frequently than adults. This is because children have smaller bladders and have less well developed muscular control. Urinary problems, such as urinary tract infections, are common in children. Symptoms of urinary problems in children include pain on passing urine, needing to pass urine more frequently than usual, cloudy urine, or unpleasant-smelling urine. Occasionally, unexplained vomiting and fever may be due to a urinary tract infection. In some children, urinary tract infections are associated with reflux, in which urine flows back towards the kidneys when the bladder is emptied. Urinary problems in a child should always be assessed promptly by your doctor.

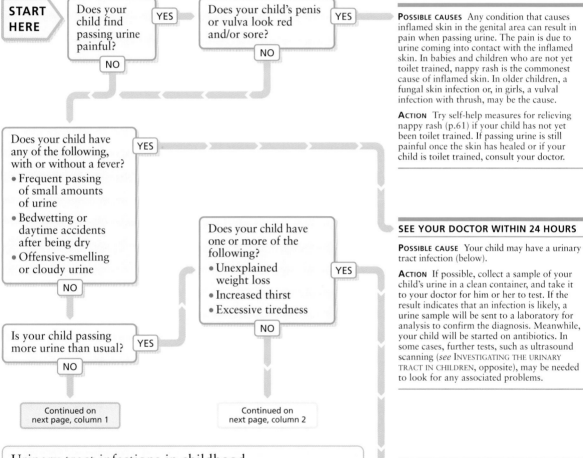

POSSIBLE CAUSES Any condition that causes inflamed skin in the genital area can result in pain when passing urine. The pain is due to urine coming into contact with the inflamed skin. In babies and children who are not yet toilet trained, nappy rash is the commonest cause of inflamed skin. In older children, a fungal skin infection or, in girls, a vulval infection with thrush, may be the cause.

ACTION Try self-help measures for relieving nappy rash (p.61) if your child has not yet been toilet trained. If passing urine is still painful once the skin has healed or if your child is toilet trained, consult your doctor.

SEE YOUR DOCTOR WITHIN 24 HOURS

POSSIBLE CAUSE Your child may have a urinary tract infection (below).

ACTION If possible, collect a sample of your child's urine in a clean container, and take it to your doctor for him or her to test. If the result indicates that an infection is likely, a urine sample will be sent to a laboratory for analysis to confirm the diagnosis. Meanwhile, your child will be started on antibiotics. In some cases, further tests, such as ultrasound scanning (*see* INVESTIGATING THE URINARY TRACT IN CHILDREN, opposite), may be needed to look for any associated problems.

Urinary tract infections in childhood

If you suspect that your child has a urinary tract infection, it is important that you bring it to your doctor's attention within 24 hours. Urinary tract infections can be more serious in children than they are in adults because they may be associated with reflux, in which urine flows back up the ureters towards the kidneys when the bladder is emptied. If untreated, reflux of infected urine can cause permanent scarring of the kidneys and impaired kidney function in later life.

Most young children who have had a urinary tract infection will need to have tests (*see* INVESTIGATING THE URINARY TRACT IN CHILDREN, opposite) to establish whether reflux is occurring and to assess kidney function. If your child is diagnosed as having reflux, he or she will be prescribed continuous, low-dose antibiotics to reduce the risk of subsequent infection and kidney damage. This treatment can often be discontinued by the time your child is 5 years old.

SEE YOUR DOCTOR WITHIN 24 HOURS

POSSIBLE CAUSE Diabetes mellitus is a possible cause of these symptoms. It is caused by insufficient production of the hormone insulin, which is needed by the body to get energy from sugar and carbohydrate foods.

ACTION Your doctor will take a blood sample to check your child's blood sugar level. If the diagnosis of diabetes is confirmed, you will be given advice on your child's diet and lifestyle (*see* DIABETES MELLITUS, p.145). Your child will also need to have drug treatment with insulin injections for the rest of his or her life.

Continued from previous page, column 1

Continued from previous page, column 2

Is your child a boy, and does his foreskin balloon when he passes urine? **YES** / **NO**

Is your child excited, anxious, or cold? **YES** / **NO**

POSSIBLE CAUSE AND ACTION It is normal to need to pass urine more frequently in times of excitement or anxiety or when exposed to cold temperatures. If your child continues to pass urine frequently after his or her situation returns to normal, consult your doctor.

CONSULT YOUR DOCTOR IF YOU ARE UNABLE TO MAKE A DIAGNOSIS FROM THIS CHART.

POSSIBLE CAUSE Your child may have phimosis, in which the opening in the foreskin is too small.

Go to chart **45** GENITAL PROBLEMS IN BOYS (p.126)

Is your child's urine discoloured? **YES** / **NO**

POSSIBLE CAUSES AND ACTION Some foods, such as beetroot, and some drugs may temporarily change the colour of urine. The colour will return to normal once the food or drug is stopped. Rarely, however, a change in colour indicates liver or kidney disease or is due to blood in the urine. If you cannot clearly identify a dietary cause, consult your doctor, taking a sample of your child's urine with you. The doctor will test it for the presence of abnormal substances, including blood.

Does your child have problems with bladder control? **YES** / **NO**

Does your child regularly wet himself or herself during the day and/or at night? **YES** / **NO**

Go to chart **44** TOILET-TRAINING PROBLEMS (p.124)

CONSULT YOUR DOCTOR IF YOU ARE UNABLE TO MAKE A DIAGNOSIS FROM THIS CHART.

Is your child reluctant or unable to pass urine? **YES** / **NO**

CONSULT YOUR DOCTOR IF YOU ARE UNABLE TO MAKE A DIAGNOSIS FROM THIS CHART.

Investigating the urinary tract in children

If your child has had a urinary tract infection (*see* URINARY TRACT INFECTIONS IN CHILDHOOD, opposite), he or she will probably be referred for further tests to check kidney and bladder function and to exclude damage from urinary reflux, in which urine flows back towards the kidneys when the bladder is emptied.

In many cases, ultrasound scanning (p.39) is all that is needed. This quick and painless procedure is performed to check that the kidneys and bladder are of normal size.

In some cases, your child may also need DMSA scanning, a procedure that provides extra information on kidney functioning. It will establish whether he or she has urinary reflux. During the procedure, a very small amount of a radioactive substance called DMSA is given to the child by an intravenous injection. After the DMSA has passed into the urinary system, detailed images of the kidneys can be taken with a gamma camera and viewed on a computer monitor. The DMSA will be excreted in the urine and will be gone within 24 hours. It will not harm your child.

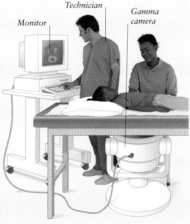

Technician — *Gamma camera* — *Monitor*

DMSA scanning
Your child will be scanned approximately 2 hours after an injection of DMSA. The gamma camera picks up radioactivity released by the kidneys and produces a picture on a monitor.

CALL YOUR DOCTOR NOW

POSSIBLE CAUSES Local soreness or severe constipation are possible causes. In some cases, a urinary infection (opposite) may be causing pain on passing urine, and your child may be reluctant to try to pass urine again. A child who feels a strong urge to pass urine but is unable to do so needs urgent medical help.

ACTION Your doctor will examine your child to try to establish the cause of the problem. He or she may suggest painkillers and suggest you encourage your child to pass urine while he or she is in a warm bath. If this fails, your child may need hospital admission.

44 Toilet-training problems

Most children gain full control over their bladder and bowel functions between the ages of 2 and 5 years. Few children have reliable control before the age of 2 years, and few have problems, apart from the occasional "accident", after the age of 5. However, the age at which an individual child masters the different skills of toilet training such as night-time control varies widely. It is not known why some children learn later than others, but it is seldom due to an unwillingness to learn.

Changes in circumstances, such as a new baby in the family or starting school, may make a child anxious and delay toilet training. Children whose parents were late to learn may also be later in learning reliable control. Unless there is a physical problem, toilet training occurs naturally, and the process cannot be speeded up by pressure from parents. Consult this chart if you are concerned about your child's ability to control his or her bladder or bowels.

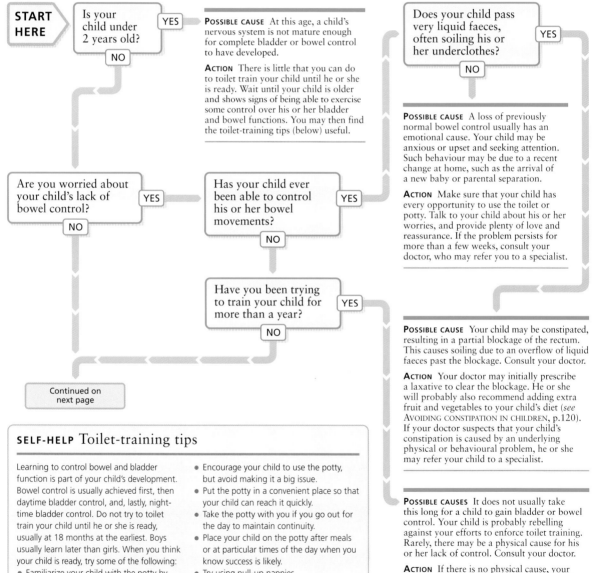

START HERE

Is your child under 2 years old? — YES

POSSIBLE CAUSE At this age, a child's nervous system is not mature enough for complete bladder or bowel control to have developed.

ACTION There is little that you can do to toilet train your child until he or she is ready. Wait until your child is older and shows signs of being able to exercise some control over his or her bladder and bowel functions. You may then find the toilet-training tips (below) useful.

Are you worried about your child's lack of bowel control? — YES

Has your child ever been able to control his or her bowel movements? — YES

Have you been trying to train your child for more than a year? — YES

Does your child pass very liquid faeces, often soiling his or her underclothes? — YES

POSSIBLE CAUSE A loss of previously normal bowel control usually has an emotional cause. Your child may be anxious or upset and seeking attention. Such behaviour may be due to a recent change at home, such as the arrival of a new baby or parental separation.

ACTION Make sure that your child has every opportunity to use the toilet or potty. Talk to your child about his or her worries, and provide plenty of love and reassurance. If the problem persists for more than a few weeks, consult your doctor, who may refer you to a specialist.

POSSIBLE CAUSE Your child may be constipated, resulting in a partial blockage of the rectum. This causes soiling due to an overflow of liquid faeces past the blockage. Consult your doctor.

ACTION Your doctor may initially prescribe a laxative to clear the blockage. He or she will probably also recommend adding extra fruit and vegetables to your child's diet (*see* AVOIDING CONSTIPATION IN CHILDREN, p.120). If your doctor suspects that your child's constipation is caused by an underlying physical or behavioural problem, he or she may refer your child to a specialist.

POSSIBLE CAUSES It does not usually take this long for a child to gain bladder or bowel control. Your child is probably rebelling against your efforts to enforce toilet training. Rarely, there may be a physical cause for his or her lack of control. Consult your doctor.

ACTION If there is no physical cause, your doctor may suggest that you have a break from toilet training. Ideally, wait until your child is keen to cooperate before trying again.

Continued on next page

SELF-HELP Toilet-training tips

Learning to control bowel and bladder function is part of your child's development. Bowel control is usually achieved first, then daytime bladder control, and, lastly, night-time bladder control. Do not try to toilet train your child until he or she is ready, usually at 18 months at the earliest. Boys usually learn later than girls. When you think your child is ready, try some of the following:

- Familiarize your child with the potty by sitting him or her on it during nappy changes or while you are on the toilet.
- Encourage your child to use the potty, but avoid making it a big issue.
- Put the potty in a convenient place so that your child can reach it quickly.
- Take the potty with you if you go out for the day to maintain continuity.
- Place your child on the potty after meals or at particular times of the day when you know success is likely.
- Try using pull-up nappies.
- Once your child is using the potty reliably, progress to using a child seat on the toilet.

Continued from previous page

Are you worried about your child's lack of bladder control? YES

NO

CONSULT YOUR DOCTOR IF YOU ARE UNABLE TO FIND A CAUSE FOR YOUR CHILD'S PROBLEM FROM THIS CHART.

SELF-HELP Overcoming bedwetting

If your child regularly wets the bed, try to be patient. Reassure your child that you are not angry and that he or she will learn to stay dry through the night. Encourage him or her to use the toilet before going to bed, and perhaps also wake your child to use the toilet when you go to bed. A chart on which you award your child a star after each dry night may help. For children over 7 years who regularly wet the bed, a pad-and-buzzer system may be advised, but such systems should only be used under medical supervision and if all other methods have failed.

Pad and buzzer system
A moisture-detecting pad is wired to a buzzer, which wakes the child as soon as he or she has wet the bed. In time, the child learns to wake before the buzzer goes off.

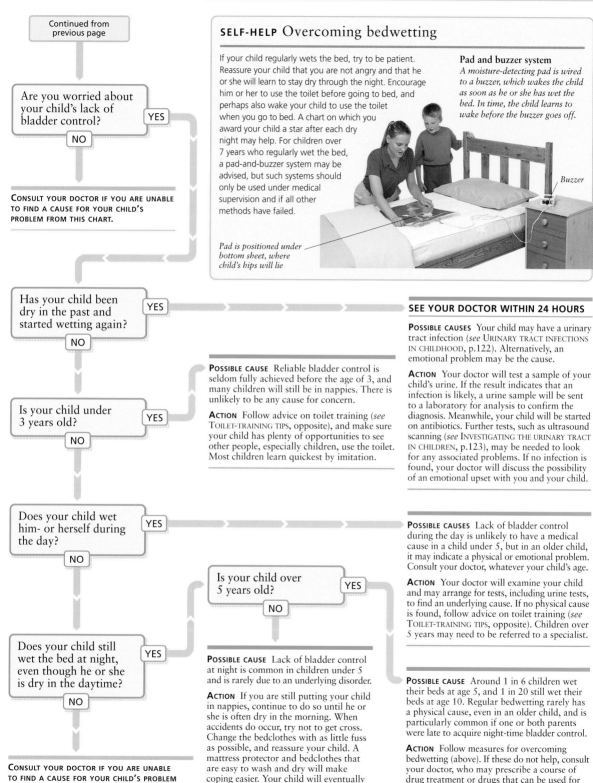

Buzzer

Pad is positioned under bottom sheet, where child's hips will lie

---

Has your child been dry in the past and started wetting again? YES

NO

Is your child under 3 years old? YES

NO

POSSIBLE CAUSE Reliable bladder control is seldom fully achieved before the age of 3, and many children will still be in nappies. There is unlikely to be any cause for concern.

ACTION Follow advice on toilet training (*see* TOILET-TRAINING TIPS, opposite), and make sure your child has plenty of opportunities to see other people, especially children, use the toilet. Most children learn quickest by imitation.

SEE YOUR DOCTOR WITHIN 24 HOURS

POSSIBLE CAUSES Your child may have a urinary tract infection (*see* URINARY TRACT INFECTIONS IN CHILDHOOD, p.122). Alternatively, an emotional problem may be the cause.

ACTION Your doctor will test a sample of your child's urine. If the result indicates that an infection is likely, a urine sample will be sent to a laboratory for analysis to confirm the diagnosis. Meanwhile, your child will be started on antibiotics. Further tests, such as ultrasound scanning (*see* INVESTIGATING THE URINARY TRACT IN CHILDREN, p.123), may be needed to look for any associated problems. If no infection is found, your doctor will discuss the possibility of an emotional upset with you and your child.

Does your child wet him- or herself during the day? YES

NO

Is your child over 5 years old? YES

NO

Does your child still wet the bed at night, even though he or she is dry in the daytime? YES

NO

POSSIBLE CAUSE Lack of bladder control at night is common in children under 5 and is rarely due to an underlying disorder.

ACTION If you are still putting your child in nappies, continue to do so until he or she is often dry in the morning. When accidents do occur, try not to get cross. Change the bedclothes with as little fuss as possible, and reassure your child. A mattress protector and bedclothes that are easy to wash and dry will make coping easier. Your child will eventually achieve night-time control.

POSSIBLE CAUSES Lack of bladder control during the day is unlikely to have a medical cause in a child under 5, but in an older child, it may indicate a physical or emotional problem. Consult your doctor, whatever your child's age.

ACTION Your doctor will examine your child and may arrange for tests, including urine tests, to find an underlying cause. If no physical cause is found, follow advice on toilet training (*see* TOILET-TRAINING TIPS, opposite). Children over 5 years may need to be referred to a specialist.

POSSIBLE CAUSE Around 1 in 6 children wet their beds at age 5, and 1 in 20 still wet their beds at age 10. Regular bedwetting rarely has a physical cause, even in an older child, and is particularly common if one or both parents were late to acquire night-time bladder control.

ACTION Follow measures for overcoming bedwetting (above). If these do not help, consult your doctor, who may prescribe a course of drug treatment or drugs that can be used for events such as an overnight school trip.

CONSULT YOUR DOCTOR IF YOU ARE UNABLE TO FIND A CAUSE FOR YOUR CHILD'S PROBLEM FROM THIS CHART.

45 Genital problems in boys

Consult this chart if your child develops a painful or swollen penis or a problem with his scrotum (the supportive bag that encloses the testes). Although most genital problems in boys are due to minor infections, you should always consult your doctor promptly if your child develops a problem in the genital area. In some cases, a delay in treatment can have serious consequences – for example, it may lead to problems with your child's fertility in the future.

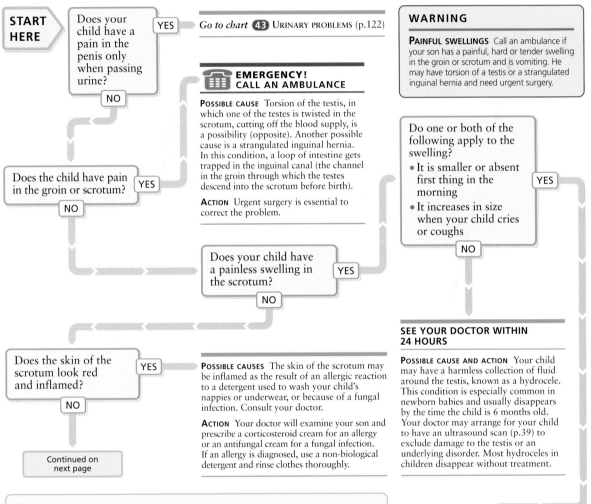

START HERE

Does your child have a pain in the penis only when passing urine?

YES → Go to chart **43** URINARY PROBLEMS (p.122)

NO

Does the child have pain in the groin or scrotum?

YES →

☎ EMERGENCY! CALL AN AMBULANCE

POSSIBLE CAUSE Torsion of the testis, in which one of the testes is twisted in the scrotum, cutting off the blood supply, is a possibility (opposite). Another possible cause is a strangulated inguinal hernia. In this condition, a loop of intestine gets trapped in the inguinal canal (the channel in the groin through which the testes descend into the scrotum before birth).

ACTION Urgent surgery is essential to correct the problem.

NO

Does your child have a painless swelling in the scrotum?

YES →

NO

Does the skin of the scrotum look red and inflamed?

YES →

POSSIBLE CAUSES The skin of the scrotum may be inflamed as the result of an allergic reaction to a detergent used to wash your child's nappies or underwear, or because of a fungal infection. Consult your doctor.

ACTION Your doctor will examine your son and prescribe a corticosteroid cream for an allergy or an antifungal cream for a fungal infection. If an allergy is diagnosed, use a non-biological detergent and rinse clothes thoroughly.

NO

Continued on next page

WARNING

PAINFUL SWELLINGS Call an ambulance if your son has a painful, hard or tender swelling in the groin or scrotum and is vomiting. He may have torsion of a testis or a strangulated inguinal hernia and need urgent surgery.

Do one or both of the following apply to the swelling?
- It is smaller or absent first thing in the morning
- It increases in size when your child cries or coughs

YES →

NO

SEE YOUR DOCTOR WITHIN 24 HOURS

POSSIBLE CAUSE AND ACTION Your child may have a harmless collection of fluid around the testis, known as a hydrocele. This condition is especially common in newborn babies and usually disappears by the time the child is 6 months old. Your doctor may arrange for your child to have an ultrasound scan (p.39) to exclude damage to the testis or an underlying disorder. Most hydroceles in children disappear without treatment.

SEE YOUR DOCTOR WITHIN 24 HOURS

POSSIBLE CAUSE Your child probably has a hernia, in which a loop of intestine bulges through a weak area in the abdominal wall. This condition is most common in babies. If the swelling becomes painful, call an ambulance.

ACTION If the diagnosis is confirmed, the weak area should be repaired to avoid the risk of a strangulated hernia, in which a loop of intestine gets trapped in the gap in the abdominal wall.

Circumcision

Circumcision is a surgical operation to remove the foreskin, which is the fold of skin that covers the tip of the penis. In the UK, most circumcisions are carried out for religious reasons. However, in some cases, circumcision may also be recommended if a child's foreskin is too tight or if a child has recurrent infections of the penis. In the past, circumcision was often performed routinely in childhood in the belief that it would improve hygiene, but this practice is no longer recommended.

In newborn boys, circumcision is most often carried out under local anaesthetic, whereas in older boys or in men it is usually performed under general anaesthetic.

During the operation, most of the foreskin is cut away. The remnant of the foreskin that remains is then stitched to the skin just behind the head of the penis, leaving the head uncovered. No dressing is needed while the wound heals. The stitches will either dissolve or fall out after a few days.

Continued from previous page

Torsion of the testis

Twisting (torsion) of the testis within the scrotum reduces or stops the blood supply to the testis. It can affect males of any age but is most common in boys around age 10. The symptoms can start during sleep or following an injury and include pain in the scrotum, groin, and/or abdomen and redness and tenderness of the scrotum. There may also be associated nausea and/or vomiting. Torsion of the testis requires urgent surgery in order to prevent permanent damage to the testis. During surgery, the blood vessels are untwisted and then both of the testes are anchored to the scrotum with stitches to prevent recurrence of the condition.

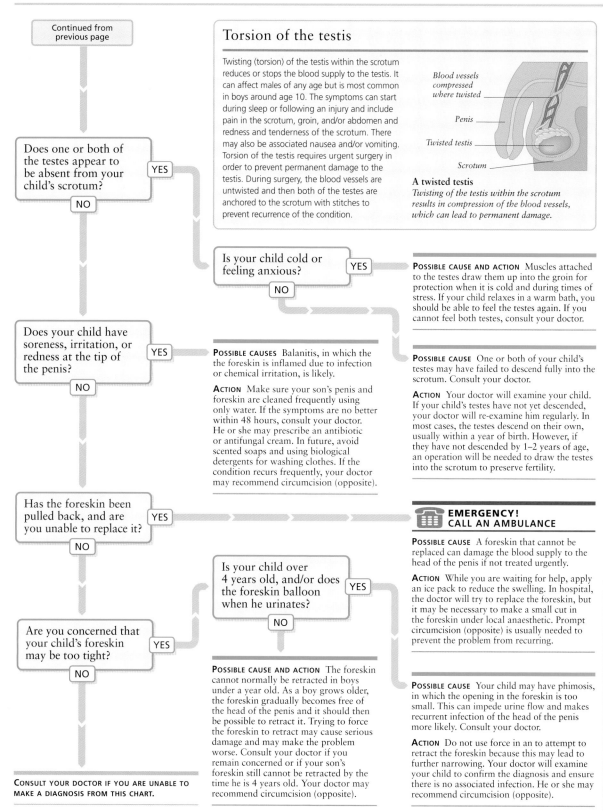

Blood vessels compressed where twisted

Penis

Twisted testis

Scrotum

A twisted testis
Twisting of the testis within the scrotum results in compression of the blood vessels, which can lead to permanent damage.

Does one or both of the testes appear to be absent from your child's scrotum? — YES

NO

Is your child cold or feeling anxious? — YES

NO

POSSIBLE CAUSE AND ACTION Muscles attached to the testes draw them up into the groin for protection when it is cold and during times of stress. If your child relaxes in a warm bath, you should be able to feel the testes again. If you cannot feel both testes, consult your doctor.

Does your child have soreness, irritation, or redness at the tip of the penis? — YES

NO

POSSIBLE CAUSES Balanitis, in which the the foreskin is inflamed due to infection or chemical irritation, is likely.

ACTION Make sure your son's penis and foreskin are cleaned frequently using only water. If the symptoms are no better within 48 hours, consult your doctor. He or she may prescribe an antibiotic or antifungal cream. In future, avoid scented soaps and using biological detergents for washing clothes. If the condition recurs frequently, your doctor may recommend circumcision (opposite).

POSSIBLE CAUSE One or both of your child's testes may have failed to descend fully into the scrotum. Consult your doctor.

ACTION Your doctor will examine your child. If your child's testes have not yet descended, your doctor will re-examine him regularly. In most cases, the testes descend on their own, usually within a year of birth. However, if they have not descended by 1–2 years of age, an operation will be needed to draw the testes into the scrotum to preserve fertility.

Has the foreskin been pulled back, and are you unable to replace it? — YES

NO

📞 **EMERGENCY!
CALL AN AMBULANCE**

POSSIBLE CAUSE A foreskin that cannot be replaced can damage the blood supply to the head of the penis if not treated urgently.

ACTION While you are waiting for help, apply an ice pack to reduce the swelling. In hospital, the doctor will try to replace the foreskin, but it may be necessary to make a small cut in the foreskin under local anaesthetic. Prompt circumcision (opposite) is usually needed to prevent the problem from recurring.

Is your child over 4 years old, and/or does the foreskin balloon when he urinates? — YES

NO

Are you concerned that your child's foreskin may be too tight? — YES

NO

POSSIBLE CAUSE AND ACTION The foreskin cannot normally be retracted in boys under a year old. As a boy grows older, the foreskin gradually becomes free of the head of the penis and it should then be possible to retract it. Trying to force the foreskin to retract may cause serious damage and may make the problem worse. Consult your doctor if you remain concerned or if your son's foreskin still cannot be retracted by the time he is 4 years old. Your doctor may recommend circumcision (opposite).

POSSIBLE CAUSE Your child may have phimosis, in which the opening in the foreskin is too small. This can impede urine flow and makes recurrent infection of the head of the penis more likely. Consult your doctor.

ACTION Do not use force in an to attempt to retract the foreskin because this may lead to further narrowing. Your doctor will examine your child to confirm the diagnosis and ensure there is no associated infection. He or she may recommend circumcision (opposite).

CONSULT YOUR DOCTOR IF YOU ARE UNABLE TO MAKE A DIAGNOSIS FROM THIS CHART.

46 Genital problems in girls

The most common genital problems in young girls are itching, inflammation of the external genital area, and, less commonly, an unusual discharge, possibly with pain on passing urine.

These symptoms may be caused by a minor infection or by irritation from toiletries or laundry products. Consult this chart if your daughter complains of any of these symptoms.

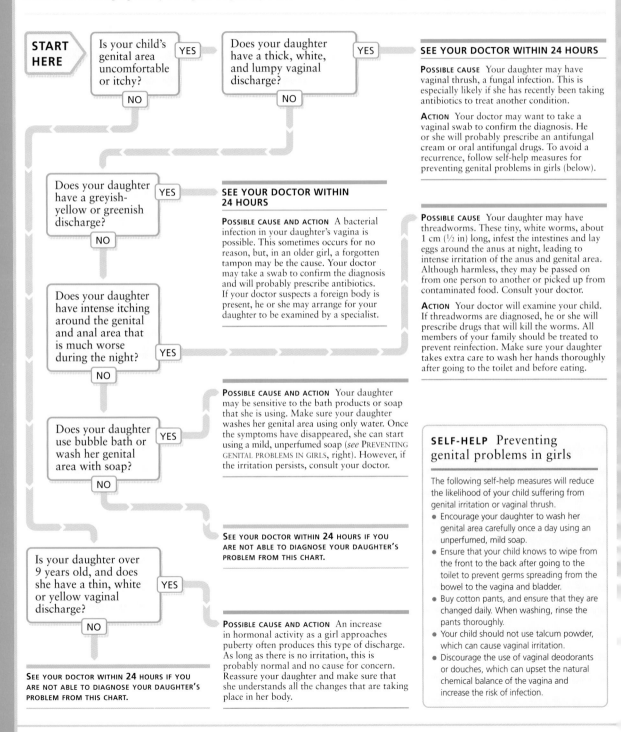

START HERE

Is your child's genital area uncomfortable or itchy? — **YES** → Does your daughter have a thick, white, and lumpy vaginal discharge? — **YES** →

NO ↓ (child's genital area)

NO ↓ (thick, white discharge)

SEE YOUR DOCTOR WITHIN 24 HOURS

POSSIBLE CAUSE Your daughter may have vaginal thrush, a fungal infection. This is especially likely if she has recently been taking antibiotics to treat another condition.

ACTION Your doctor may want to take a vaginal swab to confirm the diagnosis. He or she will probably prescribe an antifungal cream or oral antifungal drugs. To avoid a recurrence, follow self-help measures for preventing genital problems in girls (below).

Does your daughter have a greyish-yellow or greenish discharge? — **YES** →

NO ↓

SEE YOUR DOCTOR WITHIN 24 HOURS

POSSIBLE CAUSE AND ACTION A bacterial infection in your daughter's vagina is possible. This sometimes occurs for no reason, but, in an older girl, a forgotten tampon may be the cause. Your doctor may take a swab to confirm the diagnosis and will probably prescribe antibiotics. If your doctor suspects a foreign body is present, he or she may arrange for your daughter to be examined by a specialist.

POSSIBLE CAUSE Your daughter may have threadworms. These tiny, white worms, about 1 cm (½ in) long, infest the intestines and lay eggs around the anus at night, leading to intense irritation of the anus and genital area. Although harmless, they may be passed on from one person to another or picked up from contaminated food. Consult your doctor.

ACTION Your doctor will examine your child. If threadworms are diagnosed, he or she will prescribe drugs that will kill the worms. All members of your family should be treated to prevent reinfection. Make sure your daughter takes extra care to wash her hands thoroughly after going to the toilet and before eating.

Does your daughter have intense itching around the genital and anal area that is much worse during the night? — **YES** →

NO ↓

Does your daughter use bubble bath or wash her genital area with soap? — **YES** →

NO ↓

POSSIBLE CAUSE AND ACTION Your daughter may be sensitive to the bath products or soap that she is using. Make sure your daughter washes her genital area using only water. Once the symptoms have disappeared, she can start using a mild, unperfumed soap (see PREVENTING GENITAL PROBLEMS IN GIRLS, right). However, if the irritation persists, consult your doctor.

SEE YOUR DOCTOR WITHIN 24 HOURS IF YOU ARE NOT ABLE TO DIAGNOSE YOUR DAUGHTER'S PROBLEM FROM THIS CHART.

Is your daughter over 9 years old, and does she have a thin, white or yellow vaginal discharge? — **YES** →

NO ↓

POSSIBLE CAUSE AND ACTION An increase in hormonal activity as a girl approaches puberty often produces this type of discharge. As long as there is no irritation, this is probably normal and no cause for concern. Reassure your daughter and make sure that she understands all the changes that are taking place in her body.

SEE YOUR DOCTOR WITHIN 24 HOURS IF YOU ARE NOT ABLE TO DIAGNOSE YOUR DAUGHTER'S PROBLEM FROM THIS CHART.

SELF-HELP Preventing genital problems in girls

The following self-help measures will reduce the likelihood of your child suffering from genital irritation or vaginal thrush.

- Encourage your daughter to wash her genital area carefully once a day using an unperfumed, mild soap.
- Ensure that your child knows to wipe from the front to the back after going to the toilet to prevent germs spreading from the bowel to the vagina and bladder.
- Buy cotton pants, and ensure that they are changed daily. When washing, rinse the pants thoroughly.
- Your child should not use talcum powder, which can cause vaginal irritation.
- Discourage the use of vaginal deodorants or douches, which can upset the natural chemical balance of the vagina and increase the risk of infection.

47 Painful arm or leg

Consult this chart if your child complains of pain in the arms and/or legs. Parents often attribute a recurrent ache in a child's limb to growing pains (below). However, minor injuries are a more likely cause. Sprains and strains are not usually serious; however, a broken bone (fracture) needs immediate medical attention. Cramp is another common cause of limb pain, but it can be relieved by self-help: gently massage and stretch the affected muscle and apply a wrapped hot-water bottle if necessary. Any pain that has no obvious cause or that persists should be brought to your doctor's attention.

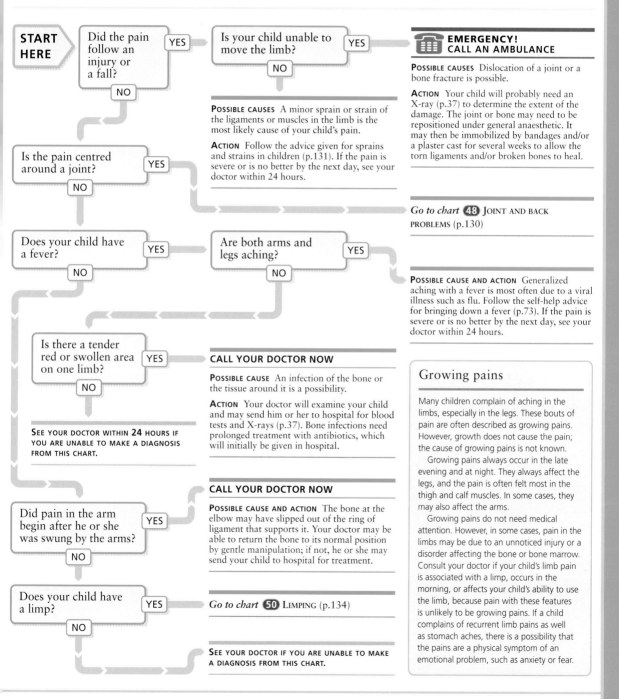

START HERE

Did the pain follow an injury or a fall? — YES → **Is your child unable to move the limb?** — YES →

NO ↓ (from injury)

NO ↓ (unable to move)

POSSIBLE CAUSES A minor sprain or strain of the ligaments or muscles in the limb is the most likely cause of your child's pain.

ACTION Follow the advice given for sprains and strains in children (p.131). If the pain is severe or is no better by the next day, see your doctor within 24 hours.

Is the pain centred around a joint? — YES →

NO ↓

Does your child have a fever? — YES → **Are both arms and legs aching?** — YES →

NO ↓   NO ↓

Is there a tender red or swollen area on one limb? — YES →

NO ↓

SEE YOUR DOCTOR WITHIN **24** HOURS IF YOU ARE UNABLE TO MAKE A DIAGNOSIS FROM THIS CHART.

Did pain in the arm begin after he or she was swung by the arms? — YES →

NO ↓

Does your child have a limp? — YES →

NO ↓

SEE YOUR DOCTOR IF YOU ARE UNABLE TO MAKE A DIAGNOSIS FROM THIS CHART.

Right column boxes

📞 **EMERGENCY! CALL AN AMBULANCE**

POSSIBLE CAUSES Dislocation of a joint or a bone fracture is possible.

ACTION Your child will probably need an X-ray (p.37) to determine the extent of the damage. The joint or bone may need to be repositioned under general anaesthetic. It may then be immobilized by bandages and/or a plaster cast for several weeks to allow the torn ligaments and/or broken bones to heal.

Go to chart **48** JOINT AND BACK PROBLEMS (p.130)

POSSIBLE CAUSE AND ACTION Generalized aching with a fever is most often due to a viral illness such as flu. Follow the self-help advice for bringing down a fever (p.73). If the pain is severe or is no better by the next day, see your doctor within 24 hours.

CALL YOUR DOCTOR NOW

POSSIBLE CAUSE An infection of the bone or the tissue around it is a possibility.

ACTION Your doctor will examine your child and may send him or her to hospital for blood tests and X-rays (p.37). Bone infections need prolonged treatment with antibiotics, which will initially be given in hospital.

CALL YOUR DOCTOR NOW

POSSIBLE CAUSE AND ACTION The bone at the elbow may have slipped out of the ring of ligament that supports it. Your doctor may be able to return the bone to its normal position by gentle manipulation; if not, he or she may send your child to hospital for treatment.

Go to chart **50** LIMPING (p.134)

Growing pains

Many children complain of aching in the limbs, especially in the legs. These bouts of pain are often described as growing pains. However, growth does not cause the pain; the cause of growing pains is not known.

Growing pains always occur in the late evening and at night. They always affect the legs, and the pain is often felt most in the thigh and calf muscles. In some cases, they may also affect the arms.

Growing pains do not need medical attention. However, in some cases, pain in the limbs may be due to an unnoticed injury or a disorder affecting the bone or bone marrow. Consult your doctor if your child's limb pain is associated with a limp, occurs in the morning, or affects your child's ability to use the limb, because pain with these features is unlikely to be growing pains. If a child complains of recurrent limb pains as well as stomach aches, there is a possibility that the pains are a physical symptom of an emotional problem, such as anxiety or fear.

48 Joint and back problems

Serious joint and back problems are uncommon in children. A painful or swollen joint is most often the result of a minor strain or sprain of the muscles and ligaments surrounding the joint. A more serious cause of joint pain or swelling is arthritis (joint inflammation). Arthritis is less common in children than in adults. However, in childhood the disease can also involve internal organs such as the heart and kidneys. Problems with the spine may be noticed for the first time in adolescence and need medical assessment. Severe back pain in a child of any age needs prompt medical attention.

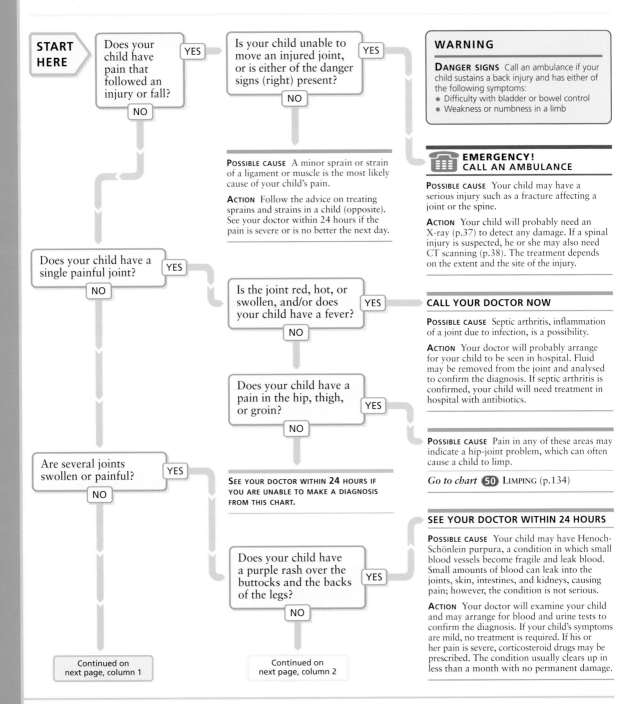

START HERE → Does your child have pain that followed an injury or fall? — **YES** → Is your child unable to move an injured joint, or is either of the danger signs (right) present? — **YES** →

NO ↓ (from first question)

NO ↓ (from second question)

POSSIBLE CAUSE A minor sprain or strain of a ligament or muscle is the most likely cause of your child's pain.

ACTION Follow the advice on treating sprains and strains in a child (opposite). See your doctor within 24 hours if the pain is severe or is no better the next day.

Does your child have a single painful joint? — **YES** →

NO ↓

Is the joint red, hot, or swollen, and/or does your child have a fever? — **YES** →

NO ↓

Does your child have a pain in the hip, thigh, or groin? — **YES** →

NO ↓

Are several joints swollen or painful? — **YES** →

NO ↓

SEE YOUR DOCTOR WITHIN **24** HOURS IF YOU ARE UNABLE TO MAKE A DIAGNOSIS FROM THIS CHART.

Does your child have a purple rash over the buttocks and the backs of the legs? — **YES** →

NO ↓

Continued on next page, column 1

Continued on next page, column 2

WARNING

DANGER SIGNS Call an ambulance if your child sustains a back injury and has either of the following symptoms:
- Difficulty with bladder or bowel control
- Weakness or numbness in a limb

📞 EMERGENCY! CALL AN AMBULANCE

POSSIBLE CAUSE Your child may have a serious injury such as a fracture affecting a joint or the spine.

ACTION Your child will probably need an X-ray (p.37) to detect any damage. If a spinal injury is suspected, he or she may also need CT scanning (p.38). The treatment depends on the extent and the site of the injury.

CALL YOUR DOCTOR NOW

POSSIBLE CAUSE Septic arthritis, inflammation of a joint due to infection, is a possibility.

ACTION Your doctor will probably arrange for your child to be seen in hospital. Fluid may be removed from the joint and analysed to confirm the diagnosis. If septic arthritis is confirmed, your child will need treatment in hospital with antibiotics.

POSSIBLE CAUSE Pain in any of these areas may indicate a hip-joint problem, which can often cause a child to limp.

Go to chart **50** LIMPING (p.134)

SEE YOUR DOCTOR WITHIN 24 HOURS

POSSIBLE CAUSE Your child may have Henoch-Schönlein purpura, a condition in which small blood vessels become fragile and leak blood. Small amounts of blood can leak into the joints, skin, intestines, and kidneys, causing pain; however, the condition is not serious.

ACTION Your doctor will examine your child and may arrange for blood and urine tests to confirm the diagnosis. If your child's symptoms are mild, no treatment is required. If his or her pain is severe, corticosteroid drugs may be prescribed. The condition usually clears up in less than a month with no permanent damage.

Continued from
previous page, column 1

Continued from
previous page, column 2

Are you concerned
that your child may
have a problem with
his or her back?

NO   **YES**

Does your child have
a fever, feel generally
unwell, and/or have
a blotchy rash?

YES   **NO**

SEE YOUR DOCTOR WITHIN 24 HOURS

POSSIBLE CAUSE AND ACTION Your child may
have systemic juvenile arthritis, in which the
immune system attacks the joints and, in some
cases, the internal organs. Your doctor will
probably refer your child to hospital for tests.
If the diagnosis is confirmed, treatment will
include nonsteroidal anti-inflammatory drugs
and, in some cases, corticosteroid drugs.

**CONSULT YOUR DOCTOR IF YOU ARE UNABLE
TO MAKE A DIAGNOSIS FROM THIS CHART.**

Has your child recently
had an infection, such
as a sore throat or a
chest infection?

YES   **NO**

SEE YOUR DOCTOR WITHIN 24 HOURS

POSSIBLE CAUSE AND ACTION Reactive arthritis,
inflammation of the joints in response to a
recent infection, is possible. Your doctor may
arrange for tests to confirm that the infection
has cleared up and may prescribe nonsteroidal
anti-inflammatory drugs. Reactive arthritis
usually improves within weeks.

Is your child woken in
the night by back pain,
or does he or she have
a stiff back on waking?

NO   **YES**

SEE YOUR DOCTOR WITHIN 24 HOURS

POSSIBLE CAUSES AND ACTION Your child may
have a serious problem such as a bone disorder
or arthritis of the spine. Your doctor will
probably arrange for X-rays (p.37) of the back
and blood tests to make a diagnosis and
determine the appropriate treatment.

SEE YOUR DOCTOR WITHIN 24 HOURS

POSSIBLE CAUSE Juvenile chronic arthritis, in
which the immune system attacks the joints
and, in some cases, the eyes, is possible.

ACTION Your child may be referred to hospital
for blood tests and a full eye examination.
Nonsteroidal anti-inflammatory drugs and
corticosteroids may be prescribed.

SELF-HELP Treating sprains and strains in a child

If your child has a sprain or strain or a deep
bruise, the appropriate treatment for the
injury can be remembered as RICE – Rest,
Ice, Compression, and Elevation (see TREATING
SPRAINS AND STRAINS, p.225). If necessary, give
your child the recommended dose of a
painkiller. If the injury is no better within
24 hours, consult your doctor.

Your child should avoid sports or any
unnecessary exercise involving the affected
part of the body until it is free from pain. If
necessary, write your child's school a note
explaining the problem.

Cold compress
*If your child has a sprain or
strain, a cold compress will
help reduce the swelling.*

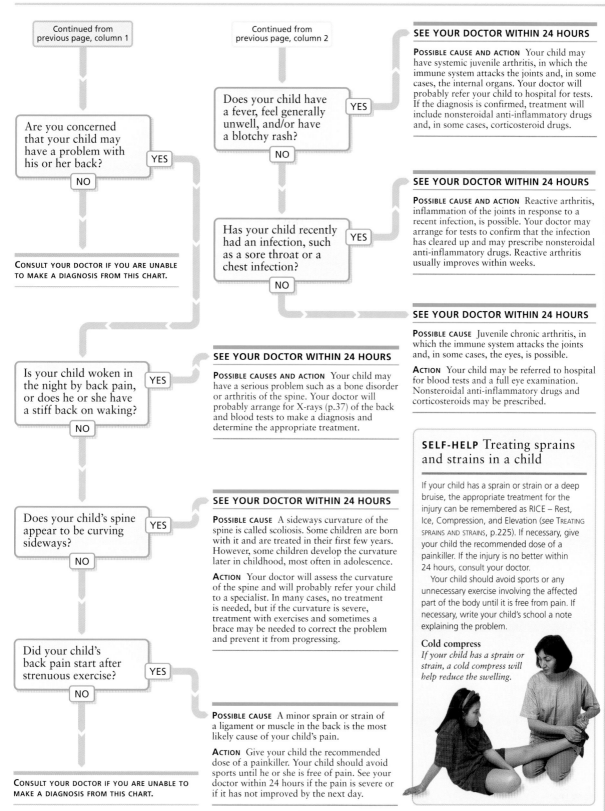

Does your child's spine
appear to be curving
sideways?

NO   **YES**

SEE YOUR DOCTOR WITHIN 24 HOURS

POSSIBLE CAUSE A sideways curvature of the
spine is called scoliosis. Some children are born
with it and are treated in their first few years.
However, some children develop the curvature
later in childhood, most often in adolescence.

ACTION Your doctor will assess the curvature
of the spine and will probably refer your child
to a specialist. In many cases, no treatment
is needed, but if the curvature is severe,
treatment with exercises and sometimes a
brace may be needed to correct the problem
and prevent it from progressing.

Did your child's
back pain start after
strenuous exercise?

NO   **YES**

POSSIBLE CAUSE A minor sprain or strain of
a ligament or muscle in the back is the most
likely cause of your child's pain.

ACTION Give your child the recommended
dose of a painkiller. Your child should avoid
sports until he or she is free of pain. See your
doctor within 24 hours if the pain is severe or
if it has not improved by the next day.

**CONSULT YOUR DOCTOR IF YOU ARE UNABLE TO
MAKE A DIAGNOSIS FROM THIS CHART.**

49 Foot problems

The bones in children's feet are soft, unlike bones in other parts of the body, and can be distorted by shoes that do not fit properly. Children's feet grow quickly, and you should check your child's shoes regularly. Children should not wear second-hand shoes. Feet can also be damaged by wearing high heels or shoes with pointed toes for any length of time.

Although wearing ill-fitting shoes may not cause symptoms at the time, it may result in foot problems later in life. Most symptoms affecting children's feet are caused by minor conditions, such as veruccas, and can be treated at home. However, if your child's foot is very painful or swollen or home treatment has been ineffective, consult your doctor.

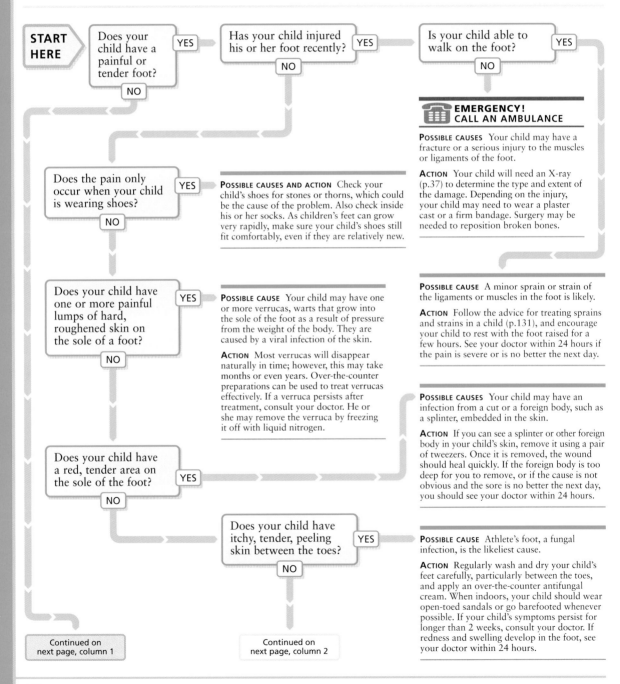

START HERE

Does your child have a painful or tender foot? — YES → **Has your child injured his or her foot recently?** — YES → **Is your child able to walk on the foot?** — YES

NO ↓ (from "painful or tender foot")

NO (from "injured recently")

NO (from "able to walk")

☎ **EMERGENCY! CALL AN AMBULANCE**

POSSIBLE CAUSES Your child may have a fracture or a serious injury to the muscles or ligaments of the foot.

ACTION Your child will need an X-ray (p.37) to determine the type and extent of the damage. Depending on the injury, your child may need to wear a plaster cast or a firm bandage. Surgery may be needed to reposition broken bones.

Does the pain only occur when your child is wearing shoes? — YES →

POSSIBLE CAUSES AND ACTION Check your child's shoes for stones or thorns, which could be the cause of the problem. Also check inside his or her socks. As children's feet can grow very rapidly, make sure your child's shoes still fit comfortably, even if they are relatively new.

NO ↓

POSSIBLE CAUSE A minor sprain or strain of the ligaments or muscles in the foot is likely.

ACTION Follow the advice for treating sprains and strains in a child (p.131), and encourage your child to rest with the foot raised for a few hours. See your doctor within 24 hours if the pain is severe or is no better the next day.

Does your child have one or more painful lumps of hard, roughened skin on the sole of a foot? — YES →

POSSIBLE CAUSE Your child may have one or more verrucas, warts that grow into the sole of the foot as a result of pressure from the weight of the body. They are caused by a viral infection of the skin.

ACTION Most verrucas will disappear naturally in time; however, this may take months or even years. Over-the-counter preparations can be used to treat verrucas effectively. If a verruca persists after treatment, consult your doctor. He or she may remove the verruca by freezing it off with liquid nitrogen.

NO ↓

POSSIBLE CAUSES Your child may have an infection from a cut or a foreign body, such as a splinter, embedded in the skin.

ACTION If you can see a splinter or other foreign body in your child's skin, remove it using a pair of tweezers. Once it is removed, the wound should heal quickly. If the foreign body is too deep for you to remove, or if the cause is not obvious and the sore is no better the next day, you should see your doctor within 24 hours.

Does your child have a red, tender area on the sole of the foot? — YES →

NO ↓

Does your child have itchy, tender, peeling skin between the toes? — YES →

POSSIBLE CAUSE Athlete's foot, a fungal infection, is the likeliest cause.

ACTION Regularly wash and dry your child's feet carefully, particularly between the toes, and apply an over-the-counter antifungal cream. When indoors, your child should wear open-toed sandals or go barefooted whenever possible. If your child's symptoms persist for longer than 2 weeks, consult your doctor. If redness and swelling develop in the foot, see your doctor within 24 hours.

NO ↓

Continued on next page, column 1

Continued on next page, column 2

Continued from previous page, column 1

Continued from previous page, column 2

POSSIBLE CAUSE An infected ingrowing toenail is a likely cause. This may be the result of cutting the toenails incorrectly or wearing shoes that are too tight. Consult your doctor.

ACTION Your doctor may prescribe antibiotics and drain any pus under a local anaesthetic. Surgery is sometimes recommended to remove part or all of the toenail (*see* REMOVAL OF AN INGROWING TOENAIL, p.232). To prevent ingrowing toenails, your child should always wear correctly fitting shoes or, if practical, open-toed sandals. Keep the affected area clean and dry, and always cut the toenails straight across rather than in a curve.

Are you concerned about the appearance of your child's feet? **NO** / **YES**

Does your child have a red, tender swelling around the big toenail? **NO** / **YES**

CONSULT YOUR DOCTOR IF YOU ARE UNABLE TO MAKE A DIAGNOSIS FROM THIS CHART.

CONSULT YOUR DOCTOR IF YOU ARE UNABLE TO MAKE A DIAGNOSIS FROM THIS CHART.

Does the whole foot including the heel turn inwards, and has it been like this since birth? **NO** / **YES**

POSSIBLE CAUSES The shape of your child's foot may be due to an abnormality in the structure of the bones in the foot or to the position of the baby's foot when it was in the uterus. It is usually noticed by a doctor when the child is born. Consult your doctor.

ACTION If the shape of the foot has resulted from its position in the uterus, it should correct itself within a few weeks of birth. If the shape of the foot is due to a structural abnormality, treatment will consist of manipulation and the use of a splint. If this has not corrected the problem by 3 years of age, an operation may be needed.

Does one or both of your child's feet turn inwards? **NO** / **YES**

POSSIBLE CAUSE AND ACTION Your child may have a condition called "intoeing". This is usually noticed when a child begins to walk and is often caused by the inward rotation of the whole leg from the hip or by bow legs, both of which are normal in some children. Consult your doctor so that the diagnosis can be confirmed. This condition rarely needs treatment. Bow legs usually correct themselves by the age of 3 years, while hip rotation usually corrects itself by the age of 8 years. In rare cases, an operation is needed to correct the problem.

Are you concerned that your child may have flat feet? **NO** / **YES**

POSSIBLE CAUSE AND ACTION Children under 3 years of age usually have flat feet because the muscles, ligaments, and bones in their feet are not yet fully developed. The fat pad in the feet of young children also adds to this appearance. There is no cause for concern at this age because a normal arch will probably develop as your child grows.

Is your child under 3 years old? **NO** / **YES**

Are your child's toes bent or curled under? **NO** / **YES**

CONSULT YOUR DOCTOR IF YOU ARE UNABLE TO MAKE A DIAGNOSIS FROM THIS CHART.

POSSIBLE CAUSES AND ACTION If your child was born with bent toes, there is probably no cause for concern. If they lead to pain or embarrassment, however, an operation to straighten the toes may be recommended when your child is older. If the condition has developed recently, your child's shoes and/or socks may be too small. Make sure your child always wears well-fitting shoes and socks.

POSSIBLE CAUSE AND ACTION Flat feet are often inherited. In this condition, ligaments in the foot are lax and only form an arch when the child stands on tiptoes. Flat feet are rarely a cause for concern and do not prevent a child from doing well in sports or cause problems in the future. Special exercises and shoe inserts are almost always ineffective and unnecessary. If your child's feet are painful or if you are worried, consult your doctor.

50 Limping

For limping due to a painful foot, see chart 49, FOOT
PROBLEMS **(p. 132).**
A limp or reluctance to walk may be the first sign of a problem
in a child who is too young to explain that something is

wrong. A minor injury that causes a limp may get better
on its own. However, any child with a limp, even a painless
one, should be seen by a doctor within 24 hours. There may
be an underlying disorder that requires prompt treatment.

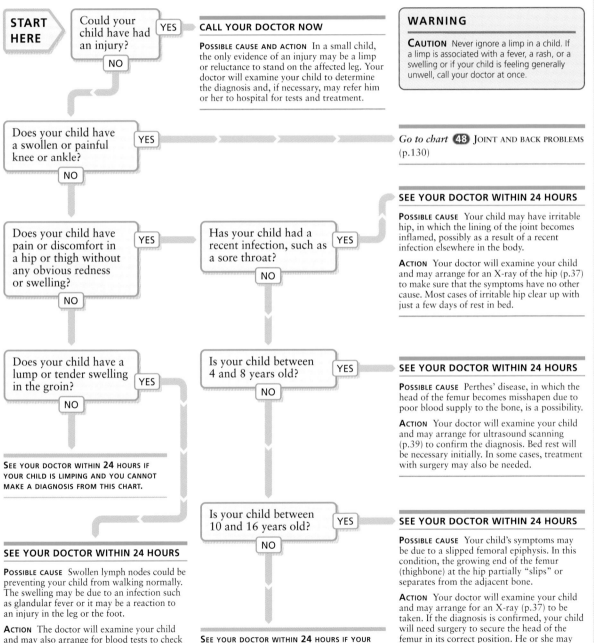

START HERE

Could your child have had an injury? — **YES** →

CALL YOUR DOCTOR NOW

POSSIBLE CAUSE AND ACTION In a small child,
the only evidence of an injury may be a limp
or reluctance to stand on the affected leg. Your
doctor will examine your child to determine
the diagnosis and, if necessary, may refer him
or her to hospital for tests and treatment.

WARNING

CAUTION Never ignore a limp in a child. If
a limp is associated with a fever, a rash, or a
swelling or if your child is feeling generally
unwell, call your doctor at once.

NO ↓

Does your child have a swollen or painful knee or ankle? — **YES** →

Go to chart **48** JOINT AND BACK PROBLEMS
(p.130)

NO ↓

Does your child have pain or discomfort in a hip or thigh without any obvious redness or swelling? — **YES** →

Has your child had a recent infection, such as a sore throat? — **YES** →

SEE YOUR DOCTOR WITHIN 24 HOURS

POSSIBLE CAUSE Your child may have irritable
hip, in which the lining of the joint becomes
inflamed, possibly as a result of a recent
infection elsewhere in the body.

ACTION Your doctor will examine your child
and may arrange for an X-ray of the hip (p.37)
to make sure that the symptoms have no other
cause. Most cases of irritable hip clear up with
just a few days of rest in bed.

NO ↓ (of infection question)

NO ↓ (of hip/thigh question)

Does your child have a lump or tender swelling in the groin? — **YES** →

Is your child between 4 and 8 years old? — **YES** →

SEE YOUR DOCTOR WITHIN 24 HOURS

POSSIBLE CAUSE Perthes' disease, in which the
head of the femur becomes misshapen due to
poor blood supply to the bone, is a possibility.

ACTION Your doctor will examine your child
and may arrange for ultrasound scanning
(p.39) to confirm the diagnosis. Bed rest will
be necessary initially. In some cases, treatment
with surgery may also be needed.

NO ↓

**SEE YOUR DOCTOR WITHIN 24 HOURS IF
YOUR CHILD IS LIMPING AND YOU CANNOT
MAKE A DIAGNOSIS FROM THIS CHART.**

Is your child between 10 and 16 years old? — **YES** →

SEE YOUR DOCTOR WITHIN 24 HOURS

POSSIBLE CAUSE Your child's symptoms may
be due to a slipped femoral epiphysis. In this
condition, the growing end of the femur
(thighbone) at the hip partially "slips" or
separates from the adjacent bone.

ACTION Your doctor will examine your child
and may arrange for an X-ray (p.37) to be
taken. If the diagnosis is confirmed, your child
will need surgery to secure the head of the
femur in its correct position. He or she may
also need surgery on the other leg to prevent
the same problem from occurring.

NO ↓

**SEE YOUR DOCTOR WITHIN 24 HOURS IF YOUR
CHILD IS LIMPING AND YOU CANNOT MAKE A
DIAGNOSIS FROM THIS CHART.**

SEE YOUR DOCTOR WITHIN 24 HOURS

POSSIBLE CAUSE Swollen lymph nodes could be
preventing your child from walking normally.
The swelling may be due to an infection such
as glandular fever or it may be a reaction to
an injury in the leg or the foot.

ACTION The doctor will examine your child
and may also arrange for blood tests to check
for infection. If an injury has become infected,
antibiotics may be needed.

51 Adolescent weight problems

An adolescent needs more calories than an adult with a manual job. The rapid increase in height that occurs in adolescence and the development of adult body proportions sometimes leads a teenager to feel either too thin or too fat. Adolescence is a time when young people are particularly sensitive about their appearance, and as a result, it is a time when eating disorders, such as anorexia nervosa, are most likely to occur. Consult this chart if you are worried about your child's weight or if your child is outside the normal range for his or her height (see GROWTH CHARTS, p.26).

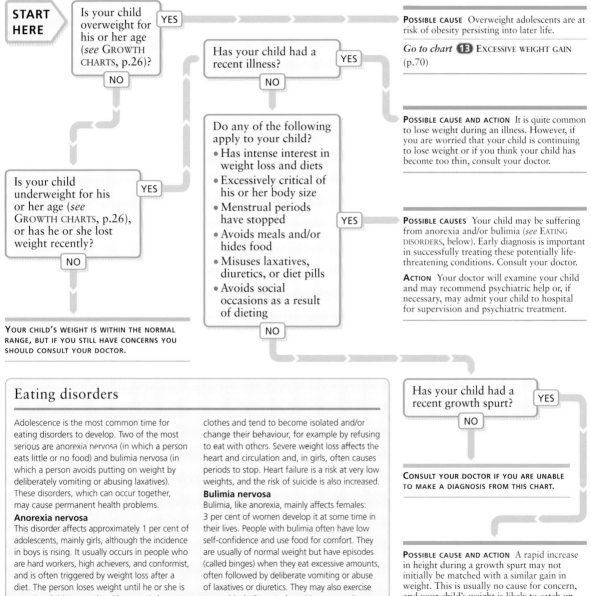

START HERE

Is your child overweight for his or her age (see GROWTH CHARTS, p.26)?

YES → **POSSIBLE CAUSE** Overweight adolescents are at risk of obesity persisting into later life.

Go to chart **13** EXCESSIVE WEIGHT GAIN (p.70)

NO

Has your child had a recent illness?

YES →

NO

POSSIBLE CAUSE AND ACTION It is quite common to lose weight during an illness. However, if you are worried that your child is continuing to lose weight or if you think your child has become too thin, consult your doctor.

Is your child underweight for his or her age (see GROWTH CHARTS, p.26), or has he or she lost weight recently?

YES →

Do any of the following apply to your child?
- Has intense interest in weight loss and diets
- Excessively critical of his or her body size
- Menstrual periods have stopped
- Avoids meals and/or hides food
- Misuses laxatives, diuretics, or diet pills
- Avoids social occasions as a result of dieting

YES →

POSSIBLE CAUSES Your child may be suffering from anorexia and/or bulimia (see EATING DISORDERS, below). Early diagnosis is important in successfully treating these potentially life-threatening conditions. Consult your doctor.

ACTION Your doctor will examine your child and may recommend psychiatric help or, if necessary, may admit your child to hospital for supervision and psychiatric treatment.

NO

YOUR CHILD'S WEIGHT IS WITHIN THE NORMAL RANGE, BUT IF YOU STILL HAVE CONCERNS YOU SHOULD CONSULT YOUR DOCTOR.

NO

Has your child had a recent growth spurt?

YES →

NO

CONSULT YOUR DOCTOR IF YOU ARE UNABLE TO MAKE A DIAGNOSIS FROM THIS CHART.

POSSIBLE CAUSE AND ACTION A rapid increase in height during a growth spurt may not initially be matched with a similar gain in weight. This is usually no cause for concern, and your child's weight is likely to catch up with his or her height over the next few months. However, if your child seems unwell or if his or her weight continues to cause you concern, you should consult your doctor.

Eating disorders

Adolescence is the most common time for eating disorders to develop. Two of the most serious are anorexia nervosa (in which a person eats little or no food) and bulimia nervosa (in which a person avoids putting on weight by deliberately vomiting or abusing laxatives). These disorders, which can occur together, may cause permanent health problems.

Anorexia nervosa
This disorder affects approximately 1 per cent of adolescents, mainly girls, although the incidence in boys is rising. It usually occurs in people who are hard workers, high achievers, and conformist, and is often triggered by weight loss after a diet. The person loses weight until he or she is emaciated. Most people with anorexia have an intense desire to be thin and see themselves as fat even when dangerously underweight. They may disguise their weight loss by wearing loose clothes and tend to become isolated and/or change their behaviour, for example by refusing to eat with others. Severe weight loss affects the heart and circulation and, in girls, often causes periods to stop. Heart failure is a risk at very low weights, and the risk of suicide is also increased.

Bulimia nervosa
Bulimia, like anorexia, mainly affects females: 3 per cent of women develop it at some time in their lives. People with bulimia often have low self-confidence and use food for comfort. They are usually of normal weight but have episodes (called binges) when they eat excessive amounts, often followed by deliberate vomiting or abuse of laxatives or diuretics. They may also exercise compulsively. Repeated vomiting causes damage to the teeth. Vomiting and the abuse of laxatives can result in chemical imbalances that may affect the internal organs, including the heart.

52 Adolescent behaviour problems

Adolescence is the transition between childhood and adulthood. The combined effects of the hormonal changes that begin at puberty and the psychological factors involved in developing independence often lead to behavioural difficulties. An adolescent is much more self-conscious than a child, and the need to fit in with the peer group becomes increasingly important. Worries about his or her changing body, performance in school, or style of clothing often cause awkwardness. Arguments or misunderstandings at home about dress, language, or general conduct are common. In many cases, offering your support and understanding without making a fuss will be all your child needs at this time. However, if you feel that your child is outside your control and may be endangering his or her health or risking conflict with the law, consult your doctor, who may be able to give advice or recommend relevant support services.

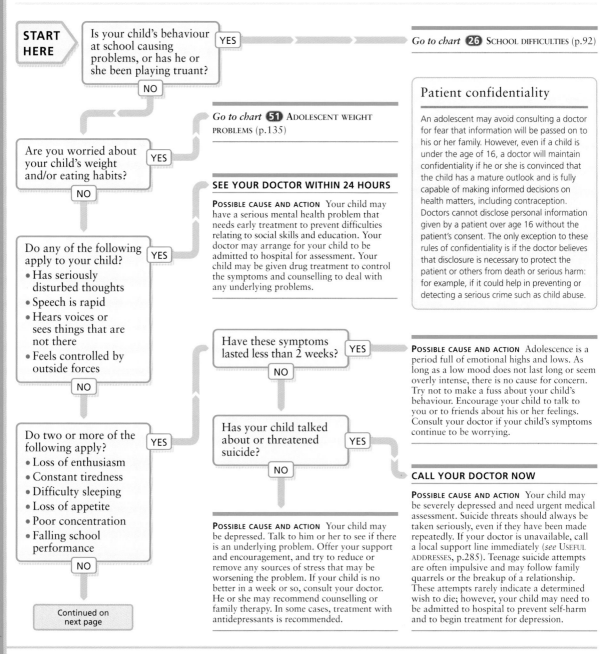

START HERE

Is your child's behaviour at school causing problems, or has he or she been playing truant?

YES → *Go to chart* **26** SCHOOL DIFFICULTIES (p.92)

NO

Are you worried about your child's weight and/or eating habits?

YES → *Go to chart* **51** ADOLESCENT WEIGHT PROBLEMS (p.135)

NO

Do any of the following apply to your child?
- Has seriously disturbed thoughts
- Speech is rapid
- Hears voices or sees things that are not there
- Feels controlled by outside forces

YES

SEE YOUR DOCTOR WITHIN 24 HOURS

POSSIBLE CAUSE AND ACTION Your child may have a serious mental health problem that needs early treatment to prevent difficulties relating to social skills and education. Your doctor may arrange for your child to be admitted to hospital for assessment. Your child may be given drug treatment to control the symptoms and counselling to deal with any underlying problems.

NO

Do two or more of the following apply?
- Loss of enthusiasm
- Constant tiredness
- Difficulty sleeping
- Loss of appetite
- Poor concentration
- Falling school performance

YES

Have these symptoms lasted less than 2 weeks?

YES → **POSSIBLE CAUSE AND ACTION** Adolescence is a period full of emotional highs and lows. As long as a low mood does not last long or seem overly intense, there is no cause for concern. Try not to make a fuss about your child's behaviour. Encourage your child to talk to you or to friends about his or her feelings. Consult your doctor if your child's symptoms continue to be worrying.

NO

Has your child talked about or threatened suicide?

YES → **CALL YOUR DOCTOR NOW**

POSSIBLE CAUSE AND ACTION Your child may be severely depressed and need urgent medical assessment. Suicide threats should always be taken seriously, even if they have been made repeatedly. If your doctor is unavailable, call a local support line immediately (*see* USEFUL ADDRESSES, p.285). Teenage suicide attempts are often impulsive and may follow family quarrels or the breakup of a relationship. These attempts rarely indicate a determined wish to die; however, your child may need to be admitted to hospital to prevent self-harm and to begin treatment for depression.

NO

POSSIBLE CAUSE AND ACTION Your child may be depressed. Talk to him or her to see if there is an underlying problem. Offer your support and encouragement, and try to reduce or remove any sources of stress that may be worsening the problem. If your child is no better in a week or so, consult your doctor. He or she may recommend counselling or family therapy. In some cases, treatment with antidepressants is recommended.

NO

Continued on next page

Patient confidentiality

An adolescent may avoid consulting a doctor for fear that information will be passed on to his or her family. However, even if a child is under the age of 16, a doctor will maintain confidentiality if he or she is convinced that the child has a mature outlook and is fully capable of making informed decisions on health matters, including contraception. Doctors cannot disclose personal information given by a patient over age 16 without the patient's consent. The only exception to these rules of confidentiality is if the doctor believes that disclosure is necessary to protect the patient or others from death or serious harm: for example, if it could help in preventing or detecting a serious crime such as child abuse.

Continued from previous page

Does your child seem particularly apprehensive or tense much of the time?

YES → Is your child worried about a problem, such as exams, difficulties with friends, or parental separation?

YES → **POSSIBLE CAUSE** Most adolescents experience periods of anxiety. This is a cause for concern only if it is severe enough to interfere with day-to-day functioning.

ACTION Talk to your child, and try to discover any underlying worries that he or she has. Offer your support and understanding. It may help to talk to your child's teachers. If your child's anxiety does not ease with time and extra support, consult your doctor. He or she may recommend counselling or family therapy.

NO

POSSIBLE CAUSE AND ACTION Your child's anxiety may be a symptom of depression. Talk to your child about his or her feelings, and offer your support and understanding. If the symptoms persist for more than 2 weeks, without an obvious cause, consult your doctor. He or she may recommend counselling or family therapy.

Do any aspects of your child's behaviour suggest drug or solvent abuse or the excess use of alcohol?

YES → **POSSIBLE CAUSE** Drug or solvent abuse (below) may be causing your child's behaviour problems.

ACTION Talk to your child, to try to find out whether he or she is using drugs or solvents. Explain the dangers of drug abuse, and try to provide your child with support. If your child is unwilling or unable to stop or denies drug use, you should consult your doctor or a self-help group (*see* USEFUL ADDRESSES, p.285).

NO

POSSIBLE CAUSE If your child is persistently antisocial or disruptive, he or she may have a conduct disorder. Consult your doctor.

ACTION Your doctor may refer your child to a specialist for assessment. Counselling or family therapy will probably be recommended. However, long-standing behaviour problems may be difficult to change.

Is your child's behaviour aggressive or violent, or is he or she breaking the law?

YES →

NO

Recognizing drug and solvent abuse

You are unlikely to discover any physical evidence that your child is taking drugs unless he or she wants you to do so. Most adolescent drug users will use the drugs they buy immediately or will be careful to hide any evidence. Behavioural changes are often the only clues. You should bear in mind, however, that most teenagers experience mood swings and other behavioural changes as a normal part of adolescence.

Although different drugs have different effects, the most common signs of regular drug or solvent abuse are:

- Behavioural changes, such as unusual mood swings, irritability, or aggressiveness
- Lying and/or secretiveness about activities
- Lethargy, sleepiness, or drowsiness
- Falling school performance
- Loss of interest in friends or usual activities
- Altered sleep patterns
- Inability to account for money spent
- Disappearance of money or belongings

If you suspect that your child is abusing drugs or solvents, choose a good time to discuss your concerns. If your child denies drug or solvent use or seems unable or unwilling to stop, consult your doctor or a self-help group (*see* USEFUL ADDRESSES, p.285).

Are you concerned that your child may be sexually active?

YES → **POSSIBLE CAUSE AND ACTION** If possible, try to talk to your child about your concerns. Regardless of your opinion about his or her actions, you should make sure that your child is aware of the risk of an unwanted pregnancy and of sexually transmitted infections (*see* SEX AND HEALTH, p.32). Your child is entitled to confidential medical care from a doctor even if he or she is under 16 (*see* PATIENT CONFIDENTIALITY, opposite).

NO

Has your child stopped following his or her treatment plan for a long-standing medical condition?

YES → **POSSIBLE CAUSE AND ACTION** A reluctance to follow the treatment plan for a long-standing disease, such as diabetes mellitus or asthma, is common in adolescents, even if they have previously been responsible. This is usually due to a child's resentment of being different from others or the need to feel in control of his or her life. Talk to your child, but do not get aggressive or angry. Explain the dangers of not taking a prescribed medication as advised. You should also consult your doctor, who may be able to help by talking to your child. He or she may recommend counselling.

NO

CONSULT YOUR DOCTOR IF YOU ARE UNABLE TO FIND AN EXPLANATION FOR YOUR CHILD'S BEHAVIOUR ON THIS CHART AND YOUR CHILD CONTINUES TO BEHAVE IN A WORRYING WAY.

53 Problems with puberty in boys

The time when a child goes through the physical changes involved in becoming an adult is known as puberty. On average, most boys start puberty at 12 years of age, but any age between 9 and 15 years is considered normal. The earliest sign of puberty is usually enlargement of the penis and testes. Other signs of puberty include the ability to ejaculate seminal fluid, the growth of body and facial hair, and deepening of the voice. In boys, the adolescent growth spurt does not tend to occur until puberty is well established. Occasionally, puberty may be associated with a temporary enlargement of breast tissue (*see* BREAST DEVELOPMENT IN MALES, below), which can be embarrassing but is no risk to health.

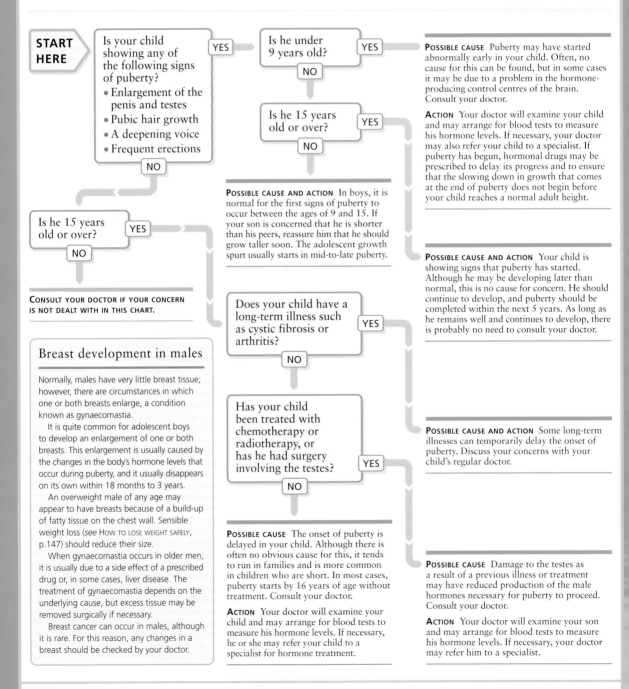

START HERE

Is your child showing any of the following signs of puberty?
- Enlargement of the penis and testes
- Pubic hair growth
- A deepening voice
- Frequent erections

YES → Is he under 9 years old?

YES → **POSSIBLE CAUSE** Puberty may have started abnormally early in your child. Often, no cause for this can be found, but in some cases it may be due to a problem in the hormone-producing control centres of the brain. Consult your doctor.

ACTION Your doctor will examine your child and may arrange for blood tests to measure his hormone levels. If necessary, your doctor may also refer your child to a specialist. If puberty has begun, hormonal drugs may be prescribed to delay its progress and to ensure that the slowing down in growth that comes at the end of puberty does not begin before your child reaches a normal adult height.

NO → Is he 15 years old or over?

YES → **POSSIBLE CAUSE AND ACTION** Your child is showing signs that puberty has started. Although he may be developing later than normal, this is no cause for concern. He should continue to develop, and puberty should be completed within the next 5 years. As long as he remains well and continues to develop, there is probably no need to consult your doctor.

NO → **POSSIBLE CAUSE AND ACTION** In boys, it is normal for the first signs of puberty to occur between the ages of 9 and 15. If your son is concerned that he is shorter than his peers, reassure him that he should grow taller soon. The adolescent growth spurt usually starts in mid-to-late puberty.

Is he 15 years old or over? **YES** →

NO →

CONSULT YOUR DOCTOR IF YOUR CONCERN IS NOT DEALT WITH IN THIS CHART.

Does your child have a long-term illness such as cystic fibrosis or arthritis?

YES →

NO →

POSSIBLE CAUSE AND ACTION Some long-term illnesses can temporarily delay the onset of puberty. Discuss your concerns with your child's regular doctor.

Has your child been treated with chemotherapy or radiotherapy, or has he had surgery involving the testes?

YES →

NO →

POSSIBLE CAUSE The onset of puberty is delayed in your child. Although there is often no obvious cause for this, it tends to run in families and is more common in children who are short. In most cases, puberty starts by 16 years of age without treatment. Consult your doctor.

ACTION Your doctor will examine your child and may arrange for blood tests to measure his hormone levels. If necessary, he or she may refer your child to a specialist for hormone treatment.

POSSIBLE CAUSE Damage to the testes as a result of a previous illness or treatment may have reduced production of the male hormones necessary for puberty to proceed. Consult your doctor.

ACTION Your doctor will examine your son and may arrange for blood tests to measure his hormone levels. If necessary, your doctor may refer him to a specialist.

Breast development in males

Normally, males have very little breast tissue; however, there are circumstances in which one or both breasts enlarge, a condition known as gynaecomastia.

It is quite common for adolescent boys to develop an enlargement of one or both breasts. This enlargement is usually caused by the changes in the body's hormone levels that occur during puberty, and it usually disappears on its own within 18 months to 3 years.

An overweight male of any age may appear to have breasts because of a build-up of fatty tissue on the chest wall. Sensible weight loss (*see* HOW TO LOSE WEIGHT SAFELY, p.147) should reduce their size.

When gynaecomastia occurs in older men, it is usually due to a side effect of a prescribed drug or, in some cases, liver disease. The treatment of gynaecomastia depends on the underlying cause, but excess tissue may be removed surgically if necessary.

Breast cancer can occur in males, although it is rare. For this reason, any changes in a breast should be checked by your doctor.

54 Problems with puberty in girls

Puberty is the time when a child goes through the physical changes involved in becoming an adult. The average age for a girl to start puberty is 11½ years, although any age between 8 and 14 years is considered normal. The first signs of puberty are the enlargement of the breasts and the growth of pubic hair, followed by armpit hair. Girls usually have a growth spurt in early puberty, and menstruation usually begins between the ages of 11 and 14. Puberty usually lasts for about 5 years, during which time all of the body features of an adult develop. Consult this chart if you are worried that your child has started puberty too early or that she seems abnormally late in reaching puberty.

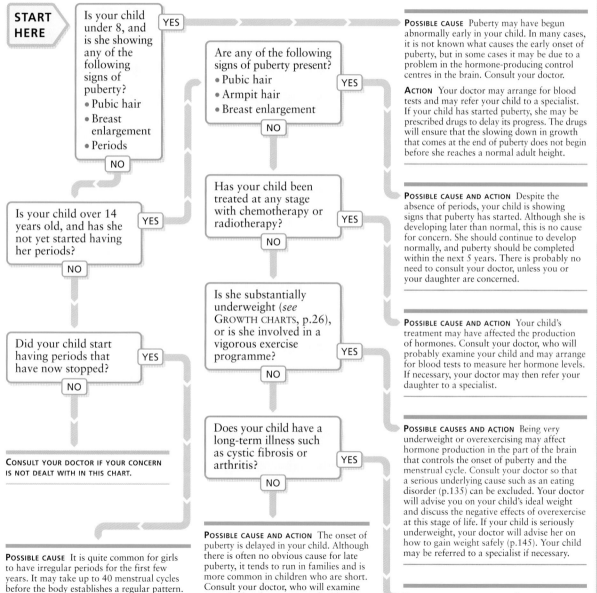

START HERE

Is your child under 8, and is she showing any of the following signs of puberty?
- Pubic hair
- Breast enlargement
- Periods

NO / YES

Are any of the following signs of puberty present?
- Pubic hair
- Armpit hair
- Breast enlargement

NO / YES

Is your child over 14 years old, and has she not yet started having her periods?

NO / YES

Has your child been treated at any stage with chemotherapy or radiotherapy?

NO / YES

Did your child start having periods that have now stopped?

NO / YES

Is she substantially underweight (see GROWTH CHARTS, p.26), or is she involved in a vigorous exercise programme?

NO / YES

Does your child have a long-term illness such as cystic fibrosis or arthritis?

NO / YES

CONSULT YOUR DOCTOR IF YOUR CONCERN IS NOT DEALT WITH IN THIS CHART.

POSSIBLE CAUSE Puberty may have begun abnormally early in your child. In many cases, it is not known what causes the early onset of puberty, but in some cases it may be due to a problem in the hormone-producing control centres in the brain. Consult your doctor.

ACTION Your doctor may arrange for blood tests and may refer your child to a specialist. If your child has started puberty, she may be prescribed drugs to delay its progress. The drugs will ensure that the slowing down in growth that comes at the end of puberty does not begin before she reaches a normal adult height.

POSSIBLE CAUSE AND ACTION Despite the absence of periods, your child is showing signs that puberty has started. Although she is developing later than normal, this is no cause for concern. She should continue to develop normally, and puberty should be completed within the next 5 years. There is probably no need to consult your doctor, unless you or your daughter are concerned.

POSSIBLE CAUSE AND ACTION Your child's treatment may have affected the production of hormones. Consult your doctor, who will probably examine your child and may arrange for blood tests to measure her hormone levels. If necessary, your doctor may then refer your daughter to a specialist.

POSSIBLE CAUSES AND ACTION Being very underweight or overexercising may affect hormone production in the part of the brain that controls the onset of puberty and the menstrual cycle. Consult your doctor so that a serious underlying cause such as an eating disorder (p.135) can be excluded. Your doctor will advise you on your child's ideal weight and discuss the negative effects of overexercise at this stage of life. If your child is seriously underweight, your doctor will advise her on how to gain weight safely (p.145). Your child may be referred to a specialist if necessary.

POSSIBLE CAUSE AND ACTION Some serious long-term illnesses can temporarily delay the onset of puberty. Discuss your concerns with your child's regular doctor.

POSSIBLE CAUSE It is quite common for girls to have irregular periods for the first few years. It may take up to 40 menstrual cycles before the body establishes a regular pattern. However, the possibility of pregnancy should always be considered.

Go to chart **130** ABSENT PERIODS (p.256)

POSSIBLE CAUSE AND ACTION The onset of puberty is delayed in your child. Although there is often no obvious cause for late puberty, it tends to run in families and is more common in children who are short. Consult your doctor, who will examine your child and may arrange for blood tests to measure her hormone levels. If necessary, he or she may then refer your child to a specialist.

55 Adolescent skin problems

The onset of adolescence often produces marked changes in the skin. Infantile eczema, which often affects younger children, may clear up altogether before or during adolescence. However, another form of eczema – contact eczema – may occur for the first time during this period. Contact eczema may result from contact with certain metals or cosmetics, causing an itchy, red rash. Other skin problems, such as psoriasis, may also develop for the first time during adolescence. However, the most noticeable skin changes during adolescence are caused by the rising levels of sex hormones. These hormones encourage the sebaceous glands in the skin to produce increasing amounts of sebum – an oily substance that helps to lubricate the skin. Not only does the increased sebaceous activity give the skin an oily appearance, but it also encourages the development of acne, which affects almost all adolescents to some extent.

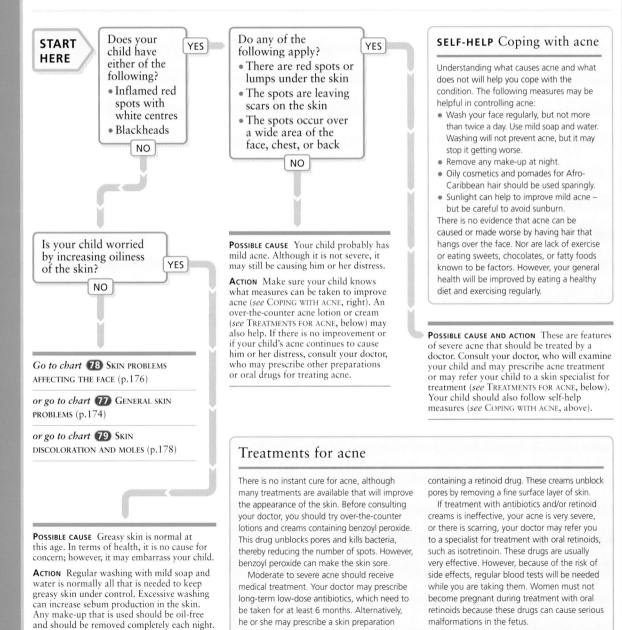

START HERE

Does your child have either of the following?
- Inflamed red spots with white centres
- Blackheads

YES → **Do any of the following apply?**
- There are red spots or lumps under the skin
- The spots are leaving scars on the skin
- The spots occur over a wide area of the face, chest, or back

NO

NO

YES

Is your child worried by increasing oiliness of the skin?

YES

NO

Go to chart 78 SKIN PROBLEMS AFFECTING THE FACE (p.176)

or go to chart 77 GENERAL SKIN PROBLEMS (p.174)

or go to chart 79 SKIN DISCOLORATION AND MOLES (p.178)

POSSIBLE CAUSE Your child probably has mild acne. Although it is not severe, it may still be causing him or her distress.

ACTION Make sure your child knows what measures can be taken to improve acne (*see* COPING WITH ACNE, right). An over-the-counter acne lotion or cream (*see* TREATMENTS FOR ACNE, below) may also help. If there is no improvement or if your child's acne continues to cause him or her distress, consult your doctor, who may prescribe other preparations or oral drugs for treating acne.

SELF-HELP Coping with acne

Understanding what causes acne and what does not will help you cope with the condition. The following measures may be helpful in controlling acne:
- Wash your face regularly, but not more than twice a day. Use mild soap and water. Washing will not prevent acne, but it may stop it getting worse.
- Remove any make-up at night.
- Oily cosmetics and pomades for Afro-Caribbean hair should be used sparingly.
- Sunlight can help to improve mild acne – but be careful to avoid sunburn.

There is no evidence that acne can be caused or made worse by having hair that hangs over the face. Nor are lack of exercise or eating sweets, chocolates, or fatty foods known to be factors. However, your general health will be improved by eating a healthy diet and exercising regularly.

POSSIBLE CAUSE AND ACTION These are features of severe acne that should be treated by a doctor. Consult your doctor, who will examine your child and may prescribe acne treatment or may refer your child to a skin specialist for treatment (*see* TREATMENTS FOR ACNE, below). Your child should also follow self-help measures (*see* COPING WITH ACNE, above).

POSSIBLE CAUSE Greasy skin is normal at this age. In terms of health, it is no cause for concern; however, it may embarrass your child.

ACTION Regular washing with mild soap and water is normally all that is needed to keep greasy skin under control. Excessive washing can increase sebum production in the skin. Any make-up that is used should be oil-free and should be removed completely each night.

Treatments for acne

There is no instant cure for acne, although many treatments are available that will improve the appearance of the skin. Before consulting your doctor, you should try over-the-counter lotions and creams containing benzoyl peroxide. This drug unblocks pores and kills bacteria, thereby reducing the number of spots. However, benzoyl peroxide can make the skin sore.

Moderate to severe acne should receive medical treatment. Your doctor may prescribe long-term low-dose antibiotics, which need to be taken for at least 6 months. Alternatively, he or she may prescribe a skin preparation containing a retinoid drug. These creams unblock pores by removing a fine surface layer of skin.

If treatment with antibiotics and/or retinoid creams is ineffective, your acne is very severe, or there is scarring, your doctor may refer you to a specialist for treatment with oral retinoids, such as isotretinoin. These drugs are usually very effective. However, because of the risk of side effects, regular blood tests will be needed while you are taking them. Women must not become pregnant during treatment with oral retinoids because these drugs can cause serious malformations in the fetus.

GENERAL

CHARTS FOR

ADULTS

56 Feeling unwell

Sometimes you may have a vague feeling of being unwell without being able to identify a specific symptom such as pain. This feeling is usually the result of a minor infection, psychological pressures, or an unhealthy lifestyle. However, you should always make an appointment to see your doctor if the feeling persists for more than a few days; there is a possibility that it may be a sign of a more serious underlying problem that requires medical treatment.

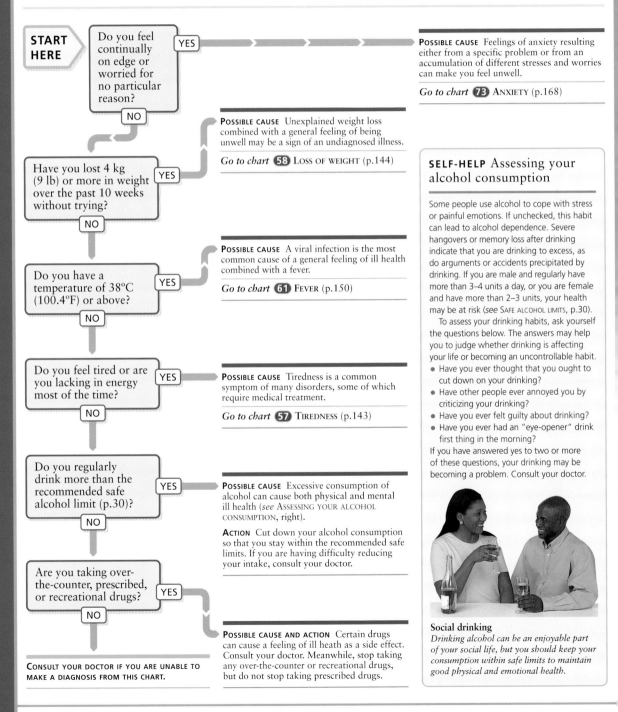

START HERE → Do you feel continually on edge or worried for no particular reason?

YES → **POSSIBLE CAUSE** Feelings of anxiety resulting either from a specific problem or from an accumulation of different stresses and worries can make you feel unwell.

Go to chart **73** ANXIETY (p.168)

NO ↓

Have you lost 4 kg (9 lb) or more in weight over the past 10 weeks without trying?

YES → **POSSIBLE CAUSE** Unexplained weight loss combined with a general feeling of being unwell may be a sign of an undiagnosed illness.

Go to chart **58** LOSS OF WEIGHT (p.144)

NO ↓

Do you have a temperature of 38°C (100.4°F) or above?

YES → **POSSIBLE CAUSE** A viral infection is the most common cause of a general feeling of ill health combined with a fever.

Go to chart **61** FEVER (p.150)

NO ↓

Do you feel tired or are you lacking in energy most of the time?

YES → **POSSIBLE CAUSE** Tiredness is a common symptom of many disorders, some of which require medical treatment.

Go to chart **57** TIREDNESS (p.143)

NO ↓

Do you regularly drink more than the recommended safe alcohol limit (p.30)?

YES → **POSSIBLE CAUSE** Excessive consumption of alcohol can cause both physical and mental ill health (*see* ASSESSING YOUR ALCOHOL CONSUMPTION, right).

ACTION Cut down your alcohol consumption so that you stay within the recommended safe limits. If you are having difficulty reducing your intake, consult your doctor.

NO ↓

Are you taking over-the-counter, prescribed, or recreational drugs?

YES → **POSSIBLE CAUSE AND ACTION** Certain drugs can cause a feeling of ill heath as a side effect. Consult your doctor. Meanwhile, stop taking any over-the-counter or recreational drugs, but do not stop taking prescribed drugs.

NO ↓

CONSULT YOUR DOCTOR IF YOU ARE UNABLE TO MAKE A DIAGNOSIS FROM THIS CHART.

SELF-HELP Assessing your alcohol consumption

Some people use alcohol to cope with stress or painful emotions. If unchecked, this habit can lead to alcohol dependence. Severe hangovers or memory loss after drinking indicate that you are drinking to excess, as do arguments or accidents precipitated by drinking. If you are male and regularly have more than 3–4 units a day, or you are female and have more than 2–3 units, your health may be at risk (*see* SAFE ALCOHOL LIMITS, p.30).

To assess your drinking habits, ask yourself the questions below. The answers may help you to judge whether drinking is affecting your life or becoming an uncontrollable habit.

- Have you ever thought that you ought to cut down on your drinking?
- Have other people ever annoyed you by criticizing your drinking?
- Have you ever felt guilty about drinking?
- Have you ever had an "eye-opener" drink first thing in the morning?

If you have answered yes to two or more of these questions, your drinking may be becoming a problem. Consult your doctor.

Social drinking
Drinking alcohol can be an enjoyable part of your social life, but you should keep your consumption within safe limits to maintain good physical and emotional health.

57 Tiredness

For problems related to sleeping, see chart 60, DIFFICULTY IN SLEEPING *(p.148).*
Tiredness is normal after physical exertion or long periods of hard work without a break. It is common after some infectious illnesses, such as flu or glandular fever, but should

have cleared up after 2 or 3 weeks. However, if there is no obvious explanation for your tiredness, if it prevents you from carrying out daily activities, or if it is prolonged, you should consult your doctor because in some cases tiredness may indicate a serious health problem.

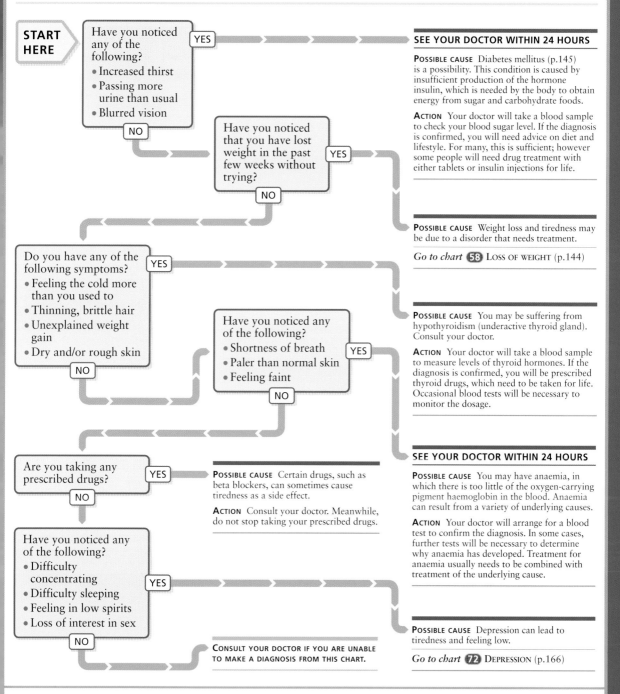

START HERE

Have you noticed any of the following?
- Increased thirst
- Passing more urine than usual
- Blurred vision

YES →

SEE YOUR DOCTOR WITHIN 24 HOURS

POSSIBLE CAUSE Diabetes mellitus (p.145) is a possibility. This condition is caused by insufficient production of the hormone insulin, which is needed by the body to obtain energy from sugar and carbohydrate foods.

ACTION Your doctor will take a blood sample to check your blood sugar level. If the diagnosis is confirmed, you will need advice on diet and lifestyle. For many, this is sufficient; however some people will need drug treatment with either tablets or insulin injections for life.

NO ↓

Have you noticed that you have lost weight in the past few weeks without trying?

YES →

POSSIBLE CAUSE Weight loss and tiredness may be due to a disorder that needs treatment.

Go to chart **58** LOSS OF WEIGHT *(p.144)*

NO ↓

Do you have any of the following symptoms?
- Feeling the cold more than you used to
- Thinning, brittle hair
- Unexplained weight gain
- Dry and/or rough skin

YES →

POSSIBLE CAUSE You may be suffering from hypothyroidism (underactive thyroid gland). Consult your doctor.

ACTION Your doctor will take a blood sample to measure levels of thyroid hormones. If the diagnosis is confirmed, you will be prescribed thyroid drugs, which need to be taken for life. Occasional blood tests will be necessary to monitor the dosage.

NO ↓

Have you noticed any of the following?
- Shortness of breath
- Paler than normal skin
- Feeling faint

YES →

SEE YOUR DOCTOR WITHIN 24 HOURS

POSSIBLE CAUSE You may have anaemia, in which there is too little of the oxygen-carrying pigment haemoglobin in the blood. Anaemia can result from a variety of underlying causes.

ACTION Your doctor will arrange for a blood test to confirm the diagnosis. In some cases, further tests will be necessary to determine why anaemia has developed. Treatment for anaemia usually needs to be combined with treatment of the underlying cause.

NO ↓

Are you taking any prescribed drugs?

YES →

POSSIBLE CAUSE Certain drugs, such as beta blockers, can sometimes cause tiredness as a side effect.

ACTION Consult your doctor. Meanwhile, do not stop taking your prescribed drugs.

NO ↓

Have you noticed any of the following?
- Difficulty concentrating
- Difficulty sleeping
- Feeling in low spirits
- Loss of interest in sex

YES →

POSSIBLE CAUSE Depression can lead to tiredness and feeling low.

Go to chart **72** DEPRESSION *(p.166)*

NO ↓

CONSULT YOUR DOCTOR IF YOU ARE UNABLE TO MAKE A DIAGNOSIS FROM THIS CHART.

58 Loss of weight

For severe weight loss in adolescents, see chart 51,
Adolescent weight problems (p.135).
Minor fluctuations in weight due to temporary changes in
your diet and/or in the amount of exercise you are taking
are normal. However, severe, unintentional weight loss,

especially if it is combined with loss of appetite or other
symptoms, may be an early warning sign of some cancers or
infections that require urgent medical attention. If you are
worried that you have lost a lot of weight and there is no
obvious cause, you should consult your doctor.

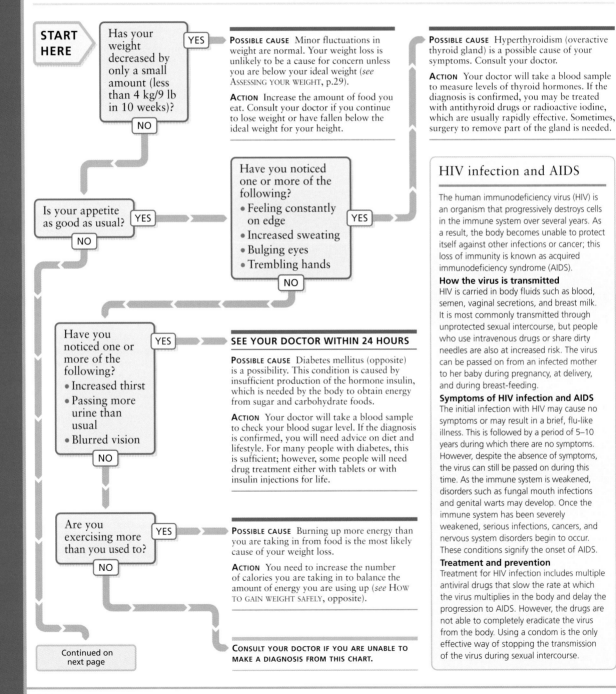

START HERE

Has your weight decreased by only a small amount (less than 4 kg/9 lb in 10 weeks)? — YES

POSSIBLE CAUSE Minor fluctuations in weight are normal. Your weight loss is unlikely to be a cause for concern unless you are below your ideal weight (*see* Assessing your weight, p.29).

ACTION Increase the amount of food you eat. Consult your doctor if you continue to lose weight or have fallen below the ideal weight for your height.

NO

Is your appetite as good as usual? — YES

NO

Have you noticed one or more of the following?
• Feeling constantly on edge
• Increased sweating
• Bulging eyes
• Trembling hands
— YES

NO

POSSIBLE CAUSE Hyperthyroidism (overactive thyroid gland) is a possible cause of your symptoms. Consult your doctor.

ACTION Your doctor will take a blood sample to measure levels of thyroid hormones. If the diagnosis is confirmed, you may be treated with antithyroid drugs or radioactive iodine, which are usually rapidly effective. Sometimes, surgery to remove part of the gland is needed.

Have you noticed one or more of the following?
• Increased thirst
• Passing more urine than usual
• Blurred vision
— YES

NO

SEE YOUR DOCTOR WITHIN 24 HOURS

POSSIBLE CAUSE Diabetes mellitus (opposite) is a possibility. This condition is caused by insufficient production of the hormone insulin, which is needed by the body to obtain energy from sugar and carbohydrate foods.

ACTION Your doctor will take a blood sample to check your blood sugar level. If the diagnosis is confirmed, you will need advice on diet and lifestyle. For many people with diabetes, this is sufficient; however, some people will need drug treatment either with tablets or with insulin injections for life.

Are you exercising more than you used to? — YES

NO

POSSIBLE CAUSE Burning up more energy than you are taking in from food is the most likely cause of your weight loss.

ACTION You need to increase the number of calories you are taking in to balance the amount of energy you are using up (*see* How to gain weight safely, opposite).

Continued on next page

CONSULT YOUR DOCTOR IF YOU ARE UNABLE TO MAKE A DIAGNOSIS FROM THIS CHART.

HIV infection and AIDS

The human immunodeficiency virus (HIV) is an organism that progressively destroys cells in the immune system over several years. As a result, the body becomes unable to protect itself against other infections or cancer; this loss of immunity is known as acquired immunodeficiency syndrome (AIDS).

How the virus is transmitted
HIV is carried in body fluids such as blood, semen, vaginal secretions, and breast milk. It is most commonly transmitted through unprotected sexual intercourse, but people who use intravenous drugs or share dirty needles are also at increased risk. The virus can be passed on from an infected mother to her baby during pregnancy, at delivery, and during breast-feeding.

Symptoms of HIV infection and AIDS
The initial infection with HIV may cause no symptoms or may result in a brief, flu-like illness. This is followed by a period of 5–10 years during which there are no symptoms. However, despite the absence of symptoms, the virus can still be passed on during this time. As the immune system is weakened, disorders such as fungal mouth infections and genital warts may develop. Once the immune system has been severely weakened, serious infections, cancers, and nervous system disorders begin to occur. These conditions signify the onset of AIDS.

Treatment and prevention
Treatment for HIV infection includes multiple antiviral drugs that slow the rate at which the virus multiplies in the body and delay the progression to AIDS. However, the drugs are not able to completely eradicate the virus from the body. Using a condom is the only effective way of stopping the transmission of the virus during sexual intercourse.

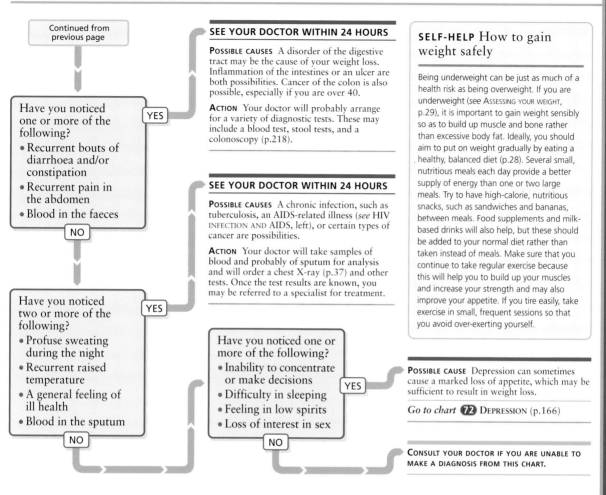

Continued from previous page

Have you noticed one or more of the following?
- Recurrent bouts of diarrhoea and/or constipation
- Recurrent pain in the abdomen
- Blood in the faeces

YES

NO

SEE YOUR DOCTOR WITHIN 24 HOURS

POSSIBLE CAUSES A disorder of the digestive tract may be the cause of your weight loss. Inflammation of the intestines or an ulcer are both possibilities. Cancer of the colon is also possible, especially if you are over 40.

ACTION Your doctor will probably arrange for a variety of diagnostic tests. These may include a blood test, stool tests, and a colonoscopy (p.218).

SEE YOUR DOCTOR WITHIN 24 HOURS

POSSIBLE CAUSES A chronic infection, such as tuberculosis, an AIDS-related illness (see HIV INFECTION AND AIDS, left), or certain types of cancer are possibilities.

ACTION Your doctor will take samples of blood and probably of sputum for analysis and will order a chest X-ray (p.37) and other tests. Once the test results are known, you may be referred to a specialist for treatment.

Have you noticed two or more of the following?
- Profuse sweating during the night
- Recurrent raised temperature
- A general feeling of ill health
- Blood in the sputum

YES

NO

Have you noticed one or more of the following?
- Inability to concentrate or make decisions
- Difficulty in sleeping
- Feeling in low spirits
- Loss of interest in sex

YES

NO

POSSIBLE CAUSE Depression can sometimes cause a marked loss of appetite, which may be sufficient to result in weight loss.

Go to chart **72** DEPRESSION (p.166)

CONSULT YOUR DOCTOR IF YOU ARE UNABLE TO MAKE A DIAGNOSIS FROM THIS CHART.

SELF-HELP How to gain weight safely

Being underweight can be just as much of a health risk as being overweight. If you are underweight (see ASSESSING YOUR WEIGHT, p.29), it is important to gain weight sensibly so as to build up muscle and bone rather than excessive body fat. Ideally, you should aim to put on weight gradually by eating a healthy, balanced diet (p.28). Several small, nutritious meals each day provide a better supply of energy than one or two large meals. Try to have high-calorie, nutritious snacks, such as sandwiches and bananas, between meals. Food supplements and milk-based drinks will also help, but these should be added to your normal diet rather than taken instead of meals. Make sure that you continue to take regular exercise because this will help you to build up your muscles and increase your strength and may also improve your appetite. If you tire easily, take exercise in small, frequent sessions so that you avoid over-exerting yourself.

Diabetes mellitus

Diabetes mellitus is a condition in which body cells are not able to absorb enough of the sugar glucose (the body's main energy source) from the blood. This inability is due to a deficiency of the hormone insulin, normally produced by the pancreas. If there is insufficient insulin, glucose accumulates in the blood and the urine. Cells have to use fats as an energy source instead of glucose, which leads to a build-up of toxic by-products. These chemical changes cause the symptoms of diabetes: thirst, excessive passing of urine, and weight loss. Diabetes mellitus affects about 3 in every 100 people; once it develops, diabetes is a life-long condition.

There are two main forms of the disorder: type 1 and type 2. In type 1 diabetes, the pancreas produces too little insulin or none at all; this form usually develops suddenly in childhood or adolescence and causes dramatic weight loss. In type 2 diabetes, the pancreas continues to produce insulin, but body cells are resistant to it. This type of diabetes is 10 times

more common than type 1. It mainly develops after the age of 40, particularly in those who are overweight. It develops gradually and symptoms may go unrecognized for years.

Complications of diabetes
High blood sugar over a prolonged period damages blood vessels throughout the body, which results in problems with the eyes, kidneys, heart, and nervous system. Treatment aims to keep blood sugar levels as normal as possible to delay the onset of complications.

Treating diabetes
Anyone with diabetes needs to eat a diet high in complex carbohydrates, such as bread, pasta, and pulses, and low in fats (particularly animal fats). Keeping fit is also an important aspect of treatment. In addition to these measures, people with type 1 diabetes need lifelong treatment with insulin injections to replace the missing hormone. The injections are self-administered and the doses have to be carefully matched to food intake. Regular monitoring of blood sugar levels

is necessary to ensure that the treatment is effective. People with type 2 diabetes may be able to control their diabetes simply by keeping fit and following the right diet, but most need to take oral drugs and a few need to have insulin injections.

People with diabetes should visit their doctor every few months so that he or she can assess the control of blood sugar levels and detect and treat any complications of the disease at an early stage.

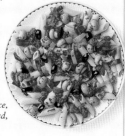

A healthy diet
If you have diabetes, make sure that your diet is high in complex carbohydrates, such as pasta, rice, cereals, and bread, and low in fats.

59 Overweight

Normally, fat accounts for between 10 and 20 per cent of the weight of a man and about 25 per cent of a woman; much more than this is unhealthy, increasing the risk of diseases such as diabetes and high blood pressure and of damage to weight-bearing joints, such as the hips or knees. Most people gradually gain a little weight as they grow older, reaching their heaviest at about age 50. Consult this chart if you weigh more than the healthy weight for your height (see ASSESSING YOUR WEIGHT, p.29) or if you have excess abdominal fat – a waist measurement of over 89 cm (35 in) for women and over 102 cm (40 in) for men. Excess fat around the abdomen is thought to be a greater risk for heart disease than fat elsewhere. Weight gain is usually due to overeating. Occasionally, there may be a medical reason.

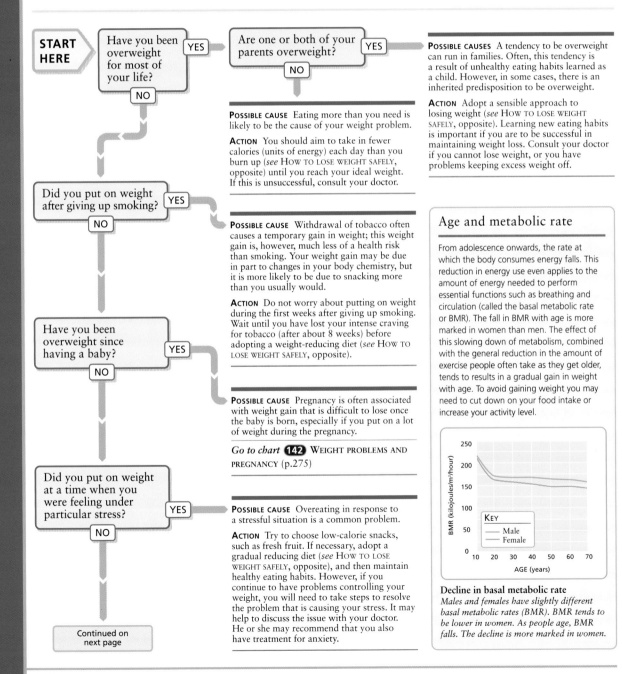

START HERE

Have you been overweight for most of your life? — YES → **Are one or both of your parents overweight?** — YES → **POSSIBLE CAUSES** A tendency to be overweight can run in families. Often, this tendency is a result of unhealthy eating habits learned as a child. However, in some cases, there is an inherited predisposition to be overweight.

ACTION Adopt a sensible approach to losing weight (see HOW TO LOSE WEIGHT SAFELY, opposite). Learning new eating habits is important if you are to be successful in maintaining weight loss. Consult your doctor if you cannot lose weight, or you have problems keeping excess weight off.

NO ↓ (from parents overweight)

POSSIBLE CAUSE Eating more than you need is likely to be the cause of your weight problem.

ACTION You should aim to take in fewer calories (units of energy) each day than you burn up (see HOW TO LOSE WEIGHT SAFELY, opposite) until you reach your ideal weight. If this is unsuccessful, consult your doctor.

NO ↓ (Have you been overweight for most of your life?)

Did you put on weight after giving up smoking? — YES →

POSSIBLE CAUSE Withdrawal of tobacco often causes a temporary gain in weight; this weight gain is, however, much less of a health risk than smoking. Your weight gain may be due in part to changes in your body chemistry, but it is more likely to be due to snacking more than you usually would.

ACTION Do not worry about putting on weight during the first weeks after giving up smoking. Wait until you have lost your intense craving for tobacco (after about 8 weeks) before adopting a weight-reducing diet (see HOW TO LOSE WEIGHT SAFELY, opposite).

NO ↓

Have you been overweight since having a baby? — YES →

POSSIBLE CAUSE Pregnancy is often associated with weight gain that is difficult to lose once the baby is born, especially if you put on a lot of weight during the pregnancy.

Go to chart **142** WEIGHT PROBLEMS AND PREGNANCY (p.275)

NO ↓

Did you put on weight at a time when you were feeling under particular stress? — YES →

POSSIBLE CAUSE Overeating in response to a stressful situation is a common problem.

ACTION Try to choose low-calorie snacks, such as fresh fruit. If necessary, adopt a gradual reducing diet (see HOW TO LOSE WEIGHT SAFELY, opposite), and then maintain healthy eating habits. However, if you continue to have problems controlling your weight, you will need to take steps to resolve the problem that is causing your stress. It may help to discuss the issue with your doctor. He or she may recommend that you also have treatment for anxiety.

NO ↓

Continued on next page

Age and metabolic rate

From adolescence onwards, the rate at which the body consumes energy falls. This reduction in energy use even applies to the amount of energy needed to perform essential functions such as breathing and circulation (called the basal metabolic rate or BMR). The fall in BMR with age is more marked in women than men. The effect of this slowing down of metabolism, combined with the general reduction in the amount of exercise people often take as they get older, tends to results in a gradual gain in weight with age. To avoid gaining weight you may need to cut down on your food intake or increase your activity level.

Decline in basal metabolic rate
Males and females have slightly different basal metabolic rates (BMR). BMR tends to be lower in women. As people age, BMR falls. The decline is more marked in women.

Continued from previous page

Did the weight gain follow a change from a physically active life to a more sedentary job or lifestyle?

NO

YES →

POSSIBLE CAUSE The energy requirements of the body vary according to the amount of exercise your daily routine involves.

ACTION Adjusting your food intake to take account of your reduced energy requirements should help you to lose the weight you have put on. This will mean changing eating habits you have developed over many years, and it may take a little while for you to become accustomed to your new diet. You should also try to incorporate physical exercise into your daily routine. This will maintain your general health and help to boost weight loss (*see* HOW TO LOSE WEIGHT SAFELY, right).

Have you noticed one or more of the following?
• Excessive tiredness
• Feeling the cold more than you used to
• Increased dryness or roughness of the skin
• Thinning, brittle hair

NO

YES →

POSSIBLE CAUSE You may be suffering from hypothyroidism (underactive thyroid gland). Consult your doctor.

ACTION Your doctor will take a blood sample to measure levels of thyroid hormones. If the diagnosis is confirmed, you will be prescribed thyroid drugs, which need to be taken for life. Your doctor will arrange occasional blood tests to monitor the drug dosage.

POSSIBLE CAUSE Certain prescribed drugs, such as corticosteroids, can cause weight gain as a side effect. Consult your doctor. Meanwhile, do not stop taking prescribed drugs.

Are you taking any prescribed drugs?

NO

YES →

POSSIBLE CAUSE Alcohol is high in calories but has no nutritional value and is probably contributing to your weight gain.

ACTION Cut down your alcohol consumption. If you have difficulty cutting down, consult your doctor for advice.

Do you regularly drink more than the recommended safe alcohol limit (p.30)?

NO

YES →

Are you over 40 years old?

NO

YES →

POSSIBLE CAUSE Eating more than you need is the likely cause of your excess weight.

ACTION Follow a sensible reducing diet (*see* HOW TO LOSE WEIGHT SAFELY, above). If after a month you have failed to lose weight, consult your doctor for advice.

SELF-HELP How to lose weight safely

The most likely cause of being overweight is a combination of overeating and lack of exercise. The best way to lose weight is to combine a reduced calorie intake with regular exercise. Set yourself a realistic, short-term target for weight loss; about 2–4 kg (4–9 lb) a month is sensible. Rapid weight-loss plans and fasting should be avoided.

Calorie reduction

The best type of weight-reducing diet is one that is low in calories but balanced so that you stay well nourished. You should try to reduce your daily calorie intake by 500–1,000 calories. The following suggestions may help:

• Cut down on fatty foods; good alternatives include wholemeal bread, potatoes, and pasta.
• Oven bake or grill rather than fry food.
• Avoid excessive snacking.
• Cut down your alcohol consumption.
• Avoid shopping for food when you are feeling hungry.

Exercise

Regular exercise benefits your general health as well as helping you to reduce weight. Exercise does not have to be strenuous, but you should aim to do 30 minutes, five times a week. Not only are calories burned up during exercise, but it also raises basal metabolic rate (BMR), the rate at which your body consumes energy when at rest to maintain basic processes such as breathing and digestion. If your BMR rises, you use up more calories, and, if you have a calorie-controlled diet, you will lose weight.

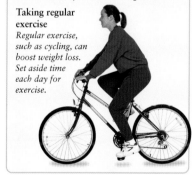

Taking regular exercise
Regular exercise, such as cycling, can boost weight loss. Set aside time each day for exercise.

POSSIBLE CAUSE Growing older is often accompanied by a gain in weight. Your weight gain is probably due to the fact you are taking less exercise at a time when your body needs less food to perform basic functions (*see* AGE AND METABOLIC RATE, opposite).

ACTION Reduce your food intake and/or increase your level of activity to restore the balance of energy intake and expenditure (*see* HOW TO LOSE WEIGHT SAFELY, above).

60 Difficulty in sleeping

It is quite common to have the odd night when you find it difficult to get to sleep or to stay asleep, and this need not cause concern. Consult this chart if you often find it hard to get to sleep or if you frequently wake during the night. Lifestyle changes can sometimes help with sleeping problems (*see* GETTING A GOOD NIGHT'S SLEEP, opposite).

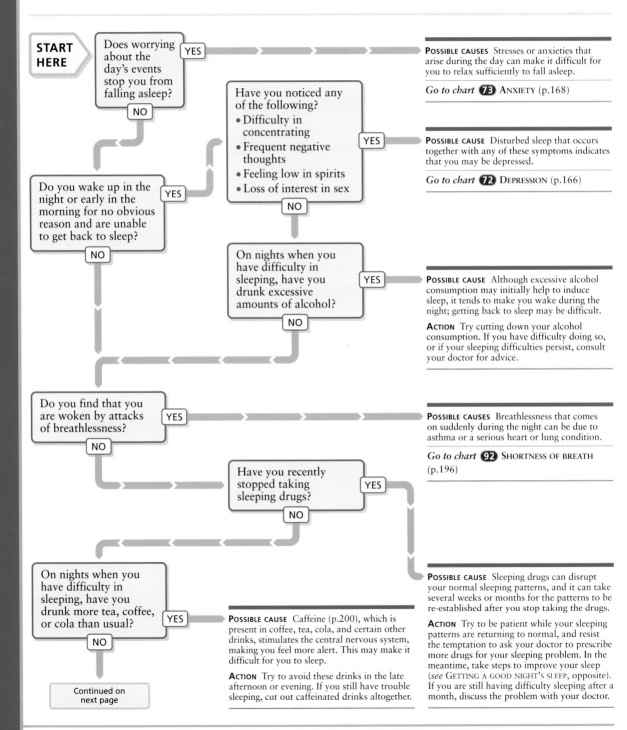

START HERE

Does worrying about the day's events stop you from falling asleep?
YES →
POSSIBLE CAUSES Stresses or anxieties that arise during the day can make it difficult for you to relax sufficiently to fall asleep.

Go to chart **73** ANXIETY (p.168)

NO

Have you noticed any of the following?
- Difficulty in concentrating
- Frequent negative thoughts
- Feeling low in spirits
- Loss of interest in sex

YES →
POSSIBLE CAUSE Disturbed sleep that occurs together with any of these symptoms indicates that you may be depressed.

Go to chart **72** DEPRESSION (p.166)

NO

Do you wake up in the night or early in the morning for no obvious reason and are unable to get back to sleep?
YES →

NO

On nights when you have difficulty in sleeping, have you drunk excessive amounts of alcohol?
YES →
POSSIBLE CAUSE Although excessive alcohol consumption may initially help to induce sleep, it tends to make you wake during the night; getting back to sleep may be difficult.

ACTION Try cutting down your alcohol consumption. If you have difficulty doing so, or if your sleeping difficulties persist, consult your doctor for advice.

NO

Do you find that you are woken by attacks of breathlessness?
YES →
POSSIBLE CAUSES Breathlessness that comes on suddenly during the night can be due to asthma or a serious heart or lung condition.

Go to chart **92** SHORTNESS OF BREATH (p.196)

NO

Have you recently stopped taking sleeping drugs?
YES →

NO

On nights when you have difficulty in sleeping, have you drunk more tea, coffee, or cola than usual?
YES →
POSSIBLE CAUSE Caffeine (p.200), which is present in coffee, tea, cola, and certain other drinks, stimulates the central nervous system, making you feel more alert. This may make it difficult for you to sleep.

ACTION Try to avoid these drinks in the late afternoon or evening. If you still have trouble sleeping, cut out caffeinated drinks altogether.

NO

POSSIBLE CAUSE Sleeping drugs can disrupt your normal sleeping patterns, and it can take several weeks or months for the patterns to be re-established after you stop taking the drugs.

ACTION Try to be patient while your sleeping patterns are returning to normal, and resist the temptation to ask your doctor to prescribe more drugs for your sleeping problem. In the meantime, take steps to improve your sleep (*see* GETTING A GOOD NIGHT'S SLEEP, opposite). If you are still having difficulty sleeping after a month, discuss the problem with your doctor.

Continued on next page

Continued from previous page

On nights when you have trouble sleeping, have you eaten a late or particularly heavy meal? YES / NO

POSSIBLE CAUSE Eating to excess or late in the evening can often make it difficult to sleep.

ACTION Try eating lighter meals or eat your last meal of the day earlier in the evening.

Are you pregnant? YES / NO

POSSIBLE CAUSE AND ACTION Your sleep problems may be related to your pregnancy. You may need to get up during the night to pass urine even early in pregnancy. Later in pregnancy, your baby's movements may disturb your sleep and your enlarged abdomen may make it difficult to get comfortable. Anxiety about the birth may also cause sleep problems. Follow the self-help measures for getting a good night's sleep during pregnancy (below). If you still cannot sleep, get up, read, or do odd jobs. Try to catch up on sleep by taking naps during the day. Discuss any worries that you have about the birth with your doctor or health visitor.

Are you taking any prescribed drugs? YES / NO

POSSIBLE CAUSE AND ACTION Some drugs, such as beta blockers, may cause sleep disturbance as a side effect. Consult your doctor. Meanwhile, do not stop taking your prescribed drugs.

Do you have a sedentary job, and do you take little physical exercise during the day? YES / NO

POSSIBLE CAUSE A lack of physical exercise during the daytime may mean that you are not sufficiently tired to fall sleep easily, even if you have had a mentally tiring day.

ACTION Try to get some form of regular exercise during the day or evening. This will make you more physically tired and may also help you to relax. Not only will regular exercise help you to sleep better, but it will also improve your general health and feeling of wellbeing (*see* How EXERCISE BENEFITS HEALTH, p.29).

Are you over 60? YES / NO

POSSIBLE CAUSE AND ACTION Most people need less sleep as they grow older; many people over 60 need only 6 hours sleep a night. For this reason, you may find that you wake earlier in the morning than you used to, or you find it difficult to fall asleep at the same time as when you were younger. Take advantage of your extra time, and try to avoid napping during the day.

CONSULT YOUR DOCTOR IF YOU ARE UNABLE TO MAKE A DIAGNOSIS FROM THIS CHART.

SELF-HELP Getting a good night's sleep

Sleep is an important factor in maintaining good health. If you are having difficulty sleeping, these suggestions may help:

- Exercise during the day to tire yourself physically and help you relax.
- Cut out coffee, tea, cola, and other drinks containing caffeine, particularly during the afternoon and evening.
- Avoid high alcohol consumption: although alcohol may make you sleepy at first, you are more likely to wake up during the night and be unable to get back to sleep.
- Try to establish regular times for going to sleep and waking up; avoid daytime naps.
- Avoid heavy meals in the evening.
- Have a warm drink such as heated up milk or camomile tea at bedtime.
- If you need to work in the evening, stop at least 1 hour before bedtime.
- Make sure that your bed is comfortable and your bedroom is well ventilated.

Taking daily exercise
Regular exercise, such as walking, will make you feel more tired and help you to sleep.

SELF-HELP Getting a good night's sleep during pregnancy

Getting a full night's undisturbed sleep may be difficult during pregnancy, especially in later pregnancy when the enlarging abdomen makes it more difficult to find a comfortable position. However, there are several measures you can take to help make sleeping easier. Before going to bed, try to relax. Have a warm bath, listen to the radio, or read until you feel sleepy. Avoid drinks containing caffeine, such as coffee and tea, especially in the evening.

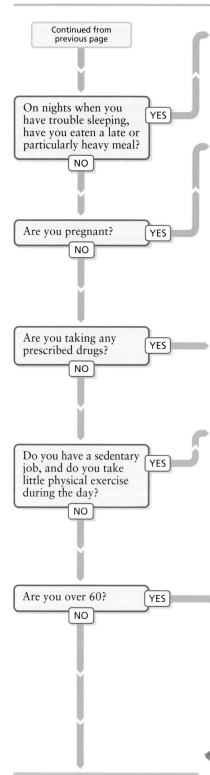

Pillow between legs

Sleeping comfortably
Try to sleep on your side with a pillow between your legs. You may also feel more comfortable if you place another pillow under your abdomen.

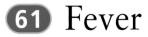

61 Fever

A fever is a body temperature higher than 38°C (100.4°F). It can be a symptom of many diseases, but it usually indicates that your body is fighting an infection. Heat exposure and certain drugs can also raise your body temperature. You may suspect that you have a fever if you feel shivery, alternately hot and cold, and you are generally unwell. To check if you do have a fever, use a thermometer to measure your temperature accurately (*see* MANAGING A FEVER, below).

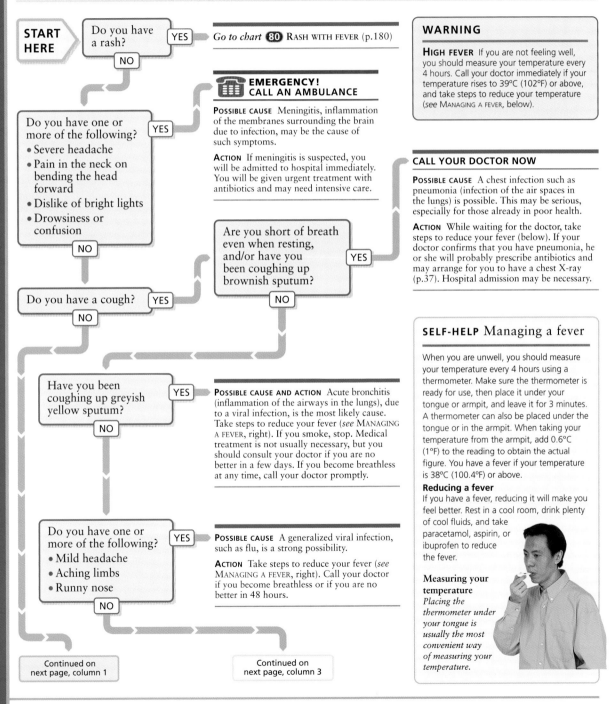

START HERE

Do you have a rash? — YES → *Go to chart* **80** RASH WITH FEVER (p.180)

NO

Do you have one or more of the following?
- Severe headache
- Pain in the neck on bending the head forward
- Dislike of bright lights
- Drowsiness or confusion

YES →

📞 **EMERGENCY! CALL AN AMBULANCE**

POSSIBLE CAUSE Meningitis, inflammation of the membranes surrounding the brain due to infection, may be the cause of such symptoms.

ACTION If meningitis is suspected, you will be admitted to hospital immediately. You will be given urgent treatment with antibiotics and may need intensive care.

NO

Do you have a cough? — YES →

Are you short of breath even when resting, and/or have you been coughing up brownish sputum? — YES →

NO

NO

Have you been coughing up greyish yellow sputum? — YES → **POSSIBLE CAUSE AND ACTION** Acute bronchitis (inflammation of the airways in the lungs), due to a viral infection, is the most likely cause. Take steps to reduce your fever (*see* MANAGING A FEVER, right). If you smoke, stop. Medical treatment is not usually necessary, but you should consult your doctor if you are no better in a few days. If you become breathless at any time, call your doctor promptly.

NO

Do you have one or more of the following?
- Mild headache
- Aching limbs
- Runny nose

YES → **POSSIBLE CAUSE** A generalized viral infection, such as flu, is a strong possibility.

ACTION Take steps to reduce your fever (*see* MANAGING A FEVER, right). Call your doctor if you become breathless or if you are no better in 48 hours.

NO

Continued on next page, column 1

Continued on next page, column 3

WARNING

HIGH FEVER If you are not feeling well, you should measure your temperature every 4 hours. Call your doctor immediately if your temperature rises to 39°C (102°F) or above, and take steps to reduce your temperature (*see* MANAGING A FEVER, below).

CALL YOUR DOCTOR NOW

POSSIBLE CAUSE A chest infection such as pneumonia (infection of the air spaces in the lungs) is possible. This may be serious, especially for those already in poor health.

ACTION While waiting for the doctor, take steps to reduce your fever (below). If your doctor confirms that you have pneumonia, he or she will probably prescribe antibiotics and may arrange for you to have a chest X-ray (p.37). Hospital admission may be necessary.

SELF-HELP Managing a fever

When you are unwell, you should measure your temperature every 4 hours using a thermometer. Make sure the thermometer is ready for use, then place it under your tongue or armpit, and leave it for 3 minutes. A thermometer can also be placed under the tongue or in the armpit. When taking your temperature from the armpit, add 0.6°C (1°F) to the reading to obtain the actual figure. You have a fever if your temperature is 38°C (100.4°F) or above.

Reducing a fever
If you have a fever, reducing it will make you feel better. Rest in a cool room, drink plenty of cool fluids, and take paracetamol, aspirin, or ibuprofen to reduce the fever.

Measuring your temperature
Placing the thermometer under your tongue is usually the most convenient way of measuring your temperature.

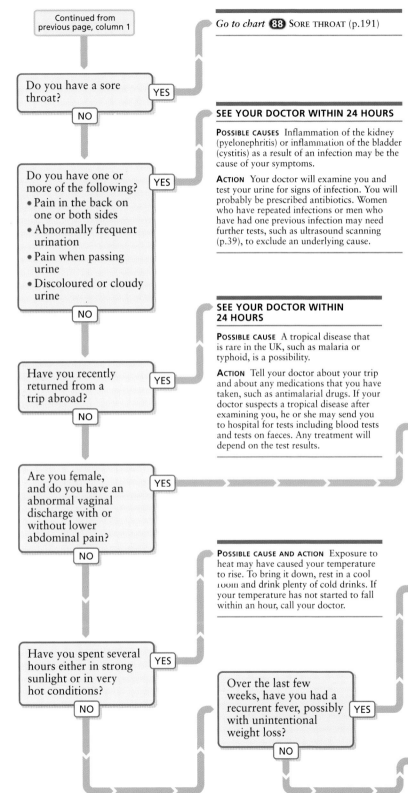

Continued from previous page, column 1

Go to chart **88** SORE THROAT (p.191)

Continued from previous page, column 2

Do you have a sore throat? **YES**

NO

SEE YOUR DOCTOR WITHIN 24 HOURS

POSSIBLE CAUSES Inflammation of the kidney (pyelonephritis) or inflammation of the bladder (cystitis) as a result of an infection may be the cause of your symptoms.

ACTION Your doctor will examine you and test your urine for signs of infection. You will probably be prescribed antibiotics. Women who have repeated infections or men who have had one previous infection may need further tests, such as ultrasound scanning (p.39), to exclude an underlying cause.

Are you coughing up blood? **YES**

NO

SEE A DOCTOR WITHIN **24** HOURS IF YOU ARE STILL FEVERISH AFTER **2** DAYS AND CANNOT MAKE A DIAGNOSIS FROM THIS CHART.

Do you have one or more of the following? **YES**
- Pain in the back on one or both sides
- Abnormally frequent urination
- Pain when passing urine
- Discoloured or cloudy urine

NO

SEE YOUR DOCTOR WITHIN 24 HOURS

POSSIBLE CAUSE You may have a serious lung disorder, such as tuberculosis or lung cancer.

ACTION Your doctor will probably arrange for initial blood and sputum tests and a chest X-ray (p.37). You may then be referred to a specialist for tests, such as bronchoscopy (p.195), which will help determine what treatment is necessary.

SEE YOUR DOCTOR WITHIN 24 HOURS

POSSIBLE CAUSE A tropical disease that is rare in the UK, such as malaria or typhoid, is a possibility.

ACTION Tell your doctor about your trip and about any medications that you have taken, such as antimalarial drugs. If your doctor suspects a tropical disease after examining you, he or she may send you to hospital for tests including blood tests and tests on faeces. Any treatment will depend on the test results.

Have you recently returned from a trip abroad? **YES**

NO

Are you female, and do you have an abnormal vaginal discharge with or without lower abdominal pain? **YES**

NO

SEE YOUR DOCTOR WITHIN 24 HOURS

POSSIBLE CAUSE Pelvic inflammatory disease, inflammation of the reproductive organs, often due to a sexually transmitted infection, may be the cause.

ACTION Your doctor will examine you and may arrange for tests to confirm the diagnosis. You will probably be given painkillers and prescribed antibiotics.

POSSIBLE CAUSE AND ACTION Exposure to heat may have caused your temperature to rise. To bring it down, rest in a cool room and drink plenty of cold drinks. If your temperature has not started to fall within an hour, call your doctor.

SEE YOUR DOCTOR WITHIN 24 HOURS

POSSIBLE CAUSE A serious disorder such as tuberculosis, cancer of the lymph nodes, or an AIDS-related illness (*see* HIV INFECTION AND AIDS, p.144) is possible.

ACTION Your doctor will examine you and will probably arrange blood and/or sputum tests. He or she may also order a chest X-ray (p.37) and other tests. You may need to be referred to a specialist for further investigations and for treatment.

Have you spent several hours either in strong sunlight or in very hot conditions? **YES**

NO

Over the last few weeks, have you had a recurrent fever, possibly with unintentional weight loss? **YES**

NO

SEE A DOCTOR WITHIN **24** HOURS IF YOU ARE STILL FEVERISH AFTER **2** DAYS AND ARE UNABLE TO MAKE A DIAGNOSIS FROM THIS CHART.

62 Excessive sweating

Sweating is one of the natural mechanisms for regulating body temperature and is the normal response to hot conditions or strenuous exercise. Some people naturally sweat more than others, so if you have always sweated profusely, there is unlikely to be anything wrong. However, sweating that is not brought on by heat or exercise or that is more profuse than you are used to may be a sign of one of a number of medical conditions.

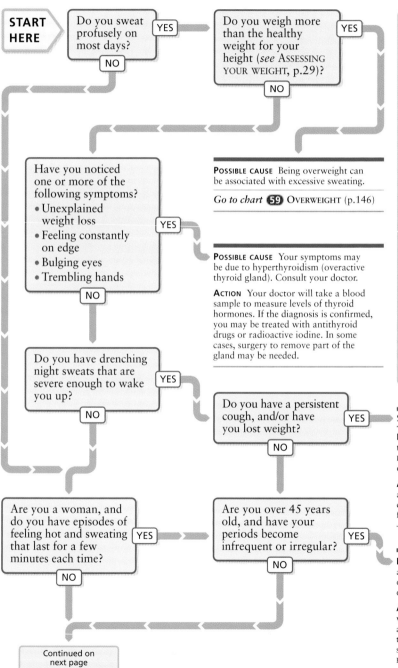

START HERE

Do you sweat profusely on most days? — YES → **Do you weigh more than the healthy weight for your height (see ASSESSING YOUR WEIGHT, p.29)?** — YES →

NO ↓   NO ↓

POSSIBLE CAUSE Being overweight can be associated with excessive sweating.

Go to chart **59** OVERWEIGHT (p.146)

Have you noticed one or more of the following symptoms?
• Unexplained weight loss
• Feeling constantly on edge
• Bulging eyes
• Trembling hands

YES →

NO ↓

POSSIBLE CAUSE Your symptoms may be due to hyperthyroidism (overactive thyroid gland). Consult your doctor.

ACTION Your doctor will take a blood sample to measure levels of thyroid hormones. If the diagnosis is confirmed, you may be treated with antithyroid drugs or radioactive iodine. In some cases, surgery to remove part of the gland may be needed.

Do you have drenching night sweats that are severe enough to wake you up? — YES →

NO ↓

Do you have a persistent cough, and/or have you lost weight? — YES →

NO ↓

Are you a woman, and do you have episodes of feeling hot and sweating that last for a few minutes each time? — YES → **Are you over 45 years old, and have your periods become infrequent or irregular?** — YES →

NO ↓   NO ↓

Continued on next page

Controlling excessive sweating

Excessive sweating can be very embarrassing, especially if it results in a noticeable body odour or causes the hands to be particularly wet and slippery. Washing regularly and wearing comfortable, loose clothing made from natural fibres that absorb sweat should help to prevent body odour. An underarm deodorant containing an antiperspirant should help to reduce the amount of sweat produced from the armpits.

If these measures do not help to combat excessive sweating, consult your pharmacist or doctor. Stronger treatments containing aluminium chloride are available over the counter. If you sweat heavily from your armpits and aluminium chloride treatments do not work, your doctor may recommend local injections of botulinum toxin, which paralyse the nerves to the sweat glands of the armpits for several months. If you still sweat heavily, particularly on your hands, your doctor may suggest that you have an operation to destroy nerves near the back of the neck that supply the sweat glands under the arms and on the palms of the hands. This operation dramatically reduces sweating in these areas.

SEE YOUR DOCTOR WITHIN 24 HOURS

POSSIBLE CAUSES A chronic infection such as tuberculosis, an AIDS-related illness (see HIV INFECTION AND AIDS, p.144), or certain types of cancer are possibilities.

ACTION After initial investigations, such as a chest X-ray (p.37) and blood tests, your doctor may refer you to a specialist for any further tests or appropriate treatment.

POSSIBLE CAUSE Sudden episodes of feeling hot and sweating, known as hot flushes, are one of the most common symptoms of the onset of the menopause (p.21).

ACTION Many women are prepared to put up with hot flushes, knowing that they will stop after a year or so. However, you may wish to consult your doctor to discuss treatments such as hormone replacement therapy (see A HEALTHY MENOPAUSE, p.257).

Continued from previous page

Do you have a temperature of 38°C (100.4°F) or above?

YES → **POSSIBLE CAUSE** Sweating is the body's response to fever and is part of the normal temperature control mechanism.

Go to chart **61** FEVER (p.150)

NO ↓

Are you female, and does the excessive sweating occur only during your periods?

YES → **POSSIBLE CAUSE AND ACTION** In some women, changes in the levels of sex hormones can cause increased sweating during menstruation. This is no cause for concern, but consult your doctor if you are worried.

NO ↓

Do you regularly drink more than the recommended safe alcohol limit (p.30)?

YES → **POSSIBLE CAUSE** Excessive alcohol consumption can be a cause of increased sweating.

ACTION Cut down your alcohol intake so that you stay within the recommended safe limit. If you are having difficulty reducing your alcohol consumption, consult your doctor for advice.

NO ↓

Are you taking any prescribed or over-the-counter drugs?

YES → **POSSIBLE CAUSE AND ACTION** Certain drugs, such as some antidepressants and aspirin, can cause excessive sweating as a side effect. Stop taking over-the-counter drugs, and consult your doctor. Meanwhile, do not stop taking your prescribed drugs.

NO ↓

Is the excessive sweating confined to your hands or feet?

YES → **POSSIBLE CAUSE** The hands and feet have a high concentration of sweat glands (left). For this reason, these parts of the body react most noticeably to a rise in temperature. However, this is not a cause for concern.

ACTION If the sweating becomes worse when you are worried or feeling anxious, learn relaxation exercises (p.32) to use in stressful situations. Wash your hands and feet regularly. If these measures do not help, consult your doctor. For severe cases of sweating of the hands, surgery to destroy the nerves that control sweating in the palms may be considered.

NO ↓

Do you notice the sweating only when you are anxious or excited?

YES → **POSSIBLE CAUSE AND ACTION** Emotional stress can easily cause an increase in sweating. This in itself is not a cause for concern, but if it happens regularly or causes embarrassment, try doing some relaxation exercises (p.32). Consult your doctor if these exercises do not help.

NO ↓

Are you in your teens?

YES → **POSSIBLE CAUSE** In adolescence, the apocrine sweat glands (*see* SWEAT GLANDS, left) become active. This is usually associated with an increase in sweating that is particularly noticeable under the arms. It is perfectly normal.

ACTION Make sure you wash regularly. You may also want to use an antiperspirant deodorant to reduce wetness and prevent body odour (*see* CONTROLLING EXCESSIVE SWEATING, opposite).

NO ↓

CONSULT YOUR DOCTOR IF YOU ARE UNABLE TO MAKE A DIAGNOSIS FROM THIS CHART AND YOUR EXCESSIVE SWEATING CONTINUES TO WORRY YOU. THERE IS, HOWEVER, UNLIKELY TO BE A SERIOUS CAUSE FOR THIS SYMPTOM.

Sweat glands

Sweat glands are found in the layer of the skin called the dermis and release moisture (sweat) through pores in the surface of the skin. There are two types of sweat glands – eccrine glands and apocrine glands – and these produce different kinds of sweat.

Eccrine glands

These glands are found all over the body and are active from birth onwards. The sweat from them is a clear, salty fluid containing various waste chemicals. This sweat evaporates on the surface of the skin to reduce body temperature as necessary. The eccrine glands may also produce sweat in response to anxiety or fear. Eccrine glands are most concentrated on the forehead, palms, and soles of the feet, and profuse sweating is likely to become apparent first in these areas.

Apocrine glands

During adolescence, apocrine glands become active. They are mainly concentrated in the armpit, in the groin, and around the nipples. These glands produce a fluid that contains fats and proteins. The scent from this type of gland is thought to play a role in attracting the opposite sex. However, if it is allowed to remain on the skin for long, it may interact with bacteria to produce body odour.

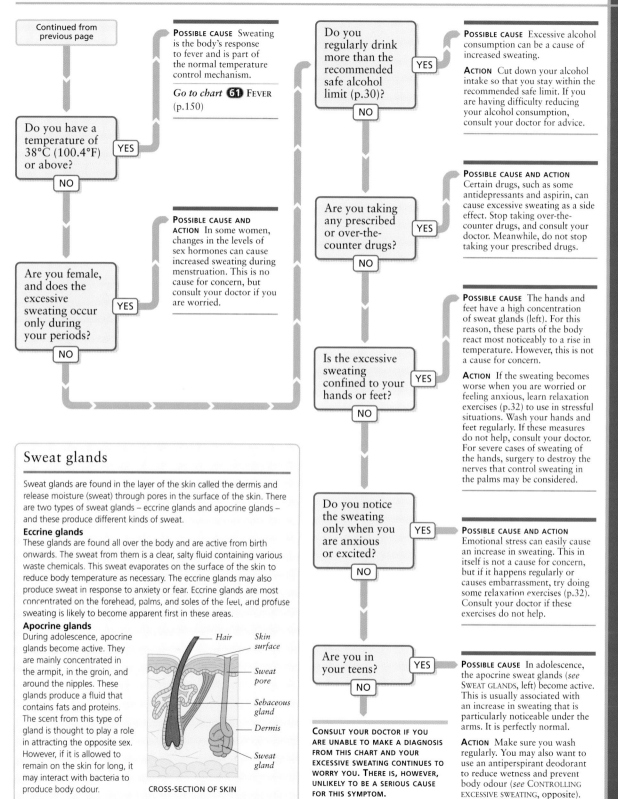

Hair
Skin surface
Sweat pore
Sebaceous gland
Dermis
Sweat gland

CROSS-SECTION OF SKIN

63 Headache

From time to time nearly everyone suffers from mild to moderate headaches that develop gradually and clear up after a few hours, leaving no after-effects. Headaches like this are extremely unlikely to be a sign of a serious underlying disorder and are usually the result of factors such as tension, tiredness, or an excessive consumption of alcohol. However, if you have a headache that is severe, lasts for more than 24 hours, is not improved by taking over-the-counter painkillers, or recurs several times during one week, you should see your doctor promptly.

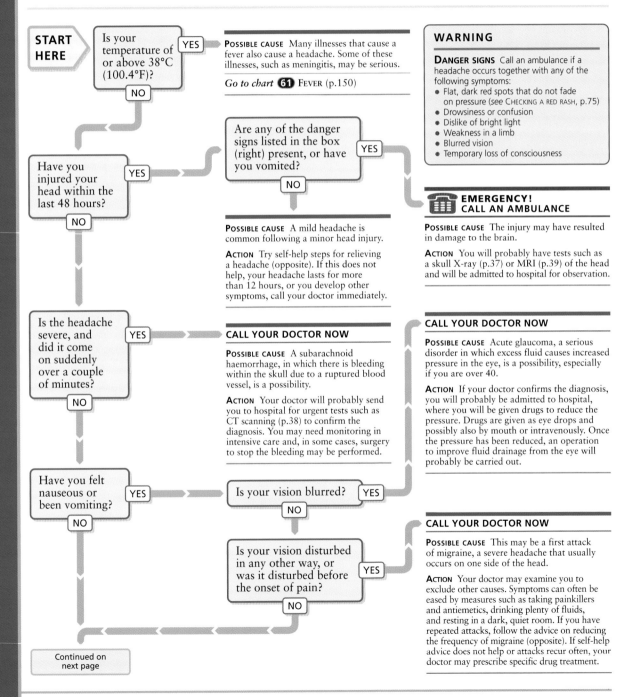

START HERE

Is your temperature of or above 38°C (100.4°F)? — YES → **POSSIBLE CAUSE** Many illnesses that cause a fever also cause a headache. Some of these illnesses, such as meningitis, may be serious.

Go to chart **61** FEVER (p.150)

NO

Have you injured your head within the last 48 hours? — YES → **Are any of the danger signs listed in the box (right) present, or have you vomited?** — YES →

NO

NO ↓

POSSIBLE CAUSE A mild headache is common following a minor head injury.

ACTION Try self-help steps for relieving a headache (opposite). If this does not help, your headache lasts for more than 12 hours, or you develop other symptoms, call your doctor immediately.

WARNING

DANGER SIGNS Call an ambulance if a headache occurs together with any of the following symptoms:
- Flat, dark red spots that do not fade on pressure (see CHECKING A RED RASH, p.75)
- Drowsiness or confusion
- Dislike of bright light
- Weakness in a limb
- Blurred vision
- Temporary loss of consciousness

EMERGENCY! CALL AN AMBULANCE

POSSIBLE CAUSE The injury may have resulted in damage to the brain.

ACTION You will probably have tests such as a skull X-ray (p.37) or MRI (p.39) of the head and will be admitted to hospital for observation.

Is the headache severe, and did it come on suddenly over a couple of minutes? — YES →

CALL YOUR DOCTOR NOW

POSSIBLE CAUSE A subarachnoid haemorrhage, in which there is bleeding within the skull due to a ruptured blood vessel, is a possibility.

ACTION Your doctor will probably send you to hospital for urgent tests such as CT scanning (p.38) to confirm the diagnosis. You may need monitoring in intensive care and, in some cases, surgery to stop the bleeding may be performed.

CALL YOUR DOCTOR NOW

POSSIBLE CAUSE Acute glaucoma, a serious disorder in which excess fluid causes increased pressure in the eye, is a possibility, especially if you are over 40.

ACTION If your doctor confirms the diagnosis, you will probably be admitted to hospital, where you will be given drugs to reduce the pressure. Drugs are given as eye drops and possibly also by mouth or intravenously. Once the pressure has been reduced, an operation to improve fluid drainage from the eye will probably be carried out.

NO

Have you felt nauseous or been vomiting? — YES → **Is your vision blurred?** — YES →

NO

NO ↓

Is your vision disturbed in any other way, or was it disturbed before the onset of pain? — YES →

NO

CALL YOUR DOCTOR NOW

POSSIBLE CAUSE This may be a first attack of migraine, a severe headache that usually occurs on one side of the head.

ACTION Your doctor may examine you to exclude other causes. Symptoms can often be eased by measures such as taking painkillers and antiemetics, drinking plenty of fluids, and resting in a dark, quiet room. If you have repeated attacks, follow the advice on reducing the frequency of migraine (opposite). If self-help advice does not help or attacks recur often, your doctor may prescribe specific drug treatment.

Continued on next page

Continued from previous page

Is the pain felt mainly in the face, and is the pain worse when you bend down? — YES

NO

SEE YOUR DOCTOR WITHIN 24 HOURS

POSSIBLE CAUSE Sinusitis (inflammation of the membranes lining the air spaces in the skull) may be the cause, especially if you have recently had a cold or a runny or blocked nose.

ACTION Your doctor will examine you. If he or she suspects sinusitis, you will be given antibiotics. In the meantime, follow the self-help measures for treating a cold (p.190).

Is the pain felt mainly in the temples, and/or are these areas tender to touch? — YES

NO

CALL YOUR DOCTOR NOW

POSSIBLE CAUSE Temporal arteritis (inflammation of the arteries in the scalp and elsewhere in the body) is a possibility. Urgent treatment may be needed to prevent the condition from affecting the arteries supplying the eyes.

ACTION Your doctor will probably prescribe corticosteroid drugs to reduce the inflammation. It may be necessary for you to have regular blood tests to confirm that the dose you are taking is sufficient to control the inflammation.

SELF-HELP Reducing the frequency of migraine

Many factors are known to trigger a migraine. You need to identify the particular ones that affect you. Keeping a migraine diary for a few weeks may help to pinpoint any triggering factors, which should then be avoided if possible. The following self-help measures may also help in reducing the frequency of your migraine attacks:

- Avoid foods such as cheese or chocolate, which are common triggering factors.
- Eat regularly, because missing a meal may trigger an attack.
- Follow a regular sleep pattern if possible, because changing it may trigger an attack.
- If stress is a trigger, try doing relaxation exercises (p.32).

Did the headache occur after you had been reading or doing close work? — YES

NO

POSSIBLE CAUSE Muscle strain in your neck, as a result of poor posture or tension from concentration, is the most likely cause of your headache.

ACTION Try self-help measures for relieving a headache (below). In order to prevent the problem from recurring, make sure that when you read, you are not sitting in an awkward position. Periodic rest from whatever you are doing will also help. If headaches do recur, either arrange for a vision test (p.185) with an optician or consult your doctor.

Are you sleeping poorly, and/or are you feeling tense or under stress? — YES

NO

POSSIBLE CAUSE AND ACTION Headaches can be caused by lack of sleep. Psychological stress often causes tension headaches. Try self-help measures for relieving a headache (left).

Go to chart **73** ANXIETY (p.168)

SELF-HELP Relieving a headache

Most headaches are not serious and are simply due to the pressures of everyday life. To ease the pain of a headache, take a break and get some fresh air. Try massaging your neck and shoulder muscles. If these measures do not help, rest in a quiet, cool, darkened room and take the recommended dose of a standard painkiller.

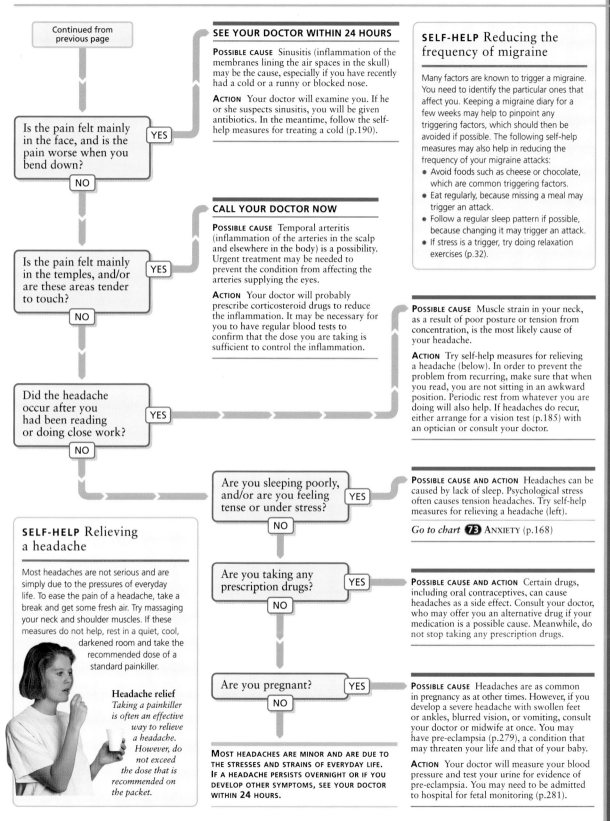

Headache relief
Taking a painkiller is often an effective way to relieve a headache. However, do not exceed the dose that is recommended on the packet.

Are you taking any prescription drugs? — YES

NO

POSSIBLE CAUSE AND ACTION Certain drugs, including oral contraceptives, can cause headaches as a side effect. Consult your doctor, who may offer you an alternative drug if your medication is a possible cause. Meanwhile, do not stop taking any prescription drugs.

Are you pregnant? — YES

NO

MOST HEADACHES ARE MINOR AND ARE DUE TO THE STRESSES AND STRAINS OF EVERYDAY LIFE. IF A HEADACHE PERSISTS OVERNIGHT OR IF YOU DEVELOP OTHER SYMPTOMS, SEE YOUR DOCTOR WITHIN 24 HOURS.

POSSIBLE CAUSE Headaches are as common in pregnancy as at other times. However, if you develop a severe headache with swollen feet or ankles, blurred vision, or vomiting, consult your doctor or midwife at once. You may have pre-eclampsia (p.279), a condition that may threaten your life and that of your baby.

ACTION Your doctor will measure your blood pressure and test your urine for evidence of pre-eclampsia. You may need to be admitted to hospital for fetal monitoring (p.281).

64 Feeling faint and passing out

People who feel faint usually experience a sensation of lightheadedness or dizziness and possibly nausea. Such feelings of faintness may sometimes progress to passing out – a brief loss of consciousness known as fainting. Feeling faint and passing out are usually caused by a sudden drop in blood pressure – as a result, for example, of emotional shock – or they may be due to an abnormally low level of sugar in the blood. Isolated episodes of feeling faint are hardly ever a cause for concern, but if you suffer repeated episodes, or if you pass out for no obvious reason, you should seek medical advice. Loss of consciousness may sometimes be due to a serious underlying medical condition.

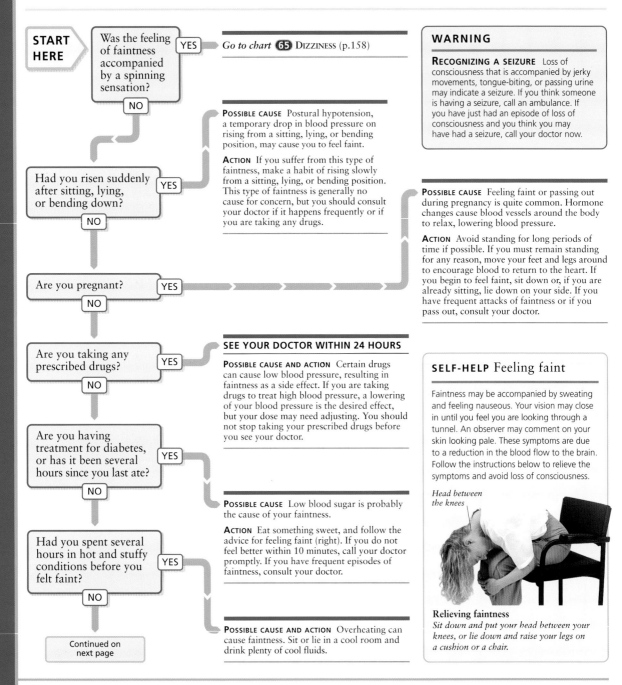

START HERE

Was the feeling of faintness accompanied by a spinning sensation?
YES → *Go to chart* **65** DIZZINESS (p.158)
NO

Had you risen suddenly after sitting, lying, or bending down?
YES →
NO

POSSIBLE CAUSE Postural hypotension, a temporary drop in blood pressure on rising from a sitting, lying, or bending position, may cause you to feel faint.

ACTION If you suffer from this type of faintness, make a habit of rising slowly from a sitting, lying, or bending position. This type of faintness is generally no cause for concern, but you should consult your doctor if it happens frequently or if you are taking any drugs.

Are you pregnant?
YES →
NO

Are you taking any prescribed drugs?
YES →
NO

SEE YOUR DOCTOR WITHIN 24 HOURS

POSSIBLE CAUSE AND ACTION Certain drugs can cause low blood pressure, resulting in faintness as a side effect. If you are taking drugs to treat high blood pressure, a lowering of your blood pressure is the desired effect, but your dose may need adjusting. You should not stop taking your prescribed drugs before you see your doctor.

Are you having treatment for diabetes, or has it been several hours since you last ate?
YES →
NO

POSSIBLE CAUSE Low blood sugar is probably the cause of your faintness.

ACTION Eat something sweet, and follow the advice for feeling faint (right). If you do not feel better within 10 minutes, call your doctor promptly. If you have frequent episodes of faintness, consult your doctor.

Had you spent several hours in hot and stuffy conditions before you felt faint?
YES →
NO

POSSIBLE CAUSE AND ACTION Overheating can cause faintness. Sit or lie in a cool room and drink plenty of cool fluids.

Continued on next page

WARNING

RECOGNIZING A SEIZURE Loss of consciousness that is accompanied by jerky movements, tongue-biting, or passing urine may indicate a seizure. If you think someone is having a seizure, call an ambulance. If you have just had an episode of loss of consciousness and you think you may have had a seizure, call your doctor now.

POSSIBLE CAUSE Feeling faint or passing out during pregnancy is quite common. Hormone changes cause blood vessels around the body to relax, lowering blood pressure.

ACTION Avoid standing for long periods of time if possible. If you must remain standing for any reason, move your feet and legs around to encourage blood to return to the heart. If you begin to feel faint, sit down or, if you are already sitting, lie down on your side. If you have frequent attacks of faintness or if you pass out, consult your doctor.

SELF-HELP Feeling faint

Faintness may be accompanied by sweating and feeling nauseous. Your vision may close in until you feel you are looking through a tunnel. An observer may comment on your skin looking pale. These symptoms are due to a reduction in the blood flow to the brain. Follow the instructions below to relieve the symptoms and avoid loss of consciousness.

Head between the knees

Relieving faintness
Sit down and put your head between your knees, or lie down and raise your legs on a cushion or a chair.

Continued from previous page

Have these symptoms now disappeared? — **YES**

NO

Do you have one or more of the following symptoms?
- Difficulty in speaking
- Disturbed vision
- Numbness, tingling, or weakness in any part of the body
- Confusion

YES

NO

Do you have any form of heart disease, and/or did you notice your heart rate speed up or slow down before the onset of faintness? — **YES**

NO

Did the faintness follow an emotional shock? — **YES**

NO

Have you noticed one or more of the following symptoms?
- Excessive tiredness
- Shortness of breath
- Paler than normal skin

YES

NO

Have you vomited blood, or have your faeces become black or bloody? — **YES**

NO

Are you aged over 50, and does turning your head or looking upward bring on a feeling of faintness? — **YES**

NO

CONSULT YOUR DOCTOR IF YOU ARE UNABLE TO MAKE A DIAGNOSIS FROM THIS CHART.

CALL YOUR DOCTOR NOW

POSSIBLE CAUSES If you are over 40, the most likely cause of your symptoms is a transient ischaemic attack (TIA), in which a blood clot temporarily blocks a blood vessel supplying the brain. In younger people, a disorder of the nervous system is a possibility.

ACTION Regardless of your age, your symptoms need urgent assessment. You may need tests such as MRI (p.39) to help to determine the cause and appropriate treatment.

☎ EMERGENCY! CALL AN AMBULANCE

POSSIBLE CAUSES If you are over 40, the most likely cause of your symptoms is a stroke, in which there is permanent damage to part of the brain due to a disruption in its blood supply. In younger people, a disorder of the nervous system is a possibility.

ACTION Regardless of your age, your symptoms need urgent assessment in hospital. You may need tests such as MRI (p.39) to help to determine the cause and appropriate treatment.

CALL YOUR DOCTOR NOW

POSSIBLE CAUSES There are a number of potentially serious conditions, such as an irregular heartbeat and heart valve problems, that reduce the output of blood from the heart, resulting in faintness and passing out.

ACTION Your doctor may arrange for you to be admitted urgently to hospital, where your condition can be monitored. You will need tests such as ECG (p.199) or a chest X-ray (p.37) to look for the cause of your faintness.

POSSIBLE CAUSE AND ACTION A sudden emotional shock can cause a fall in blood pressure, resulting in feelings of faintness. This is a normal response and does not need medical treatment. However, if it happens again, make an appointment to see your doctor.

SEE YOUR DOCTOR WITHIN 24 HOURS

POSSIBLE CAUSE Your symptoms may be due to anaemia. In this condition, there is too little of the oxygen-carrying pigment haemoglobin in the blood. Anaemia can be the result of a variety of underlying causes.

ACTION Your doctor will arrange for a blood test to confirm the diagnosis. In some cases, further tests will be necessary to determine why anaemia has developed. Treatment for the anaemia will usually need to be combined with treatment of the underlying cause.

☎ EMERGENCY! CALL AN AMBULANCE

POSSIBLE CAUSE Bleeding in the digestive tract, for example from a peptic ulcer, is a likely cause of these symptoms.

ACTION You will probably be admitted to hospital. If the bleeding was severe, you may be given a blood transfusion. You may also have tests such as endoscopy (p.209) to determine the cause of the bleeding.

POSSIBLE CAUSE Cervical spondylosis, arthritis in the bones in the neck, may be the cause. This can cause compression of blood vessels in the neck when you turn your head, leading to faintness. Consult your doctor.

ACTION If your doctor thinks your faintness is due to cervical spondylosis, you may be given a supportive collar to restrict neck movement.

Dizziness

Feeling unsteady on your feet for a moment is a common experience and need not be a matter for concern. However, true dizziness (also known as vertigo), in which there is a sensation that everything is spinning around, is not normal unless you have drunk too much alcohol or have been spinning around yourself – for example on a fairground ride. Dizziness may be a symptom of an underlying disorder and should be brought to your doctor's attention.

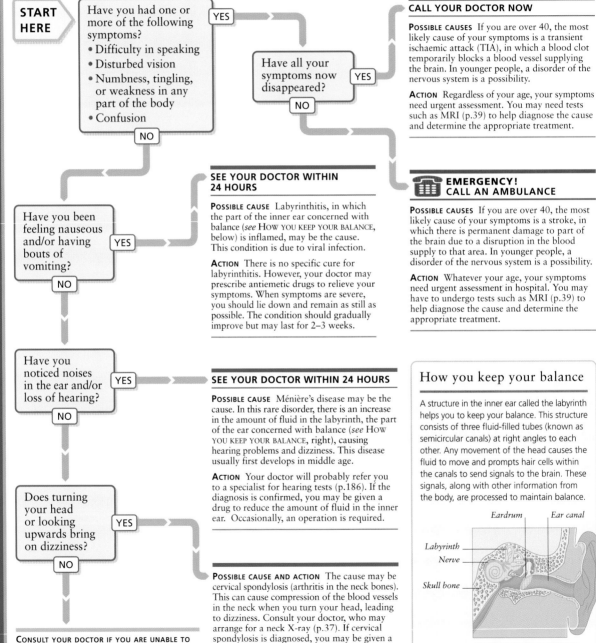

START HERE

Have you had one or more of the following symptoms?
- Difficulty in speaking
- Disturbed vision
- Numbness, tingling, or weakness in any part of the body
- Confusion

NO → **Have you been feeling nauseous and/or having bouts of vomiting?** — **YES**

NO ↓

Have you noticed noises in the ear and/or loss of hearing? — **YES**

NO ↓

Does turning your head or looking upwards bring on dizziness? — **YES**

NO ↓

CONSULT YOUR DOCTOR IF YOU ARE UNABLE TO MAKE A DIAGNOSIS FROM THIS CHART.

YES → **Have all your symptoms now disappeared?**

YES → (CALL YOUR DOCTOR NOW)

NO → (EMERGENCY! CALL AN AMBULANCE)

CALL YOUR DOCTOR NOW

POSSIBLE CAUSES If you are over 40, the most likely cause of your symptoms is a transient ischaemic attack (TIA), in which a blood clot temporarily blocks a blood vessel supplying the brain. In younger people, a disorder of the nervous system is a possibility.

ACTION Regardless of your age, your symptoms need urgent assessment. You may need tests such as MRI (p.39) to help diagnose the cause and determine the appropriate treatment.

EMERGENCY! CALL AN AMBULANCE

POSSIBLE CAUSES If you are over 40, the most likely cause of your symptoms is a stroke, in which there is permanent damage to part of the brain due to a disruption in the blood supply to that area. In younger people, a disorder of the nervous system is a possibility.

ACTION Whatever your age, your symptoms need urgent assessment in hospital. You may have to undergo tests such as MRI (p.39) to help diagnose the cause and determine the appropriate treatment.

SEE YOUR DOCTOR WITHIN 24 HOURS

POSSIBLE CAUSE Labyrinthitis, in which the part of the inner ear concerned with balance (see HOW YOU KEEP YOUR BALANCE, below) is inflamed, may be the cause. This condition is due to viral infection.

ACTION There is no specific cure for labyrinthitis. However, your doctor may prescribe antiemetic drugs to relieve your symptoms. When symptoms are severe, you should lie down and remain as still as possible. The condition should gradually improve but may last for 2–3 weeks.

SEE YOUR DOCTOR WITHIN 24 HOURS

POSSIBLE CAUSE Ménière's disease may be the cause. In this rare disorder, there is an increase in the amount of fluid in the labyrinth, the part of the ear concerned with balance (see HOW YOU KEEP YOUR BALANCE, right), causing hearing problems and dizziness. This disease usually first develops in middle age.

ACTION Your doctor will probably refer you to a specialist for hearing tests (p.186). If the diagnosis is confirmed, you may be given a drug to reduce the amount of fluid in the inner ear. Occasionally, an operation is required.

POSSIBLE CAUSE AND ACTION The cause may be cervical spondylosis (arthritis in the neck bones). This can cause compression of the blood vessels in the neck when you turn your head, leading to dizziness. Consult your doctor, who may arrange for a neck X-ray (p.37). If cervical spondylosis is diagnosed, you may be given a supportive collar to restrict neck movements.

How you keep your balance

A structure in the inner ear called the labyrinth helps you to keep your balance. This structure consists of three fluid-filled tubes (known as semicircular canals) at right angles to each other. Any movement of the head causes the fluid to move and prompts hair cells within the canals to send signals to the brain. These signals, along with other information from the body, are processed to maintain balance.

Eardrum   *Ear canal*

Labyrinth
Nerve

Skull bone

CROSS-SECTION OF THE EAR

66 Numbness and/or tingling

It is normal to experience numbness and/or tingling if you have been sitting in an awkward position. This is commonly called "pins and needles" and can occur in any part of the body. The feeling disappears as soon as you move around. Numbness or tingling that occurs without apparent cause may be due to a disorder that needs medical treatment.

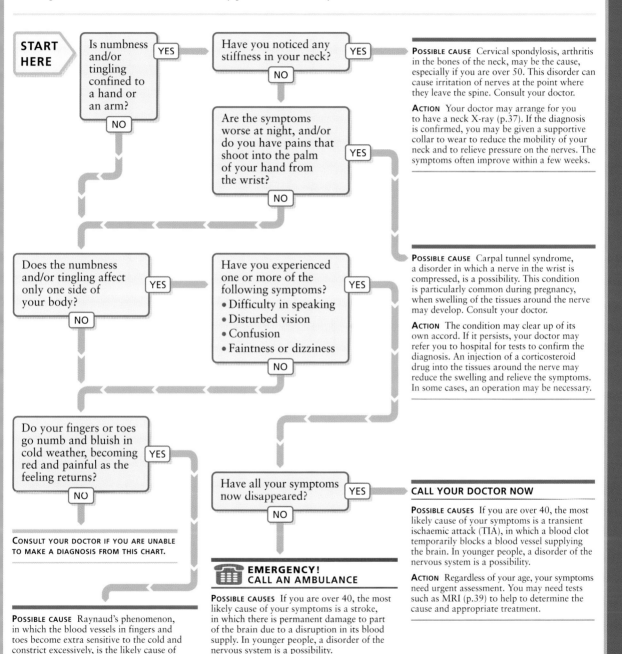

START HERE

Is numbness and/or tingling confined to a hand or an arm?
YES → **Have you noticed any stiffness in your neck?**
YES →

POSSIBLE CAUSE Cervical spondylosis, arthritis in the bones of the neck, may be the cause, especially if you are over 50. This disorder can cause irritation of nerves at the point where they leave the spine. Consult your doctor.

ACTION Your doctor may arrange for you to have a neck X-ray (p.37). If the diagnosis is confirmed, you may be given a supportive collar to wear to reduce the mobility of your neck and to relieve pressure on the nerves. The symptoms often improve within a few weeks.

NO ↓

Are the symptoms worse at night, and/or do you have pains that shoot into the palm of your hand from the wrist?
YES →

POSSIBLE CAUSE Carpal tunnel syndrome, a disorder in which a nerve in the wrist is compressed, is a possibility. This condition is particularly common during pregnancy, when swelling of the tissues around the nerve may develop. Consult your doctor.

ACTION The condition may clear up of its own accord. If it persists, your doctor may refer you to hospital for tests to confirm the diagnosis. An injection of a corticosteroid drug into the tissues around the nerve may reduce the swelling and relieve the symptoms. In some cases, an operation may be necessary.

NO (from first question) ↓

Does the numbness and/or tingling affect only one side of your body?
YES → **Have you experienced one or more of the following symptoms?**
- Difficulty in speaking
- Disturbed vision
- Confusion
- Faintness or dizziness

YES →

NO ↓

Do your fingers or toes go numb and bluish in cold weather, becoming red and painful as the feeling returns?
YES → **Have all your symptoms now disappeared?**
YES →

NO ↓

CONSULT YOUR DOCTOR IF YOU ARE UNABLE TO MAKE A DIAGNOSIS FROM THIS CHART.

POSSIBLE CAUSE Raynaud's phenomenon, in which the blood vessels in fingers and toes become extra sensitive to the cold and constrict excessively, is the likely cause of these symptoms. Consult your doctor.

ACTION Keep your hands and feet warm and dry. Do not smoke. In some cases, drug treatment or, rarely, surgery may be needed.

☎ **EMERGENCY! CALL AN AMBULANCE**

POSSIBLE CAUSES If you are over 40, the most likely cause of your symptoms is a stroke, in which there is permanent damage to part of the brain due to a disruption in its blood supply. In younger people, a disorder of the nervous system is a possibility.

ACTION Regardless of your age, your symptoms need urgent assessment in hospital. You may need tests such as MRI (p.39) to help to determine the cause and appropriate treatment.

CALL YOUR DOCTOR NOW

POSSIBLE CAUSES If you are over 40, the most likely cause of your symptoms is a transient ischaemic attack (TIA), in which a blood clot temporarily blocks a blood vessel supplying the brain. In younger people, a disorder of the nervous system is a possibility.

ACTION Regardless of your age, your symptoms need urgent assessment. You may need tests such as MRI (p.39) to help to determine the cause and appropriate treatment.

67 Forgetfulness and/or confusion

We all suffer from mild forgetfulness from time to time, especially in later life when such "absent-mindedness" is a natural part of aging. People often forget details when they have been preoccupied with other things, and this is no cause for concern. However, confusion, particularly if it comes on suddenly, or forgetfulness and confusion severe enough to disrupt everyday life, may be due to an underlying medical problem. This chart deals with sudden or severe confusion or forgetfulness that you are aware of in yourself or in someone else who may not realize they have a problem.

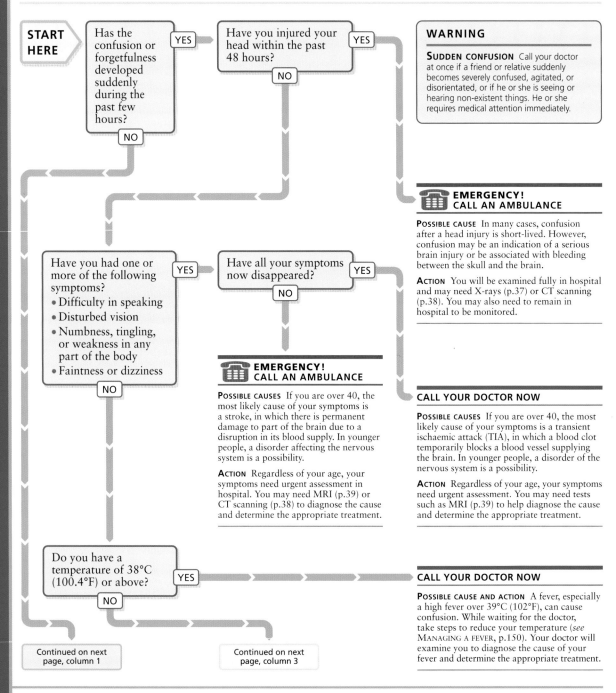

START HERE

Has the confusion or forgetfulness developed suddenly during the past few hours? — **YES** →

Have you injured your head within the past 48 hours? — **YES** →

NO

NO

WARNING

SUDDEN CONFUSION Call your doctor at once if a friend or relative suddenly becomes severely confused, agitated, or disorientated, or if he or she is seeing or hearing non-existent things. He or she requires medical attention immediately.

📞 EMERGENCY! CALL AN AMBULANCE

POSSIBLE CAUSE In many cases, confusion after a head injury is short-lived. However, confusion may be an indication of a serious brain injury or be associated with bleeding between the skull and the brain.

ACTION You will be examined fully in hospital and may need X-rays (p.37) or CT scanning (p.38). You may also need to remain in hospital to be monitored.

Have you had one or more of the following symptoms?
• Difficulty in speaking
• Disturbed vision
• Numbness, tingling, or weakness in any part of the body
• Faintness or dizziness — **YES** →

Have all your symptoms now disappeared? — **YES** →

NO

NO

📞 EMERGENCY! CALL AN AMBULANCE

POSSIBLE CAUSES If you are over 40, the most likely cause of your symptoms is a stroke, in which there is permanent damage to part of the brain due to a disruption in its blood supply. In younger people, a disorder affecting the nervous system is a possibility.

ACTION Regardless of your age, your symptoms need urgent assessment in hospital. You may need MRI (p.39) or CT scanning (p.38) to diagnose the cause and determine the appropriate treatment.

CALL YOUR DOCTOR NOW

POSSIBLE CAUSES If you are over 40, the most likely cause of your symptoms is a transient ischaemic attack (TIA), in which a blood clot temporarily blocks a blood vessel supplying the brain. In younger people, a disorder of the nervous system is a possibility.

ACTION Regardless of your age, your symptoms need urgent assessment. You may need tests such as MRI (p.39) to help diagnose the cause and determine the appropriate treatment.

Do you have a temperature of 38°C (100.4°F) or above? — **YES** →

NO

CALL YOUR DOCTOR NOW

POSSIBLE CAUSE AND ACTION A fever, especially a high fever over 39°C (102°F), can cause confusion. While waiting for the doctor, take steps to reduce your temperature (*see* MANAGING A FEVER, p.150). Your doctor will examine you to diagnose the cause of your fever and determine the appropriate treatment.

Continued on next page, column 1

Continued on next page, column 3

Continued from previous page, column 1

Have you noticed any of the following symptoms?
- Inability to concentrate or make decisions
- Difficulty in sleeping
- Feeling in low spirits
- Loss of interest in sex

YES →

POSSIBLE CAUSE Depression can cause forgetfulness and confusion, particularly in elderly people. Consult your doctor.

ACTION If your doctor confirms that you are depressed, he or she may prescribe antidepressant drugs. These drugs often improve mental functioning as well as treating depression, but they may take a few weeks to take effect.

NO ↓

Have you noticed that you have difficulty coping with everyday matters or in following complex instructions?

YES →

POSSIBLE CAUSE Progressive loss of mental function (dementia) due to a disorder such as Alzheimer's disease or recurrent small strokes is a possibility. Dementia is most likely to occur in people over the age of 65, although in rare cases the condition can affect younger people. Consult your doctor.

ACTION Your doctor will examine you and he or she may refer you to a specialist. You may need blood tests or MRI (p.39) to exclude other underlying causes. In most cases, treatments cannot reverse dementia, but drug treatments may slow deterioration. Support groups (*see* USEFUL ADDRESSES, p.285) can provide self-help information, and social services may provide practical help.

NO ↓

Continued from previous page, column 2

Are you suffering from a serious heart or lung condition?

YES →

CALL YOUR DOCTOR NOW

POSSIBLE CAUSE A sudden worsening of disorders affecting the heart or lungs may reduce the supply of oxygen to the brain, leading to confusion.

ACTION You may need to be admitted to hospital, where you will be given oxygen and drugs to stabilize your condition.

NO ↓

Are you being treated for diabetes?

YES →

POSSIBLE CAUSES Your blood sugar level may be too low, particularly if the symptoms started suddenly. Less commonly, these symptoms may be due to an abnormally high blood sugar level.

ACTION Eat or drink something very sweet. This should correct a low blood sugar level and will do you no harm if your sugar level is too high. If you are no better within 10 minutes, call your doctor immediately.

NO ↓

Are you taking any prescribed drugs?

YES →

SEE YOUR DOCTOR WITHIN 24 HOURS

POSSIBLE CAUSE AND ACTION Certain drugs may be the cause of forgetfulness or confusion as a side effect. Do not stop taking your prescribed drugs unless your doctor tells you otherwise.

NO ↓

Do you regularly drink more than the recommended safe alcohol limit (p.30)?

YES →

POSSIBLE CAUSE Excessive alcohol consumption commonly causes memory loss and confusion.

ACTION If you regularly drink enough alcohol to leave you confused, you should cut down your consumption. If you have difficulty doing so, consult your doctor for advice.

NO ↓

Do you use recreational drugs or inhale solvents?

YES →

POSSIBLE CAUSE AND ACTION Recreational drugs may cause confusion, and prolonged use can lead to irreversible brain damage. Stop using recreational drugs or inhaling solvents. If you have trouble stopping, consult your doctor, who may be able to help or may put you in contact with a counsellor or a self-help group (*see* USEFUL ADDRESSES, p.285).

NO ↓

CONSULT YOUR DOCTOR IF YOU ARE UNABLE TO MAKE A DIAGNOSIS FROM THIS CHART.

161

68 Twitching and/or trembling

Consult this chart if you experience any involuntary or uncontrolled movements. Such movements may range from slight twitching to prolonged, repeated trembling or shaking of the arms, legs, or head. Brief episodes are often simply the result of tiredness or stress and are rarely a cause for concern. Jerking movements that happen while you are falling asleep are also common and harmless. Occasionally, however, involuntary movements may be caused by problems that require medical treatment, such as excessive alcohol consumption or a neurological disorder.

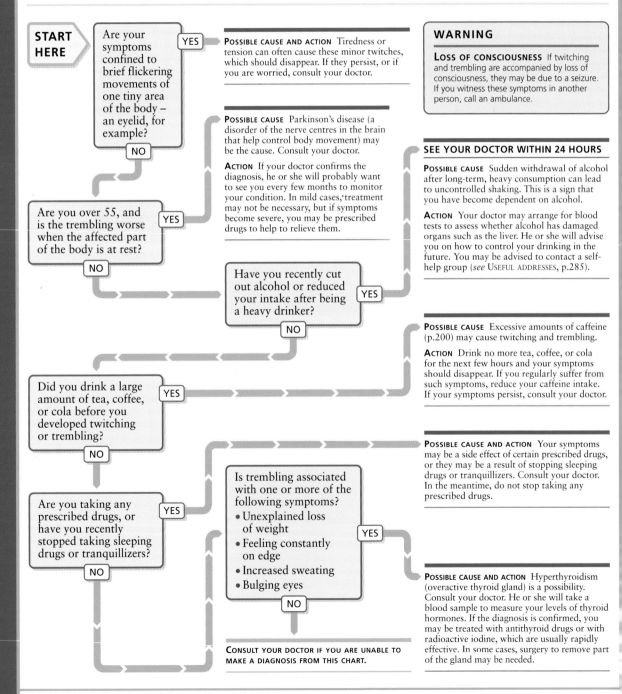

START HERE

Are your symptoms confined to brief flickering movements of one tiny area of the body – an eyelid, for example?

YES → **POSSIBLE CAUSE AND ACTION** Tiredness or tension can often cause these minor twitches, which should disappear. If they persist, or if you are worried, consult your doctor.

NO

Are you over 55, and is the trembling worse when the affected part of the body is at rest?

YES → **POSSIBLE CAUSE** Parkinson's disease (a disorder of the nerve centres in the brain that help control body movement) may be the cause. Consult your doctor.

ACTION If your doctor confirms the diagnosis, he or she will probably want to see you every few months to monitor your condition. In mild cases, treatment may not be necessary, but if symptoms become severe, you may be prescribed drugs to help to relieve them.

NO

Have you recently cut out alcohol or reduced your intake after being a heavy drinker?

YES

NO

Did you drink a large amount of tea, coffee, or cola before you developed twitching or trembling?

YES

NO

Are you taking any prescribed drugs, or have you recently stopped taking sleeping drugs or tranquillizers?

YES →

Is trembling associated with one or more of the following symptoms?
- Unexplained loss of weight
- Feeling constantly on edge
- Increased sweating
- Bulging eyes

YES

NO

NO

CONSULT YOUR DOCTOR IF YOU ARE UNABLE TO MAKE A DIAGNOSIS FROM THIS CHART.

WARNING

LOSS OF CONSCIOUSNESS If twitching and trembling are accompanied by loss of consciousness, they may be due to a seizure. If you witness these symptoms in another person, call an ambulance.

SEE YOUR DOCTOR WITHIN 24 HOURS

POSSIBLE CAUSE Sudden withdrawal of alcohol after long-term, heavy consumption can lead to uncontrolled shaking. This is a sign that you have become dependent on alcohol.

ACTION Your doctor may arrange for blood tests to assess whether alcohol has damaged organs such as the liver. He or she will advise you on how to control your drinking in the future. You may be advised to contact a self-help group (see USEFUL ADDRESSES, p.285).

POSSIBLE CAUSE Excessive amounts of caffeine (p.200) may cause twitching and trembling.

ACTION Drink no more tea, coffee, or cola for the next few hours and your symptoms should disappear. If you regularly suffer from such symptoms, reduce your caffeine intake. If your symptoms persist, consult your doctor.

POSSIBLE CAUSE AND ACTION Your symptoms may be a side effect of certain prescribed drugs, or they may be a result of stopping sleeping drugs or tranquillizers. Consult your doctor. In the meantime, do not stop taking any prescribed drugs.

POSSIBLE CAUSE AND ACTION Hyperthyroidism (overactive thyroid gland) is a possibility. Consult your doctor. He or she will take a blood sample to measure your levels of thyroid hormones. If the diagnosis is confirmed, you may be treated with antithyroid drugs or with radioactive iodine, which are usually rapidly effective. In some cases, surgery to remove part of the gland may be needed.

69 Pain in the face

For toothache, see chart 95, Teeth problems (p.202). For pain in or around the mouth, see chart 96, Mouth problems (p.204). For a headache, see chart 63, Headache (p.154). Consult this chart if you develop pain or discomfort that is limited to the area of the face and/or the forehead. Facial pain may be a dull, throbbing ache or a sharp, stabbing sensation. It is often caused by infection or inflammation of the underlying tissues or irritation of a nerve. Although pain in the face can be distressing and may require medical treatment, it is rarely a sign of a serious disorder.

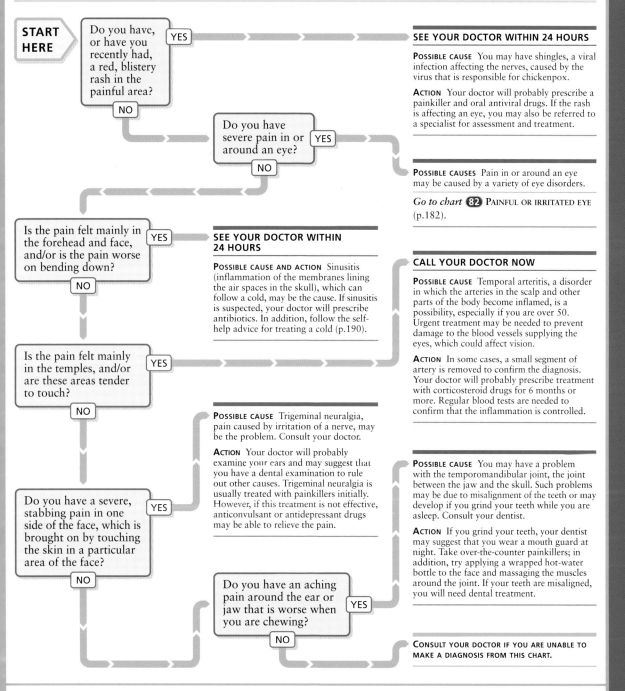

START HERE

Do you have, or have you recently had, a red, blistery rash in the painful area? — **YES** →

NO ↓

Do you have severe pain in or around an eye? — **YES** →

NO ↓

Is the pain felt mainly in the forehead and face, and/or is the pain worse on bending down? — **YES** →

NO ↓

Is the pain felt mainly in the temples, and/or are these areas tender to touch? — **YES** →

NO ↓

Do you have a severe, stabbing pain in one side of the face, which is brought on by touching the skin in a particular area of the face? — **YES** →

NO ↓

Do you have an aching pain around the ear or jaw that is worse when you are chewing? — **YES** →

NO ↓

SEE YOUR DOCTOR WITHIN 24 HOURS

POSSIBLE CAUSE You may have shingles, a viral infection affecting the nerves, caused by the virus that is responsible for chickenpox.

ACTION Your doctor will probably prescribe a painkiller and oral antiviral drugs. If the rash is affecting an eye, you may also be referred to a specialist for assessment and treatment.

POSSIBLE CAUSES Pain in or around an eye may be caused by a variety of eye disorders.

Go to chart 82 PAINFUL OR IRRITATED EYE (p.182).

CALL YOUR DOCTOR NOW

POSSIBLE CAUSE Temporal arteritis, a disorder in which the arteries in the scalp and other parts of the body become inflamed, is a possibility, especially if you are over 50. Urgent treatment may be needed to prevent damage to the blood vessels supplying the eyes, which could affect vision.

ACTION In some cases, a small segment of artery is removed to confirm the diagnosis. Your doctor will probably prescribe treatment with corticosteroid drugs for 6 months or more. Regular blood tests are needed to confirm that the inflammation is controlled.

POSSIBLE CAUSE You may have a problem with the temporomandibular joint, the joint between the jaw and the skull. Such problems may be due to misalignment of the teeth or may develop if you grind your teeth while you are asleep. Consult your dentist.

ACTION If you grind your teeth, your dentist may suggest that you wear a mouth guard at night. Take over-the-counter painkillers; in addition, try applying a wrapped hot-water bottle to the face and massaging the muscles around the joint. If your teeth are misaligned, you will need dental treatment.

SEE YOUR DOCTOR WITHIN 24 HOURS

POSSIBLE CAUSE AND ACTION Sinusitis (inflammation of the membranes lining the air spaces in the skull), which can follow a cold, may be the cause. If sinusitis is suspected, your doctor will prescribe antibiotics. In addition, follow the self-help advice for treating a cold (p.190).

POSSIBLE CAUSE Trigeminal neuralgia, pain caused by irritation of a nerve, may be the problem. Consult your doctor.

ACTION Your doctor will probably examine your ears and may suggest that you have a dental examination to rule out other causes. Trigeminal neuralgia is usually treated with painkillers initially. However, if this treatment is not effective, anticonvulsant or antidepressant drugs may be able to relieve the pain.

CONSULT YOUR DOCTOR IF YOU ARE UNABLE TO MAKE A DIAGNOSIS FROM THIS CHART.

70 Difficulty in speaking

Consult this chart if you have, or recently have had, difficulty in finding or using words or if your speech has become unclear. Such speech difficulties may be related to disorders affecting the brain, the mouth, or the facial nerves. In some cases, speech may be affected permanently, although speech therapy (below) is often beneficial.

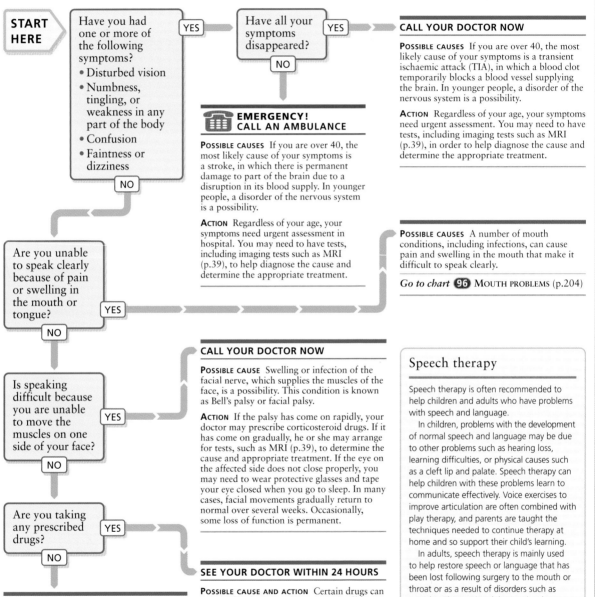

START HERE

Have you had one or more of the following symptoms?
- Disturbed vision
- Numbness, tingling, or weakness in any part of the body
- Confusion
- Faintness or dizziness

YES →

Have all your symptoms disappeared?

YES →

NO ↓

Are you unable to speak clearly because of pain or swelling in the mouth or tongue?

YES →

NO ↓

Is speaking difficult because you are unable to move the muscles on one side of your face?

YES →

NO ↓

Are you taking any prescribed drugs?

YES →

NO ↓

EMERGENCY! CALL AN AMBULANCE

POSSIBLE CAUSES If you are over 40, the most likely cause of your symptoms is a stroke, in which there is permanent damage to part of the brain due to a disruption in its blood supply. In younger people, a disorder of the nervous system is a possibility.

ACTION Regardless of your age, your symptoms need urgent assessment in hospital. You may need to have tests, including imaging tests such as MRI (p.39), to help diagnose the cause and determine the appropriate treatment.

CALL YOUR DOCTOR NOW

POSSIBLE CAUSES If you are over 40, the most likely cause of your symptoms is a transient ischaemic attack (TIA), in which a blood clot temporarily blocks a blood vessel supplying the brain. In younger people, a disorder of the nervous system is a possibility.

ACTION Regardless of your age, your symptoms need urgent assessment. You may need to have tests, including imaging tests such as MRI (p.39), in order to help diagnose the cause and determine the appropriate treatment.

POSSIBLE CAUSES A number of mouth conditions, including infections, can cause pain and swelling in the mouth that make it difficult to speak clearly.

Go to chart **96** MOUTH PROBLEMS (p.204)

CALL YOUR DOCTOR NOW

POSSIBLE CAUSE Swelling or infection of the facial nerve, which supplies the muscles of the face, is a possibility. This condition is known as Bell's palsy or facial palsy.

ACTION If the palsy has come on rapidly, your doctor may prescribe corticosteroid drugs. If it has come on gradually, he or she may arrange for tests, such as MRI (p.39), to determine the cause and appropriate treatment. If the eye on the affected side does not close properly, you may need to wear protective glasses and tape your eye closed when you go to sleep. In many cases, facial movements gradually return to normal over several weeks. Occasionally, some loss of function is permanent.

SEE YOUR DOCTOR WITHIN 24 HOURS

POSSIBLE CAUSE AND ACTION Certain drugs can cause difficulty in speaking as a side effect – for example, antianxiety drugs may cause slurred speech as a result of their action on the brain, and antidepressants may make speech more difficult by causing a dry mouth. However, you should not stop taking your prescribed drugs unless you are advised to do so by your doctor.

SEE YOUR DOCTOR WITHIN 24 HOURS

POSSIBLE CAUSE AND ACTION Unexplained difficulty in speaking may be an early sign of an underlying disorder of the brain or nervous system and needs prompt medical assessment. Your doctor may arrange for tests to diagnose the cause and determine the treatment.

Speech therapy

Speech therapy is often recommended to help children and adults who have problems with speech and language.

In children, problems with the development of normal speech and language may be due to other problems such as hearing loss, learning difficulties, or physical causes such as a cleft lip and palate. Speech therapy can help children with these problems learn to communicate effectively. Voice exercises to improve articulation are often combined with play therapy, and parents are taught the techniques needed to continue therapy at home and so support their child's learning.

In adults, speech therapy is mainly used to help restore speech or language that has been lost following surgery to the mouth or throat or as a result of disorders such as a stroke. Therapy in adults may involve relearning speech, voice exercises, or, in some cases, using electronic devices to aid speech production. If speech cannot be restored, help with communication – for example, help with the use of pictures or specialized computers – may be offered.

71 Disturbing thoughts and feelings

Consult this chart if you begin to have thoughts and feelings that worry you or that seem to you or to other people to be abnormal or unhealthy. You may be having upsetting or intrusive thoughts or you may be experiencing unfamiliar or uncontrolled emotions. If your thoughts and feelings continue to worry you, whatever your particular problem, talk to your doctor about them. He or she may be able to help you to put your feelings into context by discussing them with you. If your concerns are justified, he or she may suggest treatment or refer you to a specialized therapist.

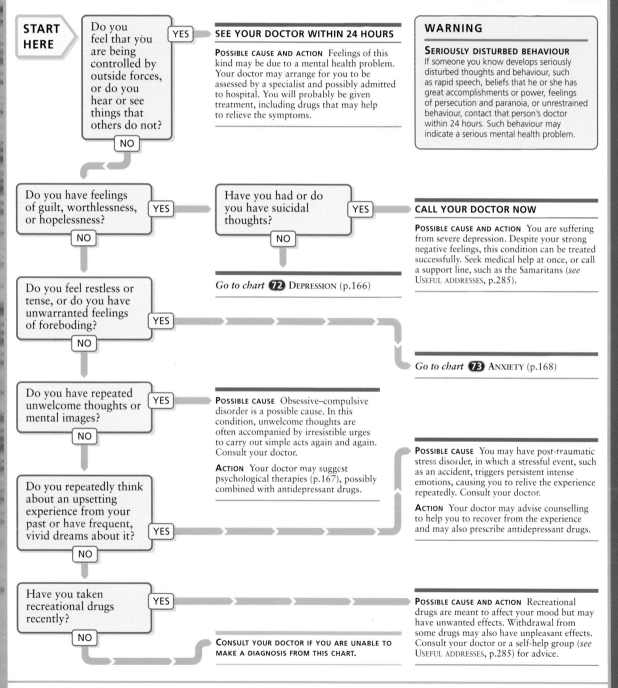

START HERE

Do you feel that you are being controlled by outside forces, or do you hear or see things that others do not? — **YES** →

SEE YOUR DOCTOR WITHIN 24 HOURS

POSSIBLE CAUSE AND ACTION Feelings of this kind may be due to a mental health problem. Your doctor may arrange for you to be assessed by a specialist and possibly admitted to hospital. You will probably be given treatment, including drugs that may help to relieve the symptoms.

NO

WARNING

SERIOUSLY DISTURBED BEHAVIOUR
If someone you know develops seriously disturbed thoughts and behaviour, such as rapid speech, beliefs that he or she has great accomplishments or power, feelings of persecution and paranoia, or unrestrained behaviour, contact that person's doctor within 24 hours. Such behaviour may indicate a serious mental health problem.

Do you have feelings of guilt, worthlessness, or hopelessness? — **YES** →

Have you had or do you have suicidal thoughts? — **YES** →

CALL YOUR DOCTOR NOW

POSSIBLE CAUSE AND ACTION You are suffering from severe depression. Despite your strong negative feelings, this condition can be treated successfully. Seek medical help at once, or call a support line, such as the Samaritans (*see* USEFUL ADDRESSES, p.285).

NO / **NO**

Go to chart **72** DEPRESSION (p.166)

Do you feel restless or tense, or do you have unwarranted feelings of foreboding? — **YES** →

Go to chart **73** ANXIETY (p.168)

NO

Do you have repeated unwelcome thoughts or mental images? — **YES** →

POSSIBLE CAUSE Obsessive–compulsive disorder is a possible cause. In this condition, unwelcome thoughts are often accompanied by irresistible urges to carry out simple acts again and again. Consult your doctor.

ACTION Your doctor may suggest psychological therapies (p.167), possibly combined with antidepressant drugs.

NO

Do you repeatedly think about an upsetting experience from your past or have frequent, vivid dreams about it? — **YES** →

POSSIBLE CAUSE You may have post-traumatic stress disorder, in which a stressful event, such as an accident, triggers persistent intense emotions, causing you to relive the experience repeatedly. Consult your doctor.

ACTION Your doctor may advise counselling to help you to recover from the experience and may also prescribe antidepressant drugs.

NO

Have you taken recreational drugs recently? — **YES** →

POSSIBLE CAUSE AND ACTION Recreational drugs are meant to affect your mood but may have unwanted effects. Withdrawal from some drugs may also have unpleasant effects. Consult your doctor or a self-help group (*see* USEFUL ADDRESSES, p.285) for advice.

NO

CONSULT YOUR DOCTOR IF YOU ARE UNABLE TO MAKE A DIAGNOSIS FROM THIS CHART.

72 Depression

Most people have minor ups and downs in mood, feeling good one day but low the next. These changes often have an identifiable cause and usually pass quickly. True depression is associated with physical symptoms including excessive tiredness, loss of weight, and sleep disturbances, such as early waking (see RECOGNIZING DEPRESSION, below). In some cases, a depressive illness follows a traumatic event, such as divorce,

bereavement, or loss of a job. In other cases, it follows a time a major life change, such as retirement. It may also be precipitated by hormonal changes at the menopause or after childbirth. However, in many cases, depression has no apparent cause, and some people have repeated episodes. Depression is a treatable disorder, and you should always see your doctor if you think you might be depressed.

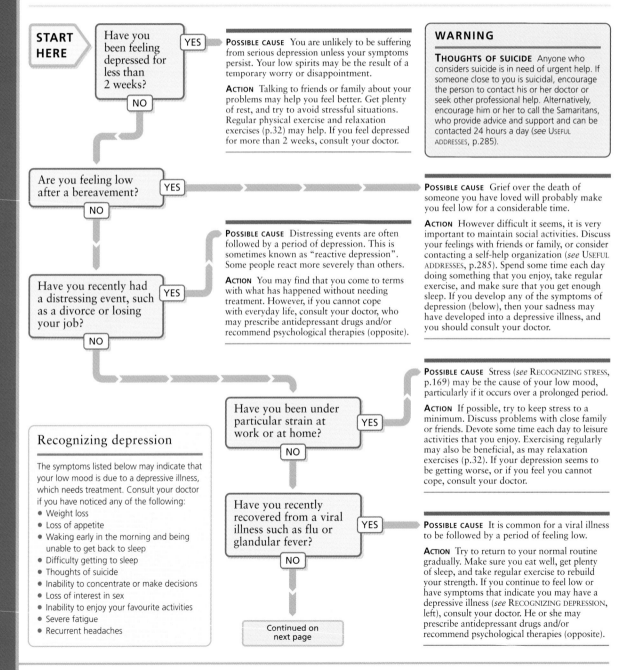

START HERE

Have you been feeling depressed for less than 2 weeks?

YES → **POSSIBLE CAUSE** You are unlikely to be suffering from serious depression unless your symptoms persist. Your low spirits may be the result of a temporary worry or disappointment.

ACTION Talking to friends or family about your problems may help you feel better. Get plenty of rest, and try to avoid stressful situations. Regular physical exercise and relaxation exercises (p.32) may help. If you feel depressed for more than 2 weeks, consult your doctor.

NO

Are you feeling low after a bereavement?

YES → **POSSIBLE CAUSE** Grief over the death of someone you have loved will probably make you feel low for a considerable time.

ACTION However difficult it seems, it is very important to maintain social activities. Discuss your feelings with friends or family, or consider contacting a self-help organization (see USEFUL ADDRESSES, p.285). Spend some time each day doing something that you enjoy, take regular exercise, and make sure that you get enough sleep. If you develop any of the symptoms of depression (below), then your sadness may have developed into a depressive illness, and you should consult your doctor.

NO

Have you recently had a distressing event, such as a divorce or losing your job?

YES → **POSSIBLE CAUSE** Distressing events are often followed by a period of depression. This is sometimes known as "reactive depression". Some people react more severely than others.

ACTION You may find that you come to terms with what has happened without needing treatment. However, if you cannot cope with everyday life, consult your doctor, who may prescribe antidepressant drugs and/or recommend psychological therapies (opposite).

NO

Have you been under particular strain at work or at home?

YES → **POSSIBLE CAUSE** Stress (see RECOGNIZING STRESS, p.169) may be the cause of your low mood, particularly if it occurs over a prolonged period.

ACTION If possible, try to keep stress to a minimum. Discuss problems with close family or friends. Devote some time each day to leisure activities that you enjoy. Exercising regularly may also be beneficial, as may relaxation exercises (p.32). If your depression seems to be getting worse, or if you feel you cannot cope, consult your doctor.

NO

Have you recently recovered from a viral illness such as flu or glandular fever?

YES → **POSSIBLE CAUSE** It is common for a viral illness to be followed by a period of feeling low.

ACTION Try to return to your normal routine gradually. Make sure you eat well, get plenty of sleep, and take regular exercise to rebuild your strength. If you continue to feel low or have symptoms that indicate you may have a depressive illness (see RECOGNIZING DEPRESSION, left), consult your doctor. He or she may prescribe antidepressant drugs and/or recommend psychological therapies (opposite).

NO

Continued on next page

WARNING

THOUGHTS OF SUICIDE Anyone who considers suicide is in need of urgent help. If someone close to you is suicidal, encourage the person to contact his or her doctor or seek other professional help. Alternatively, encourage him or her to call the Samaritans, who provide advice and support and can be contacted 24 hours a day (see USEFUL ADDRESSES, p.285).

Recognizing depression

The symptoms listed below may indicate that your low mood is due to a depressive illness, which needs treatment. Consult your doctor if you have noticed any of the following:

- Weight loss
- Loss of appetite
- Waking early in the morning and being unable to get back to sleep
- Difficulty getting to sleep
- Thoughts of suicide
- Inability to concentrate or make decisions
- Loss of interest in sex
- Inability to enjoy your favourite activities
- Severe fatigue
- Recurrent headaches

Continued from previous page

Have you recently had a serious illness or accident? — YES →

NO ↓

POSSIBLE CAUSES A serious physical illness, such as a heart attack, or a major accident may often be followed by depression. This may slow down your physical recovery. Consult your doctor.

ACTION Your doctor will talk to you about your current health and will explain that this is a common reaction. You may be prescribed antidepressant drugs and/or your doctor may recommend psychological therapies (below).

POSSIBLE CAUSE Regularly drinking too much alcohol may lead to depression. You should also be aware of why you drink. Some people may use alcohol to help them cope with stress or unrecognized depression. Drinking too much may be compounding the problem.

ACTION Cut down the amount of alcohol you drink. If you find this difficult, or you continue to feel depressed, consult your doctor for advice.

Do you regularly drink more than the recommended safe alcohol limit (p.30)? — YES →

NO ↓

Are you using, or have you ever used, recreational drugs? — YES →

NO ↓

POSSIBLE CAUSE Many recreational drugs can cause profound psychological disturbances, both during use and after withdrawal. Some drugs can cause problems even years later.

ACTION If you still take recreational drugs, stop now. If you find you cannot stop or are still having problems after you have stopped, consult your doctor, who may be able to help or may put you in contact with a counsellor or self-help group (*see* USEFUL ADDRESSES, p.285).

Are you taking any prescribed drugs? — YES →

NO ↓

POSSIBLE CAUSE AND ACTION Certain drugs, such as antihypertensives (drugs used to treat high blood pressure) and oral contraceptives, can cause depression as a side effect. Consult your doctor. Meanwhile, do not stop taking your prescribed drugs.

Are you male? — YES →

NO ↓

IF YOU ARE UNABLE TO FIND AN EXPLANATION FOR YOUR FEELINGS FROM THIS CHART, CONSULT YOUR DOCTOR BECAUSE YOU MAY BE SUFFERING FROM A DEPRESSIVE ILLNESS.

Have you recently had a baby? — YES →

NO ↓

Go to chart **150** DEPRESSION AFTER CHILDBIRTH (p.284)

Do you often feel low just before your period is due? — YES →

NO ↓

POSSIBLE CAUSE AND ACTION Premenstrual syndrome, a collection of symptoms that may include low spirits and is caused by hormone changes, is likely. Follow self-help measures (*see* PREMENSTRUAL SYNDROME, p.253). If your symptoms do not improve, consult your doctor.

Are you menopausal, or have you recently passed the menopause? — YES →

NO ↓

IF YOU ARE UNABLE TO FIND AN EXPLANATION FOR YOUR FEELINGS FROM THIS CHART, CONSULT YOUR DOCTOR BECAUSE YOU MAY BE SUFFERING FROM A DEPRESSIVE ILLNESS.

POSSIBLE CAUSE AND ACTION Hormonal changes around the menopause may cause depression. Such feelings may be exaggerated by concerns over the approach of old age and loss of fertility and by stressful events such as children leaving home. Consult your doctor, who may suggest hormone replacement therapy (*see* A HEALTHY MENOPAUSE, p.257) around the time of the menopause. In some cases, antidepressant drugs may be needed.

Psychological therapies

There are a variety of psychological therapies available, some of which explore a person's past, while others focus on current behaviour or thought processes. All involve a therapist who usually encourages you to talk about your feelings and fears, while he or she provides help and advice.

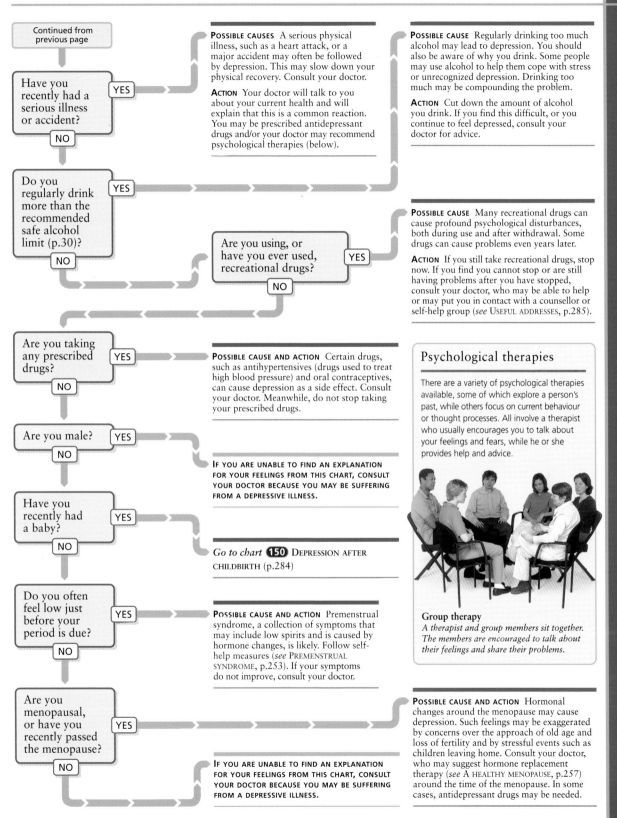

Group therapy
A therapist and group members sit together. The members are encouraged to talk about their feelings and share their problems.

73 Anxiety

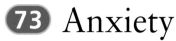

If you are suffering from anxiety, you will probably feel apprehensive and tense and be unable to concentrate, think clearly, or sleep well. You may have a sense of foreboding for no obvious reason or have repetitive worrying thoughts. Some people also have physical symptoms such as headaches, excessive sweating, chest pains, palpitations, abdominal cramps, and a general feeling of tiredness. Anxiety is a

natural reaction to stress, and it is normal to feel anxious if, for example, you are worried about money or family matters or if you have exams coming up. Such anxiety may help you to deal with stressful events and can help to improve your performance in certain situations. However, anxiety is not normal if it comes on without an apparent cause or if it is so severe that you can no longer cope with everyday life.

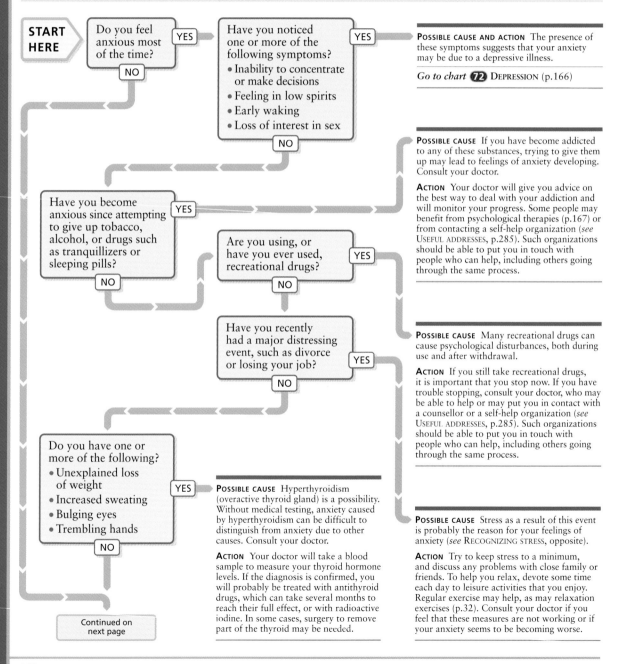

START HERE

Do you feel anxious most of the time? — YES → **Have you noticed one or more of the following symptoms?**
- Inability to concentrate or make decisions
- Feeling in low spirits
- Early waking
- Loss of interest in sex

YES → **POSSIBLE CAUSE AND ACTION** The presence of these symptoms suggests that your anxiety may be due to a depressive illness.

Go to chart **72** DEPRESSION (p.166)

NO ↓ (from symptoms box)

NO ↓ (from Do you feel anxious box)

Have you become anxious since attempting to give up tobacco, alcohol, or drugs such as tranquillizers or sleeping pills? — YES →

POSSIBLE CAUSE If you have become addicted to any of these substances, trying to give them up may lead to feelings of anxiety developing. Consult your doctor.

ACTION Your doctor will give you advice on the best way to deal with your addiction and will monitor your progress. Some people may benefit from psychological therapies (p.167) or from contacting a self-help organization (*see* USEFUL ADDRESSES, p.285). Such organizations should be able to put you in touch with people who can help, including others going through the same process.

NO ↓

Are you using, or have you ever used, recreational drugs? — YES →

NO ↓

POSSIBLE CAUSE Many recreational drugs can cause psychological disturbances, both during use and after withdrawal.

ACTION If you still take recreational drugs, it is important that you stop now. If you have trouble stopping, consult your doctor, who may be able to help or may put you in contact with a counsellor or a self-help organization (*see* USEFUL ADDRESSES, p.285). Such organizations should be able to put you in touch with people who can help, including others going through the same process.

Have you recently had a major distressing event, such as divorce or losing your job? — YES →

NO ↓

Do you have one or more of the following?
- Unexplained loss of weight
- Increased sweating
- Bulging eyes
- Trembling hands

YES →

POSSIBLE CAUSE Hyperthyroidism (overactive thyroid gland) is a possibility. Without medical testing, anxiety caused by hyperthyroidism can be difficult to distinguish from anxiety due to other causes. Consult your doctor.

ACTION Your doctor will take a blood sample to measure your thyroid hormone levels. If the diagnosis is confirmed, you will probably be treated with antithyroid drugs, which can take several months to reach their full effect, or with radioactive iodine. In some cases, surgery to remove part of the thyroid may be needed.

POSSIBLE CAUSE Stress as a result of this event is probably the reason for your feelings of anxiety (*see* RECOGNIZING STRESS, opposite).

ACTION Try to keep stress to a minimum, and discuss any problems with close family or friends. To help you relax, devote some time each day to leisure activities that you enjoy. Regular exercise may help, as may relaxation exercises (p.32). Consult your doctor if you feel that these measures are not working or if your anxiety seems to be becoming worse.

NO ↓

Continued on next page

Continued from previous page

Recognizing stress

Stress is a normal part of life for many people and has a beneficial effect under certain circumstances, readying the body for action. The normal stress response causes the release of epinephrine (adrenaline), which increases heart rate and maximizes blood flow to the muscles in preparation for action. These responses are beneficial if stress is released. However, prolonged or excessive stress can result in a range of symptoms, including chest pain, stomach upsets, headaches, tiredness,

insomnia, and anxiety. Having a series of infections, such as colds, or getting recurrent mouth ulcers is often a sign of stress as stress tends to depress the immune system. Stress can also result in flare-ups of existing disorders such as eczema. In the long term, stress may seriously damage health; it can, for example, contribute to high blood pressure, which increases the risk of heart attack. It is therefore important that you learn to recognize signs of stress and take action to deal with it (*see* STRESS, p.32).

Do you have any worries related to sex? YES

POSSIBLE CAUSES Anxiety about sex is common, particularly during early adult life. A specific difficulty affecting you or your partner, such as premature ejaculation or a fear of pregnancy or contracting a sexually transmitted disease, can be a source of anxiety. Worries about sexual orientation (p.247) may also cause anxiety. In later life, anxiety may be related to decreasing sexual activity or worries about attractiveness (*see* SEX IN LATER LIFE, p.266).

ACTION If you have a regular partner, you should discuss your feelings with him or her. Talking about sex openly (*see* COMMUNICATING YOUR SEXUAL NEEDS, p.269) is often the best way to deal with anxiety. If you are unable to communicate satisfactorily or if you do not have a regular partner with whom you can talk, consult your doctor. He or she may be able to advise you or may suggest that you receive counselling (*see* SEX COUNSELLING, p.247).

NO

Do you only feel anxious in certain social situations – for instance, meeting people or going to parties? YES

POSSIBLE CAUSE In some situations, a degree of anxiety is natural, and the problem usually improves with experience. If your anxiety is so severe that you avoid certain types of social interaction, consult your doctor.

ACTION Your doctor may be able to teach you coping strategies for dealing with social situations, or he or she may refer you to a counsellor for help. If your anxiety is severe, drug treatment with beta blockers or some types of antidepressant may be helpful.

NO

Do you feel anxious only when confronted with specific objects or if you are prevented from doing things in your usual way? YES

POSSIBLE CAUSES Your anxiety may be caused by a phobia, which is an irrational fear of a specific object or situation – for example, you may be afraid of spiders. Otherwise, you may have obsessive–compulsive disorder, in which you feel an irresistible need to behave in a certain fashion, even though you may know that it is not necessary – for example, you may feel the need to repeatedly wash your hands and become excessively anxious if you are unable to do so. Consult your doctor.

ACTION Your doctor will ask you about your feelings. He or she may advise psychological therapies (p.167) or drug treatment for your anxiety. Most people can learn to manage their fears and anxiety so that they do not affect their lives on a day-to day basis.

NO

SELF-HELP Coping with a panic attack

Rapid breathing during a panic attack reduces carbon dioxide levels in the blood and may lead to frightening physical symptoms, such as palpitations and muscle spasms. You can control the symptoms by breathing into and out of a paper bag. When you do this, you rebreathe carbon dioxide, restoring your blood levels. Place the bag over your mouth, and breathe in and out 10 times. Then, remove the bag and breathe normally for 15 seconds. Repeat this process until your breathing rate is back to normal.

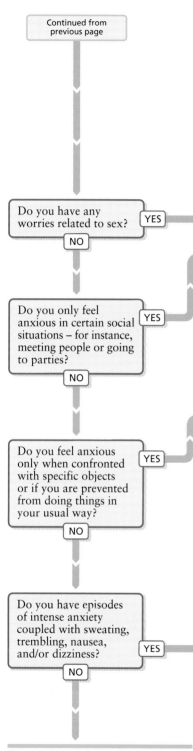

Rebreathing from a bag
Hold a paper bag tightly over the mouth, and breathe in and out slowly.

Do you have episodes of intense anxiety coupled with sweating, trembling, nausea, and/or dizziness? YES

SEE YOUR DOCTOR WITHIN 24 HOURS

POSSIBLE CAUSE You may be having panic attacks, in which feelings of intense anxiety are coupled with alarming physical symptoms. Panic attacks are unpredictable and usually have no obvious cause.

ACTION It is important to see your doctor as soon as possible so that he or she can confirm the diagnosis and rule out a physical cause for your symptoms. If you are having panic attacks, you may need treatment with psychological therapies (p.167). Follow self-help measures for coping with panic attacks (right).

NO

CONSULT YOUR DOCTOR IF YOU ARE UNABLE TO FIND A CAUSE FOR YOUR ANXIETY FROM THIS CHART AND/OR UNEXPLAINED ANXIETY PERSISTS FOR MORE THAN A FEW DAYS.

74 Lumps and swellings

For breast lumps, see chart 128, BREAST PROBLEMS (p.252).
For lumps and swellings in the scrotum, see chart 123,
TESTES AND SCROTUM PROBLEMS (p.244).
Consult this chart if you develop one or more swellings or lumps beneath the surface of the skin. In some cases,

a swelling is due to enlargement of a lymph gland in response to an infection. However, multiple swellings that last longer than about a month may be the result of an underlying disorder. Always consult your doctor if you have one or more painless or persistent lumps or swellings.

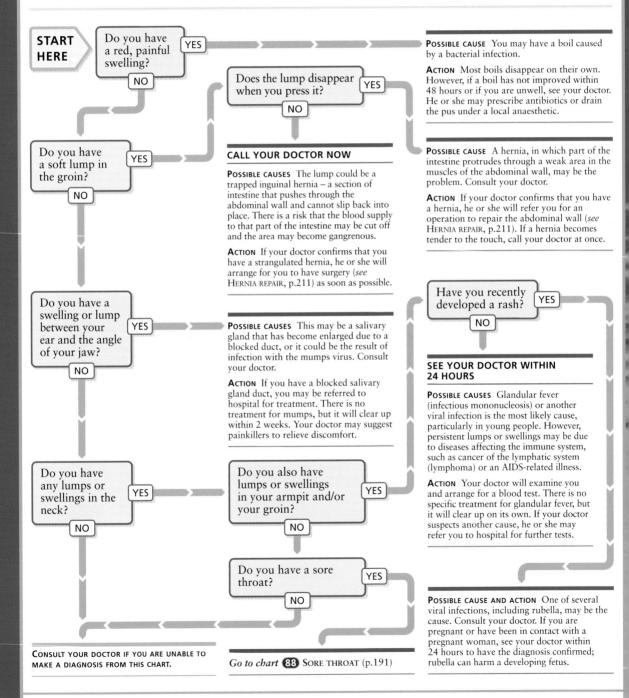

START HERE → Do you have a red, painful swelling? — **YES** → **POSSIBLE CAUSE** You may have a boil caused by a bacterial infection.

ACTION Most boils disappear on their own. However, if a boil has not improved within 48 hours or if you are unwell, see your doctor. He or she may prescribe antibiotics or drain the pus under a local anaesthetic.

Do you have a red, painful swelling? — **NO**

Does the lump disappear when you press it? — **YES** →

Does the lump disappear when you press it? — **NO**

POSSIBLE CAUSE A hernia, in which part of the intestine protrudes through a weak area in the muscles of the abdominal wall, may be the problem. Consult your doctor.

ACTION If your doctor confirms that you have a hernia, he or she will refer you for an operation to repair the abdominal wall (*see* HERNIA REPAIR, p.211). If a hernia becomes tender to the touch, call your doctor at once.

Do you have a soft lump in the groin? — **YES** →

CALL YOUR DOCTOR NOW

POSSIBLE CAUSES The lump could be a trapped inguinal hernia – a section of intestine that pushes through the abdominal wall and cannot slip back into place. There is a risk that the blood supply to that part of the intestine may be cut off and the area may become gangrenous.

ACTION If your doctor confirms that you have a strangulated hernia, he or she will arrange for you to have surgery (*see* HERNIA REPAIR, p.211) as soon as possible.

Do you have a soft lump in the groin? — **NO**

Have you recently developed a rash? — **YES** →

Have you recently developed a rash? — **NO**

Do you have a swelling or lump between your ear and the angle of your jaw? — **YES** →

POSSIBLE CAUSES This may be a salivary gland that has become enlarged due to a blocked duct, or it could be the result of infection with the mumps virus. Consult your doctor.

ACTION If you have a blocked salivary gland duct, you may be referred to hospital for treatment. There is no treatment for mumps, but it will clear up within 2 weeks. Your doctor may suggest painkillers to relieve discomfort.

Do you have a swelling or lump between your ear and the angle of your jaw? — **NO**

SEE YOUR DOCTOR WITHIN 24 HOURS

POSSIBLE CAUSES Glandular fever (infectious mononucleosis) or another viral infection is the most likely cause, particularly in young people. However, persistent lumps or swellings may be due to diseases affecting the immune system, such as cancer of the lymphatic system (lymphoma) or an AIDS-related illness.

ACTION Your doctor will examine you and arrange for a blood test. There is no specific treatment for glandular fever, but it will clear up on its own. If your doctor suspects another cause, he or she may refer you to hospital for further tests.

Do you have any lumps or swellings in the neck? — **YES** →

Do you also have lumps or swellings in your armpit and/or your groin? — **YES** →

Do you also have lumps or swellings in your armpit and/or your groin? — **NO**

Do you have any lumps or swellings in the neck? — **NO**

Do you have a sore throat? — **YES** →

Do you have a sore throat? — **NO**

POSSIBLE CAUSE AND ACTION One of several viral infections, including rubella, may be the cause. Consult your doctor. If you are pregnant or have been in contact with a pregnant woman, see your doctor within 24 hours to have the diagnosis confirmed; rubella can harm a developing fetus.

CONSULT YOUR DOCTOR IF YOU ARE UNABLE TO MAKE A DIAGNOSIS FROM THIS CHART.

Go to chart **88** SORE THROAT (p.191)

75 Itching

For itching confined to the scalp, see chart 76, HAIR AND SCALP PROBLEMS (p.172). For itching confined to the anus, see chart 107, ANAL PROBLEMS (p.219).
Itching (irritation of the skin that leads to an intense desire to scratch) may be caused by an infection or by an allergic reaction to a particular substance. In other cases, itching can be a feature of a skin disorder or may even indicate an underlying disease or psychological stress. Loss of natural oils in the skin as a result of aging or from excessive washing may cause dryness and itching of the skin.

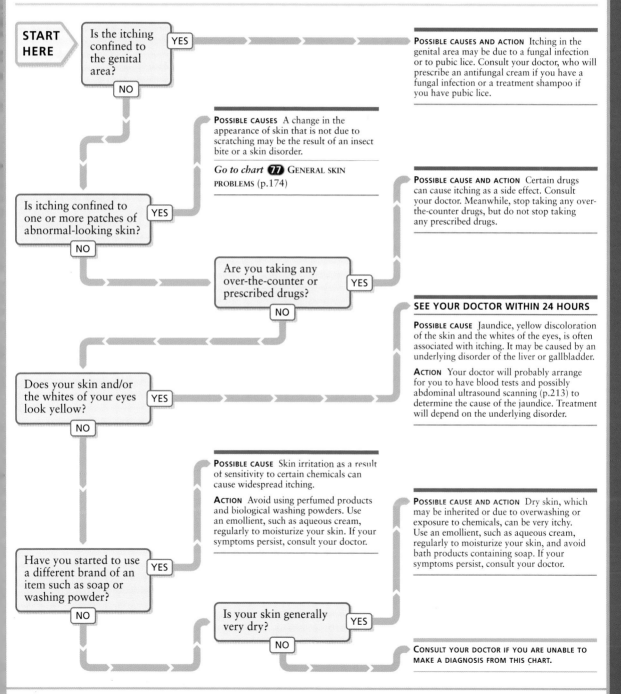

START HERE

Is the itching confined to the genital area?
YES → **POSSIBLE CAUSES AND ACTION** Itching in the genital area may be due to a fungal infection or to pubic lice. Consult your doctor, who will prescribe an antifungal cream if you have a fungal infection or a treatment shampoo if you have pubic lice.
NO ↓

Is itching confined to one or more patches of abnormal-looking skin?
YES → **POSSIBLE CAUSES** A change in the appearance of skin that is not due to scratching may be the result of an insect bite or a skin disorder.

Go to chart 77 GENERAL SKIN PROBLEMS (p.174)
NO ↓

Are you taking any over-the-counter or prescribed drugs?
YES → **POSSIBLE CAUSE AND ACTION** Certain drugs can cause itching as a side effect. Consult your doctor. Meanwhile, stop taking any over-the-counter drugs, but do not stop taking any prescribed drugs.
NO ↓

Does your skin and/or the whites of your eyes look yellow?
YES → **SEE YOUR DOCTOR WITHIN 24 HOURS**

POSSIBLE CAUSE Jaundice, yellow discoloration of the skin and the whites of the eyes, is often associated with itching. It may be caused by an underlying disorder of the liver or gallbladder.

ACTION Your doctor will probably arrange for you to have blood tests and possibly abdominal ultrasound scanning (p.213) to determine the cause of the jaundice. Treatment will depend on the underlying disorder.
NO ↓

Have you started to use a different brand of an item such as soap or washing powder?
YES → **POSSIBLE CAUSE** Skin irritation as a result of sensitivity to certain chemicals can cause widespread itching.

ACTION Avoid using perfumed products and biological washing powders. Use an emollient, such as aqueous cream, regularly to moisturize your skin. If your symptoms persist, consult your doctor.
NO ↓

Is your skin generally very dry?
YES → **POSSIBLE CAUSE AND ACTION** Dry skin, which may be inherited or due to overwashing or exposure to chemicals, can be very itchy. Use an emollient, such as aqueous cream, regularly to moisturize your skin, and avoid bath products containing soap. If your symptoms persist, consult your doctor.
NO →

CONSULT YOUR DOCTOR IF YOU ARE UNABLE TO MAKE A DIAGNOSIS FROM THIS CHART.

76 Hair and scalp problems

Fine hairs grow on most areas of the body. The hair on the head is usually far thicker and problems affecting its growth are therefore very noticeable. Your hair colour and type (straight, wavy, or curly) are inherited, but the condition of your hair may be affected by your overall state of health and factors such as your diet and age. This chart deals with some of the more common problems affecting the hair on the head and the condition of the scalp.

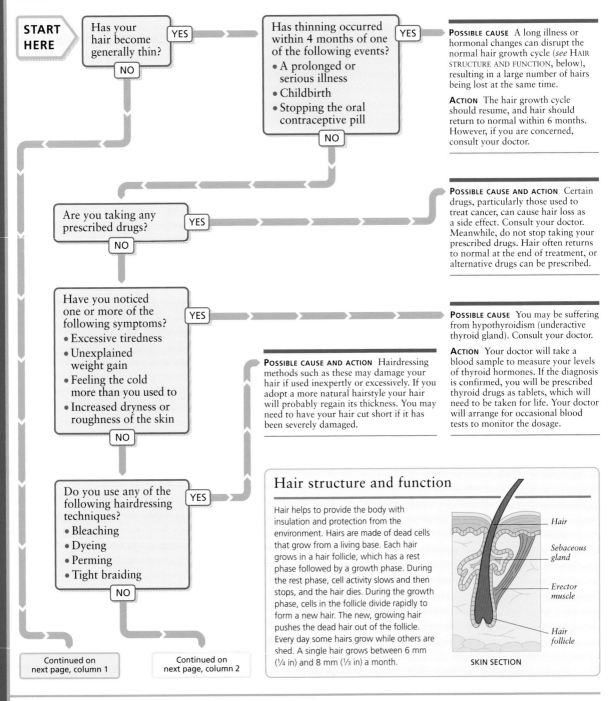

START HERE

Has your hair become generally thin? — YES → **Has thinning occurred within 4 months of one of the following events?**
- A prolonged or serious illness
- Childbirth
- Stopping the oral contraceptive pill

YES → **POSSIBLE CAUSE** A long illness or hormonal changes can disrupt the normal hair growth cycle (*see* HAIR STRUCTURE AND FUNCTION, below), resulting in a large number of hairs being lost at the same time.

ACTION The hair growth cycle should resume, and hair should return to normal within 6 months. However, if you are concerned, consult your doctor.

NO

Are you taking any prescribed drugs? — YES →

POSSIBLE CAUSE AND ACTION Certain drugs, particularly those used to treat cancer, can cause hair loss as a side effect. Consult your doctor. Meanwhile, do not stop taking your prescribed drugs. Hair often returns to normal at the end of treatment, or alternative drugs can be prescribed.

NO

Have you noticed one or more of the following symptoms?
- Excessive tiredness
- Unexplained weight gain
- Feeling the cold more than you used to
- Increased dryness or roughness of the skin

YES →

POSSIBLE CAUSE You may be suffering from hypothyroidism (underactive thyroid gland). Consult your doctor.

ACTION Your doctor will take a blood sample to measure your levels of thyroid hormones. If the diagnosis is confirmed, you will be prescribed thyroid drugs as tablets, which will need to be taken for life. Your doctor will arrange for occasional blood tests to monitor the dosage.

POSSIBLE CAUSE AND ACTION Hairdressing methods such as these may damage your hair if used inexpertly or excessively. If you adopt a more natural hairstyle your hair will probably regain its thickness. You may need to have your hair cut short if it has been severely damaged.

NO

Do you use any of the following hairdressing techniques?
- Bleaching
- Dyeing
- Perming
- Tight braiding

YES →

NO

Hair structure and function

Hair helps to provide the body with insulation and protection from the environment. Hairs are made of dead cells that grow from a living base. Each hair grows in a hair follicle, which has a rest phase followed by a growth phase. During the rest phase, cell activity slows and then stops, and the hair dies. During the growth phase, cells in the follicle divide rapidly to form a new hair. The new, growing hair pushes the dead hair out of the follicle. Every day some hairs grow while others are shed. A single hair grows between 6 mm (¼ in) and 8 mm (⅓ in) a month.

Hair

Sebaceous gland

Erector muscle

Hair follicle

SKIN SECTION

Continued on next page, column 1

Continued on next page, column 2

Hair transplant

Baldness can be treated surgically by several different methods of hair transplantation. In the method shown, skin and hair are taken from a donor site, often at the back of the scalp or behind the ears. The removed hairs and their attached follicles are then inserted in the bald area (the recipient site). A mild sedative is usually given, and both sites are anaesthetized. The transplanted hairs will fall out shortly after the transplant, but new hair starts to grow from the transplanted follicles 3 weeks to 3 months later.

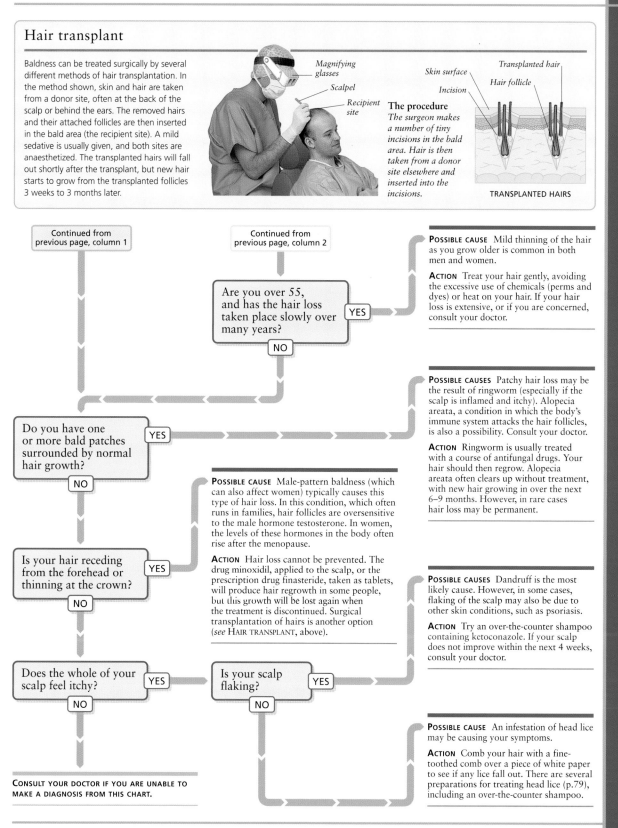

Magnifying glasses

Scalpel

Recipient site

The procedure
The surgeon makes a number of tiny incisions in the bald area. Hair is then taken from a donor site elsewhere and inserted into the incisions.

Skin surface

Incision

Transplanted hair

Hair follicle

TRANSPLANTED HAIRS

Continued from previous page, column 1

Continued from previous page, column 2

Are you over 55, and has the hair loss taken place slowly over many years? — YES

POSSIBLE CAUSE Mild thinning of the hair as you grow older is common in both men and women.

ACTION Treat your hair gently, avoiding the excessive use of chemicals (perms and dyes) or heat on your hair. If your hair loss is extensive, or if you are concerned, consult your doctor.

NO

Do you have one or more bald patches surrounded by normal hair growth? — YES

POSSIBLE CAUSES Patchy hair loss may be the result of ringworm (especially if the scalp is inflamed and itchy). Alopecia areata, a condition in which the body's immune system attacks the hair follicles, is also a possibility. Consult your doctor.

ACTION Ringworm is usually treated with a course of antifungal drugs. Your hair should then regrow. Alopecia areata often clears up without treatment, with new hair growing in over the next 6–9 months. However, in rare cases hair loss may be permanent.

NO

POSSIBLE CAUSE Male-pattern baldness (which can also affect women) typically causes this type of hair loss. In this condition, which often runs in families, hair follicles are oversensitive to the male hormone testosterone. In women, the levels of these hormones in the body often rise after the menopause.

ACTION Hair loss cannot be prevented. The drug minoxidil, applied to the scalp, or the prescription drug finasteride, taken as tablets, will produce hair regrowth in some people, but this growth will be lost again when the treatment is discontinued. Surgical transplantation of hairs is another option (*see* HAIR TRANSPLANT, above).

Is your hair receding from the forehead or thinning at the crown? — YES

NO

POSSIBLE CAUSES Dandruff is the most likely cause. However, in some cases, flaking of the scalp may also be due to other skin conditions, such as psoriasis.

ACTION Try an over-the-counter shampoo containing ketoconazole. If your scalp does not improve within the next 4 weeks, consult your doctor.

Does the whole of your scalp feel itchy? — YES

NO

Is your scalp flaking? — YES

NO

POSSIBLE CAUSE An infestation of head lice may be causing your symptoms.

ACTION Comb your hair with a fine-toothed comb over a piece of white paper to see if any lice fall out. There are several preparations for treating head lice (p.79), including an over-the-counter shampoo.

CONSULT YOUR DOCTOR IF YOU ARE UNABLE TO MAKE A DIAGNOSIS FROM THIS CHART.

77 General skin problems

For itching in skin that appears normal, see chart 75, ITCHING **(p.171)**.

Short-term skin problems are often the result of a minor injury or a superficial infection and are easily treated. Many skin conditions can be distressing if they persist or affect visible areas of skin, but most do not pose a serious risk to health. It is important, however, that potentially fatal conditions, such as skin cancer, are recognized and treated early.

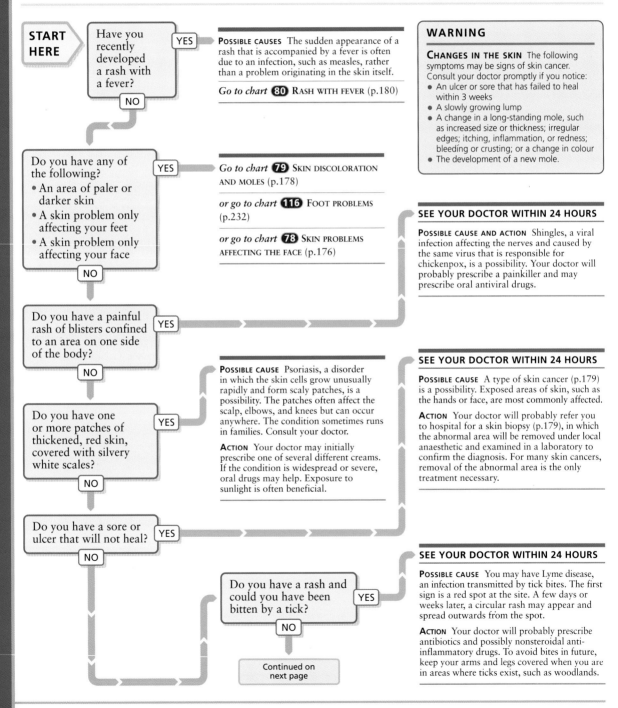

START HERE

Have you recently developed a rash with a fever? — YES → **POSSIBLE CAUSES** The sudden appearance of a rash that is accompanied by a fever is often due to an infection, such as measles, rather than a problem originating in the skin itself.

Go to chart 80 RASH WITH FEVER (p.180)

NO

Do you have any of the following?
- **An area of paler or darker skin**
- **A skin problem only affecting your feet**
- **A skin problem only affecting your face**
— YES → *Go to chart* 79 SKIN DISCOLORATION AND MOLES (p.178)

or go to chart 116 FOOT PROBLEMS (p.232)

or go to chart 78 SKIN PROBLEMS AFFECTING THE FACE (p.176)

NO

Do you have a painful rash of blisters confined to an area on one side of the body? — YES →

NO

Do you have one or more patches of thickened, red skin, covered with silvery white scales? — YES →

NO

Do you have a sore or ulcer that will not heal? — YES →

NO

Do you have a rash and could you have been bitten by a tick? — YES →

NO

Continued on next page

WARNING

CHANGES IN THE SKIN The following symptoms may be signs of skin cancer. Consult your doctor promptly if you notice:
- An ulcer or sore that has failed to heal within 3 weeks
- A slowly growing lump
- A change in a long-standing mole, such as increased size or thickness; irregular edges; itching, inflammation, or redness; bleeding or crusting; or a change in colour
- The development of a new mole.

SEE YOUR DOCTOR WITHIN 24 HOURS

POSSIBLE CAUSE AND ACTION Shingles, a viral infection affecting the nerves and caused by the same virus that is responsible for chickenpox, is a possibility. Your doctor will probably prescribe a painkiller and may prescribe oral antiviral drugs.

SEE YOUR DOCTOR WITHIN 24 HOURS

POSSIBLE CAUSE A type of skin cancer (p.179) is a possibility. Exposed areas of skin, such as the hands or face, are most commonly affected.

ACTION Your doctor will probably refer you to hospital for a skin biopsy (p.179), in which the abnormal area will be removed under local anaesthetic and examined in a laboratory to confirm the diagnosis. For many skin cancers, removal of the abnormal area is the only treatment necessary.

POSSIBLE CAUSE Psoriasis, a disorder in which the skin cells grow unusually rapidly and form scaly patches, is a possibility. The patches often affect the scalp, elbows, and knees but can occur anywhere. The condition sometimes runs in families. Consult your doctor.

ACTION Your doctor may initially prescribe one of several different creams. If the condition is widespread or severe, oral drugs may help. Exposure to sunlight is often beneficial.

SEE YOUR DOCTOR WITHIN 24 HOURS

POSSIBLE CAUSE You may have Lyme disease, an infection transmitted by tick bites. The first sign is a red spot at the site. A few days or weeks later, a circular rash may appear and spread outwards from the spot.

ACTION Your doctor will probably prescribe antibiotics and possibly nonsteroidal anti-inflammatory drugs. To avoid bites in future, keep your arms and legs covered when you are in areas where ticks exist, such as woodlands.

Continued from previous page

Do you have one or more areas of itchy, abnormal-looking skin?
NO / YES

Are you taking any over-the-counter or prescribed drugs?
NO / YES

CONSULT YOUR DOCTOR IF YOU ARE UNABLE TO MAKE A DIAGNOSIS FROM THIS CHART.

POSSIBLE CAUSE AND ACTION Some drugs commonly cause a rash, and others, such as penicillin, may only cause a rash in people who are allergic to them. If the rash has developed suddenly, call your doctor before the next dose of any prescribed drugs is due. Otherwise, make an appointment with your doctor. Meanwhile, stop taking any over-the-counter drugs.

Are these areas raised, red lumps?
YES / NO

POSSIBLE CAUSES You may have urticaria, also known as hives. This condition may occur as an allergic reaction to a particular type of food, such as shellfish, but, in many cases, no cause can be found. Insect bites, such as flea or mosquito bites, are another possibility.

ACTION If the itching is severe, over-the-counter antihistamine creams or tablets should provide relief. In most cases, urticaria clears up within hours and insect bites clear up within a few days. If urticaria recurs, you should consult your doctor. Tests may be needed to look for an underlying cause.

Does the rash mainly affect your hands, and do you spend a lot of time with your hands in water or do you handle chemicals?
YES / NO

POSSIBLE CAUSE You probably have irritant hand eczema (dermatitis). This is a common problem for people who work in occupations such as hairdressing and cleaning, where hands are frequently in water or exposed to chemicals.

ACTION Try to keep your hands out of water. If this is not possible or if you are using chemicals, wear cotton-lined rubber gloves. Use a barrier cream or an emollient, such as aqueous cream, frequently throughout the day, and wash your hands with mild soap. If these measures do not help, consult your doctor, who may prescribe a corticosteroid cream to relieve the itching and irritation.

Does the area of itching clear up and then recur, and is it always in the same place?
YES / NO

POSSIBLE CAUSE Allergic contact dermatitis, in which inflammation of the skin occurs in response to contact with a particular substance, is possible. Nickel, found in earrings and in the studs in jeans, is a common cause, although a wide variety of substances can cause allergic contact dermatitis.

ACTION If you can identify the cause and avoid it, the condition will probably clear up without any treatment. If you are unsure why the condition is occurring, consult your doctor, who may refer you to hospital for tests to identify the cause.

Do the abnormal areas of skin have clearly defined, scaly edges?
YES / NO

POSSIBLE CAUSES You may have a fungal infection such as ringworm. Warm, moist areas, such as the groin or the armpit, are most likely to be affected. Alternatively, a type of eczema, known as discoid eczema, is a possibility, particularly if the affected areas are on the limbs. Consult your doctor.

ACTION Your doctor may want to take skin scrapings to see if fungi are present. If they are, treatment is with antifungal cream or tablets. If eczema is the cause, you will be prescribed corticosteroid cream.

Do you have intense itching, with or without grey lines between your fingers and/or on your wrists?
YES / NO

SEE YOUR DOCTOR WITHIN 24 HOURS

POSSIBLE CAUSE Scabies, a parasitic infection, may be causing your symptoms. Scabies mites burrow under the skin between the fingers and can cause a widespread rash. Scabies is very contagious and often affects a whole family.

ACTION Your doctor will probably prescribe a treatment lotion, which you will need to apply to the whole of your body as directed. Everyone else in the household will need to be treated at the same time, and clothing and bedding also need to be washed. The mites should die within 3 days of treatment, but the itching may continue for up to 2 weeks.

POSSIBLE CAUSE You may have atopic eczema. This condition often appears first during childhood, and can flare up during adulthood.

ACTION An over-the-counter corticosteroid cream will probably relieve the irritation. Use an emollient, such as aqueous cream, to keep the skin from becoming dry. If these measures do not help, consult your doctor.

78 Skin problems affecting the face

Consult this chart if you have a skin problem confined to the face. The skin of the face can be affected by conditions that rarely appear on other parts of the body, such as cold sores. Facial skin may also be at risk of damage from external factors that are not as likely to affect other areas of the body. For example, the face is exposed to weather conditions such as sunlight, cold, and wind, and in women, cosmetics are a common cause of skin irritation and allergy. Abnormal areas of skin on the face are more noticeable than on other parts of the body and may therefore be more distressing.

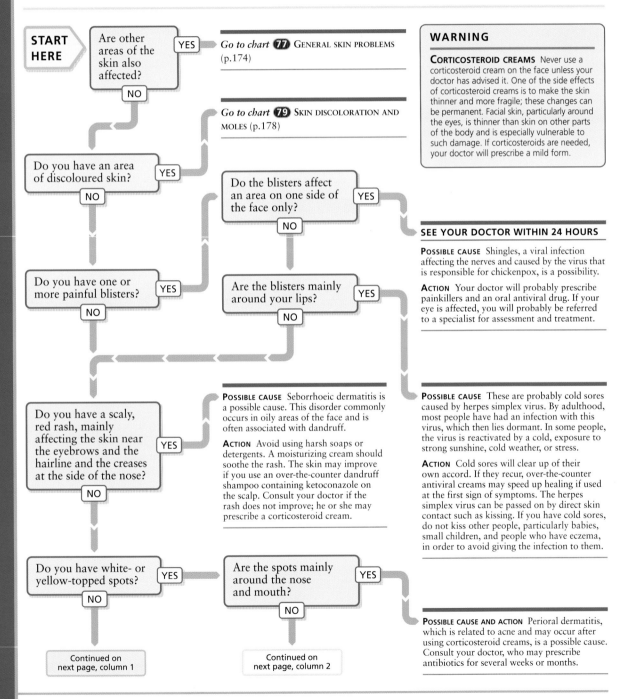

START HERE

Are other areas of the skin also affected?
YES → *Go to chart* **77** GENERAL SKIN PROBLEMS (p.174)
NO

Go to chart **79** SKIN DISCOLORATION AND MOLES (p.178)

Do you have an area of discoloured skin?
YES
NO

Do the blisters affect an area on one side of the face only?
YES
NO

Do you have one or more painful blisters?
YES
NO

Are the blisters mainly around your lips?
YES
NO

Do you have a scaly, red rash, mainly affecting the skin near the eyebrows and the hairline and the creases at the side of the nose?
YES
NO

Do you have white- or yellow-topped spots?
YES
NO

Are the spots mainly around the nose and mouth?
YES
NO

WARNING

CORTICOSTEROID CREAMS Never use a corticosteroid cream on the face unless your doctor has advised it. One of the side effects of corticosteroid creams is to make the skin thinner and more fragile; these changes can be permanent. Facial skin, particularly around the eyes, is thinner than skin on other parts of the body and is especially vulnerable to such damage. If corticosteroids are needed, your doctor will prescribe a mild form.

SEE YOUR DOCTOR WITHIN 24 HOURS

POSSIBLE CAUSE Shingles, a viral infection affecting the nerves and caused by the virus that is responsible for chickenpox, is a possibility.

ACTION Your doctor will probably prescribe painkillers and an oral antiviral drug. If your eye is affected, you will probably be referred to a specialist for assessment and treatment.

POSSIBLE CAUSE Seborrhoeic dermatitis is a possible cause. This disorder commonly occurs in oily areas of the face and is often associated with dandruff.

ACTION Avoid using harsh soaps or detergents. A moisturizing cream should soothe the rash. The skin may improve if you use an over-the-counter dandruff shampoo containing ketoconazole on the scalp. Consult your doctor if the rash does not improve; he or she may prescribe a corticosteroid cream.

POSSIBLE CAUSE These are probably cold sores caused by herpes simplex virus. By adulthood, most people have had an infection with this virus, which then lies dormant. In some people, the virus is reactivated by a cold, exposure to strong sunshine, cold weather, or stress.

ACTION Cold sores will clear up of their own accord. If they recur, over-the-counter antiviral creams may speed up healing if used at the first sign of symptoms. The herpes simplex virus can be passed on by direct skin contact such as kissing. If you have cold sores, do not kiss other people, particularly babies, small children, and people who have eczema, in order to avoid giving the infection to them.

POSSIBLE CAUSE AND ACTION Perioral dermatitis, which is related to acne and may occur after using corticosteroid creams, is a possible cause. Consult your doctor, who may prescribe antibiotics for several weeks or months.

Continued on next page, column 1

Continued on next page, column 2

Continued from previous page, column 1

Continued from previous page, column 2

Do you have a growth with a raised pearly edge, with or without a central depression or ulcer? **YES** / **NO**

Do you also have blackheads and/or tender, red spots? **YES** / **NO**

POSSIBLE CAUSE AND ACTION Acne, which occurs when hair follicles are blocked by sebum (an oily substance secreted by skin glands), is likely. It usually starts during adolescence but often persists into adulthood. Try self-help measures (*see* COPING WITH ACNE, p.140) and over-the-counter treatments for acne (p.140). If these steps do not help, consult your doctor.

Does your face become easily flushed – for example when you have been drinking alcohol or when you enter a warm room? **YES** / **NO**

POSSIBLE CAUSE Basal cell carcinoma, a type of skin cancer (p.179), is a possible cause. Consult your doctor.

ACTION Your doctor will probably refer you to hospital for a skin biopsy (p.179), in which the abnormal area is removed under a local anaesthetic and examined in a laboratory to confirm the diagnosis. Because the abnormal area has been removed, further treatment is not usually needed.

Do you have an ulcer that will not heal? **YES** / **NO**

CONSULT YOUR DOCTOR IF YOU ARE UNABLE TO MAKE A DIAGNOSIS FROM THIS CHART.

Is the affected skin red and swollen, and do you have a high temperature? **YES** / **NO**

POSSIBLE CAUSE Squamous cell carcinoma, a type of skin cancer (p.179), is a possibility. Consult your doctor.

ACTION Your doctor will probably refer you to hospital for a skin biopsy (p.179), in which the abnormal area is removed under a local anaesthetic and examined in a laboratory to confirm the diagnosis. You may not need any further treatment if all of the abnormal area has been removed. In some cases, further surgery may be necessary.

POSSIBLE CAUSE Rosacea, a condition similar to acne, is possible. It usually develops between the ages of 40 and 60 and is often worst on the cheeks and nose. Consult your doctor.

ACTION Your doctor may prescribe antibiotic tablets or cream to be used for several weeks or months. You should avoid excessive exposure to the sun and cut down your alcohol intake, because they may make the condition worse.

CALL YOUR DOCTOR NOW

Does the problem seem related to cosmetics or perfumed products? **YES** / **NO**

POSSIBLE CAUSE Erysipelas, a bacterial infection of the facial skin and the underlying tissues, is a possible cause. If not treated, this condition can spread, resulting in a serious blood infection known as septicaemia.

ACTION If the diagnosis is confirmed, your doctor will probably prescribe oral antibiotics. If the infection is severe, you may need to be admitted to hospital so that you can be given treatment with intravenous antibiotics.

POSSIBLE CAUSE AND ACTION You may be allergic to a new product, or you may have recently become allergic to a product you have been using for some time. Stop using all the products that could be responsible; the skin should return to normal in a few days. You can then reintroduce one item every few days so that the cause of the problem can be identified.

Have you been taking any over-the-counter or prescribed drugs? **YES** / **NO**

POSSIBLE CAUSE AND ACTION Certain drugs increase the sensitivity of skin to sunlight and can cause a reaction confined to the face. Stop taking any over-the-counter drugs, and consult your doctor. Meanwhile, continue taking any prescribed drugs.

CONSULT YOUR DOCTOR IF YOU ARE UNABLE TO MAKE A DIAGNOSIS FROM THIS CHART.

79 Skin discoloration and moles

For birthmarks, see chart 8, SKIN PROBLEMS IN BABIES (p.60). Consult this chart if areas of your skin have become darker or paler than the surrounding skin or if you are worried about a new mole or changes in a mole. Although changes in skin colour are most often due to exposure to the sun, you may have a skin condition that needs medical attention. Too much exposure to the sun can cause the skin to burn and increases the risk of developing skin cancer in later life.

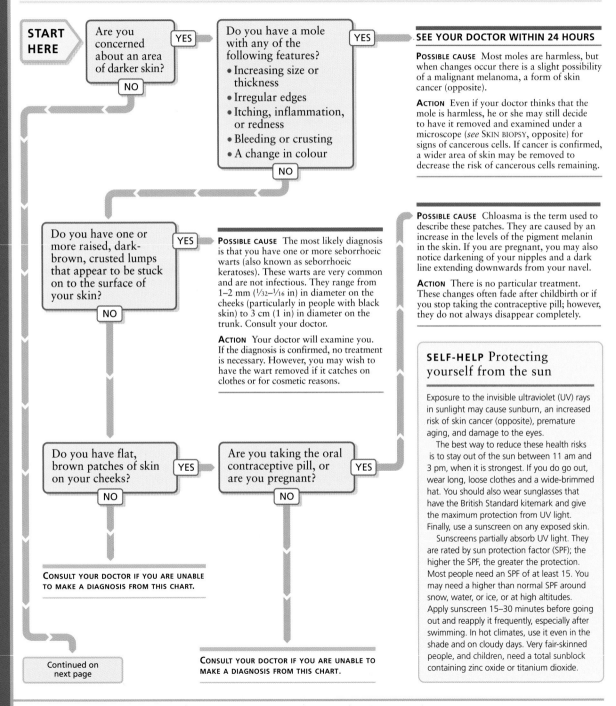

START HERE

Are you concerned about an area of darker skin? → YES → **Do you have a mole with any of the following features?**
- Increasing size or thickness
- Irregular edges
- Itching, inflammation, or redness
- Bleeding or crusting
- A change in colour

→ YES →

SEE YOUR DOCTOR WITHIN 24 HOURS

POSSIBLE CAUSE Most moles are harmless, but when changes occur there is a slight possibility of a malignant melanoma, a form of skin cancer (opposite).

ACTION Even if your doctor thinks that the mole is harmless, he or she may still decide to have it removed and examined under a microscope (*see* SKIN BIOPSY, opposite) for signs of cancerous cells. If cancer is confirmed, a wider area of skin may be removed to decrease the risk of cancerous cells remaining.

POSSIBLE CAUSE Chloasma is the term used to describe these patches. They are caused by an increase in the levels of the pigment melanin in the skin. If you are pregnant, you may also notice darkening of your nipples and a dark line extending downwards from your navel.

ACTION There is no particular treatment. These changes often fade after childbirth or if you stop taking the contraceptive pill; however, they do not always disappear completely.

Do you have one or more raised, dark-brown, crusted lumps that appear to be stuck on to the surface of your skin? → YES →

POSSIBLE CAUSE The most likely diagnosis is that you have one or more seborrhoeic warts (also known as seborrhoeic keratoses). These warts are very common and are not infectious. They range from 1–2 mm (1/32–1/16 in) in diameter on the cheeks (particularly in people with black skin) to 3 cm (1 in) in diameter on the trunk. Consult your doctor.

ACTION Your doctor will examine you. If the diagnosis is confirmed, no treatment is necessary. However, you may wish to have the wart removed if it catches on clothes or for cosmetic reasons.

SELF-HELP Protecting yourself from the sun

Exposure to the invisible ultraviolet (UV) rays in sunlight may cause sunburn, an increased risk of skin cancer (opposite), premature aging, and damage to the eyes.

The best way to reduce these health risks is to stay out of the sun between 11 am and 3 pm, when it is strongest. If you do go out, wear long, loose clothes and a wide-brimmed hat. You should also wear sunglasses that have the British Standard kitemark and give the maximum protection from UV light. Finally, use a sunscreen on any exposed skin.

Sunscreens partially absorb UV light. They are rated by sun protection factor (SPF); the higher the SPF, the greater the protection. Most people need an SPF of at least 15. You may need a higher than normal SPF around snow, water, or ice, or at high altitudes. Apply sunscreen 15–30 minutes before going out and reapply it frequently, especially after swimming. In hot climates, use it even in the shade and on cloudy days. Very fair-skinned people, and children, need a total sunblock containing zinc oxide or titanium dioxide.

Do you have flat, brown patches of skin on your cheeks? → YES →

Are you taking the oral contraceptive pill, or are you pregnant? → YES →

CONSULT YOUR DOCTOR IF YOU ARE UNABLE TO MAKE A DIAGNOSIS FROM THIS CHART.

CONSULT YOUR DOCTOR IF YOU ARE UNABLE TO MAKE A DIAGNOSIS FROM THIS CHART.

Continued on next page

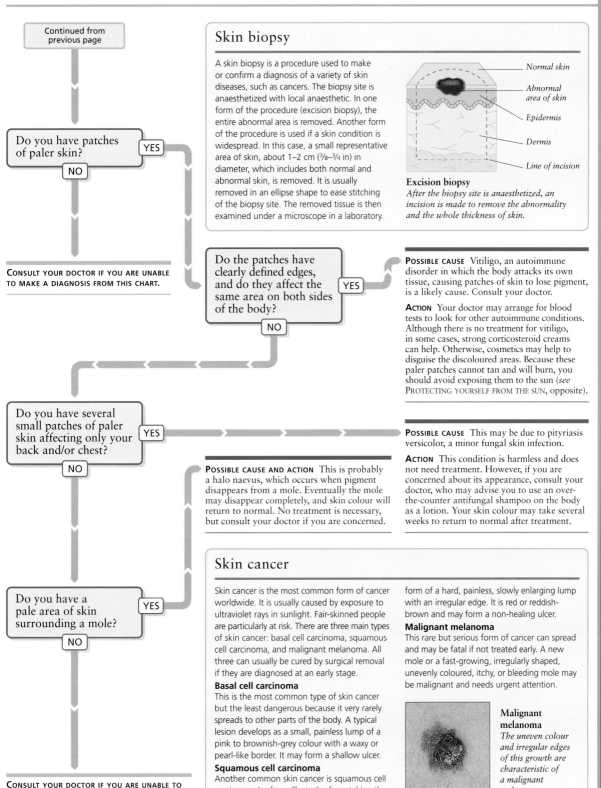

Continued from previous page

Do you have patches of paler skin? — YES

NO

CONSULT YOUR DOCTOR IF YOU ARE UNABLE TO MAKE A DIAGNOSIS FROM THIS CHART.

Do you have several small patches of paler skin affecting only your back and/or chest? — YES

NO

Do you have a pale area of skin surrounding a mole? — YES

NO

CONSULT YOUR DOCTOR IF YOU ARE UNABLE TO MAKE A DIAGNOSIS FROM THIS CHART.

Skin biopsy

A skin biopsy is a procedure used to make or confirm a diagnosis of a variety of skin diseases, such as cancers. The biopsy site is anaesthetized with local anaesthetic. In one form of the procedure (excision biopsy), the entire abnormal area is removed. Another form of the procedure is used if a skin condition is widespread. In this case, a small representative area of skin, about 1–2 cm (3/8–3/4 in) in diameter, which includes both normal and abnormal skin, is removed. It is usually removed in an ellipse shape to ease stitching of the biopsy site. The removed tissue is then examined under a microscope in a laboratory.

Normal skin
Abnormal area of skin
Epidermis
Dermis
Line of incision

Excision biopsy
After the biopsy site is anaesthetized, an incision is made to remove the abnormality and the whole thickness of skin.

Do the patches have clearly defined edges, and do they affect the same area on both sides of the body? — YES

NO

POSSIBLE CAUSE Vitiligo, an autoimmune disorder in which the body attacks its own tissue, causing patches of skin to lose pigment, is a likely cause. Consult your doctor.

ACTION Your doctor may arrange for blood tests to look for other autoimmune conditions. Although there is no treatment for vitiligo, in some cases, strong corticosteroid creams can help. Otherwise, cosmetics may help to disguise the discoloured areas. Because these paler patches cannot tan and will burn, you should avoid exposing them to the sun (*see* PROTECTING YOURSELF FROM THE SUN, opposite).

POSSIBLE CAUSE This may be due to pityriasis versicolor, a minor fungal skin infection.

ACTION This condition is harmless and does not need treatment. However, if you are concerned about its appearance, consult your doctor, who may advise you to use an over-the-counter antifungal shampoo on the body as a lotion. Your skin colour may take several weeks to return to normal after treatment.

POSSIBLE CAUSE AND ACTION This is probably a halo naevus, which occurs when pigment disappears from a mole. Eventually the mole may disappear completely, and skin colour will return to normal. No treatment is necessary, but consult your doctor if you are concerned.

Skin cancer

Skin cancer is the most common form of cancer worldwide. It is usually caused by exposure to ultraviolet rays in sunlight. Fair-skinned people are particularly at risk. There are three main types of skin cancer: basal cell carcinoma, squamous cell carcinoma, and malignant melanoma. All three can usually be cured by surgical removal if they are diagnosed at an early stage.

Basal cell carcinoma
This is the most common type of skin cancer but the least dangerous because it very rarely spreads to other parts of the body. A typical lesion develops as a small, painless lump of a pink to brownish-grey colour with a waxy or pearl-like border. It may form a shallow ulcer.

Squamous cell carcinoma
Another common skin cancer is squamous cell carcinoma. It often affects the face, taking the form of a hard, painless, slowly enlarging lump with an irregular edge. It is red or reddish-brown and may form a non-healing ulcer.

Malignant melanoma
This rare but serious form of cancer can spread and may be fatal if not treated early. A new mole or a fast-growing, irregularly shaped, unevenly coloured, itchy, or bleeding mole may be malignant and needs urgent attention.

Malignant melanoma
The uneven colour and irregular edges of this growth are characteristic of a malignant melanoma.

80 Rash with fever

Consult this chart if you have widespread spots or discoloured areas of skin and a temperature of 38°C (100.4°F) or above. You may have an infectious disease. These diseases may be more likely to cause complications in adults than in children. To find out if you have a fever, measure your temperature with a thermometer (*see* MANAGING A FEVER, p.150).

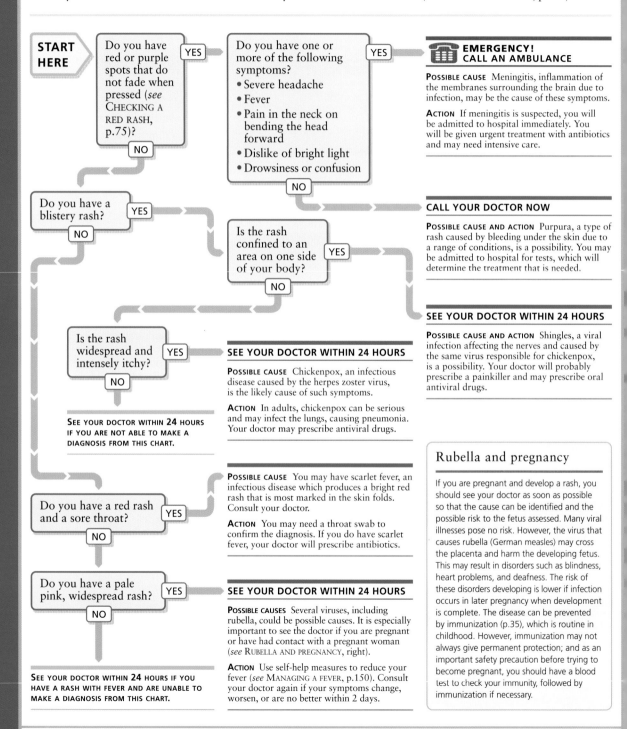

START HERE

Do you have red or purple spots that do not fade when pressed (*see* CHECKING A RED RASH, p.75)? — **YES** → Do you have one or more of the following symptoms?
- Severe headache
- Fever
- Pain in the neck on bending the head forward
- Dislike of bright light
- Drowsiness or confusion

NO

Do you have one or more of the following symptoms? — **YES**

NO

EMERGENCY! CALL AN AMBULANCE

POSSIBLE CAUSE Meningitis, inflammation of the membranes surrounding the brain due to infection, may be the cause of these symptoms.

ACTION If meningitis is suspected, you will be admitted to hospital immediately. You will be given urgent treatment with antibiotics and may need intensive care.

Do you have a blistery rash? — **YES**

NO

Is the rash confined to an area on one side of your body? — **YES**

NO

CALL YOUR DOCTOR NOW

POSSIBLE CAUSE AND ACTION Purpura, a type of rash caused by bleeding under the skin due to a range of conditions, is a possibility. You may be admitted to hospital for tests, which will determine the treatment that is needed.

Is the rash widespread and intensely itchy? — **YES**

NO

SEE YOUR DOCTOR WITHIN 24 HOURS IF YOU ARE NOT ABLE TO MAKE A DIAGNOSIS FROM THIS CHART.

SEE YOUR DOCTOR WITHIN 24 HOURS

POSSIBLE CAUSE Chickenpox, an infectious disease caused by the herpes zoster virus, is the likely cause of such symptoms.

ACTION In adults, chickenpox can be serious and may infect the lungs, causing pneumonia. Your doctor may prescribe antiviral drugs.

SEE YOUR DOCTOR WITHIN 24 HOURS

POSSIBLE CAUSE AND ACTION Shingles, a viral infection affecting the nerves and caused by the same virus responsible for chickenpox, is a possibility. Your doctor will probably prescribe a painkiller and may prescribe oral antiviral drugs.

Do you have a red rash and a sore throat? — **YES**

NO

POSSIBLE CAUSE You may have scarlet fever, an infectious disease which produces a bright red rash that is most marked in the skin folds. Consult your doctor.

ACTION You may need a throat swab to confirm the diagnosis. If you do have scarlet fever, your doctor will prescribe antibiotics.

Do you have a pale pink, widespread rash? — **YES**

NO

SEE YOUR DOCTOR WITHIN 24 HOURS

POSSIBLE CAUSES Several viruses, including rubella, could be possible causes. It is especially important to see the doctor if you are pregnant or have had contact with a pregnant woman (*see* RUBELLA AND PREGNANCY, right).

ACTION Use self-help measures to reduce your fever (*see* MANAGING A FEVER, p.150). Consult your doctor again if your symptoms change, worsen, or are no better within 2 days.

SEE YOUR DOCTOR WITHIN 24 HOURS IF YOU HAVE A RASH WITH FEVER AND ARE UNABLE TO MAKE A DIAGNOSIS FROM THIS CHART.

Rubella and pregnancy

If you are pregnant and develop a rash, you should see your doctor as soon as possible so that the cause can be identified and the possible risk to the fetus assessed. Many viral illnesses pose no risk. However, the virus that causes rubella (German measles) may cross the placenta and harm the developing fetus. This may result in disorders such as blindness, heart problems, and deafness. The risk of these disorders developing is lower if infection occurs in later pregnancy when development is complete. The disease can be prevented by immunization (p.35), which is routine in childhood. However, immunization may not always give permanent protection; and as an important safety precaution before trying to become pregnant, you should have a blood test to check your immunity, followed by immunization if necessary.

81 Nail problems

Nails are made of hard, dead tissue called keratin, which protects the sensitive tips of the fingers and toes from damage. Common problems affecting the nails include distortion of the nail and painful or inflamed skin around the nail. The most common causes of misshapen nails are injury and fungal infections. However, most widespread skin conditions, including psoriasis and eczema, can also affect the growth and appearance of the nails. It takes between 6 months and 1 year for a nail to replace itself, so treatment for nail problems often needs to be continued for some time.

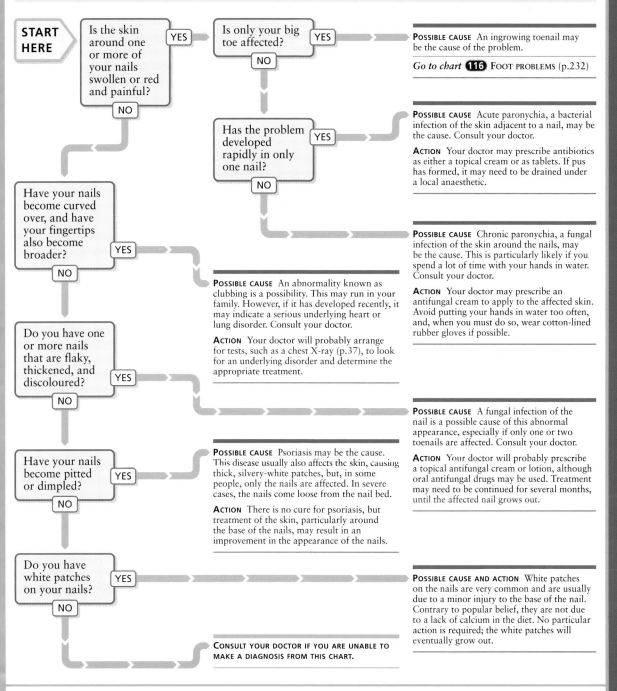

START HERE

Is the skin around one or more of your nails swollen or red and painful?

YES → **Is only your big toe affected?**

YES → **POSSIBLE CAUSE** An ingrowing toenail may be the cause of the problem.

Go to chart **116** FOOT PROBLEMS (p.232)

NO ↓

Has the problem developed rapidly in only one nail?

YES → **POSSIBLE CAUSE** Acute paronychia, a bacterial infection of the skin adjacent to a nail, may be the cause. Consult your doctor.

ACTION Your doctor may prescribe antibiotics as either a topical cream or as tablets. If pus has formed, it may need to be drained under a local anaesthetic.

NO ↓

POSSIBLE CAUSE Chronic paronychia, a fungal infection of the skin around the nails, may be the cause. This is particularly likely if you spend a lot of time with your hands in water. Consult your doctor.

ACTION Your doctor may prescribe an antifungal cream to apply to the affected skin. Avoid putting your hands in water too often, and, when you must do so, wear cotton-lined rubber gloves if possible.

NO (from start) ↓

Have your nails become curved over, and have your fingertips also become broader?

YES → **POSSIBLE CAUSE** An abnormality known as clubbing is a possibility. This may run in your family. However, if it has developed recently, it may indicate a serious underlying heart or lung disorder. Consult your doctor.

ACTION Your doctor will probably arrange for tests, such as a chest X-ray (p.37), to look for an underlying disorder and determine the appropriate treatment.

NO ↓

Do you have one or more nails that are flaky, thickened, and discoloured?

YES → **POSSIBLE CAUSE** A fungal infection of the nail is a possible cause of this abnormal appearance, especially if only one or two toenails are affected. Consult your doctor.

ACTION Your doctor will probably prescribe a topical antifungal cream or lotion, although oral antifungal drugs may be used. Treatment may need to be continued for several months, until the affected nail grows out.

NO ↓

Have your nails become pitted or dimpled?

YES → **POSSIBLE CAUSE** Psoriasis may be the cause. This disease usually also affects the skin, causing thick, silvery-white patches, but, in some people, only the nails are affected. In severe cases, the nails come loose from the nail bed.

ACTION There is no cure for psoriasis, but treatment of the skin, particularly around the base of the nails, may result in an improvement in the appearance of the nails.

NO ↓

Do you have white patches on your nails?

YES → **POSSIBLE CAUSE AND ACTION** White patches on the nails are very common and are usually due to a minor injury to the base of the nail. Contrary to popular belief, they are not due to a lack of calcium in the diet. No particular action is required; the white patches will eventually grow out.

NO ↓

CONSULT YOUR DOCTOR IF YOU ARE UNABLE TO MAKE A DIAGNOSIS FROM THIS CHART.

82 Painful or irritated eye

For blurred vision, see chart 83, DISTURBED OR IMPAIRED VISION *(p.184).*

In most cases, a painful or irritated eye is due to a relatively minor problem and, unless you wear contact lenses, may not need professional attention. However, an eye problem that persists or impairs vision should always be seen by a doctor. A red, painless area in the white of the eye is probably a burst blood vessel and should clear up on its own.

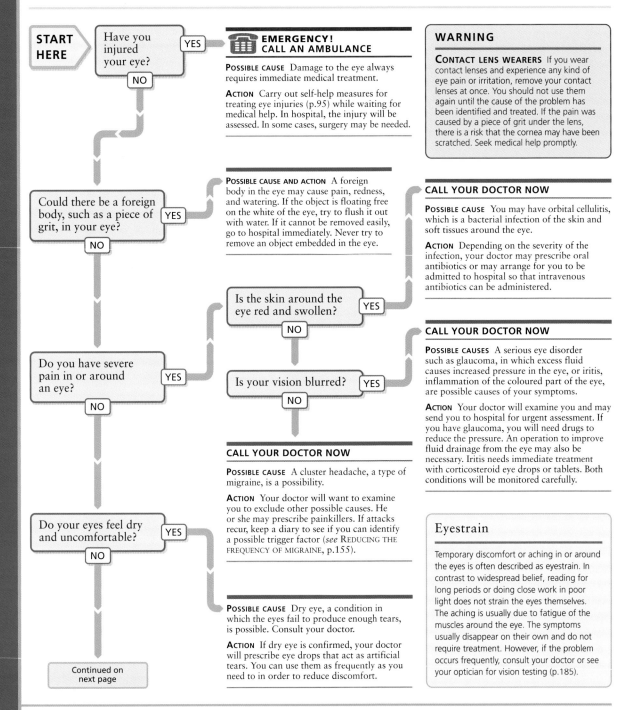

START HERE → **Have you injured your eye?** — YES →

☎ **EMERGENCY! CALL AN AMBULANCE**

POSSIBLE CAUSE Damage to the eye always requires immediate medical treatment.

ACTION Carry out self-help measures for treating eye injuries (p.95) while waiting for medical help. In hospital, the injury will be assessed. In some cases, surgery may be needed.

NO ↓

Could there be a foreign body, such as a piece of grit, in your eye? — YES →

POSSIBLE CAUSE AND ACTION A foreign body in the eye may cause pain, redness, and watering. If the object is floating free on the white of the eye, try to flush it out with water. If it cannot be removed easily, go to hospital immediately. Never try to remove an object embedded in the eye.

NO ↓

Do you have severe pain in or around an eye? — YES →

Is the skin around the eye red and swollen? — YES →

CALL YOUR DOCTOR NOW

POSSIBLE CAUSE You may have orbital cellulitis, which is a bacterial infection of the skin and soft tissues around the eye.

ACTION Depending on the severity of the infection, your doctor may prescribe oral antibiotics or may arrange for you to be admitted to hospital so that intravenous antibiotics can be administered.

NO ↓

Is your vision blurred? — YES →

CALL YOUR DOCTOR NOW

POSSIBLE CAUSES A serious eye disorder such as glaucoma, in which excess fluid causes increased pressure in the eye, or iritis, inflammation of the coloured part of the eye, are possible causes of your symptoms.

ACTION Your doctor will examine you and may send you to hospital for urgent assessment. If you have glaucoma, you will need drugs to reduce the pressure. An operation to improve fluid drainage from the eye may also be necessary. Iritis needs immediate treatment with corticosteroid eye drops or tablets. Both conditions will be monitored carefully.

NO ↓

CALL YOUR DOCTOR NOW

POSSIBLE CAUSE A cluster headache, a type of migraine, is a possibility.

ACTION Your doctor will want to examine you to exclude other possible causes. He or she may prescribe painkillers. If attacks recur, keep a diary to see if you can identify a possible trigger factor (*see* REDUCING THE FREQUENCY OF MIGRAINE, p.155).

NO ↓

Do your eyes feel dry and uncomfortable? — YES →

POSSIBLE CAUSE Dry eye, a condition in which the eyes fail to produce enough tears, is possible. Consult your doctor.

ACTION If dry eye is confirmed, your doctor will prescribe eye drops that act as artificial tears. You can use them as frequently as you need to in order to reduce discomfort.

NO ↓

Continued on next page

WARNING

CONTACT LENS WEARERS If you wear contact lenses and experience any kind of eye pain or irritation, remove your contact lenses at once. You should not use them again until the cause of the problem has been identified and treated. If the pain was caused by a piece of grit under the lens, there is a risk that the cornea may have been scratched. Seek medical help promptly.

Eyestrain

Temporary discomfort or aching in or around the eyes is often described as eyestrain. In contrast to widespread belief, reading for long periods or doing close work in poor light does not strain the eyes themselves. The aching is usually due to fatigue of the muscles around the eye. The symptoms usually disappear on their own and do not require treatment. However, if the problem occurs frequently, consult your doctor or see your optician for vision testing (p.185).

Continued from previous page

SELF-HELP Avoiding contact lens problems

Most people who wear contact lenses do so to correct their vision and have few problems with them. If your eyes become irritated while wearing or after wearing contact lenses, you may have an allergy to the cleaning or soaking solutions. To prevent potentially serious eye infections, use strict hygiene when cleaning non-disposable lenses, and never moisten contact lenses with saliva. If not treated promptly, an infection may result in permanent damage to your vision. If you wear contact lenses, always consult your pharmacist before using any over-the-counter eye drops because some may be incompatible with contact lenses.

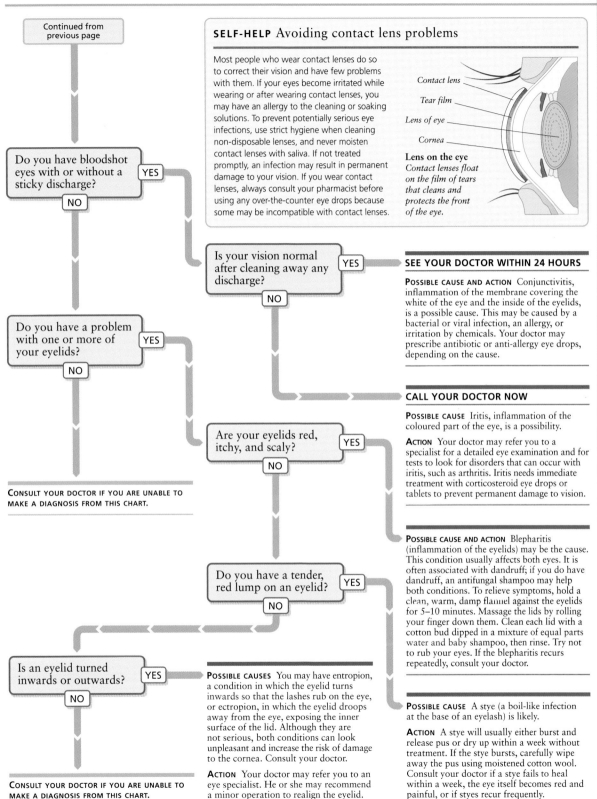

Contact lens
Tear film
Lens of eye
Cornea

Lens on the eye
Contact lenses float on the film of tears that cleans and protects the front of the eye.

Do you have bloodshot eyes with or without a sticky discharge? — YES
NO

Is your vision normal after cleaning away any discharge? — YES
NO

SEE YOUR DOCTOR WITHIN 24 HOURS

POSSIBLE CAUSE AND ACTION Conjunctivitis, inflammation of the membrane covering the white of the eye and the inside of the eyelids, is a possible cause. This may be caused by a bacterial or viral infection, an allergy, or irritation by chemicals. Your doctor may prescribe antibiotic or anti-allergy eye drops, depending on the cause.

Do you have a problem with one or more of your eyelids? — YES
NO

Are your eyelids red, itchy, and scaly? — YES
NO

CALL YOUR DOCTOR NOW

POSSIBLE CAUSE Iritis, inflammation of the coloured part of the eye, is a possibility.

ACTION Your doctor may refer you to a specialist for a detailed eye examination and for tests to look for disorders that can occur with iritis, such as arthritis. Iritis needs immediate treatment with corticosteroid eye drops or tablets to prevent permanent damage to vision.

CONSULT YOUR DOCTOR IF YOU ARE UNABLE TO MAKE A DIAGNOSIS FROM THIS CHART.

POSSIBLE CAUSE AND ACTION Blepharitis (inflammation of the eyelids) may be the cause. This condition usually affects both eyes. It is often associated with dandruff; if you do have dandruff, an antifungal shampoo may help both conditions. To relieve symptoms, hold a clean, warm, damp flannel against the eyelids for 5–10 minutes. Massage the lids by rolling your finger down them. Clean each lid with a cotton bud dipped in a mixture of equal parts water and baby shampoo, then rinse. Try not to rub your eyes. If the blepharitis recurs repeatedly, consult your doctor.

Do you have a tender, red lump on an eyelid? — YES
NO

Is an eyelid turned inwards or outwards? — YES
NO

POSSIBLE CAUSES You may have entropion, a condition in which the eyelid turns inwards so that the lashes rub on the eye, or ectropion, in which the eyelid droops away from the eye, exposing the inner surface of the lid. Although they are not serious, both conditions can look unpleasant and increase the risk of damage to the cornea. Consult your doctor.

ACTION Your doctor may refer you to an eye specialist. He or she may recommend a minor operation to realign the eyelid.

POSSIBLE CAUSE A stye (a boil-like infection at the base of an eyelash) is likely.

ACTION A stye will usually either burst and release pus or dry up within a week without treatment. If the stye bursts, carefully wipe away the pus using moistened cotton wool. Consult your doctor if a stye fails to heal within a week, the eye itself becomes red and painful, or if styes recur frequently.

CONSULT YOUR DOCTOR IF YOU ARE UNABLE TO MAKE A DIAGNOSIS FROM THIS CHART.

83 Disturbed or impaired vision

This chart deals with any change in your vision, including blurring, double vision, seeing flashing lights or floating spots, and loss of part or all of your field of vision. Any such change in vision should be brought to your doctor's attention to rule out the possibility of a serious nervous system or eye disorder, some of which could damage your sight. Successful treatment of many of these disorders may depend on detecting the disease in its early stages.

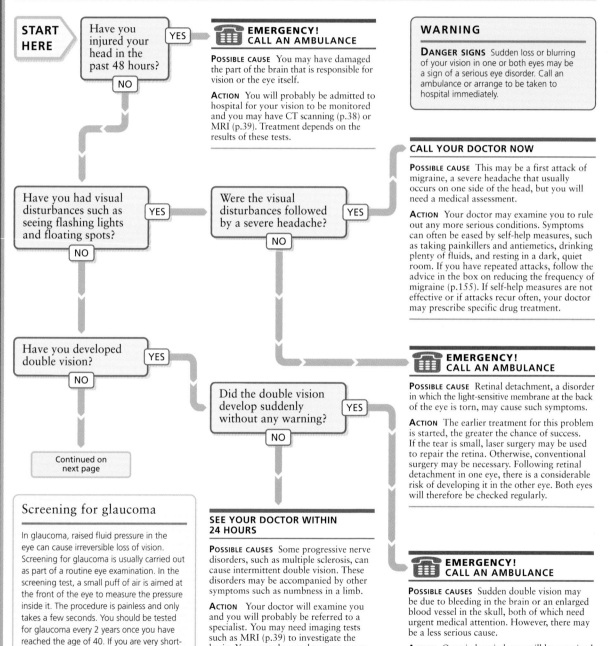

START HERE

Have you injured your head in the past 48 hours? — YES →

☎ EMERGENCY! CALL AN AMBULANCE

POSSIBLE CAUSE You may have damaged the part of the brain that is responsible for vision or the eye itself.

ACTION You will probably be admitted to hospital for your vision to be monitored and you may have CT scanning (p.38) or MRI (p.39). Treatment depends on the results of these tests.

NO ↓

WARNING

DANGER SIGNS Sudden loss or blurring of your vision in one or both eyes may be a sign of a serious eye disorder. Call an ambulance or arrange to be taken to hospital immediately.

Have you had visual disturbances such as seeing flashing lights and floating spots? — YES →

Were the visual disturbances followed by a severe headache? — YES →

CALL YOUR DOCTOR NOW

POSSIBLE CAUSE This may be a first attack of migraine, a severe headache that usually occurs on one side of the head, but you will need a medical assessment.

ACTION Your doctor may examine you to rule out any more serious conditions. Symptoms can often be eased by self-help measures, such as taking painkillers and antiemetics, drinking plenty of fluids, and resting in a dark, quiet room. If you have repeated attacks, follow the advice in the box on reducing the frequency of migraine (p.155). If self-help measures are not effective or if attacks recur often, your doctor may prescribe specific drug treatment.

NO ↓ (visual disturbances)

NO ↓ (severe headache)

Have you developed double vision? — YES →

☎ EMERGENCY! CALL AN AMBULANCE

POSSIBLE CAUSE Retinal detachment, a disorder in which the light-sensitive membrane at the back of the eye is torn, may cause such symptoms.

ACTION The earlier treatment for this problem is started, the greater the chance of success. If the tear is small, laser surgery may be used to repair the retina. Otherwise, conventional surgery may be necessary. Following retinal detachment in one eye, there is a considerable risk of developing it in the other eye. Both eyes will therefore be checked regularly.

NO ↓

Did the double vision develop suddenly without any warning? — YES →

NO ↓

Continued on next page

Screening for glaucoma

In glaucoma, raised fluid pressure in the eye can cause irreversible loss of vision. Screening for glaucoma is usually carried out as part of a routine eye examination. In the screening test, a small puff of air is aimed at the front of the eye to measure the pressure inside it. The procedure is painless and only takes a few seconds. You should be tested for glaucoma every 2 years once you have reached the age of 40. If you are very short-sighted or if glaucoma runs in your family, testing should start at an earlier age.

SEE YOUR DOCTOR WITHIN 24 HOURS

POSSIBLE CAUSES Some progressive nerve disorders, such as multiple sclerosis, can cause intermittent double vision. These disorders may be accompanied by other symptoms such as numbness in a limb.

ACTION Your doctor will examine you and you will probably be referred to a specialist. You may need imaging tests such as MRI (p.39) to investigate the brain. You may also need tests to assess the optic nerves supplying the eyes. Treatment depends on the results.

☎ EMERGENCY! CALL AN AMBULANCE

POSSIBLE CAUSES Sudden double vision may be due to bleeding in the brain or an enlarged blood vessel in the skull, both of which need urgent medical attention. However, there may be a less serious cause.

ACTION Once in hospital, you will be examined and may have CT scanning (p.38) to look for the cause and determine the appropriate treatment.

Continued from previous page

Has your vision become blurred? **YES**

NO

CONSULT YOUR DOCTOR IF YOU ARE UNABLE TO MAKE A DIAGNOSIS FROM THIS CHART.

Vision testing

You should have your vision tested every 2 years, especially once you are over 40. The most common test gauges the sharpness of your distance vision by assessing how well you can read letters lined up in decreasing size on a Snellen chart. Your ability to focus on near objects may also be measured by asking you to read very small print on a chart held at normal reading distance. These tests show whether you need corrective lenses, and, if so, which ones. In addition, your optician will examine your eyes to look for disorders such as diabetes and high blood pressure, which can cause changes in the back of the eye before general symptoms develop. You may also be tested for glaucoma (see SCREENING FOR GLAUCOMA, opposite).

Phoropter

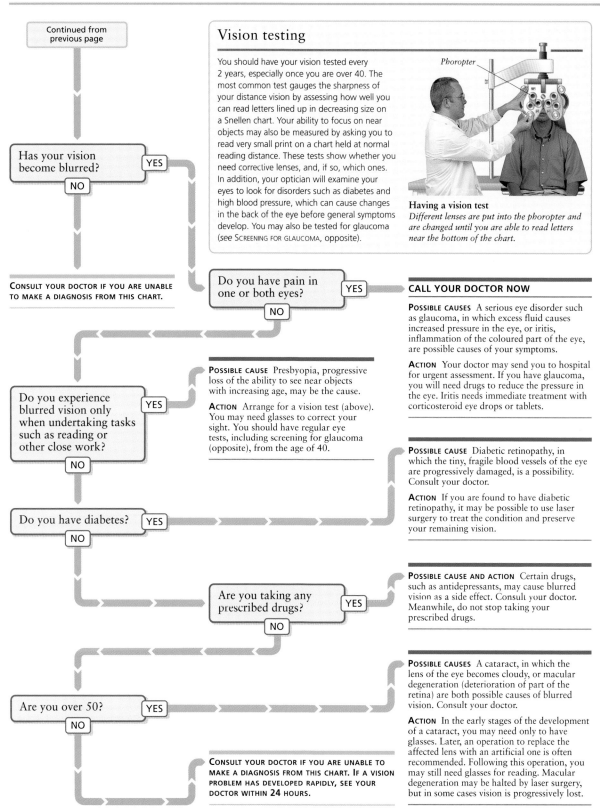

Having a vision test
Different lenses are put into the phoropter and are changed until you are able to read letters near the bottom of the chart.

Do you have pain in one or both eyes? **YES**

NO

Do you experience blurred vision only when undertaking tasks such as reading or other close work? **YES**

NO

POSSIBLE CAUSE Presbyopia, progressive loss of the ability to see near objects with increasing age, may be the cause.

ACTION Arrange for a vision test (above). You may need glasses to correct your sight. You should have regular eye tests, including screening for glaucoma (opposite), from the age of 40.

Do you have diabetes? **YES**

NO

Are you taking any prescribed drugs? **YES**

NO

Are you over 50? **YES**

NO

CONSULT YOUR DOCTOR IF YOU ARE UNABLE TO MAKE A DIAGNOSIS FROM THIS CHART. IF A VISION PROBLEM HAS DEVELOPED RAPIDLY, SEE YOUR DOCTOR WITHIN **24** HOURS.

CALL YOUR DOCTOR NOW

POSSIBLE CAUSES A serious eye disorder such as glaucoma, in which excess fluid causes increased pressure in the eye, or iritis, inflammation of the coloured part of the eye, are possible causes of your symptoms.

ACTION Your doctor may send you to hospital for urgent assessment. If you have glaucoma, you will need drugs to reduce the pressure in the eye. Iritis needs immediate treatment with corticosteroid eye drops or tablets.

POSSIBLE CAUSE Diabetic retinopathy, in which the tiny, fragile blood vessels of the eye are progressively damaged, is a possibility. Consult your doctor.

ACTION If you are found to have diabetic retinopathy, it may be possible to use laser surgery to treat the condition and preserve your remaining vision.

POSSIBLE CAUSE AND ACTION Certain drugs, such as antidepressants, may cause blurred vision as a side effect. Consult your doctor. Meanwhile, do not stop taking your prescribed drugs.

POSSIBLE CAUSES A cataract, in which the lens of the eye becomes cloudy, or macular degeneration (deterioration of part of the retina) are both possible causes of blurred vision. Consult your doctor.

ACTION In the early stages of the development of a cataract, you may need only to have glasses. Later, an operation to replace the affected lens with an artificial one is often recommended. Following this operation, you may still need glasses for reading. Macular degeneration may be halted by laser surgery, but in some cases vision is progressively lost.

84 Hearing problems

Deterioration in the ability to hear some or all sounds may come on gradually over a period of several months or years or may occur suddenly over a matter of hours or days. In many cases, hearing loss is the result of an ear infection or a wax blockage and can be treated easily. Hearing loss is also a common feature of aging. However, if you suddenly develop severe hearing loss in one or both ears for no obvious reason, always consult your doctor.

START HERE

Do you have an earache?

YES → *Go to chart* **86** EARACHE (p.189)

NO

Did the hearing loss start during or immediately after an aeroplane flight?

YES →

POSSIBLE CAUSE Barotrauma, damage to the eardrum resulting from a pressure difference between the middle and outer ear, is possible, especially if you already had a blocked nose.

ACTION Try gently blowing through your nose while pinching the nostrils closed to restore your hearing to normal. If the hearing loss persists for more than 24 hours, consult your doctor. Follow the advice on preventing ear problems caused by flying (p.189) in future.

NO

Is there a greenish-yellow discharge from the ear?

YES →

POSSIBLE CAUSE An infection of the outer ear canal, resulting in discharge blocking the canal, may be the cause, particularly if you feel pain when pulling on the ear lobe. Alternatively, you may have a middle ear infection and a perforated eardrum. Consult your doctor.

ACTION Depending on the type of infection, your doctor may prescribe ear drops containing an antibiotic or antifungal drug and/or a corticosteroid drug. If the infection is severe, or you have a middle ear infection, you may be given oral antibiotics. Your doctor may also clean the ear canal to remove debris.

NO

Have you had a runny or blocked nose, or a sore throat in the past week?

YES →

POSSIBLE CAUSE A cold or hay fever may result in blockage of the eustachian tube, which connects the middle ear to the throat. This may account for your hearing problem.

ACTION This is usually no cause for concern and should clear up without treatment within a week. Try steam inhalation (p.190). Consult your doctor if your symptoms do not improve.

NO

Have you experienced attacks of dizziness, during which everything around you seems to spin, and do you also have noises in the ear?

YES →

POSSIBLE CAUSE Ménière's disease may be the problem. This is a relatively uncommon disorder in which there is an increase in the amount of fluid in the inner ear (*see* HOW YOU KEEP YOUR BALANCE, p.158). The problem is most common in middle age.

ACTION Your doctor will probably arrange for you to undergo tests in hospital to confirm the diagnosis. If you have Ménière's disease, you may be given drugs to relieve nausea and vertigo and to reduce the amount of fluid in the inner ear. Your doctor may also advise you to cut down your intake of salt and alcohol, which may help reduce the frequency of future attacks. Very occasionally, surgery is recommended.

NO

Continued on next page

Hearing tests

Preliminary hearing tests assess the type of hearing loss you might have.

Audiometry measures the degree of hearing loss. Sounds of increasing volume and at different frequencies are transmitted to one ear at a time through headphones.

Tympanometry shows whether the eardrum moves normally when sounds hit it. A probe with a sound generator, microphone, and air pump is placed in the ear canal. Sounds are played while the air pressure is varied and the pattern of the sound waves reflected by the eardrum is recorded.

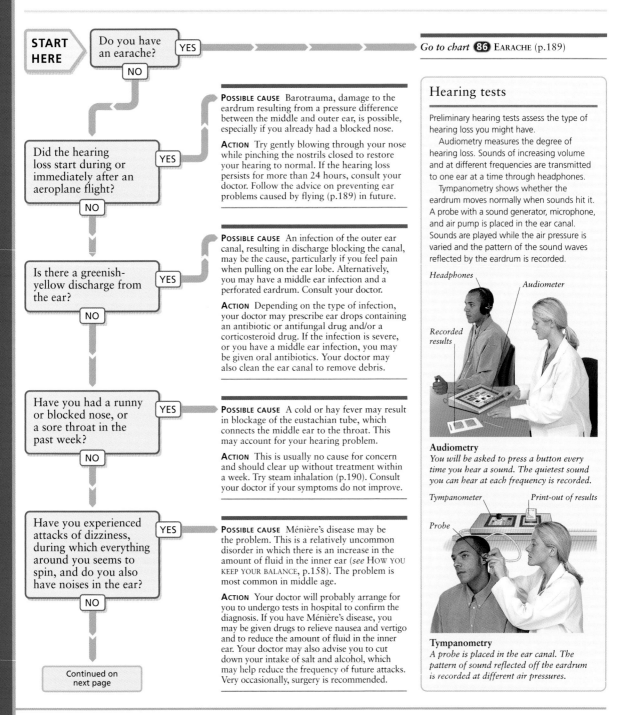

Headphones

Audiometer

Recorded results

Audiometry
You will be asked to press a button every time you hear a sound. The quietest sound you can hear at each frequency is recorded.

Tympanometer

Print-out of results

Probe

Tympanometry
A probe is placed in the ear canal. The pattern of sound reflected off the eardrum is recorded at different air pressures.

Continued from previous page

Do any of the following apply?
- You regularly listen to loud music
- You are exposed to loud noise at work
- You have been exposed to loud noise very recently

YES →

NO ↓

POSSIBLE CAUSE Brief exposure to loud noise can cause temporary hearing loss and ringing noises in the ears. However, repeated exposure to loud noise, even if the noise does not cause discomfort, can cause permanent loss of hearing.

ACTION If you have temporary hearing loss caused by a short exposure to excessive noise, your hearing should return to normal within hours. If you have been regularly exposed to loud noises and you are concerned about your hearing, consult your doctor. He or she will probably arrange for hearing tests (opposite) to be performed. To prevent your hearing deteriorating further, follow the advice for preventing noise-induced hearing loss (below).

Are you taking any prescribed or over-the-counter drugs?

YES →

NO ↓

POSSIBLE CAUSE Certain drugs, such as aspirin and some antibiotics, can cause hearing problems as a side effect. Stop taking any over-the-counter drugs, but continue taking prescribed medicines until you see your doctor.

Has your hearing been getting worse over a period of several weeks or more?

YES →

NO ↓

CONSULT YOUR DOCTOR IF YOU ARE UNABLE TO MAKE A DIAGNOSIS FROM THIS CHART.

Are you over 50 years of age?

YES →

NO ↓

POSSIBLE CAUSES Presbycusis, gradual loss of hearing as you get older, is a common cause of this symptom, but wax blockage may also be a possibility. Consult your doctor.

ACTION Your doctor will examine your ears and may refer you for hearing tests (opposite). If you have age-related hearing loss, you will probably be offered a hearing aid (above). If wax blockage is the problem, your doctor may suggest trying over-the-counter ear drops or may arrange for your ears to be syringed.

Have other members of your family also suffered from gradual hearing loss?

YES →

NO ↓

Hearing aids

Hearing aids amplify sounds, improving hearing in people with most types of hearing loss. All types of hearing aids have a tiny microphone, amplifier, and speaker, which are all powered by a battery. In older hearing aids, these parts are often housed in a small case that is worn behind the ear. However, newer hearing aids are much smaller and can fit entirely within the ear canal. The range of sounds that is amplified by a hearing aid is usually tailored to an individual's own pattern of hearing loss.

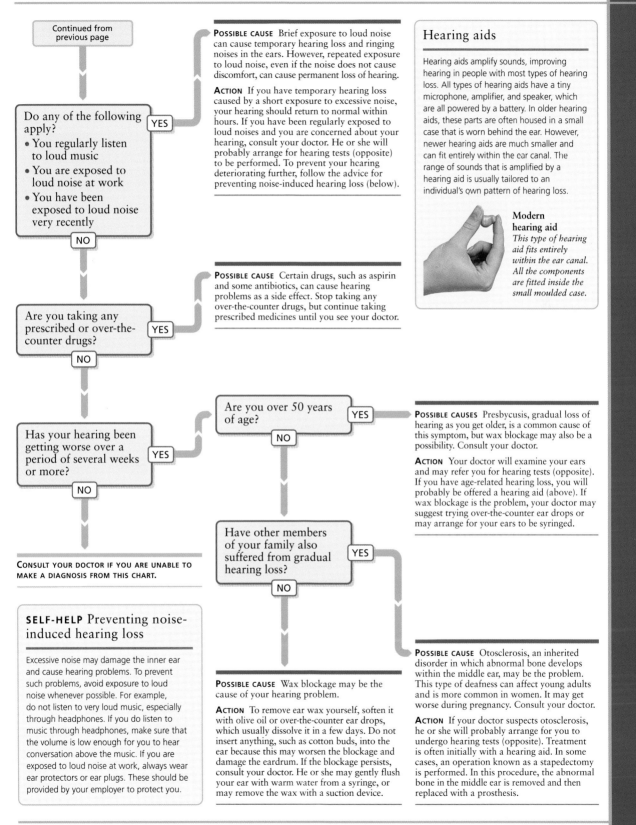

Modern hearing aid *This type of hearing aid fits entirely within the ear canal. All the components are fitted inside the small moulded case.*

SELF-HELP Preventing noise-induced hearing loss

Excessive noise may damage the inner ear and cause hearing problems. To prevent such problems, avoid exposure to loud noise whenever possible. For example, do not listen to very loud music, especially through headphones. If you do listen to music through headphones, make sure that the volume is low enough for you to hear conversation above the music. If you are exposed to loud noise at work, always wear ear protectors or ear plugs. These should be provided by your employer to protect you.

POSSIBLE CAUSE Wax blockage may be the cause of your hearing problem.

ACTION To remove ear wax yourself, soften it with olive oil or over-the-counter ear drops, which usually dissolve it in a few days. Do not insert anything, such as cotton buds, into the ear because this may worsen the blockage and damage the eardrum. If the blockage persists, consult your doctor. He or she may gently flush your ear with warm water from a syringe, or may remove the wax with a suction device.

POSSIBLE CAUSE Otosclerosis, an inherited disorder in which abnormal bone develops within the middle ear, may be the problem. This type of deafness can affect young adults and is more common in women. It may get worse during pregnancy. Consult your doctor.

ACTION If your doctor suspects otosclerosis, he or she will probably arrange for you to undergo hearing tests (opposite). Treatment is often initially with a hearing aid. In some cases, an operation known as a stapedectomy is performed. In this procedure, the abnormal bone in the middle ear is removed and then replaced with a prosthesis.

85 Noises in the ear

Hearing noises inside your ear, such as buzzing, ringing, or hissing, is known as tinnitus. Some people have brief episodes of tinnitus that are not due to an ear disorder and

that clear up without needing medical treatment. Others have persistent tinnitus that is not only distressing but may also indicate an ear problem that should be investigated.

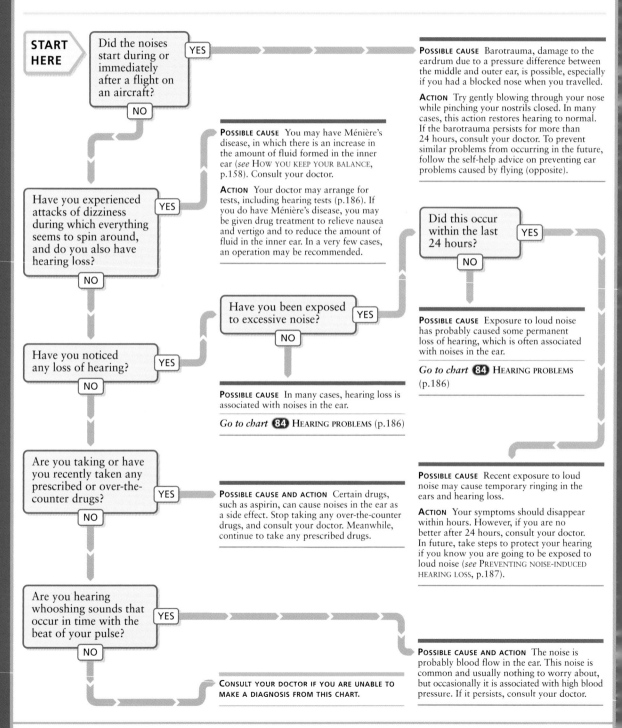

START HERE

Did the noises start during or immediately after a flight on an aircraft?   YES

NO

POSSIBLE CAUSE Barotrauma, damage to the eardrum due to a pressure difference between the middle and outer ear, is possible, especially if you had a blocked nose when you travelled.

ACTION Try gently blowing through your nose while pinching your nostrils closed. In many cases, this action restores hearing to normal. If the barotrauma persists for more than 24 hours, consult your doctor. To prevent similar problems from occurring in the future, follow the self-help advice on preventing ear problems caused by flying (opposite).

Have you experienced attacks of dizziness during which everything seems to spin around, and do you also have hearing loss?   YES

NO

POSSIBLE CAUSE You may have Ménière's disease, in which there is an increase in the amount of fluid formed in the inner ear (*see* HOW YOU KEEP YOUR BALANCE, p.158). Consult your doctor.

ACTION Your doctor may arrange for tests, including hearing tests (p.186). If you do have Ménière's disease, you may be given drug treatment to relieve nausea and vertigo and to reduce the amount of fluid in the inner ear. In a very few cases, an operation may be recommended.

Did this occur within the last 24 hours?   YES

NO

Have you been exposed to excessive noise?   YES

NO

POSSIBLE CAUSE Exposure to loud noise has probably caused some permanent loss of hearing, which is often associated with noises in the ear.

Go to chart **84** HEARING PROBLEMS (p.186)

Have you noticed any loss of hearing?   YES

NO

POSSIBLE CAUSE In many cases, hearing loss is associated with noises in the ear.

Go to chart **84** HEARING PROBLEMS (p.186)

Are you taking or have you recently taken any prescribed or over-the-counter drugs?   YES

NO

POSSIBLE CAUSE AND ACTION Certain drugs, such as aspirin, can cause noises in the ear as a side effect. Stop taking any over-the-counter drugs, and consult your doctor. Meanwhile, continue to take any prescribed drugs.

POSSIBLE CAUSE Recent exposure to loud noise may cause temporary ringing in the ears and hearing loss.

ACTION Your symptoms should disappear within hours. However, if you are no better after 24 hours, consult your doctor. In future, take steps to protect your hearing if you know you are going to be exposed to loud noise (*see* PREVENTING NOISE-INDUCED HEARING LOSS, p.187).

Are you hearing whooshing sounds that occur in time with the beat of your pulse?   YES

NO

CONSULT YOUR DOCTOR IF YOU ARE UNABLE TO MAKE A DIAGNOSIS FROM THIS CHART.

POSSIBLE CAUSE AND ACTION The noise is probably blood flow in the ear. This noise is common and usually nothing to worry about, but occasionally it is associated with high blood pressure. If it persists, consult your doctor.

86 Earache

Earache may vary from a dull, throbbing sensation to a sharp, severe, stabbing pain. Although it is very common in childhood, it occurs much less frequently in adults. The pain is often due to infection of the ear canal or of the middle ear behind the eardrum. Sometimes, earache may require medical attention and, in some cases, treatment with antibiotics.

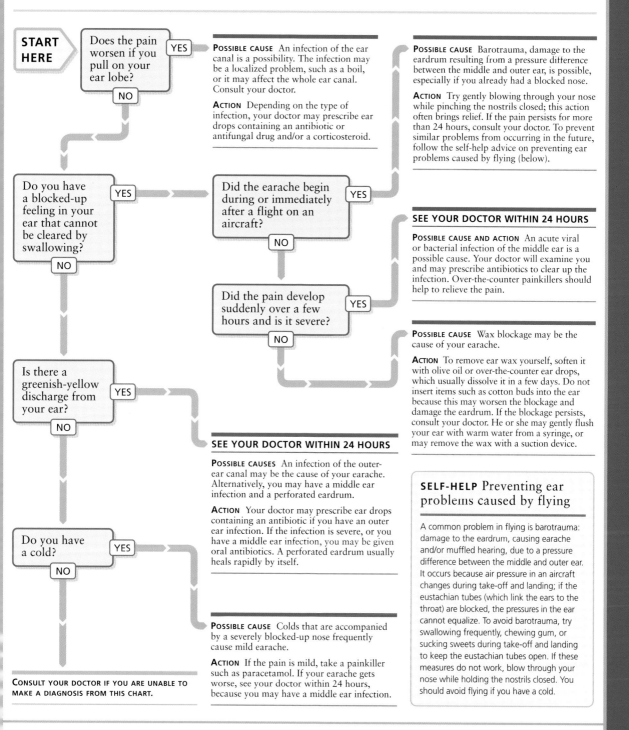

START HERE

Does the pain worsen if you pull on your ear lobe? — YES

POSSIBLE CAUSE An infection of the ear canal is a possibility. The infection may be a localized problem, such as a boil, or it may affect the whole ear canal. Consult your doctor.

ACTION Depending on the type of infection, your doctor may prescribe ear drops containing an antibiotic or antifungal drug and/or a corticosteroid.

NO

Do you have a blocked-up feeling in your ear that cannot be cleared by swallowing? — YES

Did the earache begin during or immediately after a flight on an aircraft? — YES

POSSIBLE CAUSE Barotrauma, damage to the eardrum resulting from a pressure difference between the middle and outer ear, is possible, especially if you already had a blocked nose.

ACTION Try gently blowing through your nose while pinching the nostrils closed; this action often brings relief. If the pain persists for more than 24 hours, consult your doctor. To prevent similar problems from occurring in the future, follow the self-help advice on preventing ear problems caused by flying (below).

NO

NO

SEE YOUR DOCTOR WITHIN 24 HOURS

POSSIBLE CAUSE AND ACTION An acute viral or bacterial infection of the middle ear is a possible cause. Your doctor will examine you and may prescribe antibiotics to clear up the infection. Over-the-counter painkillers should help to relieve the pain.

Did the pain develop suddenly over a few hours and is it severe? — YES

NO

Is there a greenish-yellow discharge from your ear? — YES

POSSIBLE CAUSE Wax blockage may be the cause of your earache.

ACTION To remove ear wax yourself, soften it with olive oil or over-the-counter ear drops, which usually dissolve it in a few days. Do not insert items such as cotton buds into the ear because this may worsen the blockage and damage the eardrum. If the blockage persists, consult your doctor. He or she may gently flush your ear with warm water from a syringe, or may remove the wax with a suction device.

NO

SEE YOUR DOCTOR WITHIN 24 HOURS

POSSIBLE CAUSES An infection of the outer-ear canal may be the cause of your earache. Alternatively, you may have a middle ear infection and a perforated eardrum.

ACTION Your doctor may prescribe ear drops containing an antibiotic if you have an outer ear infection. If the infection is severe, or you have a middle ear infection, you may be given oral antibiotics. A perforated eardrum usually heals rapidly by itself.

Do you have a cold? — YES

NO

POSSIBLE CAUSE Colds that are accompanied by a severely blocked-up nose frequently cause mild earache.

ACTION If the pain is mild, take a painkiller such as paracetamol. If your earache gets worse, see your doctor within 24 hours, because you may have a middle ear infection.

CONSULT YOUR DOCTOR IF YOU ARE UNABLE TO MAKE A DIAGNOSIS FROM THIS CHART.

SELF-HELP Preventing ear problems caused by flying

A common problem in flying is barotrauma: damage to the eardrum, causing earache and/or muffled hearing, due to a pressure difference between the middle and outer ear. It occurs because air pressure in an aircraft changes during take-off and landing; if the eustachian tubes (which link the ears to the throat) are blocked, the pressures in the ear cannot equalize. To avoid barotrauma, try swallowing frequently, chewing gum, or sucking sweets during take-off and landing to keep the eustachian tubes open. If these measures do not work, blow through your nose while holding the nostrils closed. You should avoid flying if you have a cold.

87 Runny or blocked nose

Most people have a blocked or runny nose at least once a year. The usual cause of these symptoms is irritation of the lining of the nose. This irritation can be caused by a viral infection, such as a cold, or it can result from an allergic reaction, such as hay fever (seasonal allergic rhinitis). Nosebleeds (below) may have a specific cause, such as injury or forceful nose blowing, but they may occur spontaneously. They can be serious in people over the age of 50.

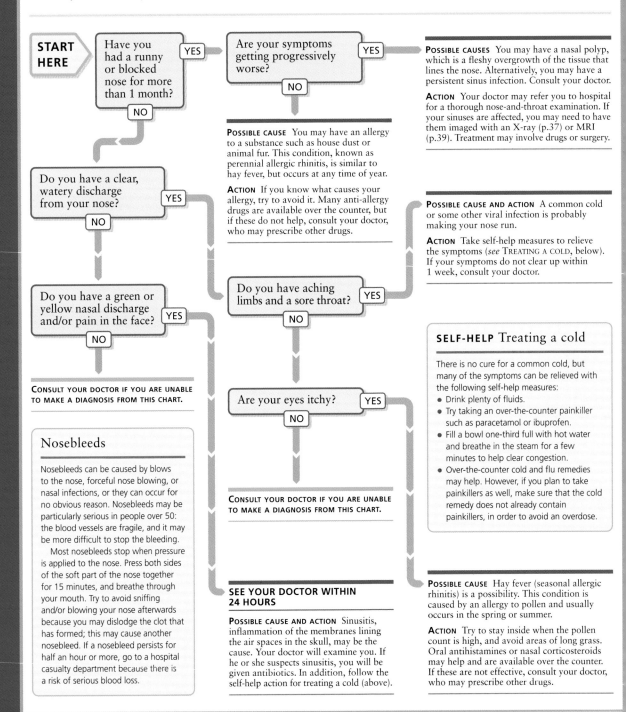

START HERE

Have you had a runny or blocked nose for more than 1 month? — YES → **Are your symptoms getting progressively worse?** — YES → **POSSIBLE CAUSES** You may have a nasal polyp, which is a fleshy overgrowth of the tissue that lines the nose. Alternatively, you may have a persistent sinus infection. Consult your doctor.

ACTION Your doctor may refer you to hospital for a thorough nose-and-throat examination. If your sinuses are affected, you may need to have them imaged with an X-ray (p.37) or MRI (p.39). Treatment may involve drugs or surgery.

Are your symptoms getting progressively worse? — NO

POSSIBLE CAUSE You may have an allergy to a substance such as house dust or animal fur. This condition, known as perennial allergic rhinitis, is similar to hay fever, but occurs at any time of year.

ACTION If you know what causes your allergy, try to avoid it. Many anti-allergy drugs are available over the counter, but if these do not help, consult your doctor, who may prescribe other drugs.

Have you had a runny or blocked nose for more than 1 month? — NO

Do you have a clear, watery discharge from your nose? — YES

POSSIBLE CAUSE AND ACTION A common cold or some other viral infection is probably making your nose run.

ACTION Take self-help measures to relieve the symptoms (see TREATING A COLD, below). If your symptoms do not clear up within 1 week, consult your doctor.

Do you have a clear, watery discharge from your nose? — NO

Do you have aching limbs and a sore throat? — YES

Do you have aching limbs and a sore throat? — NO

SELF-HELP Treating a cold

There is no cure for a common cold, but many of the symptoms can be relieved with the following self-help measures:
- Drink plenty of fluids.
- Try taking an over-the-counter painkiller such as paracetamol or ibuprofen.
- Fill a bowl one-third full with hot water and breathe in the steam for a few minutes to help clear congestion.
- Over-the-counter cold and flu remedies may help. However, if you plan to take painkillers as well, make sure that the cold remedy does not already contain painkillers, in order to avoid an overdose.

Do you have a green or yellow nasal discharge and/or pain in the face? — YES

Do you have a green or yellow nasal discharge and/or pain in the face? — NO

CONSULT YOUR DOCTOR IF YOU ARE UNABLE TO MAKE A DIAGNOSIS FROM THIS CHART.

Are your eyes itchy? — YES

Are your eyes itchy? — NO

CONSULT YOUR DOCTOR IF YOU ARE UNABLE TO MAKE A DIAGNOSIS FROM THIS CHART.

Nosebleeds

Nosebleeds can be caused by blows to the nose, forceful nose blowing, or nasal infections, or they can occur for no obvious reason. Nosebleeds may be particularly serious in people over 50: the blood vessels are fragile, and it may be more difficult to stop the bleeding.

Most nosebleeds stop when pressure is applied to the nose. Press both sides of the soft part of the nose together for 15 minutes, and breathe through your mouth. Try to avoid sniffing and/or blowing your nose afterwards because you may dislodge the clot that has formed; this may cause another nosebleed. If a nosebleed persists for half an hour or more, go to a hospital casualty department because there is a risk of serious blood loss.

SEE YOUR DOCTOR WITHIN 24 HOURS

POSSIBLE CAUSE AND ACTION Sinusitis, inflammation of the membranes lining the air spaces in the skull, may be the cause. Your doctor will examine you. If he or she suspects sinusitis, you will be given antibiotics. In addition, follow the self-help action for treating a cold (above).

POSSIBLE CAUSE Hay fever (seasonal allergic rhinitis) is a possibility. This condition is caused by an allergy to pollen and usually occurs in the spring or summer.

ACTION Try to stay inside when the pollen count is high, and avoid areas of long grass. Oral antihistamines or nasal corticosteroids may help and are available over the counter. If these are not effective, consult your doctor, who may prescribe other drugs.

88 Sore throat

Most people suffer from a painful, rough, or raw feeling in the throat from time to time. A sore throat usually clears up within a few days and is most commonly due to a minor infection, such as a cold, or irritation from smoke. Swallowing something sharp, such as a fish bone, can scratch the throat. The cause of the soreness in this case is usually obvious.

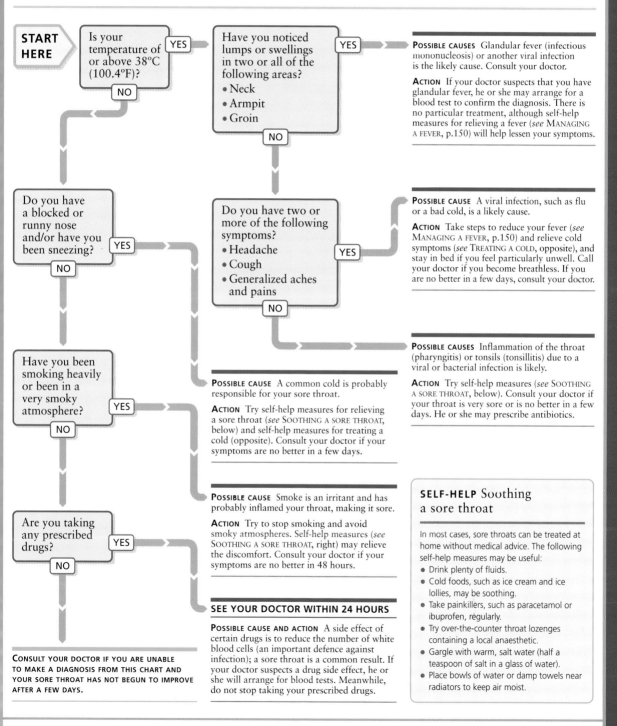

START HERE

Is your temperature of or above 38°C (100.4°F)? — **YES** → **Have you noticed lumps or swellings in two or all of the following areas?**
- Neck
- Armpit
- Groin

YES →

POSSIBLE CAUSES Glandular fever (infectious mononucleosis) or another viral infection is the likely cause. Consult your doctor.

ACTION If your doctor suspects that you have glandular fever, he or she may arrange for a blood test to confirm the diagnosis. There is no particular treatment, although self-help measures for relieving a fever (*see* MANAGING A FEVER, p.150) will help lessen your symptoms.

NO ↓ (from lumps question)

Do you have two or more of the following symptoms?
- Headache
- Cough
- Generalized aches and pains

YES →

POSSIBLE CAUSE A viral infection, such as flu or a bad cold, is a likely cause.

ACTION Take steps to reduce your fever (*see* MANAGING A FEVER, p.150) and relieve cold symptoms (*see* TREATING A COLD, opposite), and stay in bed if you feel particularly unwell. Call your doctor if you become breathless. If you are no better in a few days, consult your doctor.

NO ↓

POSSIBLE CAUSES Inflammation of the throat (pharyngitis) or tonsils (tonsillitis) due to a viral or bacterial infection is likely.

ACTION Try self-help measures (*see* SOOTHING A SORE THROAT, below). Consult your doctor if your throat is very sore or is no better in a few days. He or she may prescribe antibiotics.

NO (from temperature question) ↓

Do you have a blocked or runny nose and/or have you been sneezing? — **YES** →

POSSIBLE CAUSE A common cold is probably responsible for your sore throat.

ACTION Try self-help measures for relieving a sore throat (*see* SOOTHING A SORE THROAT, below) and self-help measures for treating a cold (opposite). Consult your doctor if your symptoms are no better in a few days.

NO ↓

Have you been smoking heavily or been in a very smoky atmosphere? — **YES** →

POSSIBLE CAUSE Smoke is an irritant and has probably inflamed your throat, making it sore.

ACTION Try to stop smoking and avoid smoky atmospheres. Self-help measures (*see* SOOTHING A SORE THROAT, right) may relieve the discomfort. Consult your doctor if your symptoms are no better in 48 hours.

NO ↓

Are you taking any prescribed drugs? — **YES** →

SEE YOUR DOCTOR WITHIN 24 HOURS

POSSIBLE CAUSE AND ACTION A side effect of certain drugs is to reduce the number of white blood cells (an important defence against infection); a sore throat is a common result. If your doctor suspects a drug side effect, he or she will arrange for blood tests. Meanwhile, do not stop taking your prescribed drugs.

NO ↓

CONSULT YOUR DOCTOR IF YOU ARE UNABLE TO MAKE A DIAGNOSIS FROM THIS CHART AND YOUR SORE THROAT HAS NOT BEGUN TO IMPROVE AFTER A FEW DAYS.

SELF-HELP Soothing a sore throat

In most cases, sore throats can be treated at home without medical advice. The following self-help measures may be useful:
- Drink plenty of fluids.
- Cold foods, such as ice cream and ice lollies, may be soothing.
- Take painkillers, such as paracetamol or ibuprofen, regularly.
- Try over-the-counter throat lozenges containing a local anaesthetic.
- Gargle with warm, salt water (half a teaspoon of salt in a glass of water).
- Place bowls of water or damp towels near radiators to keep air moist.

89 Hoarseness or loss of voice

Hoarseness, huskiness, or loss of voice is almost always due to laryngitis – inflammation and swelling of the vocal cords. In most cases, the cause of the inflammation is a viral infection or overuse of the voice; symptoms can be relieved by using self-help measures, and there is no need to consult your doctor. However, persistent or recurrent hoarseness or loss or change of voice may have a serious cause, and, in these cases, you should always consult your doctor.

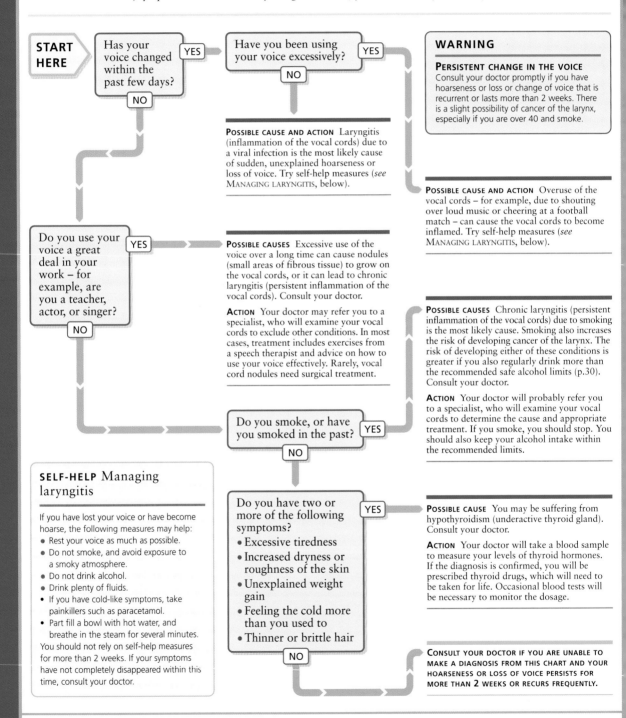

START HERE

Has your voice changed within the past few days?
YES / NO

Have you been using your voice excessively?
YES / NO

POSSIBLE CAUSE AND ACTION Laryngitis (inflammation of the vocal cords) due to a viral infection is the most likely cause of sudden, unexplained hoarseness or loss of voice. Try self-help measures (*see* MANAGING LARYNGITIS, below).

WARNING

PERSISTENT CHANGE IN THE VOICE
Consult your doctor promptly if you have hoarseness or loss or change of voice that is recurrent or lasts more than 2 weeks. There is a slight possibility of cancer of the larynx, especially if you are over 40 and smoke.

POSSIBLE CAUSE AND ACTION Overuse of the vocal cords – for example, due to shouting over loud music or cheering at a football match – can cause the vocal cords to become inflamed. Try self-help measures (*see* MANAGING LARYNGITIS, below).

Do you use your voice a great deal in your work – for example, are you a teacher, actor, or singer?
YES / NO

POSSIBLE CAUSES Excessive use of the voice over a long time can cause nodules (small areas of fibrous tissue) to grow on the vocal cords, or it can lead to chronic laryngitis (persistent inflammation of the vocal cords). Consult your doctor.

ACTION Your doctor may refer you to a specialist, who will examine your vocal cords to exclude other conditions. In most cases, treatment includes exercises from a speech therapist and advice on how to use your voice effectively. Rarely, vocal cord nodules need surgical treatment.

POSSIBLE CAUSES Chronic laryngitis (persistent inflammation of the vocal cords) due to smoking is the most likely cause. Smoking also increases the risk of developing cancer of the larynx. The risk of developing either of these conditions is greater if you also regularly drink more than the recommended safe alcohol limits (p.30). Consult your doctor.

ACTION Your doctor will probably refer you to a specialist, who will examine your vocal cords to determine the cause and appropriate treatment. If you smoke, you should stop. You should also keep your alcohol intake within the recommended limits.

Do you smoke, or have you smoked in the past?
YES / NO

SELF-HELP Managing laryngitis

If you have lost your voice or have become hoarse, the following measures may help:
- Rest your voice as much as possible.
- Do not smoke, and avoid exposure to a smoky atmosphere.
- Do not drink alcohol.
- Drink plenty of fluids.
- If you have cold-like symptoms, take painkillers such as paracetamol.
- Part fill a bowl with hot water, and breathe in the steam for several minutes.

You should not rely on self-help measures for more than 2 weeks. If your symptoms have not completely disappeared within this time, consult your doctor.

Do you have two or more of the following symptoms?
- Excessive tiredness
- Increased dryness or roughness of the skin
- Unexplained weight gain
- Feeling the cold more than you used to
- Thinner or brittle hair

YES / NO

POSSIBLE CAUSE You may be suffering from hypothyroidism (underactive thyroid gland). Consult your doctor.

ACTION Your doctor will take a blood sample to measure your levels of thyroid hormones. If the diagnosis is confirmed, you will be prescribed thyroid drugs, which will need to be taken for life. Occasional blood tests will be necessary to monitor the dosage.

CONSULT YOUR DOCTOR IF YOU ARE UNABLE TO MAKE A DIAGNOSIS FROM THIS CHART AND YOUR HOARSENESS OR LOSS OF VOICE PERSISTS FOR MORE THAN 2 WEEKS OR RECURS FREQUENTLY.

90 Wheezing

Wheezing is a whistling or rasping sound made when you breathe out. It is usually due to narrowing of the airways as a result of inflammation caused by infection, asthma, or smoking. Rarely, wheezing is due to a small foreign body or a tumour partially blocking an airway. If you suddenly start to wheeze or are short of breath, get medical help at once.

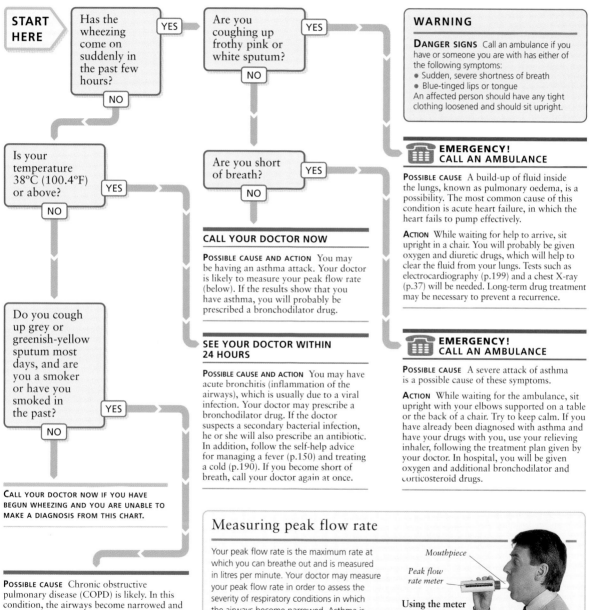

START HERE

Has the wheezing come on suddenly in the past few hours?
- **YES** → **Are you coughing up frothy pink or white sputum?**
  - **YES** → (see WARNING / EMERGENCY)
  - **NO** → **Are you short of breath?**
    - **YES** → (see EMERGENCY)
    - **NO** → **CALL YOUR DOCTOR NOW**
- **NO** → **Is your temperature 38°C (100.4°F) or above?**
  - **YES** → **SEE YOUR DOCTOR WITHIN 24 HOURS**
  - **NO** → **Do you cough up grey or greenish-yellow sputum most days, and are you a smoker or have you smoked in the past?**
    - **YES** → (POSSIBLE CAUSE: COPD)
    - **NO** → **CALL YOUR DOCTOR NOW IF YOU HAVE BEGUN WHEEZING AND YOU ARE UNABLE TO MAKE A DIAGNOSIS FROM THIS CHART.**

WARNING

DANGER SIGNS Call an ambulance if you have or someone you are with has either of the following symptoms:
- Sudden, severe shortness of breath
- Blue-tinged lips or tongue

An affected person should have any tight clothing loosened and should sit upright.

☎ EMERGENCY! CALL AN AMBULANCE

POSSIBLE CAUSE A build-up of fluid inside the lungs, known as pulmonary oedema, is a possibility. The most common cause of this condition is acute heart failure, in which the heart fails to pump effectively.

ACTION While waiting for help to arrive, sit upright in a chair. You will probably be given oxygen and diuretic drugs, which will help to clear the fluid from your lungs. Tests such as electrocardiography (p.199) and a chest X-ray (p.37) will be needed. Long-term drug treatment may be necessary to prevent a recurrence.

☎ EMERGENCY! CALL AN AMBULANCE

POSSIBLE CAUSE A severe attack of asthma is a possible cause of these symptoms.

ACTION While waiting for the ambulance, sit upright with your elbows supported on a table or the back of a chair. Try to keep calm. If you have already been diagnosed with asthma and have your drugs with you, use your relieving inhaler, following the treatment plan given by your doctor. In hospital, you will be given oxygen and additional bronchodilator and corticosteroid drugs.

CALL YOUR DOCTOR NOW

POSSIBLE CAUSE AND ACTION You may be having an asthma attack. Your doctor is likely to measure your peak flow rate (below). If the results show that you have asthma, you will probably be prescribed a bronchodilator drug.

SEE YOUR DOCTOR WITHIN 24 HOURS

POSSIBLE CAUSE AND ACTION You may have acute bronchitis (inflammation of the airways), which is usually due to a viral infection. Your doctor may prescribe a bronchodilator drug. If the doctor suspects a secondary bacterial infection, he or she will also prescribe an antibiotic. In addition, follow the self-help advice for managing a fever (p.150) and treating a cold (p.190). If you become short of breath, call your doctor again at once.

POSSIBLE CAUSE Chronic obstructive pulmonary disease (COPD) is likely. In this condition, the airways become narrowed and produce excess mucus, and the air sacs in the lungs are damaged. Consult your doctor.

ACTION Although the damage is irreversible, your doctor may prescribe a bronchodilator drug to help relieve symptoms. You must stop smoking to prevent the condition worsening.

Measuring peak flow rate

Your peak flow rate is the maximum rate at which you can breathe out and is measured in litres per minute. Your doctor may measure your peak flow rate in order to assess the severity of respiratory conditions in which the airways become narrowed. Asthma is commonly diagnosed and monitored by measuring peak flow rate. You may be given a peak flow rate meter to use at home so that you can check your condition regularly and adjust your treatment as necessary.

Mouthpiece

Peak flow rate meter

Using the meter
Take a full breath, and breathe out as hard as you can. The pointer on the meter shows the result.

91 Coughing

Coughing is the body's response to irritation or inflammation in the lungs or the throat; the cough may either produce sputum or be "dry". The most common causes of coughing are colds, smoking, asthma, or inhaling a foreign body. Sometimes, however, a persistent cough may signal a more serious respiratory disorder, such as a tumour.

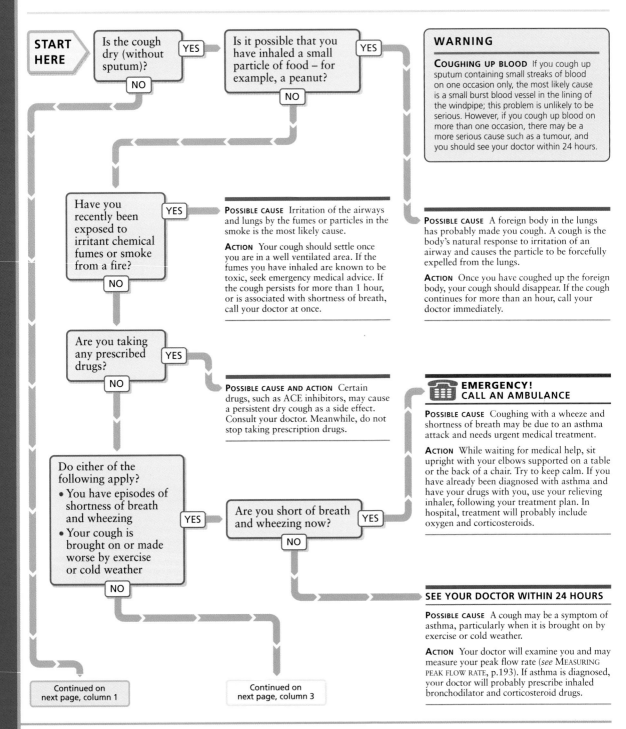

START HERE

Is the cough dry (without sputum)?
YES →
NO ↓

Is it possible that you have inhaled a small particle of food – for example, a peanut?
YES →
NO ↓

WARNING

COUGHING UP BLOOD If you cough up sputum containing small streaks of blood on one occasion only, the most likely cause is a small burst blood vessel in the lining of the windpipe; this problem is unlikely to be serious. However, if you cough up blood on more than one occasion, there may be a more serious cause such as a tumour, and you should see your doctor within 24 hours.

Have you recently been exposed to irritant chemical fumes or smoke from a fire?
YES →
NO ↓

POSSIBLE CAUSE Irritation of the airways and lungs by the fumes or particles in the smoke is the most likely cause.

ACTION Your cough should settle once you are in a well ventilated area. If the fumes you have inhaled are known to be toxic, seek emergency medical advice. If the cough persists for more than 1 hour, or is associated with shortness of breath, call your doctor at once.

POSSIBLE CAUSE A foreign body in the lungs has probably made you cough. A cough is the body's natural response to irritation of an airway and causes the particle to be forcefully expelled from the lungs.

ACTION Once you have coughed up the foreign body, your cough should disappear. If the cough continues for more than an hour, call your doctor immediately.

Are you taking any prescribed drugs?
YES →
NO ↓

POSSIBLE CAUSE AND ACTION Certain drugs, such as ACE inhibitors, may cause a persistent dry cough as a side effect. Consult your doctor. Meanwhile, do not stop taking prescription drugs.

EMERGENCY! CALL AN AMBULANCE

POSSIBLE CAUSE Coughing with a wheeze and shortness of breath may be due to an asthma attack and needs urgent medical treatment.

ACTION While waiting for medical help, sit upright with your elbows supported on a table or the back of a chair. Try to keep calm. If you have already been diagnosed with asthma and have your drugs with you, use your relieving inhaler, following your treatment plan. In hospital, treatment will probably include oxygen and corticosteroids.

Do either of the following apply?
- **You have episodes of shortness of breath and wheezing**
- **Your cough is brought on or made worse by exercise or cold weather**
YES →
NO ↓

Are you short of breath and wheezing now?
YES →
NO ↓

SEE YOUR DOCTOR WITHIN 24 HOURS

POSSIBLE CAUSE A cough may be a symptom of asthma, particularly when it is brought on by exercise or cold weather.

ACTION Your doctor will examine you and may measure your peak flow rate (see MEASURING PEAK FLOW RATE, p.193). If asthma is diagnosed, your doctor will probably prescribe inhaled bronchodilator and corticosteroid drugs.

Continued on next page, column 1

Continued on next page, column 3

Continued from previous page, column 1

Are you short of breath? **YES**

NO

Continued from previous page, column 2

Has the cough started within the past week? **YES**

NO

POSSIBLE CAUSE AND ACTION You may have acute bronchitis or another viral infection such as a common cold. Take painkillers and try steam inhalation (p.190). If you smoke, you should stop. Call your doctor if you become short of breath. Otherwise, consult your doctor if you are no better in a few days.

Do you have pain in the centre of your chest, and does it get worse when you bend over or lie down? **YES**

NO

Is your cough associated with any of the following?
• Weight loss
• Coughing up blood
• Persistent hoarse voice
• Night sweats

YES

NO

CALL YOUR DOCTOR NOW

POSSIBLE CAUSE A chest infection such as pneumonia (infection of the air sacs in the lungs) is possible.

ACTION If you have a fever, take steps to reduce it (*see* MANAGING A FEVER, p.150). If your doctor confirms that you have pneumonia, he or she will probably prescribe antibiotics and may arrange for you to have a chest X-ray (p.37). Hospital admission is sometimes necessary.

CONSULT YOUR DOCTOR IF YOU ARE UNABLE TO MAKE A DIAGNOSIS FROM THIS CHART.

POSSIBLE CAUSE Gastro-oesophageal reflux disease, in which the acid stomach contents are regurgitated back up the oesophagus, may be the cause of your cough, as some regurgitated matter can enter the lungs. Consult your doctor.

ACTION Your doctor will advise you on how to reduce the risk of gastro-oesophageal reflux disease (*see* COPING WITH GASTRO-OESOPHAGEAL REFLUX DISEASE, p.205). If the symptoms do not improve with these measures, your doctor may prescribe an ulcer-healing drug in order to reduce the production of stomach acid.

Do you cough up thick, greyish sputum most days, and do you smoke, or have you smoked in the past? **YES**

NO

SEE YOUR DOCTOR WITHIN 24 HOURS

POSSIBLE CAUSE You may have a serious lung disorder such as tuberculosis or lung cancer.

ACTION Your doctor will probably arrange for blood and sputum tests and a chest X-ray (p.37). Depending on the results, you may then be referred to a specialist for tests such as bronchoscopy (below).

CONSULT YOUR DOCTOR IF YOU ARE UNABLE TO MAKE A DIAGNOSIS FROM THIS CHART.

POSSIBLE CAUSE Chronic obstructive pulmonary disease (COPD) is likely. In this condition the airways become narrowed and produce excess mucus and the air sacs in the lungs are damaged. Consult your doctor.

ACTION The damage is irreversible, but your doctor may prescribe bronchodilators to help relieve your symptoms. You must stop smoking to prevent the condition becoming any worse.

Bronchoscopy

Bronchoscopy can be used to diagnose lung disorders, such as lung cancer. In most cases, a flexible bronchoscope is passed through the nose or mouth down into the lungs to view the bronchi (airways). Before the procedure, you will be given a local anaesthetic spray to numb the back of your throat or nose and/or offered mild sedation. Sometimes, surgical instruments can also be passed down through the bronchoscope to remove tissue samples or carry out treatments during the procedure.

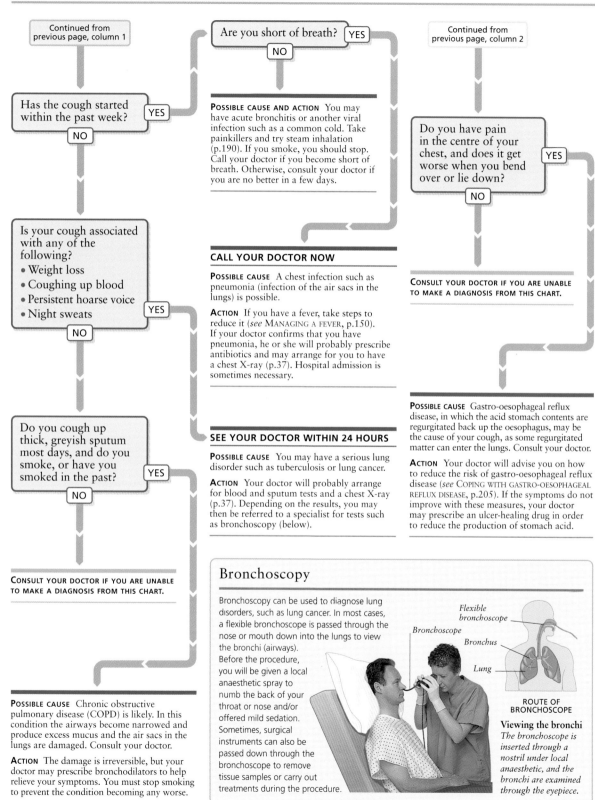

Flexible bronchoscope

Bronchoscope

Bronchus

Lung

ROUTE OF BRONCHOSCOPE

Viewing the bronchi
The bronchoscope is inserted through a nostril under local anaesthetic, and the bronchi are examined through the eyepiece.

92 Shortness of breath

It is normal to become short of breath after strenuous exercise. Pregnant women and people who are overweight become short of breath most easily. However, if you are breathing rapidly or you are "puffing" at rest or after very gentle exercise, you may have a problem affecting the heart or respiratory system. Because such problems may be serious and threaten the oxygen supply to the tissues, it is very important to seek medical advice without delay if you become short of breath for no apparent reason. A sudden shortness of breath and an inability to make any sound that comes on while eating is probably due to choking and needs urgent first-aid treatment.

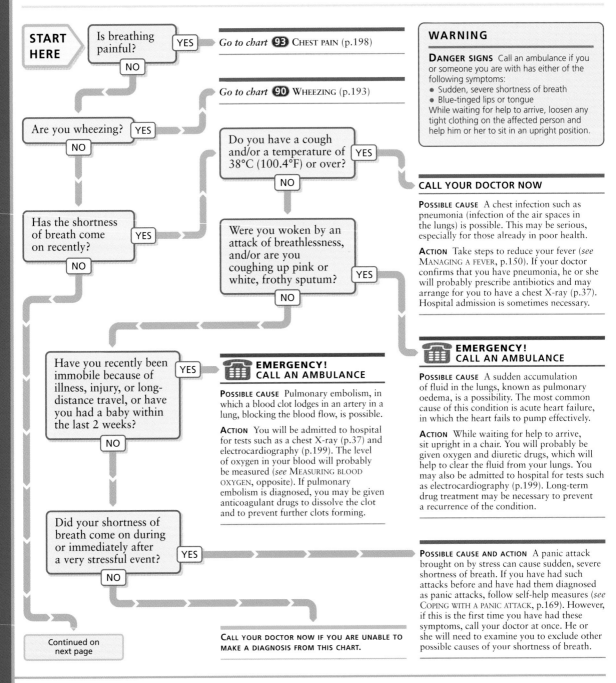

START HERE → **Is breathing painful?** — YES → Go to chart **93** CHEST PAIN (p.198)

NO

Go to chart **90** WHEEZING (p.193)

Are you wheezing? — YES

NO

Do you have a cough and/or a temperature of 38°C (100.4°F) or over? — YES

NO

Has the shortness of breath come on recently? — YES

NO

Were you woken by an attack of breathlessness, and/or are you coughing up pink or white, frothy sputum? — YES

NO

Have you recently been immobile because of illness, injury, or long-distance travel, or have you had a baby within the last 2 weeks? — YES

NO

Did your shortness of breath come on during or immediately after a very stressful event? — YES

NO

Continued on next page

WARNING

DANGER SIGNS Call an ambulance if you or someone you are with has either of the following symptoms:
- Sudden, severe shortness of breath
- Blue-tinged lips or tongue

While waiting for help to arrive, loosen any tight clothing on the affected person and help him or her to sit in an upright position.

CALL YOUR DOCTOR NOW

POSSIBLE CAUSE A chest infection such as pneumonia (infection of the air spaces in the lungs) is possible. This may be serious, especially for those already in poor health.

ACTION Take steps to reduce your fever (see MANAGING A FEVER, p.150). If your doctor confirms that you have pneumonia, he or she will probably prescribe antibiotics and may arrange for you to have a chest X-ray (p.37). Hospital admission is sometimes necessary.

EMERGENCY! CALL AN AMBULANCE

POSSIBLE CAUSE A sudden accumulation of fluid in the lungs, known as pulmonary oedema, is a possibility. The most common cause of this condition is acute heart failure, in which the heart fails to pump effectively.

ACTION While waiting for help to arrive, sit upright in a chair. You will probably be given oxygen and diuretic drugs, which will help to clear the fluid from your lungs. You may also be admitted to hospital for tests such as electrocardiography (p.199). Long-term drug treatment may be necessary to prevent a recurrence of the condition.

POSSIBLE CAUSE AND ACTION A panic attack brought on by stress can cause sudden, severe shortness of breath. If you have had such attacks before and have had them diagnosed as panic attacks, follow self-help measures (see COPING WITH A PANIC ATTACK, p.169). However, if this is the first time you have had these symptoms, call your doctor at once. He or she will need to examine you to exclude other possible causes of your shortness of breath.

EMERGENCY! CALL AN AMBULANCE

POSSIBLE CAUSE Pulmonary embolism, in which a blood clot lodges in an artery in a lung, blocking the blood flow, is possible.

ACTION You will be admitted to hospital for tests such as a chest X-ray (p.37) and electrocardiography (p.199). The level of oxygen in your blood will probably be measured (see MEASURING BLOOD OXYGEN, opposite). If pulmonary embolism is diagnosed, you may be given anticoagulant drugs to dissolve the clot and to prevent further clots forming.

CALL YOUR DOCTOR NOW IF YOU ARE UNABLE TO MAKE A DIAGNOSIS FROM THIS CHART.

Continued from previous page

Do you cough up thick, greyish sputum on most days? — YES → **Do you work or have you worked in a dusty atmosphere – for example, in a mine or quarry?** — YES →

POSSIBLE CAUSE An occupational lung disease, such as pneumoconiosis, in which the lungs are progressively damaged by inhaled particles, may be the cause. Consult your doctor.

ACTION Your doctor will ask you about your current and past occupations. He or she will also arrange for a chest X-ray (p.37) and lung function tests to assess how well your lungs are working. If you smoke, you should stop. In severe cases, you may have to consider a change of employment.

NO ↓ (from cough question)

NO ↓ (from dusty atmosphere question)

POSSIBLE CAUSE Chronic obstructive pulmonary disease (COPD) is likely, especially if you smoke or have smoked in the past. In this condition, the airways become narrowed and produce excess mucus, and the air sacs in the lungs are damaged. Consult your doctor.

ACTION Although the damage is irreversible, your doctor may prescribe bronchodilator drugs to help relieve your symptoms. If you smoke, you must stop to prevent the condition from worsening.

SEE YOUR DOCTOR WITHIN 24 HOURS

POSSIBLE CAUSE A gradual accumulation of fluid in the lungs and in other tissues is probably the cause of your symptoms. This problem is most commonly due to heart failure (in which the heart fails to pump effectively), especially in people over 60 years of age. It can also result from a kidney or liver disorder.

ACTION Your doctor will examine you. Regardless of the underlying cause, he or she may prescribe drugs, including diuretics, which will help clear excess fluid. You will need other tests, including blood tests and electrocardiography (p.199), to establish the underlying cause and appropriate treatment.

Are your ankles swollen? — YES →

NO ↓

Does your work or hobby involve regular contact with grain or other crops and/or caged birds or animals? — YES →

POSSIBLE CAUSE A lung disorder known as extrinsic allergic alveolitis, in which the air sacs in the lungs become inflamed in response to certain inhaled substances, is a possibility. The disorder can sometimes cause a fever. Consult your doctor.

ACTION Your doctor will probably arrange for diagnostic tests, including a chest X-ray (p.37) and skin tests to look for sensitivity to different substances. If the diagnosis is confirmed, you will probably be advised to avoid further exposure to the substance causing the reaction. If this is not possible, you may have to consider changing your job or hobby. You may be given corticosteroid drugs to reduce the inflammation.

NO ↓

Have you noticed any of the following symptoms with the shortness of breath?
- Excessive tiredness
- Feeling faint or passing out
- Paler than normal skin

— YES →

SEE YOUR DOCTOR WITHIN 24 HOURS

POSSIBLE CAUSE You may have anaemia, in which there is too little of the oxygen-carrying pigment haemoglobin in the blood. Anaemia can result from a variety of underlying causes. Consult your doctor.

ACTION Your doctor will arrange for a blood test to confirm the diagnosis. In some cases, further tests will be necessary to determine why anaemia has developed. Treatment for anaemia will usually need to be combined with treatment of the underlying cause.

NO ↓

SEE YOUR DOCTOR WITHIN 24 HOURS IF YOU ARE UNABLE TO MAKE A DIAGNOSIS FROM THIS CHART.

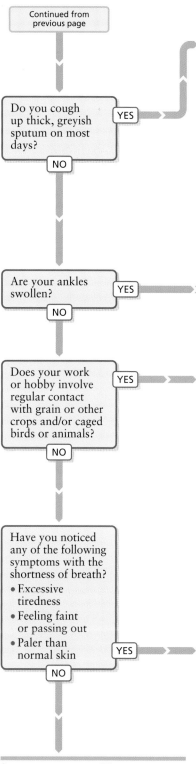

Measuring blood oxygen

Tests that measure the amount of oxygen in the blood show how efficiently the lungs are working and are used to help diagnose and monitor lung disorders such as pneumonia and pulmonary embolism. Blood oxygen levels can be measured by taking a blood sample from an artery, usually in the wrist. However, an easier and painless method is pulse oximetry, which indirectly measures the concentration of oxygen in blood in the tissues. The pulse oximeter is clipped over the fingertip and shines a light through the tissues. Changes in the amount of light absorbed by the tissues are detected and displayed on a monitor. Tissues containing oxygen-rich blood absorb more light than those in which the blood is low in oxygen.

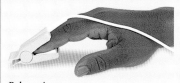

Pulse oximetry
The pulse oximeter is clipped over a fingertip. It shines light through the tissues of the finger and measures how much light is absorbed, which indicates the blood oxygen level.

93 Chest pain

Pain in the chest (anywhere between the neck and the bottom of the ribcage) may be alarming but usually does not have a serious cause. Most chest pain is due to minor disorders such as muscle strain or indigestion. Severe, crushing, central chest pain, or pain that is associated with breathlessness, an irregular heartbeat, nausea, sweating, or faintness, may be a sign of a serious disorder of the heart or lungs and may need emergency treatment.

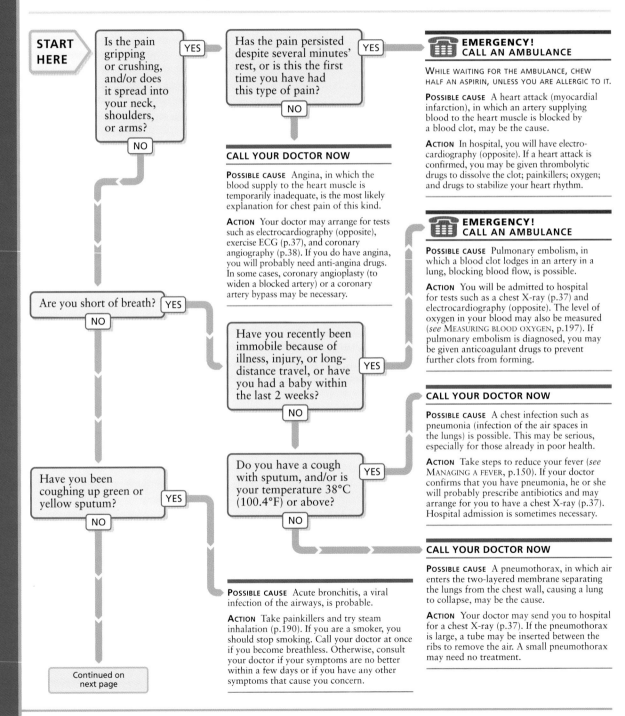

START HERE

Is the pain gripping or crushing, and/or does it spread into your neck, shoulders, or arms? — YES → **Has the pain persisted despite several minutes' rest, or is this the first time you have had this type of pain?** — YES →

EMERGENCY! CALL AN AMBULANCE

WHILE WAITING FOR THE AMBULANCE, CHEW HALF AN ASPIRIN, UNLESS YOU ARE ALLERGIC TO IT.

POSSIBLE CAUSE A heart attack (myocardial infarction), in which an artery supplying blood to the heart muscle is blocked by a blood clot, may be the cause.

ACTION In hospital, you will have electrocardiography (opposite). If a heart attack is confirmed, you may be given thrombolytic drugs to dissolve the clot; painkillers; oxygen; and drugs to stabilize your heart rhythm.

(Has the pain persisted...) — NO →

CALL YOUR DOCTOR NOW

POSSIBLE CAUSE Angina, in which the blood supply to the heart muscle is temporarily inadequate, is the most likely explanation for chest pain of this kind.

ACTION Your doctor may arrange for tests such as electrocardiography (opposite), exercise ECG (p.37), and coronary angiography (p.38). If you do have angina, you will probably need anti-angina drugs. In some cases, coronary angioplasty (to widen a blocked artery) or a coronary artery bypass may be necessary.

(Is the pain gripping...) — NO ↓

Are you short of breath? — YES →

Have you recently been immobile because of illness, injury, or long-distance travel, or have you had a baby within the last 2 weeks? — YES →

EMERGENCY! CALL AN AMBULANCE

POSSIBLE CAUSE Pulmonary embolism, in which a blood clot lodges in an artery in a lung, blocking blood flow, is possible.

ACTION You will be admitted to hospital for tests such as a chest X-ray (p.37) and electrocardiography (opposite). The level of oxygen in your blood may also be measured (*see* MEASURING BLOOD OXYGEN, p.197). If pulmonary embolism is diagnosed, you may be given anticoagulant drugs to prevent further clots from forming.

(Have you recently been immobile...) — NO ↓

Do you have a cough with sputum, and/or is your temperature 38°C (100.4°F) or above? — YES →

CALL YOUR DOCTOR NOW

POSSIBLE CAUSE A chest infection such as pneumonia (infection of the air spaces in the lungs) is possible. This may be serious, especially for those already in poor health.

ACTION Take steps to reduce your fever (*see* MANAGING A FEVER, p.150). If your doctor confirms that you have pneumonia, he or she will probably prescribe antibiotics and may arrange for you to have a chest X-ray (p.37). Hospital admission is sometimes necessary.

(Are you short of breath?) — NO ↓

Have you been coughing up green or yellow sputum? — YES →

(Do you have a cough...) — NO →

CALL YOUR DOCTOR NOW

POSSIBLE CAUSE A pneumothorax, in which air enters the two-layered membrane separating the lungs from the chest wall, causing a lung to collapse, may be the cause.

ACTION Your doctor may send you to hospital for a chest X-ray (p.37). If the pneumothorax is large, a tube may be inserted between the ribs to remove the air. A small pneumothorax may need no treatment.

(Have you been coughing up green or yellow sputum?) — NO ↓

POSSIBLE CAUSE Acute bronchitis, a viral infection of the airways, is probable.

ACTION Take painkillers and try steam inhalation (p.190). If you are a smoker, you should stop smoking. Call your doctor at once if you become breathless. Otherwise, consult your doctor if your symptoms are no better within a few days or if you have any other symptoms that cause you concern.

Continued on next page

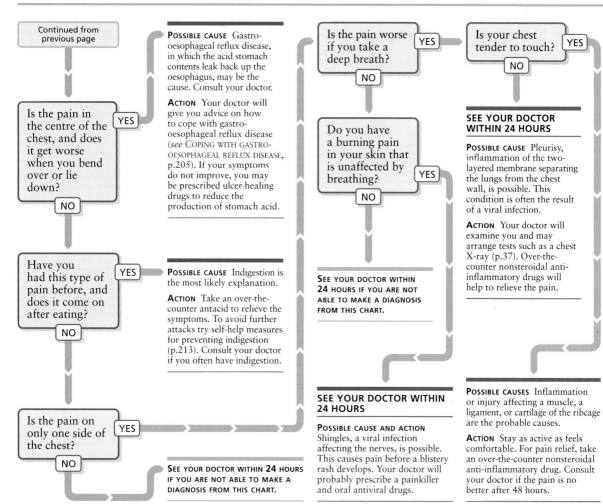

Continued from previous page

Is the pain in the centre of the chest, and does it get worse when you bend over or lie down?
NO / YES

YES → **POSSIBLE CAUSE** Gastro-oesophageal reflux disease, in which the acid stomach contents leak back up the oesophagus, may be the cause. Consult your doctor.

ACTION Your doctor will give you advice on how to cope with gastro-oesophageal reflux disease (*see* COPING WITH GASTRO-OESOPHAGEAL REFLUX DISEASE, p.205). If your symptoms do not improve, you may be prescribed ulcer-healing drugs to reduce the production of stomach acid.

Have you had this type of pain before, and does it come on after eating?
NO / YES

YES → **POSSIBLE CAUSE** Indigestion is the most likely explanation.

ACTION Take an over-the-counter antacid to relieve the symptoms. To avoid further attacks try self-help measures for preventing indigestion (p.213). Consult your doctor if you often have indigestion.

Is the pain on only one side of the chest?
NO / YES

SEE YOUR DOCTOR WITHIN 24 HOURS IF YOU ARE NOT ABLE TO MAKE A DIAGNOSIS FROM THIS CHART.

Is the pain worse if you take a deep breath?
NO / YES

Do you have a burning pain in your skin that is unaffected by breathing?
NO / YES

SEE YOUR DOCTOR WITHIN 24 HOURS IF YOU ARE NOT ABLE TO MAKE A DIAGNOSIS FROM THIS CHART.

SEE YOUR DOCTOR WITHIN 24 HOURS

POSSIBLE CAUSE AND ACTION Shingles, a viral infection affecting the nerves, is possible. This causes pain before a blistery rash develops. Your doctor will probably prescribe a painkiller and oral antiviral drugs.

Is your chest tender to touch?
NO / YES

SEE YOUR DOCTOR WITHIN 24 HOURS

POSSIBLE CAUSE Pleurisy, inflammation of the two-layered membrane separating the lungs from the chest wall, is possible. This condition is often the result of a viral infection.

ACTION Your doctor will examine you and may arrange tests such as a chest X-ray (p.37). Over-the-counter anti-inflammatory drugs will help to relieve the pain.

POSSIBLE CAUSES Inflammation or injury affecting a muscle, a ligament, or cartilage of the ribcage are the probable causes.

ACTION Stay as active as feels comfortable. For pain relief, take an over-the-counter nonsteroidal anti-inflammatory drug. Consult your doctor if the pain is no better after 48 hours.

Electrocardiography

Electrocardiography (ECG) is used to record the electrical activity produced by the heart as it beats. The procedure is frequently used to investigate the cause of chest pain and to diagnose abnormal heart rhythms. Electrodes are attached to the skin of the chest, wrists, and ankles and transmit the electrical activity of the heart to an ECG machine. This records the transmitted information as a trace on a moving graph paper or a screen. Each of the traces shows electrical activity in a different area of the heart. The test usually takes several minutes to complete, is safe, and causes no discomfort.

During the procedure
Small electrodes are attached to your chest, wrists, and ankles. Signals picked up by each electrode produces a trace.

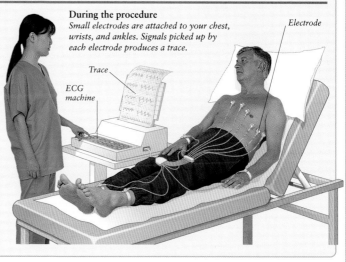

Electrode

Trace

ECG machine

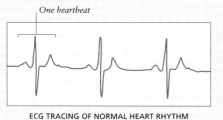

One heartbeat

ECG TRACING OF NORMAL HEART RHYTHM

94 Palpitations

Palpitations are an awareness of unusually rapid, strong, or irregular beating of the heart. It is normal for the heart rate to speed up during strenuous exercise, and you may feel your heart "thumping" for some minutes afterwards. This is usually no cause for concern. In most cases, palpitations that occur at rest are caused by the effect of drugs such as

caffeine or nicotine or may simply be due to anxiety. However, in a small proportion of people, palpitations that occur at rest are a symptom of an underlying illness. If you have recurrent palpitations that have no obvious cause or that are associated with chest pain or shortness of breath, you should always seek medical advice.

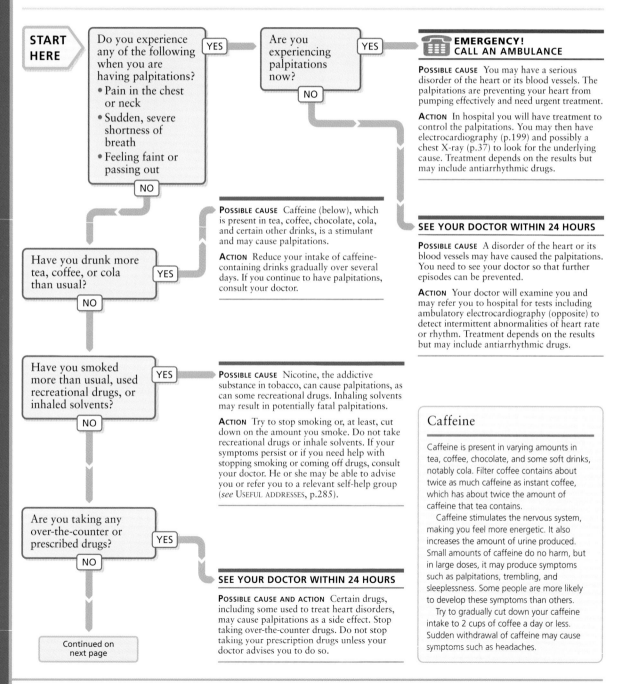

START HERE

Do you experience any of the following when you are having palpitations?
- Pain in the chest or neck
- Sudden, severe shortness of breath
- Feeling faint or passing out

YES →

Are you experiencing palpitations now?

YES →

EMERGENCY! CALL AN AMBULANCE

POSSIBLE CAUSE You may have a serious disorder of the heart or its blood vessels. The palpitations are preventing your heart from pumping effectively and need urgent treatment.

ACTION In hospital you will have treatment to control the palpitations. You may then have electrocardiography (p.199) and possibly a chest X-ray (p.37) to look for the underlying cause. Treatment depends on the results but may include antiarrhythmic drugs.

NO

SEE YOUR DOCTOR WITHIN 24 HOURS

POSSIBLE CAUSE A disorder of the heart or its blood vessels may have caused the palpitations. You need to see your doctor so that further episodes can be prevented.

ACTION Your doctor will examine you and may refer you to hospital for tests including ambulatory electrocardiography (opposite) to detect intermittent abnormalities of heart rate or rhythm. Treatment depends on the results but may include antiarrhythmic drugs.

NO

Have you drunk more tea, coffee, or cola than usual?

YES →

POSSIBLE CAUSE Caffeine (below), which is present in tea, coffee, chocolate, cola, and certain other drinks, is a stimulant and may cause palpitations.

ACTION Reduce your intake of caffeine-containing drinks gradually over several days. If you continue to have palpitations, consult your doctor.

NO

Have you smoked more than usual, used recreational drugs, or inhaled solvents?

YES →

POSSIBLE CAUSE Nicotine, the addictive substance in tobacco, can cause palpitations, as can some recreational drugs. Inhaling solvents may result in potentially fatal palpitations.

ACTION Try to stop smoking or, at least, cut down on the amount you smoke. Do not take recreational drugs or inhale solvents. If your symptoms persist or if you need help with stopping smoking or coming off drugs, consult your doctor. He or she may be able to advise you or refer you to a relevant self-help group (*see* USEFUL ADDRESSES, p.285).

NO

Caffeine

Caffeine is present in varying amounts in tea, coffee, chocolate, and some soft drinks, notably cola. Filter coffee contains about twice as much caffeine as instant coffee, which has about twice the amount of caffeine that tea contains.

Caffeine stimulates the nervous system, making you feel more energetic. It also increases the amount of urine produced. Small amounts of caffeine do no harm, but in large doses, it may produce symptoms such as palpitations, trembling, and sleeplessness. Some people are more likely to develop these symptoms than others.

Try to gradually cut down your caffeine intake to 2 cups of coffee a day or less. Sudden withdrawal of caffeine may cause symptoms such as headaches.

Are you taking any over-the-counter or prescribed drugs?

YES →

SEE YOUR DOCTOR WITHIN 24 HOURS

POSSIBLE CAUSE AND ACTION Certain drugs, including some used to treat heart disorders, may cause palpitations as a side effect. Stop taking over-the-counter drugs. Do not stop taking your prescription drugs unless your doctor advises you to do so.

NO

Continued on next page

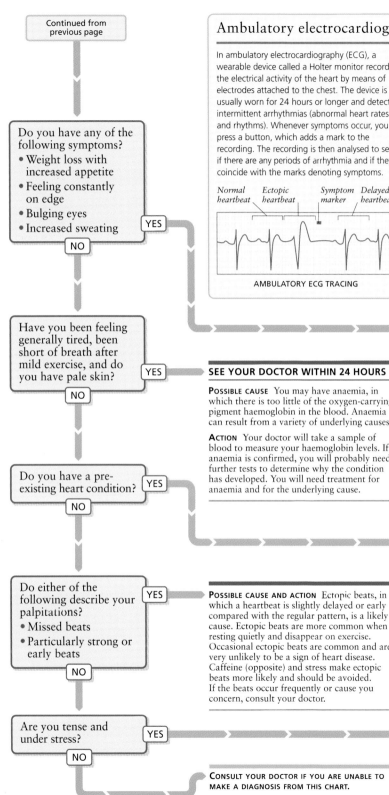

Continued from previous page

Do you have any of the following symptoms?
- Weight loss with increased appetite
- Feeling constantly on edge
- Bulging eyes
- Increased sweating

YES →

NO ↓

Have you been feeling generally tired, been short of breath after mild exercise, and do you have pale skin?

YES →

NO ↓

Do you have a pre-existing heart condition?

YES →

NO ↓

Do either of the following describe your palpitations?
- Missed beats
- Particularly strong or early beats

YES →

NO ↓

Are you tense and under stress?

YES →

NO ↓

Ambulatory electrocardiography

In ambulatory electrocardiography (ECG), a wearable device called a Holter monitor records the electrical activity of the heart by means of electrodes attached to the chest. The device is usually worn for 24 hours or longer and detects intermittent arrhythmias (abnormal heart rates and rhythms). Whenever symptoms occur, you press a button, which adds a mark to the recording. The recording is then analysed to see if there are any periods of arrhythmia and if they coincide with the marks denoting symptoms.

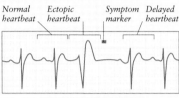

Normal heartbeat   Ectopic heartbeat   Symptom marker   Delayed heartbeat

AMBULATORY ECG TRACING

Shoulder strap

Electrode

Symptom marker button

Monitor

Using a Holter monitor
The device is worn under clothing. This trace (left) produced by the device shows an early abnormal beat (ectopic beat), which coincides with a symptom marker.

SEE YOUR DOCTOR WITHIN 24 HOURS

POSSIBLE CAUSE You may have anaemia, in which there is too little of the oxygen-carrying pigment haemoglobin in the blood. Anaemia can result from a variety of underlying causes.

ACTION Your doctor will take a sample of blood to measure your haemoglobin levels. If anaemia is confirmed, you will probably need further tests to determine why the condition has developed. You will need treatment for anaemia and for the underlying cause.

POSSIBLE CAUSE AND ACTION Ectopic beats, in which a heartbeat is slightly delayed or early compared with the regular pattern, is a likely cause. Ectopic beats are more common when resting quietly and disappear on exercise. Occasional ectopic beats are common and are very unlikely to be a sign of heart disease. Caffeine (opposite) and stress make ectopic beats more likely and should be avoided. If the beats occur frequently or cause you concern, consult your doctor.

CONSULT YOUR DOCTOR IF YOU ARE UNABLE TO MAKE A DIAGNOSIS FROM THIS CHART.

POSSIBLE CAUSE Hyperthyroidism (overactive thyroid gland) is a possible cause of these symptoms. Consult your doctor.

ACTION Your doctor will take a blood sample to measure levels of thyroid hormones. If the diagnosis is confirmed, you may be treated with antithyroid drugs or radioactive iodine. In some cases, surgery to remove part of the gland may be needed.

CALL YOUR DOCTOR NOW

POSSIBLE CAUSE The palpitations may indicate that your condition has worsened. Whatever the cause, the palpitations will put additional strain on your heart and require investigation.

ACTION Your doctor will arrange for you to have tests such as electrocardiography (p.199) and a chest X-ray (p.37). Treatment will depend on the results, but you may be prescribed antiarrhythmic drugs.

POSSIBLE CAUSE AND ACTION Anxiety can increase your awareness of your heartbeat, as well as increase the heart rate itself. Try to keep stress to a minimum and use relaxation techniques (p.32). If these measures do not help, consult your doctor.

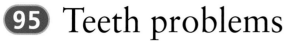 95 Teeth problems

For pain affecting other parts of the mouth, see chart 96, MOUTH PROBLEMS (p.204).

Teeth are at constant risk of decay because bacteria act on sugars in our diet to create acids that erode the surface of the teeth. If untreated, decay can spread to the centre of the teeth. The same conditions that cause decay can also cause gum

disorders and are often associated with poor dental hygiene (*see* CARING FOR YOUR TEETH AND GUMS, opposite). You should see your dentist every 6–12 months. If you have a heart valve disorder, tell your dentist; you will need to have antibiotics before dental treatment. Let your dentist know if you are pregnant so that any X-rays can be postponed.

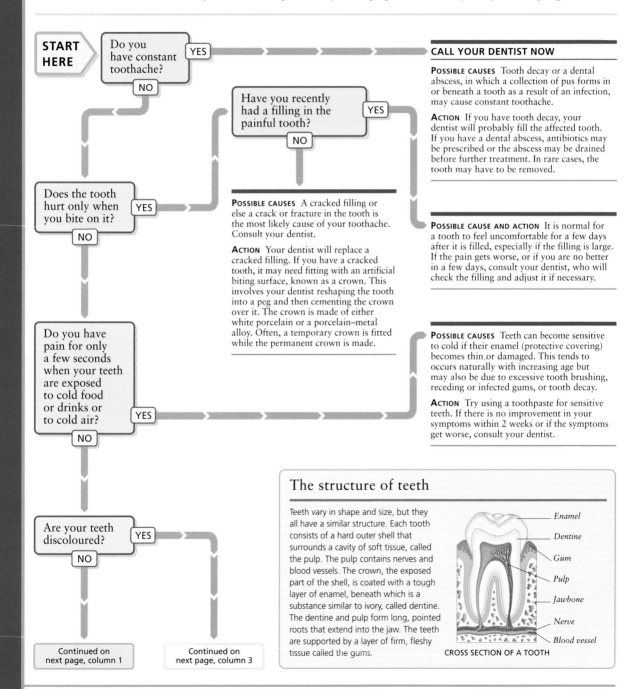

START HERE

Do you have constant toothache? — YES

CALL YOUR DENTIST NOW

POSSIBLE CAUSES Tooth decay or a dental abscess, in which a collection of pus forms in or beneath a tooth as a result of an infection, may cause constant toothache.

ACTION If you have tooth decay, your dentist will probably fill the affected tooth. If you have a dental abscess, antibiotics may be prescribed or the abscess may be drained before further treatment. In rare cases, the tooth may have to be removed.

NO

Have you recently had a filling in the painful tooth? — YES

NO

Does the tooth hurt only when you bite on it? — YES

NO

POSSIBLE CAUSES A cracked filling or else a crack or fracture in the tooth is the most likely cause of your toothache. Consult your dentist.

ACTION Your dentist will replace a cracked filling. If you have a cracked tooth, it may need fitting with an artificial biting surface, known as a crown. This involves your dentist reshaping the tooth into a peg and then cementing the crown over it. The crown is made of either white porcelain or a porcelain–metal alloy. Often, a temporary crown is fitted while the permanent crown is made.

POSSIBLE CAUSE AND ACTION It is normal for a tooth to feel uncomfortable for a few days after it is filled, especially if the filling is large. If the pain gets worse, or if you are no better in a few days, consult your dentist, who will check the filling and adjust it if necessary.

Do you have pain for only a few seconds when your teeth are exposed to cold food or drinks or to cold air? — YES

NO

POSSIBLE CAUSES Teeth can become sensitive to cold if their enamel (protective covering) becomes thin or damaged. This tends to occurs naturally with increasing age but may also be due to excessive tooth brushing, receding or infected gums, or tooth decay.

ACTION Try using a toothpaste for sensitive teeth. If there is no improvement in your symptoms within 2 weeks or if the symptoms get worse, consult your dentist.

Are your teeth discoloured? — YES

NO

The structure of teeth

Teeth vary in shape and size, but they all have a similar structure. Each tooth consists of a hard outer shell that surrounds a cavity of soft tissue, called the pulp. The pulp contains nerves and blood vessels. The crown, the exposed part of the shell, is coated with a tough layer of enamel, beneath which is a substance similar to ivory, called dentine. The dentine and pulp form long, pointed roots that extend into the jaw. The teeth are supported by a layer of firm, fleshy tissue called the gums.

Enamel
Dentine
Gum
Pulp
Jawbone
Nerve
Blood vessel

CROSS SECTION OF A TOOTH

Continued on next page, column 1

Continued on next page, column 3

SELF-HELP Caring for your teeth and gums

Daily care is vital to maintain dental health. You need to limit your intake of foods and drinks containing sugar because these contribute to tooth decay. You should also brush and floss your teeth regularly to prevent food particles from building up on your teeth and so reduce the risk of tooth decay and gum disease.

Brush your teeth at least twice a day, or, if possible, after every meal. Use a soft electric or manual toothbrush with a small head and a fluoride toothpaste. Brush for at least 2 minutes, cleaning all the surfaces of your teeth, especially where they meet the gum. Next, use dental floss or tape to clean between the teeth, removing food particles that a brush cannot reach.

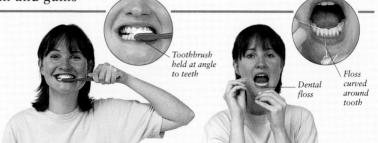

Toothbrush held at angle to teeth

Floss curved around tooth

Dental floss

Brushing your teeth
Brush your teeth in small circular motions, using a small-headed toothbrush held at an angle to the teeth. Make sure you clean each tooth.

Using dental floss
Keeping the floss taut, guide it between the teeth. Gently scrape the side of the tooth, working away from the gum.

Continued from previous page, column 1

Do you have pain or discomfort around one or more of your back teeth?
YES
NO

POSSIBLE CAUSE You may have a problem with one of your wisdom teeth, such as inflammation of the gum over an unerupted tooth. Consult your dentist.

ACTION Your dentist may take an X-ray of your mouth to look at the position of your wisdom teeth within the jaw. If a tooth is causing pain, it may need to be extracted, but most problems get better on their own.

Are your gums tender and/or bleeding?
YES
NO

POSSIBLE CAUSES You may have gingivitis, the most common type of gum disease. In this condition, the gums become inflamed, often as a result of poor oral hygiene. Rarely, painless bleeding from gums can be due to a blood disorder. Consult your dentist.

ACTION Your dentist will probably scale and polish your teeth and advise you on oral hygiene (*see* CARING FOR YOUR TEETH AND GUMS, above). If your symptoms are severe, you may be prescribed antibiotics. You may need blood tests if gingivitis is not the cause.

Does your jaw ache when you wake up in the mornings, or do you grind your teeth at night?
YES
NO

POSSIBLE CAUSE AND ACTION It is quite common for people to grind their teeth during sleep, particularly if they are stressed or anxious. Prolonged grinding can damage the teeth, causing cracks to develop or wearing away the surface. Consult your dentist, who may provide you with a mouth guard to protect your teeth while you sleep.

CONSULT YOUR DENTIST IF YOU ARE UNABLE TO MAKE A DIAGNOSIS FROM THIS CHART.

Continued from previous page, column 2

Is the discoloration in discrete patches?
YES
NO

POSSIBLE CAUSE Teeth may be stained by smoking or drinking tea or coffee. Poor oral hygiene can also cause discoloration.

ACTION Stop smoking and cut down your intake of tea and coffee. Brush and floss your teeth regularly (*see* CARING FOR YOUR TEETH AND GUMS, above). If these measures do not help, consult your dentist or oral hygienist, who will scale and polish your teeth.

POSSIBLE CAUSES Discoloration can occur if certain drugs are given to children while their teeth are developing. Excessive fluoride intake, possibly due to too high a dose of fluoride tablets or drops, may also cause patchy discoloration. Consult your dentist.

ACTION Your dentist may recommend a cosmetic coating that can be bonded to the front of the affected teeth.

96 Mouth problems

For problems with the skin around the mouth, see chart 78,
SKIN PROBLEMS AFFECTING THE FACE (p.176).
A sore mouth or tongue is most commonly due to a minor
injury. For example, biting your tongue or cheek may cause
a painful area. Such injuries should heal within a week.
Minor infections are another relatively common cause of

soreness in the mouth. Occasionally, a widespread skin
condition or an intestinal disorder such as Crohn's disease
may also affect the mouth, causing sore areas to develop. It
is important that you keep your mouth and gums healthy by
maintaining good oral hygiene (*see* CARING FOR YOUR TEETH
AND GUMS, p.203) and having regular dental check-ups.

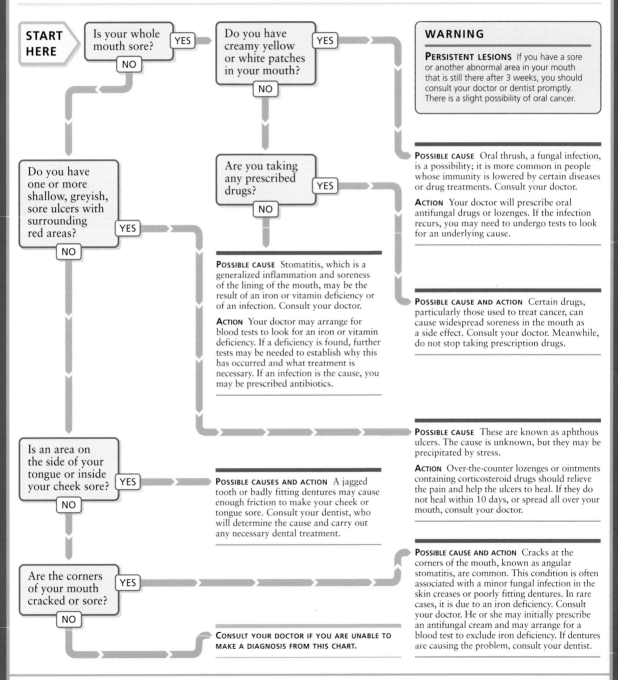

START HERE

Is your whole mouth sore? — YES → **Do you have creamy yellow or white patches in your mouth?** — YES →
NO / NO

WARNING

PERSISTENT LESIONS If you have a sore
or another abnormal area in your mouth
that is still there after 3 weeks, you should
consult your doctor or dentist promptly.
There is a slight possibility of oral cancer.

Do you have one or more shallow, greyish, sore ulcers with surrounding red areas? — YES
NO

Are you taking any prescribed drugs? — YES
NO

POSSIBLE CAUSE Oral thrush, a fungal infection,
is a possibility; it is more common in people
whose immunity is lowered by certain diseases
or drug treatments. Consult your doctor.

ACTION Your doctor will prescribe oral
antifungal drugs or lozenges. If the infection
recurs, you may need to undergo tests to look
for an underlying cause.

POSSIBLE CAUSE Stomatitis, which is a
generalized inflammation and soreness
of the lining of the mouth, may be the
result of an iron or vitamin deficiency or
of an infection. Consult your doctor.

ACTION Your doctor may arrange for
blood tests to look for an iron or vitamin
deficiency. If a deficiency is found, further
tests may be needed to establish why this
has occurred and what treatment is
necessary. If an infection is the cause, you
may be prescribed antibiotics.

POSSIBLE CAUSE AND ACTION Certain drugs,
particularly those used to treat cancer, can
cause widespread soreness in the mouth as
a side effect. Consult your doctor. Meanwhile,
do not stop taking prescription drugs.

Is an area on the side of your tongue or inside your cheek sore? — YES
NO

POSSIBLE CAUSES AND ACTION A jagged
tooth or badly fitting dentures may cause
enough friction to make your cheek or
tongue sore. Consult your dentist, who
will determine the cause and carry out
any necessary dental treatment.

POSSIBLE CAUSE These are known as aphthous
ulcers. The cause is unknown, but they may be
precipitated by stress.

ACTION Over-the-counter lozenges or ointments
containing corticosteroid drugs should relieve
the pain and help the ulcers to heal. If they do
not heal within 10 days, or spread all over your
mouth, consult your doctor.

Are the corners of your mouth cracked or sore? — YES
NO

**CONSULT YOUR DOCTOR IF YOU ARE UNABLE TO
MAKE A DIAGNOSIS FROM THIS CHART.**

POSSIBLE CAUSE AND ACTION Cracks at the
corners of the mouth, known as angular
stomatitis, are common. This condition is often
associated with a minor fungal infection in the
skin creases or poorly fitting dentures. In rare
cases, it is due to an iron deficiency. Consult
your doctor. He or she may initially prescribe
an antifungal cream and may arrange for a
blood test to exclude iron deficiency. If dentures
are causing the problem, consult your dentist.

97 Difficulty in swallowing

Difficulty in swallowing is most often due to a sore throat caused by an infection and usually clears up within a few days. However, difficulty in swallowing or pain that is not related to a sore throat may be due to a disorder of the oesophagus, the tube that leads from the throat to the stomach. In this case, you should seek medical advice.

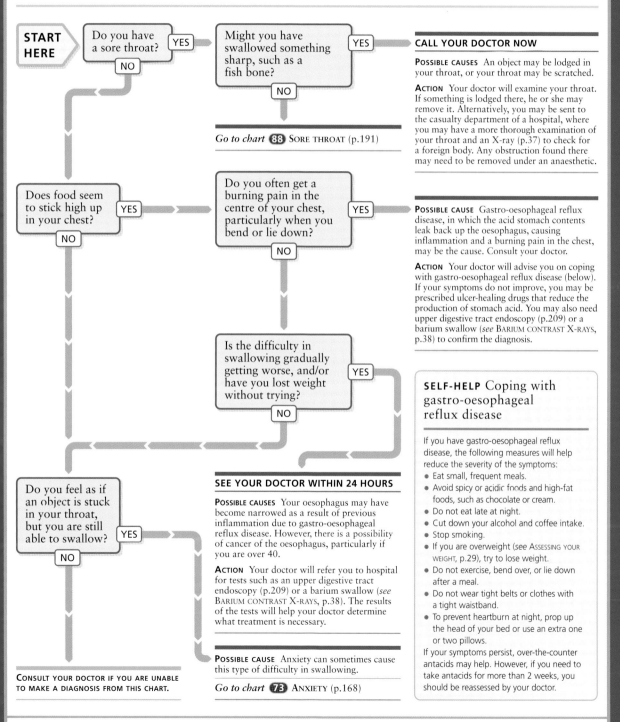

START HERE → **Do you have a sore throat?** — YES → **Might you have swallowed something sharp, such as a fish bone?** — YES →

Do you have a sore throat? — NO ↓

Might you have swallowed something sharp, such as a fish bone? — NO ↓
Go to chart **88** SORE THROAT (p.191)

Does food seem to stick high up in your chest? — YES → **Do you often get a burning pain in the centre of your chest, particularly when you bend or lie down?** — YES →

Does food seem to stick high up in your chest? — NO ↓

Do you often get a burning pain in the centre of your chest, particularly when you bend or lie down? — NO ↓

Is the difficulty in swallowing gradually getting worse, and/or have you lost weight without trying? — YES →

Is the difficulty in swallowing gradually getting worse, and/or have you lost weight without trying? — NO ↓

Do you feel as if an object is stuck in your throat, but you are still able to swallow? — YES →

Do you feel as if an object is stuck in your throat, but you are still able to swallow? — NO ↓

CONSULT YOUR DOCTOR IF YOU ARE UNABLE TO MAKE A DIAGNOSIS FROM THIS CHART.

CALL YOUR DOCTOR NOW

POSSIBLE CAUSES An object may be lodged in your throat, or your throat may be scratched.

ACTION Your doctor will examine your throat. If something is lodged there, he or she may remove it. Alternatively, you may be sent to the casualty department of a hospital, where you may have a more thorough examination of your throat and an X-ray (p.37) to check for a foreign body. Any obstruction found there may need to be removed under an anaesthetic.

POSSIBLE CAUSE Gastro-oesophageal reflux disease, in which the acid stomach contents leak back up the oesophagus, causing inflammation and a burning pain in the chest, may be the cause. Consult your doctor.

ACTION Your doctor will advise you on coping with gastro-oesophageal reflux disease (below). If your symptoms do not improve, you may be prescribed ulcer-healing drugs that reduce the production of stomach acid. You may also need upper digestive tract endoscopy (p.209) or a barium swallow (*see* BARIUM CONTRAST X-RAYS, p.38) to confirm the diagnosis.

SELF-HELP Coping with gastro-oesophageal reflux disease

If you have gastro-oesophageal reflux disease, the following measures will help reduce the severity of the symptoms:
- Eat small, frequent meals.
- Avoid spicy or acidic foods and high-fat foods, such as chocolate or cream.
- Do not eat late at night.
- Cut down your alcohol and coffee intake.
- Stop smoking.
- If you are overweight (*see* ASSESSING YOUR WEIGHT, p.29), try to lose weight.
- Do not exercise, bend over, or lie down after a meal.
- Do not wear tight belts or clothes with a tight waistband.
- To prevent heartburn at night, prop up the head of your bed or use an extra one or two pillows.

If your symptoms persist, over-the-counter antacids may help. However, if you need to take antacids for more than 2 weeks, you should be reassessed by your doctor.

SEE YOUR DOCTOR WITHIN 24 HOURS

POSSIBLE CAUSES Your oesophagus may have become narrowed as a result of previous inflammation due to gastro-oesophageal reflux disease. However, there is a possibility of cancer of the oesophagus, particularly if you are over 40.

ACTION Your doctor will refer you to hospital for tests such as an upper digestive tract endoscopy (p.209) or a barium swallow (*see* BARIUM CONTRAST X-RAYS, p.38). The results of the tests will help your doctor determine what treatment is necessary.

POSSIBLE CAUSE Anxiety can sometimes cause this type of difficulty in swallowing.

Go to chart **73** ANXIETY (p.168)

98 Vomiting

Vomiting is often the result of irritation of the stomach from infection or over-indulgence in rich food or alcohol, but it may also follow a disturbance elsewhere in the digestive tract. Occasionally, a disorder affecting the nerve signals from the brain or from the balance mechanism in the inner ear can produce vomiting. People who have recurrent migraine attacks recognize the familiar symptoms of headache with nausea and/or vomiting, but in other cases of vomiting accompanied by severe headache or when vomiting occurs with acute abdominal pain, urgent medical attention is needed.

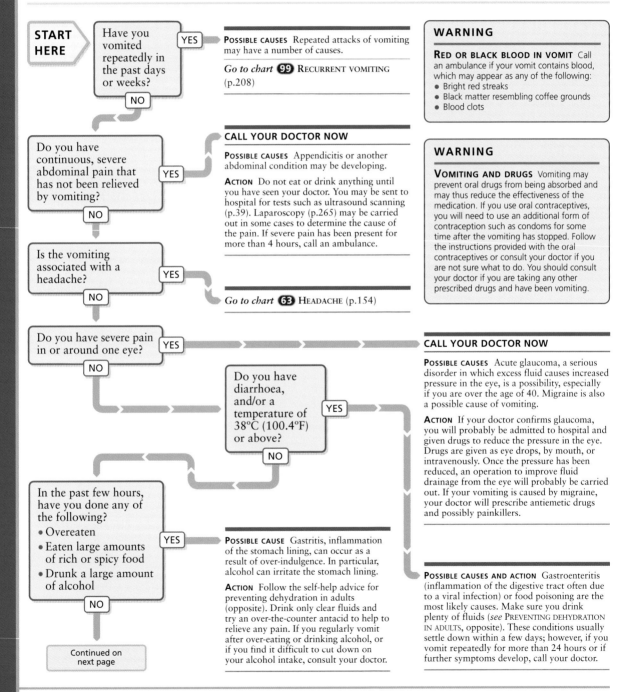

START HERE

Have you vomited repeatedly in the past days or weeks? — YES →

POSSIBLE CAUSES Repeated attacks of vomiting may have a number of causes.

Go to chart **99** RECURRENT VOMITING (p.208)

NO ↓

Do you have continuous, severe abdominal pain that has not been relieved by vomiting? — YES →

CALL YOUR DOCTOR NOW

POSSIBLE CAUSES Appendicitis or another abdominal condition may be developing.

ACTION Do not eat or drink anything until you have seen your doctor. You may be sent to hospital for tests such as ultrasound scanning (p.39). Laparoscopy (p.265) may be carried out in some cases to determine the cause of the pain. If severe pain has been present for more than 4 hours, call an ambulance.

NO ↓

Is the vomiting associated with a headache? — YES →

Go to chart **63** HEADACHE (p.154)

NO ↓

Do you have severe pain in or around one eye? — YES →

NO ↓

Do you have diarrhoea, and/or a temperature of 38°C (100.4°F) or above? — YES →

NO ↓

In the past few hours, have you done any of the following?
- Overeaten
- Eaten large amounts of rich or spicy food
- Drunk a large amount of alcohol

— YES →

POSSIBLE CAUSE Gastritis, inflammation of the stomach lining, can occur as a result of over-indulgence. In particular, alcohol can irritate the stomach lining.

ACTION Follow the self-help advice for preventing dehydration in adults (opposite). Drink only clear fluids and try an over-the-counter antacid to help to relieve any pain. If you regularly vomit after over-eating or drinking alcohol, or if you find it difficult to cut down on your alcohol intake, consult your doctor.

NO ↓

Continued on next page

WARNING

RED OR BLACK BLOOD IN VOMIT Call an ambulance if your vomit contains blood, which may appear as any of the following:
- Bright red streaks
- Black matter resembling coffee grounds
- Blood clots

WARNING

VOMITING AND DRUGS Vomiting may prevent oral drugs from being absorbed and may thus reduce the effectiveness of the medication. If you use oral contraceptives, you will need to use an additional form of contraception such as condoms for some time after the vomiting has stopped. Follow the instructions provided with the oral contraceptives or consult your doctor if you are not sure what to do. You should consult your doctor if you are taking any other prescribed drugs and have been vomiting.

CALL YOUR DOCTOR NOW

POSSIBLE CAUSES Acute glaucoma, a serious disorder in which excess fluid causes increased pressure in the eye, is a possibility, especially if you are over the age of 40. Migraine is also a possible cause of vomiting.

ACTION If your doctor confirms glaucoma, you will probably be admitted to hospital and given drugs to reduce the pressure in the eye. Drugs are given as eye drops, by mouth, or intravenously. Once the pressure has been reduced, an operation to improve fluid drainage from the eye will probably be carried out. If your vomiting is caused by migraine, your doctor will prescribe antiemetic drugs and possibly painkillers.

POSSIBLE CAUSES AND ACTION Gastroenteritis (inflammation of the digestive tract often due to a viral infection) or food poisoning are the most likely causes. Make sure you drink plenty of fluids (*see* PREVENTING DEHYDRATION IN ADULTS, opposite). These conditions usually settle down within a few days; however, if you vomit repeatedly for more than 24 hours or if further symptoms develop, call your doctor.

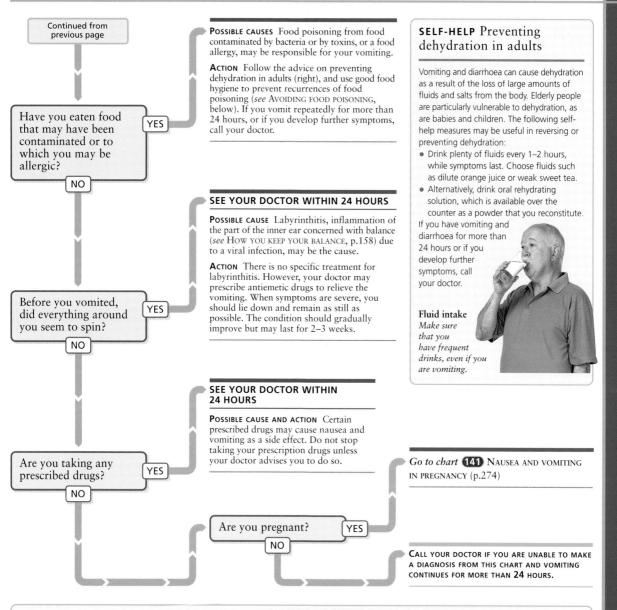

Continued from previous page

Have you eaten food that may have been contaminated or to which you may be allergic?

YES

NO

POSSIBLE CAUSES Food poisoning from food contaminated by bacteria or by toxins, or a food allergy, may be responsible for your vomiting.

ACTION Follow the advice on preventing dehydration in adults (right), and use good food hygiene to prevent recurrences of food poisoning (*see* AVOIDING FOOD POISONING, below). If you vomit repeatedly for more than 24 hours, or if you develop further symptoms, call your doctor.

SEE YOUR DOCTOR WITHIN 24 HOURS

POSSIBLE CAUSE Labyrinthitis, inflammation of the part of the inner ear concerned with balance (*see* HOW YOU KEEP YOUR BALANCE, p.158) due to a viral infection, may be the cause.

ACTION There is no specific treatment for labyrinthitis. However, your doctor may prescribe antiemetic drugs to relieve the vomiting. When symptoms are severe, you should lie down and remain as still as possible. The condition should gradually improve but may last for 2–3 weeks.

Before you vomited, did everything around you seem to spin?

YES

NO

SEE YOUR DOCTOR WITHIN 24 HOURS

POSSIBLE CAUSE AND ACTION Certain prescribed drugs may cause nausea and vomiting as a side effect. Do not stop taking your prescription drugs unless your doctor advises you to do so.

Are you taking any prescribed drugs?

YES

NO

Are you pregnant?

YES

NO

Go to chart **141** NAUSEA AND VOMITING IN PREGNANCY (p.274)

CALL YOUR DOCTOR IF YOU ARE UNABLE TO MAKE A DIAGNOSIS FROM THIS CHART AND VOMITING CONTINUES FOR MORE THAN 24 HOURS.

SELF-HELP Preventing dehydration in adults

Vomiting and diarrhoea can cause dehydration as a result of the loss of large amounts of fluids and salts from the body. Elderly people are particularly vulnerable to dehydration, as are babies and children. The following self-help measures may be useful in reversing or preventing dehydration:

- Drink plenty of fluids every 1–2 hours, while symptoms last. Choose fluids such as dilute orange juice or weak sweet tea.
- Alternatively, drink oral rehydrating solution, which is available over the counter as a powder that you reconstitute.

If you have vomiting and diarrhoea for more than 24 hours or if you develop further symptoms, call your doctor.

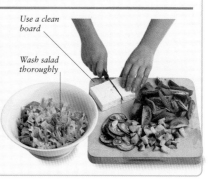

Fluid intake
Make sure that you have frequent drinks, even if you are vomiting.

SELF-HELP Avoiding food poisoning

Food poisoning is usually caused by eating food contaminated with bacteria or toxins and may be avoided by taking the following measures:

- Regularly clean work surfaces with disinfectant and hot water.
- Wash your hands thoroughly before and after handling food.
- Use separate chopping boards for raw meat, cooked meat, and vegetables, and clean each board thoroughly after use.
- Make sure the refrigerator is set at the recommended temperature.
- Always use food by the expiry date.

- Put chilled food in the refrigerator as soon as possible after purchase.
- Store raw meat and fish away from other foods inside the refrigerator.
- Once left-over food has cooled, cover or wrap it properly and store it in the refrigerator.
- Defrost frozen food before cooking it, and never refreeze thawed food.

Safe food preparation
Always wash fresh fruit and vegetables before preparing them. Chopping boards should be washed in hot soapy water after use.

Use a clean board

Wash salad thoroughly

99 Recurrent vomiting

For isolated attacks of vomiting, see chart 98, VOMITING (p.206). For vomiting during pregnancy, see chart 141, NAUSEA AND VOMITING IN PREGNANCY (p.274). Consult this chart if you have vomited or felt nauseated repeatedly over a number of days or weeks. Recurrent

vomiting can be caused by inflammation of the stomach lining or by an ulcer. Lifestyle factors such as irregular meals or excess alcohol can make the symptoms worse. Recurrent vomiting associated with weight loss or abdominal pain may have a serious cause, and you should consult your doctor.

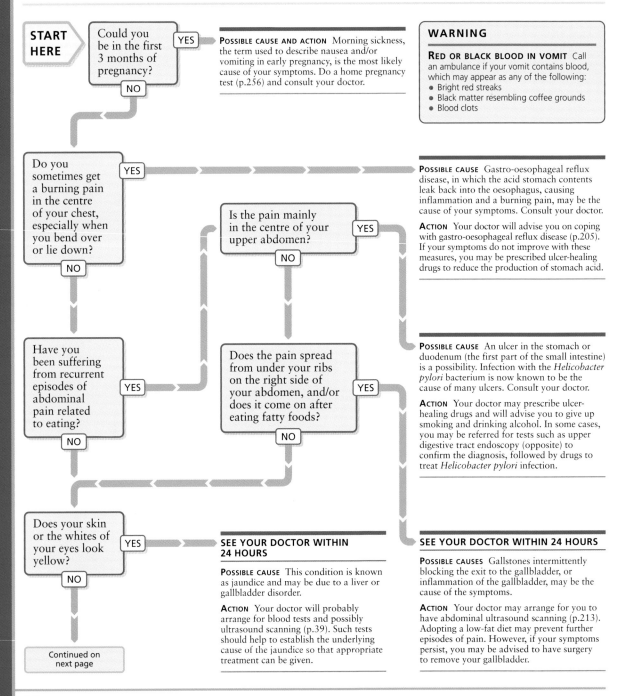

START HERE

Could you be in the first 3 months of pregnancy? YES → **POSSIBLE CAUSE AND ACTION** Morning sickness, the term used to describe nausea and/or vomiting in early pregnancy, is the most likely cause of your symptoms. Do a home pregnancy test (p.256) and consult your doctor.

NO

WARNING

RED OR BLACK BLOOD IN VOMIT Call an ambulance if your vomit contains blood, which may appear as any of the following:
● Bright red streaks
● Black matter resembling coffee grounds
● Blood clots

Do you sometimes get a burning pain in the centre of your chest, especially when you bend over or lie down? YES →

NO

Is the pain mainly in the centre of your upper abdomen? YES →

NO

POSSIBLE CAUSE Gastro-oesophageal reflux disease, in which the acid stomach contents leak back into the oesophagus, causing inflammation and a burning pain, may be the cause of your symptoms. Consult your doctor.

ACTION Your doctor will advise you on coping with gastro-oesophageal reflux disease (p.205). If your symptoms do not improve with these measures, you may be prescribed ulcer-healing drugs to reduce the production of stomach acid.

Have you been suffering from recurrent episodes of abdominal pain related to eating? YES →

NO

Does the pain spread from under your ribs on the right side of your abdomen, and/or does it come on after eating fatty foods? YES →

NO

POSSIBLE CAUSE An ulcer in the stomach or duodenum (the first part of the small intestine) is a possibility. Infection with the *Helicobacter pylori* bacterium is now known to be the cause of many ulcers. Consult your doctor.

ACTION Your doctor may prescribe ulcer-healing drugs and will advise you to give up smoking and drinking alcohol. In some cases, you may be referred for tests such as upper digestive tract endoscopy (opposite) to confirm the diagnosis, followed by drugs to treat *Helicobacter pylori* infection.

Does your skin or the whites of your eyes look yellow? YES →

NO

SEE YOUR DOCTOR WITHIN 24 HOURS

POSSIBLE CAUSE This condition is known as jaundice and may be due to a liver or gallbladder disorder.

ACTION Your doctor will probably arrange for blood tests and possibly ultrasound scanning (p.39). Such tests should help to establish the underlying cause of the jaundice so that appropriate treatment can be given.

SEE YOUR DOCTOR WITHIN 24 HOURS

POSSIBLE CAUSES Gallstones intermittently blocking the exit to the gallbladder, or inflammation of the gallbladder, may be the cause of the symptoms.

ACTION Your doctor may arrange for you to have abdominal ultrasound scanning (p.213). Adopting a low-fat diet may prevent further episodes of pain. However, if your symptoms persist, you may be advised to have surgery to remove your gallbladder.

Continued on next page

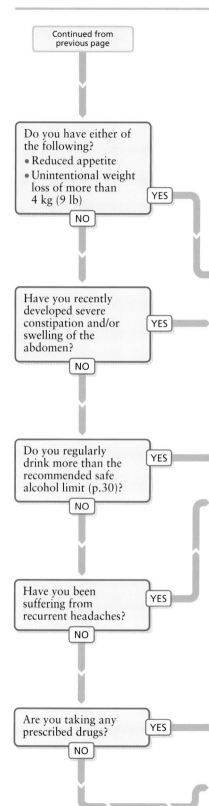

Continued from previous page

Do you have either of the following?
- Reduced appetite
- Unintentional weight loss of more than 4 kg (9 lb)

YES

NO

Have you recently developed severe constipation and/or swelling of the abdomen?

YES

NO

Do you regularly drink more than the recommended safe alcohol limit (p.30)?

YES

NO

Have you been suffering from recurrent headaches?

YES

NO

Are you taking any prescribed drugs?

YES

NO

Upper digestive tract endoscopy

Endoscopy of the upper digestive tract involves passing a flexible viewing tube through the mouth to examine the inside of the oesophagus, stomach, and duodenum (first part of the small intestine) to look for disorders such as ulcers. Your throat may be sprayed with a local anaesthetic and/or you may be sedated. The procedure usually takes around 15 minutes. Samples for analysis can be taken during the procedure.

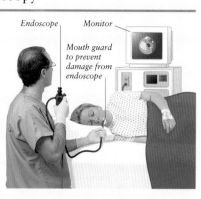

Endoscope   Monitor

Mouth guard to prevent damage from endoscope

Viewing the digestive tract
The doctor can inspect the lining of the digestive tract, which is displayed on the monitor as the endoscope is moved around.

CALL YOUR DOCTOR NOW

POSSIBLE CAUSE A blockage in the intestine could be the cause of your symptoms.

ACTION Your doctor will examine you and may send you to hospital for tests such as X-rays (p.37). If the vomiting is severe, you may be given fluids intravenously instead of by mouth. In some cases, surgery may be needed to relieve the blockage.

SEE YOUR DOCTOR WITHIN 24 HOURS

POSSIBLE CAUSE A condition that causes increased pressure on the brain, such as a tumour, may be the cause. However, such conditions are rare, and recurrent attacks of vomiting associated with headaches are more likely to be due to migraine.

ACTION If you have not previously been diagnosed as having migraine, your doctor will examine you to exclude other causes. He or she may also refer you to hospital for MRI scanning (p.39) of the brain. If migraine is the cause of your symptoms, follow the advice on relieving a headache (p.155) and reducing the frequency of migraine (p.155).

CONSULT YOUR DOCTOR IF YOU ARE UNABLE TO MAKE A DIAGNOSIS FROM THIS CHART.

SEE YOUR DOCTOR WITHIN 24 HOURS

POSSIBLE CAUSES An ulcer in the stomach or duodenum (the first part of the small intestine) is the most likely cause of your symptoms, but there is a slight possibility of stomach cancer.

ACTION Your doctor will probably arrange for you to have upper digestive tract endoscopy (above). Ulcers are usually treated with a course of antibiotics to kill the *Helicobacter pylori* bacteria that are responsible for the majority of these ulcers. Stomach cancer usually needs to be treated surgically.

POSSIBLE CAUSE Chronic gastritis (persistent inflammation of the stomach lining) is a possibility. This disorder is aggravated by excessive alcohol intake. Consult your doctor.

ACTION Your doctor will advise you to cut down your alcohol intake to within the recommended limits. He or she may also prescribe antacids. Eat small, regular meals and, if you smoke, stop. If your symptoms persist, your doctor may refer you for upper digestive tract endoscopy (above).

SEE YOUR DOCTOR WITHIN 24 HOURS

POSSIBLE CAUSE AND ACTION Certain drugs can cause recurrent vomiting as a side effect. Do not stop taking your prescribed drugs without your doctor's advice. Remember that vomiting can reduce the effectiveness of certain drugs (*see* VOMITING AND DRUGS, p.206).

100 Abdominal pain

Many cases of abdominal pain are short-lived and are due simply to eating or drinking too much or too quickly. However, pain in the abdomen may also be due to a disorder affecting the digestive system, urinary system, or, in women, the reproductive system. Any abdominal pain that is severe or persistent should receive prompt medical attention.

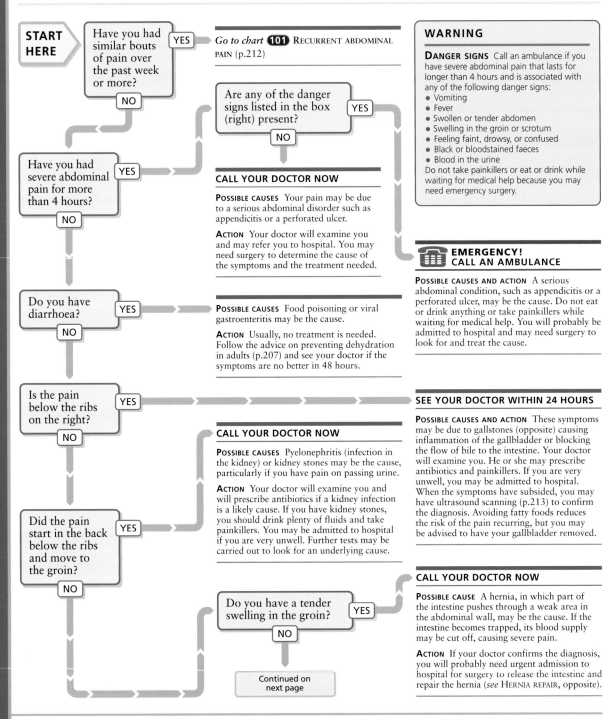

START HERE → Have you had similar bouts of pain over the past week or more?

YES → *Go to chart* **101** RECURRENT ABDOMINAL PAIN (p.212)

NO ↓

Have you had severe abdominal pain for more than 4 hours?

NO ↓

Do you have diarrhoea?

NO ↓

Is the pain below the ribs on the right?

NO ↓

Did the pain start in the back below the ribs and move to the groin?

NO ↓

Are any of the danger signs listed in the box (right) present?

YES →

NO ↓

CALL YOUR DOCTOR NOW

POSSIBLE CAUSES Your pain may be due to a serious abdominal disorder such as appendicitis or a perforated ulcer.

ACTION Your doctor will examine you and may refer you to hospital. You may need surgery to determine the cause of the symptoms and the treatment needed.

(Have you had severe abdominal pain for more than 4 hours?) **YES** →

(Do you have diarrhoea?) **YES** →

POSSIBLE CAUSES Food poisoning or viral gastroenteritis may be the cause.

ACTION Usually, no treatment is needed. Follow the advice on preventing dehydration in adults (p.207) and see your doctor if the symptoms are no better in 48 hours.

(Is the pain below the ribs on the right?) **YES** →

CALL YOUR DOCTOR NOW

POSSIBLE CAUSES Pyelonephritis (infection in the kidney) or kidney stones may be the cause, particularly if you have pain on passing urine.

ACTION Your doctor will examine you and will prescribe antibiotics if a kidney infection is a likely cause. If you have kidney stones, you should drink plenty of fluids and take painkillers. You may be admitted to hospital if you are very unwell. Further tests may be carried out to look for an underlying cause.

(Did the pain start in the back below the ribs and move to the groin?) **YES** →

Do you have a tender swelling in the groin?

YES →

NO ↓

Continued on next page

WARNING

DANGER SIGNS Call an ambulance if you have severe abdominal pain that lasts for longer than 4 hours and is associated with any of the following danger signs:
- Vomiting
- Fever
- Swollen or tender abdomen
- Swelling in the groin or scrotum
- Feeling faint, drowsy, or confused
- Black or bloodstained faeces
- Blood in the urine

Do not take painkillers or eat or drink while waiting for medical help because you may need emergency surgery.

☎ EMERGENCY! CALL AN AMBULANCE

POSSIBLE CAUSES AND ACTION A serious abdominal condition, such as appendicitis or a perforated ulcer, may be the cause. Do not eat or drink anything or take painkillers while waiting for medical help. You will probably be admitted to hospital and may need surgery to look for and treat the cause.

SEE YOUR DOCTOR WITHIN 24 HOURS

POSSIBLE CAUSES AND ACTION These symptoms may be due to gallstones (opposite) causing inflammation of the gallbladder or blocking the flow of bile to the intestine. Your doctor will examine you. He or she may prescribe antibiotics and painkillers. If you are very unwell, you may be admitted to hospital. When the symptoms have subsided, you may have ultrasound scanning (p.213) to confirm the diagnosis. Avoiding fatty foods reduces the risk of the pain recurring, but you may be advised to have your gallbladder removed.

CALL YOUR DOCTOR NOW

POSSIBLE CAUSE A hernia, in which part of the intestine pushes through a weak area in the abdominal wall, may be the cause. If the intestine becomes trapped, its blood supply may be cut off, causing severe pain.

ACTION If your doctor confirms the diagnosis, you will probably need urgent admission to hospital for surgery to release the intestine and repair the hernia (*see* HERNIA REPAIR, opposite).

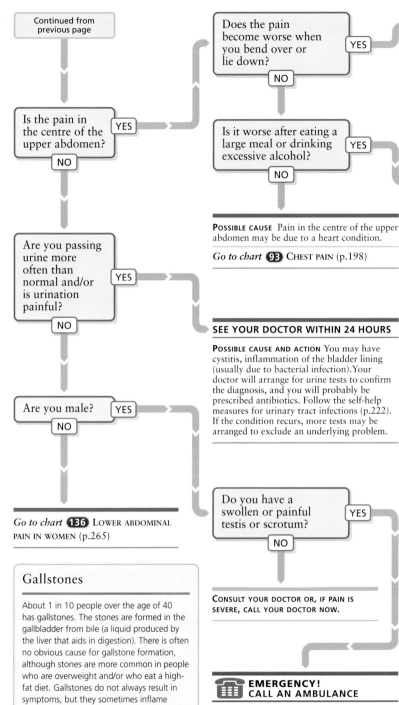

Continued from previous page

Is the pain in the centre of the upper abdomen? — YES

NO

Are you passing urine more often than normal and/or is urination painful? — YES

NO

Are you male? — YES

NO

Go to chart **136** LOWER ABDOMINAL PAIN IN WOMEN (p.265)

Does the pain become worse when you bend over or lie down? — YES

NO

Is it worse after eating a large meal or drinking excessive alcohol? — YES

NO

POSSIBLE CAUSE Pain in the centre of the upper abdomen may be due to a heart condition.

Go to chart **93** CHEST PAIN (p.198)

SEE YOUR DOCTOR WITHIN 24 HOURS

POSSIBLE CAUSE AND ACTION You may have cystitis, inflammation of the bladder lining (usually due to bacterial infection). Your doctor will arrange for urine tests to confirm the diagnosis, and you will probably be prescribed antibiotics. Follow the self-help measures for urinary tract infections (p.222). If the condition recurs, more tests may be arranged to exclude an underlying problem.

Do you have a swollen or painful testis or scrotum? — YES

NO

CONSULT YOUR DOCTOR OR, IF PAIN IS SEVERE, CALL YOUR DOCTOR NOW.

EMERGENCY! CALL AN AMBULANCE

POSSIBLE CAUSE AND ACTION You may have torsion of the testis (p.127), in which a testis is twisted in the scrotum, cutting off the blood supply. This can cause pain in the abdomen as well as in the scrotum. Torsion requires urgent surgery to untwist the testis and restore blood flow. Both testes are then stitched to the inside of the scrotum to prevent a recurrence.

POSSIBLE CAUSE Gastro-oesophageal reflux disease, in which the acid stomach contents leak back up the oesophagus, may be the cause. This condition causes inflammation of the oesophagus and a burning pain in the chest. Consult your doctor.

ACTION Your doctor will advise you on coping with gastro-oesophageal reflux disease (p.205). If your symptoms do not improve, you may be prescribed ulcer-healing drugs to reduce the production of stomach acid.

POSSIBLE CAUSES Chronic gastritis (persistent inflammation of the lining of the stomach) or indigestion, often due to overeating, are the most likely causes. Chronic gastritis may be aggravated by drinking alcohol.

ACTION Try to eat small, regular meals and cut down on your alcohol intake (*see* SAFE ALCOHOL LIMITS, p.30). Antacids may help to relieve the pain. Consult your doctor if antacids do not ease the pain, or if attacks of pain occur frequently.

Hernia repair

When part of an organ, usually the intestine, protrudes through a weakened muscle, it forms a hernia. Common types of hernia include inguinal and femoral hernias, both of which occur in the groin. The illustrations below show repair of an inguinal hernia, a simple operation done under a local or general anaesthetic. First, the intestine is eased back into place. The weakened area is then repaired: usually, a piece of synthetic mesh is positioned just over or under the area and secured with stitches or staples.

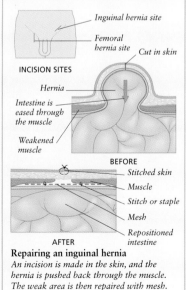

INCISION SITES

Inguinal hernia site

Femoral hernia site

Cut in skin

Hernia

Intestine is eased through the muscle

Weakened muscle

BEFORE

Stitched skin

Muscle

Stitch or staple

Mesh

Repositioned intestine

AFTER

Repairing an inguinal hernia
An incision is made in the skin, and the hernia is pushed back through the muscle. The weak area is then repaired with mesh.

Gallstones

About 1 in 10 people over the age of 40 has gallstones. The stones are formed in the gallbladder from bile (a liquid produced by the liver that aids in digestion). There is often no obvious cause for gallstone formation, although stones are more common in people who are overweight and/or who eat a high-fat diet. Gallstones do not always result in symptoms, but they sometimes inflame the gallbladder or block its exit so that bile cannot be emptied into the intestine. In both these cases, the result may be episodes of abdominal pain, nausea, and vomiting. The frequency of these painful episodes may be reduced by eating a low-fat diet, but in some cases the gallbladder needs to be removed.

101 Recurrent abdominal pain

For an isolated attack of abdominal pain, see chart 100, ABDOMINAL PAIN (p.210).

Consult this chart if you have had several episodes of pain in the abdomen (between the ribcage and the groin) over a number of days or weeks. Most recurrent abdominal pain is

the result of minor digestive disorders and can be relieved by a change in eating habits. If the pain persists, you should consult your doctor, even if you think you know what is causing the pain, so that he or she can eliminate the slight possibility of a serious underlying problem.

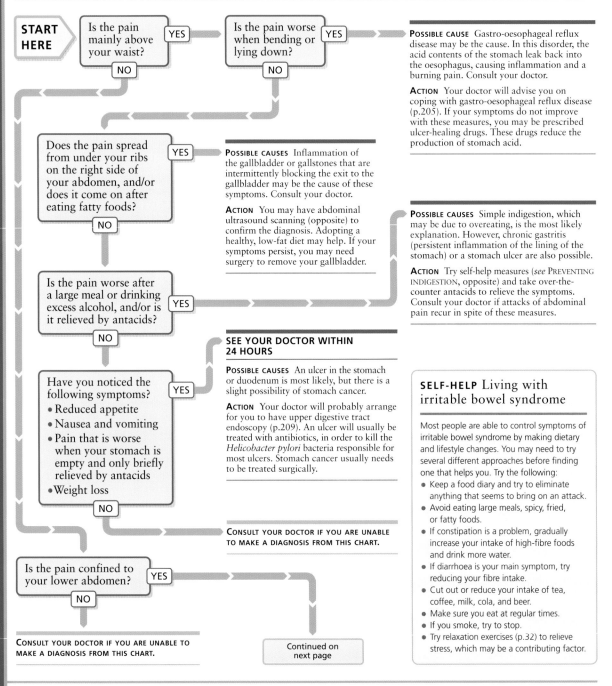

START HERE

Is the pain mainly above your waist? YES → **Is the pain worse when bending or lying down?** YES →

NO ↓   NO ↓

POSSIBLE CAUSE Gastro-oesophageal reflux disease may be the cause. In this disorder, the acid contents of the stomach leak back into the oesophagus, causing inflammation and a burning pain. Consult your doctor.

ACTION Your doctor will advise you on coping with gastro-oesophageal reflux disease (p.205). If your symptoms do not improve with these measures, you may be prescribed ulcer-healing drugs. These drugs reduce the production of stomach acid.

Does the pain spread from under your ribs on the right side of your abdomen, and/or does it come on after eating fatty foods? YES →

NO ↓

POSSIBLE CAUSES Inflammation of the gallbladder or gallstones that are intermittently blocking the exit to the gallbladder may be the cause of these symptoms. Consult your doctor.

ACTION You may have abdominal ultrasound scanning (opposite) to confirm the diagnosis. Adopting a healthy, low-fat diet may help. If your symptoms persist, you may need surgery to remove your gallbladder.

POSSIBLE CAUSES Simple indigestion, which may be due to overeating, is the most likely explanation. However, chronic gastritis (persistent inflammation of the lining of the stomach) or a stomach ulcer are also possible.

ACTION Try self-help measures (*see* PREVENTING INDIGESTION, opposite) and take over-the-counter antacids to relieve the symptoms. Consult your doctor if attacks of abdominal pain recur in spite of these measures.

Is the pain worse after a large meal or drinking excess alcohol, and/or is it relieved by antacids? YES →

NO ↓

Have you noticed the following symptoms?
- Reduced appetite
- Nausea and vomiting
- Pain that is worse when your stomach is empty and only briefly relieved by antacids
- Weight loss

YES →

NO ↓

SEE YOUR DOCTOR WITHIN 24 HOURS

POSSIBLE CAUSES An ulcer in the stomach or duodenum is most likely, but there is a slight possibility of stomach cancer.

ACTION Your doctor will probably arrange for you to have upper digestive tract endoscopy (p.209). An ulcer will usually be treated with antibiotics, in order to kill the *Helicobacter pylori* bacteria responsible for most ulcers. Stomach cancer usually needs to be treated surgically.

SELF-HELP Living with irritable bowel syndrome

Most people are able to control symptoms of irritable bowel syndrome by making dietary and lifestyle changes. You may need to try several different approaches before finding one that helps you. Try the following:
- Keep a food diary and try to eliminate anything that seems to bring on an attack.
- Avoid eating large meals, spicy, fried, or fatty foods.
- If constipation is a problem, gradually increase your intake of high-fibre foods and drink more water.
- If diarrhoea is your main symptom, try reducing your fibre intake.
- Cut out or reduce your intake of tea, coffee, milk, cola, and beer.
- Make sure you eat at regular times.
- If you smoke, try to stop.
- Try relaxation exercises (p.32) to relieve stress, which may be a contributing factor.

CONSULT YOUR DOCTOR IF YOU ARE UNABLE TO MAKE A DIAGNOSIS FROM THIS CHART.

Is the pain confined to your lower abdomen? YES →

NO ↓

CONSULT YOUR DOCTOR IF YOU ARE UNABLE TO MAKE A DIAGNOSIS FROM THIS CHART.

Continued on next page

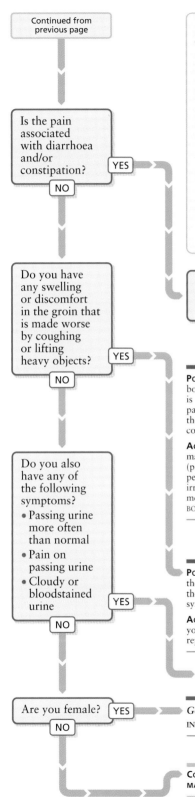

Continued from
previous page

Is the pain
associated
with diarrhoea
and/or
constipation?

YES

NO

Do you have
any swelling
or discomfort
in the groin that
is worse
by coughing
or lifting
heavy objects?

YES

NO

Do you also
have any of
the following
symptoms?
• Passing urine
more often
than normal
• Pain on
passing urine
• Cloudy or
bloodstained
urine

YES

NO

Are you female?

YES

NO

Abdominal ultrasound scanning

In ultrasound scanning (p.39), a device called a transducer emits high-frequency sound waves and receives their echoes to produce images of internal organs. Ultrasound scanning of the abdomen is often used to investigate the liver, the gallbladder, and the kidneys. To produce good contact between the transducer and the abdomen, gel is placed on the skin over the area to be examined. The radiographer moves the transducer over the area, using gentle pressure, and images from it are displayed on a monitor. The procedure is painless and safe.

During the procedure
The hand-held transducer is moved over the skin of the abdomen. The images displayed on the monitor are continually updated.

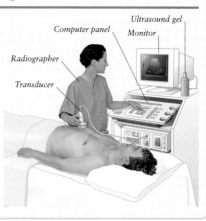

Computer panel
Ultrasound gel
Monitor
Radiographer
Transducer

Have you lost weight,
and/or do you have
blood in your faeces?

YES

NO

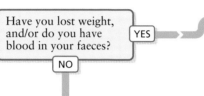

POSSIBLE CAUSE You probably have irritable bowel syndrome, a disorder in which there is a combination of intermittent abdominal pain, constipation, and/or diarrhoea. However, there is a slight possibility of cancer of the colon. Consult your doctor.

ACTION Your doctor will examine you and may arrange for tests such as colonoscopy (p.218) to rule out cancer of the colon. Most people are able to control the symptoms of irritable bowel syndrome using the self-help measures described (*see* LIVING WITH IRRITABLE BOWEL SYNDROME, opposite).

POSSIBLE CAUSE A hernia, in which part of the intestine pushes through a weak area in the abdominal wall, may be the cause of these symptoms. Consult your doctor.

ACTION If your doctor confirms the diagnosis, you will probably need to have an operation to repair the hernia (p.211).

Go to chart **136** LOWER ABDOMINAL PAIN IN WOMEN (p.265)

CONSULT YOUR DOCTOR IF YOU ARE UNABLE TO MAKE A DIAGNOSIS FROM THIS CHART.

SEE YOUR DOCTOR WITHIN 24 HOURS

POSSIBLE CAUSES Ulcerative colitis and Crohn's disease, disorders in which areas of the intestine become inflamed, are possible causes. However, there is a possibility of cancer of the colon.

ACTION You will probably be referred to hospital for tests such as colonoscopy (p.218) to establish the cause. Inflammation of the intestines may be treated with corticosteroid drugs. If cancer of the colon is the cause, it will be treated with surgery.

SEE YOUR DOCTOR WITHIN 24 HOURS

POSSIBLE CAUSES A urinary tract infection is likely. However, the possibility of a more serious condition, such as a bladder stone or a tumour, needs to be ruled out.

ACTION Your doctor will arrange for urine tests to confirm the diagnosis. If you have an infection, you will probably be prescribed antibiotics. Drink plenty of fluids and take painkillers to relieve the symptoms. If there is no infection, you will need ultrasound scanning (p.39) and may have intravenous urography (p.223) to determine the correct treatment.

SELF-HELP Preventing indigestion

The following measures may be helpful in preventing bouts of indigestion:
• Eat at regular intervals without rushing.
• Avoid eating large meals late at night.
• Cut down on alcohol, coffee, and tea.
• Avoid eating rich, fatty foods.
• Keep a food diary and avoid foods that trigger indigestion.
• Avoid medicines that irritate the stomach, such as aspirin.

102 Swollen abdomen

An enlarged abdomen is most often due to excess weight that builds up over a period of years. Abdominal swelling that develops over a relatively short time is usually caused by excess wind in the intestines or by a disorder of the urinary system. In women, abdominal swelling may also be due to a disorder of the reproductive organs or to pregnancy.

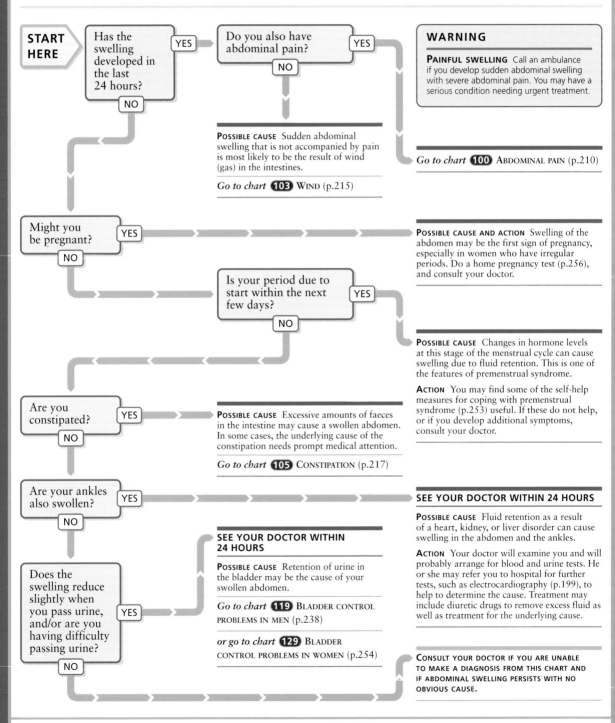

START HERE

Has the swelling developed in the last 24 hours?
YES → **Do you also have abdominal pain?**
- YES →

  WARNING

  PAINFUL SWELLING Call an ambulance if you develop sudden abdominal swelling with severe abdominal pain. You may have a serious condition needing urgent treatment.

  Go to chart **100** ABDOMINAL PAIN (p.210)

- NO →

  POSSIBLE CAUSE Sudden abdominal swelling that is not accompanied by pain is most likely to be the result of wind (gas) in the intestines.

  Go to chart **103** WIND (p.215)

NO ↓

Might you be pregnant?
YES →

POSSIBLE CAUSE AND ACTION Swelling of the abdomen may be the first sign of pregnancy, especially in women who have irregular periods. Do a home pregnancy test (p.256), and consult your doctor.

NO ↓

Is your period due to start within the next few days?
- YES →

  POSSIBLE CAUSE Changes in hormone levels at this stage of the menstrual cycle can cause swelling due to fluid retention. This is one of the features of premenstrual syndrome.

  ACTION You may find some of the self-help measures for coping with premenstrual syndrome (p.253) useful. If these do not help, or if you develop additional symptoms, consult your doctor.

- NO ↓

Are you constipated?
YES →

POSSIBLE CAUSE Excessive amounts of faeces in the intestine may cause a swollen abdomen. In some cases, the underlying cause of the constipation needs prompt medical attention.

Go to chart **105** CONSTIPATION (p.217)

NO ↓

Are your ankles also swollen?
YES →

SEE YOUR DOCTOR WITHIN 24 HOURS

POSSIBLE CAUSE Fluid retention as a result of a heart, kidney, or liver disorder can cause swelling in the abdomen and the ankles.

ACTION Your doctor will examine you and will probably arrange for blood and urine tests. He or she may refer you to hospital for further tests, such as electrocardiography (p.199), to help to determine the cause. Treatment may include diuretic drugs to remove excess fluid as well as treatment for the underlying cause.

NO ↓

Does the swelling reduce slightly when you pass urine, and/or are you having difficulty passing urine?
- YES →

  SEE YOUR DOCTOR WITHIN 24 HOURS

  POSSIBLE CAUSE Retention of urine in the bladder may be the cause of your swollen abdomen.

  Go to chart **119** BLADDER CONTROL PROBLEMS IN MEN (p.238)

  or go to chart **129** BLADDER CONTROL PROBLEMS IN WOMEN (p.254)

- NO ↓

  CONSULT YOUR DOCTOR IF YOU ARE UNABLE TO MAKE A DIAGNOSIS FROM THIS CHART AND IF ABDOMINAL SWELLING PERSISTS WITH NO OBVIOUS CAUSE.

103 Wind

Excess wind (gas) in the digestive system can cause discomfort and a bloated feeling. Expelling the gas through either the mouth (belching) or the anus generally relieves these symptoms. Wind is often caused by swallowing air while eating. It may also occur when certain foods are not broken down properly in the intestines; the food residues then ferment, producing gas. High-fibre foods such as cabbage are common causes of wind, although some people are affected by other types of food, such as dairy products. Usually, wind is nothing to worry about, but you should consult your doctor if you suddenly develop problems with wind without having had a change in your diet.

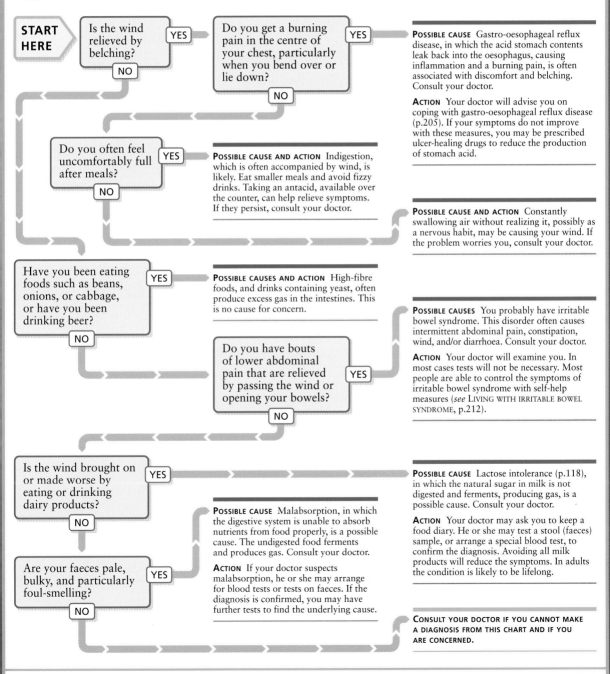

START HERE

Is the wind relieved by belching? — YES → **Do you get a burning pain in the centre of your chest, particularly when you bend over or lie down?** — YES →

POSSIBLE CAUSE Gastro-oesophageal reflux disease, in which the acid stomach contents leak back into the oesophagus, causing inflammation and a burning pain, is often associated with discomfort and belching. Consult your doctor.

ACTION Your doctor will advise you on coping with gastro-oesophageal reflux disease (p.205). If your symptoms do not improve with these measures, you may be prescribed ulcer-healing drugs to reduce the production of stomach acid.

NO ↓ (from burning pain)

Do you often feel uncomfortably full after meals? — YES →

POSSIBLE CAUSE AND ACTION Indigestion, which is often accompanied by wind, is likely. Eat smaller meals and avoid fizzy drinks. Taking an antacid, available over the counter, can help relieve symptoms. If they persist, consult your doctor.

POSSIBLE CAUSE AND ACTION Constantly swallowing air without realizing it, possibly as a nervous habit, may be causing your wind. If the problem worries you, consult your doctor.

Have you been eating foods such as beans, onions, or cabbage, or have you been drinking beer? — YES →

POSSIBLE CAUSES AND ACTION High-fibre foods, and drinks containing yeast, often produce excess gas in the intestines. This is no cause for concern.

Do you have bouts of lower abdominal pain that are relieved by passing the wind or opening your bowels? — YES →

POSSIBLE CAUSES You probably have irritable bowel syndrome. This disorder often causes intermittent abdominal pain, constipation, wind, and/or diarrhoea. Consult your doctor.

ACTION Your doctor will examine you. In most cases tests will not be necessary. Most people are able to control the symptoms of irritable bowel syndrome with self-help measures (*see* LIVING WITH IRRITABLE BOWEL SYNDROME, p.212).

Is the wind brought on or made worse by eating or drinking dairy products? — YES →

POSSIBLE CAUSE Lactose intolerance (p.118), in which the natural sugar in milk is not digested and ferments, producing gas, is a possible cause. Consult your doctor.

ACTION Your doctor may ask you to keep a food diary. He or she may test a stool (faeces) sample, or arrange a special blood test, to confirm the diagnosis. Avoiding all milk products will reduce the symptoms. In adults the condition is likely to be lifelong.

Are your faeces pale, bulky, and particularly foul-smelling? — YES →

POSSIBLE CAUSE Malabsorption, in which the digestive system is unable to absorb nutrients from food properly, is a possible cause. The undigested food ferments and produces gas. Consult your doctor.

ACTION If your doctor suspects malabsorption, he or she may arrange for blood tests or tests on faeces. If the diagnosis is confirmed, you may have further tests to find the underlying cause.

CONSULT YOUR DOCTOR IF YOU CANNOT MAKE A DIAGNOSIS FROM THIS CHART AND IF YOU ARE CONCERNED.

104 Diarrhoea

Diarrhoea is the frequent passing of unusually loose or watery faeces. It is often accompanied by cramping pains in the lower abdomen. In the UK, most attacks of diarrhoea result from viral infections and last for less than 48 hours. Diarrhoea is rarely serious, and usually no treatment is needed other than ensuring that you drink plenty of fluids in order to avoid dehydration. However, you should see your doctor if diarrhoea lasts more than 48 hours or if you have frequent episodes of diarrhoea. Also see your doctor if you have diarrhoea and your job involves handling food.

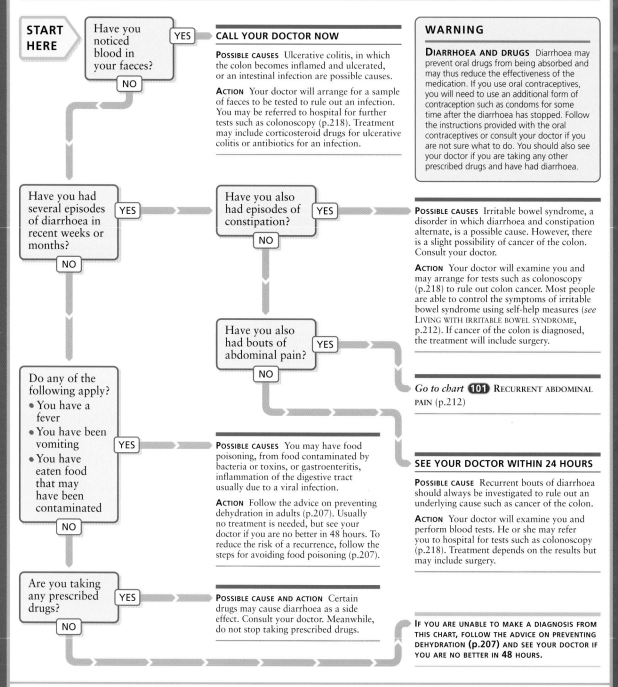

START HERE

Have you noticed blood in your faeces?

YES →

CALL YOUR DOCTOR NOW

POSSIBLE CAUSES Ulcerative colitis, in which the colon becomes inflamed and ulcerated, or an intestinal infection are possible causes.

ACTION Your doctor will arrange for a sample of faeces to be tested to rule out an infection. You may be referred to hospital for further tests such as colonoscopy (p.218). Treatment may include corticosteroid drugs for ulcerative colitis or antibiotics for an infection.

NO

Have you had several episodes of diarrhoea in recent weeks or months?

YES →

Have you also had episodes of constipation?

YES →

POSSIBLE CAUSES Irritable bowel syndrome, a disorder in which diarrhoea and constipation alternate, is a possible cause. However, there is a slight possibility of cancer of the colon. Consult your doctor.

ACTION Your doctor will examine you and may arrange for tests such as colonoscopy (p.218) to rule out colon cancer. Most people are able to control the symptoms of irritable bowel syndrome using self-help measures (*see* LIVING WITH IRRITABLE BOWEL SYNDROME, p.212). If cancer of the colon is diagnosed, the treatment will include surgery.

NO

Have you also had bouts of abdominal pain?

YES →

Go to chart **101** RECURRENT ABDOMINAL PAIN (p.212)

NO

NO

Do any of the following apply?
- You have a fever
- You have been vomiting
- You have eaten food that may have been contaminated

YES →

POSSIBLE CAUSES You may have food poisoning, from food contaminated by bacteria or toxins, or gastroenteritis, inflammation of the digestive tract usually due to a viral infection.

ACTION Follow the advice on preventing dehydration in adults (p.207). Usually no treatment is needed, but see your doctor if you are no better in 48 hours. To reduce the risk of a recurrence, follow the steps for avoiding food poisoning (p.207).

NO

Are you taking any prescribed drugs?

YES →

POSSIBLE CAUSE AND ACTION Certain drugs may cause diarrhoea as a side effect. Consult your doctor. Meanwhile, do not stop taking prescribed drugs.

NO

WARNING

DIARRHOEA AND DRUGS Diarrhoea may prevent oral drugs from being absorbed and may thus reduce the effectiveness of the medication. If you use oral contraceptives, you will need to use an additional form of contraception such as condoms for some time after the diarrhoea has stopped. Follow the instructions provided with the oral contraceptives or consult your doctor if you are not sure what to do. You should also see your doctor if you are taking any other prescribed drugs and have had diarrhoea.

SEE YOUR DOCTOR WITHIN 24 HOURS

POSSIBLE CAUSE Recurrent bouts of diarrhoea should always be investigated to rule out an underlying cause such as cancer of the colon.

ACTION Your doctor will examine you and perform blood tests. He or she may refer you to hospital for tests such as colonoscopy (p.218). Treatment depends on the results but may include surgery.

IF YOU ARE UNABLE TO MAKE A DIAGNOSIS FROM THIS CHART, FOLLOW THE ADVICE ON PREVENTING DEHYDRATION (p.207) AND SEE YOUR DOCTOR IF YOU ARE NO BETTER IN 48 HOURS.

105 Constipation

Some people open their bowels once or twice a day; others do so less frequently. If you have fewer bowel movements than usual, or if your faeces are small and hard, you are constipated. The cause is often a lack of fluid or fibre-rich foods in the diet. Constipation is also common in pregnancy because hormone changes cause intestinal muscles to relax. If you are constipated for longer than 2 weeks, consult your doctor so that cancer of the colon can be ruled out.

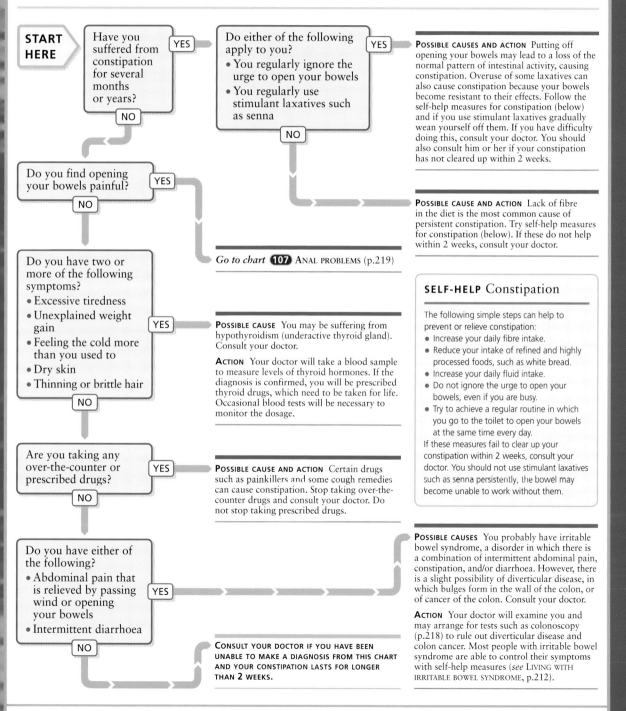

START HERE

Have you suffered from constipation for several months or years? — YES → **Do either of the following apply to you?**
- You regularly ignore the urge to open your bowels
- You regularly use stimulant laxatives such as senna

— YES → **POSSIBLE CAUSES AND ACTION** Putting off opening your bowels may lead to a loss of the normal pattern of intestinal activity, causing constipation. Overuse of some laxatives can also cause constipation because your bowels become resistant to their effects. Follow the self-help measures for constipation (below) and if you use stimulant laxatives gradually wean yourself off them. If you have difficulty doing this, consult your doctor. You should also consult him or her if your constipation has not cleared up within 2 weeks.

NO ↓ (from "Do either of the following")

POSSIBLE CAUSE AND ACTION Lack of fibre in the diet is the most common cause of persistent constipation. Try self-help measures for constipation (below). If these do not help within 2 weeks, consult your doctor.

Do you find opening your bowels painful? — YES →

Go to chart **107** ANAL PROBLEMS (p.219)

NO ↓

Do you have two or more of the following symptoms?
- Excessive tiredness
- Unexplained weight gain
- Feeling the cold more than you used to
- Dry skin
- Thinning or brittle hair

— YES → **POSSIBLE CAUSE** You may be suffering from hypothyroidism (underactive thyroid gland). Consult your doctor.

ACTION Your doctor will take a blood sample to measure levels of thyroid hormones. If the diagnosis is confirmed, you will be prescribed thyroid drugs, which need to be taken for life. Occasional blood tests will be necessary to monitor the dosage.

NO ↓

Are you taking any over-the-counter or prescribed drugs? — YES → **POSSIBLE CAUSE AND ACTION** Certain drugs such as painkillers and some cough remedies can cause constipation. Stop taking over-the-counter drugs and consult your doctor. Do not stop taking prescribed drugs.

NO ↓

Do you have either of the following?
- Abdominal pain that is relieved by passing wind or opening your bowels
- Intermittent diarrhoea

— YES → **POSSIBLE CAUSES** You probably have irritable bowel syndrome, a disorder in which there is a combination of intermittent abdominal pain, constipation, and/or diarrhoea. However, there is a slight possibility of diverticular disease, in which bulges form in the wall of the colon, or of cancer of the colon. Consult your doctor.

ACTION Your doctor will examine you and may arrange for tests such as colonoscopy (p.218) to rule out diverticular disease and colon cancer. Most people with irritable bowel syndrome are able to control their symptoms with self-help measures (*see* LIVING WITH IRRITABLE BOWEL SYNDROME, p.212).

NO ↓

CONSULT YOUR DOCTOR IF YOU HAVE BEEN UNABLE TO MAKE A DIAGNOSIS FROM THIS CHART AND YOUR CONSTIPATION LASTS FOR LONGER THAN 2 WEEKS.

SELF-HELP Constipation

The following simple steps can help to prevent or relieve constipation:
- Increase your daily fibre intake.
- Reduce your intake of refined and highly processed foods, such as white bread.
- Increase your daily fluid intake.
- Do not ignore the urge to open your bowels, even if you are busy.
- Try to achieve a regular routine in which you go to the toilet to open your bowels at the same time every day.

If these measures fail to clear up your constipation within 2 weeks, consult your doctor. You should not use stimulant laxatives such as senna persistently; the bowel may become unable to work without them.

106 Abnormal-looking faeces

Most minor changes in the colour and consistency of your faeces are due to a recent change in diet or a temporary digestive upset. However, if the faeces are significantly darker or lighter in colour than usual, or if they are streaked with blood, this may indicate a potentially serious disorder of the digestive system that requires medical attention.

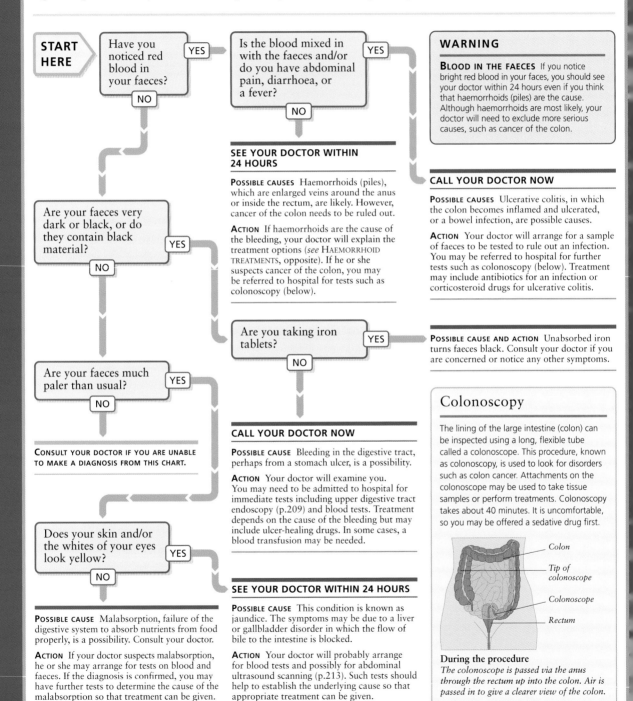

START HERE

Have you noticed red blood in your faeces? — YES → **Is the blood mixed in with the faeces and/or do you have abdominal pain, diarrhoea, or a fever?** — YES →

NO ↓ NO ↓

WARNING

BLOOD IN THE FAECES If you notice bright red blood in your faces, you should see your doctor within 24 hours even if you think that the cause. Although haemorrhoids (piles) are most likely, your doctor will need to exclude more serious causes, such as cancer of the colon.

SEE YOUR DOCTOR WITHIN 24 HOURS

POSSIBLE CAUSES Haemorrhoids (piles), which are enlarged veins around the anus or inside the rectum, are likely. However, cancer of the colon needs to be ruled out.

ACTION If haemorrhoids are the cause of the bleeding, your doctor will explain the treatment options (see HAEMORRHOID TREATMENTS, opposite). If he or she suspects cancer of the colon, you may be referred to hospital for tests such as colonoscopy (below).

CALL YOUR DOCTOR NOW

POSSIBLE CAUSES Ulcerative colitis, in which the colon becomes inflamed and ulcerated, or a bowel infection, are possible causes.

ACTION Your doctor will arrange for a sample of faeces to be tested to rule out an infection. You may be referred to hospital for further tests such as colonoscopy (below). Treatment may include antibiotics for an infection or corticosteroid drugs for ulcerative colitis.

Are your faeces very dark or black, or do they contain black material? — YES →

NO ↓

Are you taking iron tablets? — YES → **POSSIBLE CAUSE AND ACTION** Unabsorbed iron turns faeces black. Consult your doctor if you are concerned or notice any other symptoms.

NO ↓

Are your faeces much paler than usual? — YES →

NO ↓

CONSULT YOUR DOCTOR IF YOU ARE UNABLE TO MAKE A DIAGNOSIS FROM THIS CHART.

CALL YOUR DOCTOR NOW

POSSIBLE CAUSE Bleeding in the digestive tract, perhaps from a stomach ulcer, is a possibility.

ACTION Your doctor will examine you. You may need to be admitted to hospital for immediate tests including upper digestive tract endoscopy (p.209) and blood tests. Treatment depends on the cause of the bleeding but may include ulcer-healing drugs. In some cases, a blood transfusion may be needed.

Colonoscopy

The lining of the large intestine (colon) can be inspected using a long, flexible tube called a colonoscope. This procedure, known as colonoscopy, is used to look for disorders such as colon cancer. Attachments on the colonoscope may be used to take tissue samples or perform treatments. Colonoscopy takes about 40 minutes. It is uncomfortable, so you may be offered a sedative drug first.

Does your skin and/or the whites of your eyes look yellow? — YES →

NO ↓

SEE YOUR DOCTOR WITHIN 24 HOURS

POSSIBLE CAUSE This condition is known as jaundice. The symptoms may be due to a liver or gallbladder disorder in which the flow of bile to the intestine is blocked.

ACTION Your doctor will probably arrange for blood tests and possibly for abdominal ultrasound scanning (p.213). Such tests should help to establish the underlying cause so that appropriate treatment can be given.

POSSIBLE CAUSE Malabsorption, failure of the digestive system to absorb nutrients from food properly, is a possibility. Consult your doctor.

ACTION If your doctor suspects malabsorption, he or she may arrange for tests on blood and faeces. If the diagnosis is confirmed, you may have further tests to determine the cause of the malabsorption so that treatment can be given.

Colon
Tip of colonoscope
Colonoscope
Rectum

During the procedure
The colonoscope is passed via the anus through the rectum up into the colon. Air is passed in to give a clearer view of the colon.

107 Anal problems

The anus is the last part of the digestive tract and links the rectum to the outside of the body. The anus contains a ring of powerful muscles that keep it closed except when passing faeces. The most common symptoms affecting the anus are itching and pain, which are not usually signs of a serious disorder. Bleeding should always be assessed by your doctor.

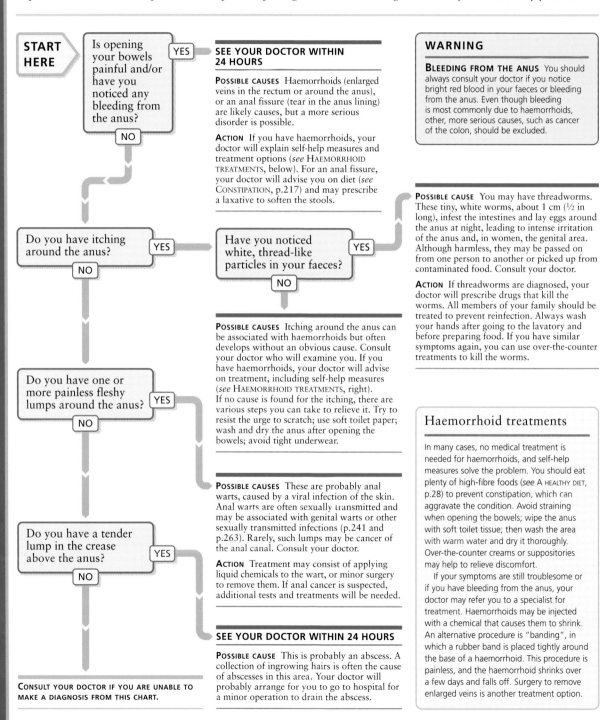

START HERE

Is opening your bowels painful and/or have you noticed any bleeding from the anus? — YES

SEE YOUR DOCTOR WITHIN 24 HOURS

POSSIBLE CAUSES Haemorrhoids (enlarged veins in the rectum or around the anus), or an anal fissure (tear in the anus lining) are likely causes, but a more serious disorder is possible.

ACTION If you have haemorrhoids, your doctor will explain self-help measures and treatment options (*see* HAEMORRHOID TREATMENTS, below). For an anal fissure, your doctor will advise you on diet (*see* CONSTIPATION, p.217) and may prescribe a laxative to soften the stools.

NO

Do you have itching around the anus? — YES

Have you noticed white, thread-like particles in your faeces? — YES

POSSIBLE CAUSE You may have threadworms. These tiny, white worms, about 1 cm (½ in long), infest the intestines and lay eggs around the anus at night, leading to intense irritation of the anus and, in women, the genital area. Although harmless, they may be passed on from one person to another or picked up from contaminated food. Consult your doctor.

ACTION If threadworms are diagnosed, your doctor will prescribe drugs that kill the worms. All members of your family should be treated to prevent reinfection. Always wash your hands after going to the lavatory and before preparing food. If you have similar symptoms again, you can use over-the-counter treatments to kill the worms.

NO

NO

POSSIBLE CAUSES Itching around the anus can be associated with haemorrhoids but often develops without an obvious cause. Consult your doctor who will examine you. If you have haemorrhoids, your doctor will advise on treatment, including self-help measures (*see* HAEMORRHOID TREATMENTS, right). If no cause is found for the itching, there are various steps you can take to relieve it. Try to resist the urge to scratch; use soft toilet paper; wash and dry the anus after opening the bowels; avoid tight underwear.

Do you have one or more painless fleshy lumps around the anus? — YES

NO

POSSIBLE CAUSES These are probably anal warts, caused by a viral infection of the skin. Anal warts are often sexually transmitted and may be associated with genital warts or other sexually transmitted infections (p.241 and p.263). Rarely, such lumps may be cancer of the anal canal. Consult your doctor.

ACTION Treatment may consist of applying liquid chemicals to the wart, or minor surgery to remove them. If anal cancer is suspected, additional tests and treatments will be needed.

Do you have a tender lump in the crease above the anus? — YES

NO

SEE YOUR DOCTOR WITHIN 24 HOURS

POSSIBLE CAUSE This is probably an abscess. A collection of ingrowing hairs is often the cause of abscesses in this area. Your doctor will probably arrange for you to go to hospital for a minor operation to drain the abscess.

CONSULT YOUR DOCTOR IF YOU ARE UNABLE TO MAKE A DIAGNOSIS FROM THIS CHART.

WARNING

BLEEDING FROM THE ANUS You should always consult your doctor if you notice bright red blood in your faeces or bleeding from the anus. Even though bleeding is most commonly due to haemorrhoids, other, more serious causes, such as cancer of the colon, should be excluded.

Haemorrhoid treatments

In many cases, no medical treatment is needed for haemorrhoids, and self-help measures solve the problem. You should eat plenty of high-fibre foods (see A HEALTHY DIET, p.28) to prevent constipation, which can aggravate the condition. Avoid straining when opening the bowels; wipe the anus with soft toilet tissue; then wash the area with warm water and dry it thoroughly. Over-the-counter creams or suppositories may help to relieve discomfort.

If your symptoms are still troublesome or if you have bleeding from the anus, your doctor may refer you to a specialist for treatment. Haemorrhoids may be injected with a chemical that causes them to shrink. An alternative procedure is "banding", in which a rubber band is placed tightly around the base of a haemorrhoid. This procedure is painless, and the haemorrhoid shrinks over a few days and falls off. Surgery to remove enlarged veins is another treatment option.

108 General urinary problems

Consult this chart for problems such as a change in the number of times you need to pass urine or the amount of urine produced. In some cases, these variations may be due simply to drinking large amounts of coffee or tea or to anxiety. However, a change may be caused by a bladder or kidney problem or a disorder of the nerves to the urinary tract.

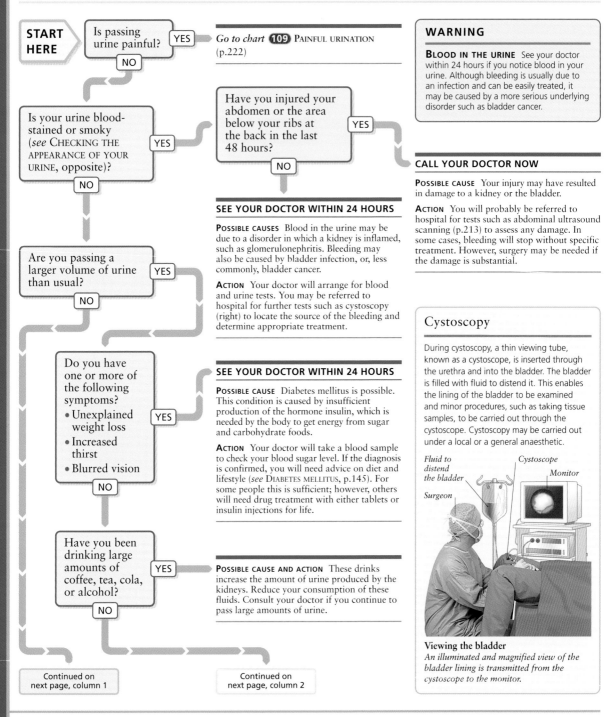

START HERE → **Is passing urine painful?** — YES → *Go to chart* **109** PAINFUL URINATION (p.222)

NO ↓

Is your urine blood-stained or smoky (*see* CHECKING THE APPEARANCE OF YOUR URINE, opposite)? — YES →

Have you injured your abdomen or the area below your ribs at the back in the last 48 hours? — YES →

NO ↓

NO ↓

SEE YOUR DOCTOR WITHIN 24 HOURS

POSSIBLE CAUSES Blood in the urine may be due to a disorder in which a kidney is inflamed, such as glomerulonephritis. Bleeding may also be caused by bladder infection, or, less commonly, bladder cancer.

ACTION Your doctor will arrange for blood and urine tests. You may be referred to hospital for further tests such as cystoscopy (right) to locate the source of the bleeding and determine appropriate treatment.

Are you passing a larger volume of urine than usual? — YES →

NO ↓

SEE YOUR DOCTOR WITHIN 24 HOURS

POSSIBLE CAUSE Diabetes mellitus is possible. This condition is caused by insufficient production of the hormone insulin, which is needed by the body to get energy from sugar and carbohydrate foods.

ACTION Your doctor will take a blood sample to check your blood sugar level. If the diagnosis is confirmed, you will need advice on diet and lifestyle (*see* DIABETES MELLITUS, p.145). For some people this is sufficient; however, others will need drug treatment with either tablets or insulin injections for life.

Do you have one or more of the following symptoms?
- Unexplained weight loss
- Increased thirst
- Blurred vision
— YES →

NO ↓

Have you been drinking large amounts of coffee, tea, cola, or alcohol? — YES →

POSSIBLE CAUSE AND ACTION These drinks increase the amount of urine produced by the kidneys. Reduce your consumption of these fluids. Consult your doctor if you continue to pass large amounts of urine.

NO ↓

Continued on next page, column 1

Continued on next page, column 2

WARNING

BLOOD IN THE URINE See your doctor within 24 hours if you notice blood in your urine. Although bleeding is usually due to an infection and can be easily treated, it may be caused by a more serious underlying disorder such as bladder cancer.

CALL YOUR DOCTOR NOW

POSSIBLE CAUSE Your injury may have resulted in damage to a kidney or the bladder.

ACTION You will probably be referred to hospital for tests such as abdominal ultrasound scanning (p.213) to assess any damage. In some cases, bleeding will stop without specific treatment. However, surgery may be needed if the damage is substantial.

Cystoscopy

During cystoscopy, a thin viewing tube, known as a cystoscope, is inserted through the urethra and into the bladder. The bladder is filled with fluid to distend it. This enables the lining of the bladder to be examined and minor procedures, such as taking tissue samples, to be carried out through the cystoscope. Cystoscopy may be carried out under a local or a general anaesthetic.

Viewing the bladder
An illuminated and magnified view of the bladder lining is transmitted from the cystoscope to the monitor.

Continued from previous page, column 1

Continued from previous page, column 2

POSSIBLE CAUSE AND ACTION Drugs such as diuretics are prescribed for conditions such as heart failure, to increase the amount of urine passed. Other drugs can also cause you to pass more urine than usual as a side effect. Stop taking any over-the-counter drugs, and consult your doctor. Meanwhile, do not stop taking any prescribed drugs.

Are you passing urine more frequently than usual?
YES
NO

Are you currently taking any over-the-counter or prescribed drugs?
YES
NO

POSSIBLE CAUSE If you are not drinking excessive amounts of liquids, a kidney or hormone disorder may be the cause. Consult your doctor.

ACTION Your doctor will examine you and arrange for blood and urine tests. You may be referred to hospital for further tests, such as ultrasound scanning (p.39) of the kidneys, which will help to confirm the cause and determine the appropriate treatment.

Might you be or are you pregnant?
YES
NO

POSSIBLE CAUSE AND ACTION Passing urine frequently is a common symptom in early pregnancy and is nothing to worry about. If you are not sure whether you are pregnant, do a home pregnancy test (p.256) and consult your doctor.

POSSIBLE CAUSES You may have a small or oversensitive bladder. Alternatively, the exit from the bladder may be partially blocked by a bladder stone. In men, an enlarged prostate gland may be the cause. Consult your doctor.

Do you have a strong urge to pass urine with little urine passed?
YES
NO

ACTION Your doctor will test your urine and may arrange for ultrasound scanning (p.39), cystoscopy (opposite), or tests to study the pressures in your bladder (*see* URODYNAMIC STUDIES, p.254). If you have an oversensitive or small bladder, your doctor may advise you on self-help measures to control your symptoms, or prescribe drugs. Surgery may be necessary to remove bladder stones. An enlarged prostate gland may be treated with either drugs or surgery (*see* PROSTATECTOMY, p.239).

Do you feel particularly anxious, or do your symptoms occur when you are under stress?
YES
NO

POSSIBLE CAUSE Anxiety commonly causes an urge to pass urine, even when the bladder is not completely full.

Go to chart **73** ANXIETY (p.168)

Go to chart **119** BLADDER CONTROL PROBLEMS IN MEN (p.238)

Are you male?
YES
NO

Go to chart **129** BLADDER CONTROL PROBLEMS IN WOMEN (p.254)

Do you have difficulty in controlling your bladder?
YES
NO

Checking the appearance of your urine

The appearance of urine varies. It is often darker in the morning than later in the day. A temporary colour change may be due to some drugs and foods, such as beetroot. However, a change in your urine may indicate a disorder. Very dark urine may be a sign of liver disease, and red or cloudy urine may be due to bleeding or infection in the kidney or bladder. If you are not sure whether a change in the appearance of your urine is normal, consult your doctor.

Clear, straw-coloured urine

Normal urine
Unless passed first thing in the morning, urine is normally clear, pale, and straw-coloured.

CONSULT YOUR DOCTOR IF YOU ARE UNABLE TO MAKE A DIAGNOSIS FROM THIS CHART.

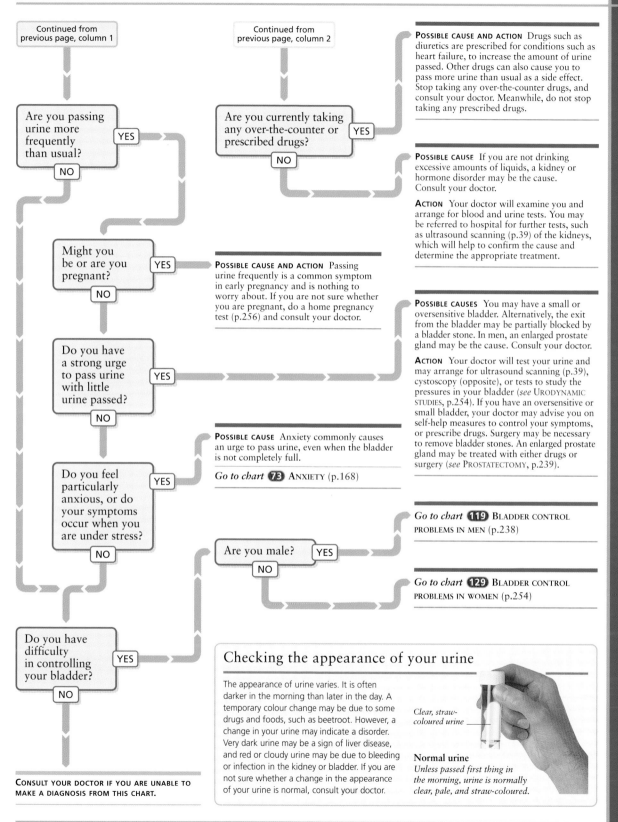

109 Painful urination

Pain or discomfort while passing urine is usually caused by inflammation of the lower urinary tract, often due to infection. In women, pain when passing urine may be due to inflammation in the genital area. Painful urination may sometimes be accompanied by cloudy or blood-stained urine (*see* CHECKING THE APPEARANCE OF YOUR URINE, p.221).

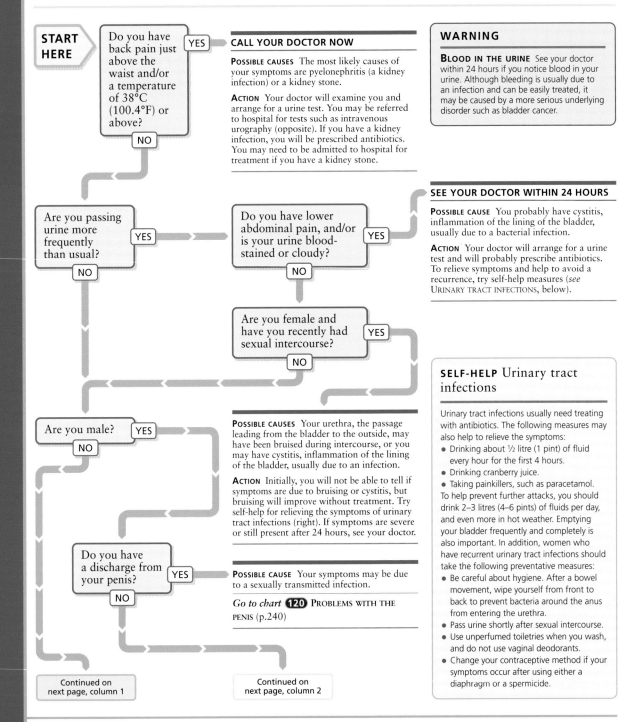

START HERE

Do you have back pain just above the waist and/or a temperature of 38°C (100.4°F) or above?
YES →

NO ↓

CALL YOUR DOCTOR NOW

POSSIBLE CAUSES The most likely causes of your symptoms are pyelonephritis (a kidney infection) or a kidney stone.

ACTION Your doctor will examine you and arrange for a urine test. You may be referred to hospital for tests such as intravenous urography (opposite). If you have a kidney infection, you will be prescribed antibiotics. You may need to be admitted to hospital for treatment if you have a kidney stone.

Are you passing urine more frequently than usual?
YES →

NO ↓

Do you have lower abdominal pain, and/or is your urine blood-stained or cloudy?
YES →

NO ↓

Are you female and have you recently had sexual intercourse?
YES →

NO ↓

Are you male?
YES →

NO ↓

Do you have a discharge from your penis?
YES →

NO ↓

SEE YOUR DOCTOR WITHIN 24 HOURS

POSSIBLE CAUSE You probably have cystitis, inflammation of the lining of the bladder, usually due to a bacterial infection.

ACTION Your doctor will arrange for a urine test and will probably prescribe antibiotics. To relieve symptoms and help to avoid a recurrence, try self-help measures (*see* URINARY TRACT INFECTIONS, below).

POSSIBLE CAUSES Your urethra, the passage leading from the bladder to the outside, may have been bruised during intercourse, or you may have cystitis, inflammation of the lining of the bladder, usually due to an infection.

ACTION Initially, you will not be able to tell if symptoms are due to bruising or cystitis, but bruising will improve without treatment. Try self-help for relieving the symptoms of urinary tract infections (right). If symptoms are severe or still present after 24 hours, see your doctor.

POSSIBLE CAUSE Your symptoms may be due to a sexually transmitted infection.

Go to chart **120** PROBLEMS WITH THE PENIS (p.240)

WARNING

BLOOD IN THE URINE See your doctor within 24 hours if you notice blood in your urine. Although bleeding is usually due to an infection and can be easily treated, it may be caused by a more serious underlying disorder such as bladder cancer.

SELF-HELP Urinary tract infections

Urinary tract infections usually need treating with antibiotics. The following measures may also help to relieve the symptoms:
- Drinking about ½ litre (1 pint) of fluid every hour for the first 4 hours.
- Drinking cranberry juice.
- Taking painkillers, such as paracetamol.

To help prevent further attacks, you should drink 2–3 litres (4–6 pints) of fluids per day, and even more in hot weather. Emptying your bladder frequently and completely is also important. In addition, women who have recurrent urinary tract infections should take the following preventative measures:
- Be careful about hygiene. After a bowel movement, wipe yourself from front to back to prevent bacteria around the anus from entering the urethra.
- Pass urine shortly after sexual intercourse.
- Use unperfumed toiletries when you wash, and do not use vaginal deodorants.
- Change your contraceptive method if your symptoms occur after using either a diaphragm or a spermicide.

Continued on next page, column 1

Continued on next page, column 2

Continued from previous page, column 1

Continued from previous page, column 2

Do you have pain between your legs? **YES** → **NO**

POSSIBLE CAUSE Prostatitis, inflammation of the prostate gland, usually as a result of a bacterial infection, is a likely cause. In some cases, the infection may be sexually transmitted (*see* SEXUALLY TRANSMITTED INFECTIONS IN MEN, p.241). Consult your doctor.

ACTION Your doctor will examine you and, if a sexually transmitted infection is likely, may refer you to a genito-urinary medicine (GUM) clinic. You will probably be prescribed antibiotics and advised to drink plenty of fluids.

Have you noticed soreness or itching in the genital area? **YES** → **NO**

Do you have blisters or shallow ulcers on the tip of your penis? **YES** → **NO**

POSSIBLE CAUSE You may have genital herpes (*see* SEXUALLY TRANSMITTED INFECTIONS IN MEN, p.241). This condition can cause pain if urine comes into contact with the ulcers. Consult your doctor.

ACTION Your doctor will examine you, and, if genital herpes is a possibility, he or she may refer you to a genito-urinary medicine (GUM) clinic. If the diagnosis is confirmed, you may be prescribed antiviral drugs. Over-the-counter painkillers may help to relieve the pain. This condition can sometimes recur, but subsequent attacks are usually less severe.

CONSULT YOUR DOCTOR IF YOU ARE UNABLE TO MAKE A DIAGNOSIS FROM THIS CHART.

CONSULT YOUR DOCTOR IF YOU ARE UNABLE TO MAKE A DIAGNOSIS FROM THIS CHART.

Do you have an abnormal vaginal discharge? **YES** → **NO**

POSSIBLE CAUSE A vulval or vaginal infection can cause pain when urine is passed.

Go to chart **134** ABNORMAL VAGINAL DISCHARGE (p.262)

Do you have blisters or shallow ulcers in the genital area? **YES** → **NO**

CONSULT YOUR DOCTOR IF YOU ARE UNABLE TO MAKE A DIAGNOSIS FROM THIS CHART.

POSSIBLE CAUSE You may have genital herpes (*see* SEXUALLY TRANSMITTED INFECTIONS IN WOMEN, p.263). This condition can cause pain if urine comes into contact with the ulcers. Consult your doctor.

ACTION Your doctor will examine you, and, if genital herpes is a possibility, he or she may refer you to a genito-urinary medicine (GUM) clinic. If the diagnosis is confirmed, you may be prescribed antiviral drugs. Over-the-counter painkillers may help to relieve the pain. This condition can sometimes recur, but subsequent attacks are usually less severe.

Intravenous urography

Intravenous urography (IVU) is an X-ray imaging procedure (p.37), which is used to look for disorders of the urinary tract, such as kidney stones. An iodine-based contrast medium, which shows up on X-rays, is injected into a vein in your arm. The contrast medium travels through the circulation to the kidneys, where it is filtered from the blood into the urine. It then passes from the kidneys to the ureters and the bladder. Several X-rays are taken at intervals to show the contrast medium outlining these organs. The procedure is painless, and it usually takes less than 1 hour in total.

During the procedure
While you lie on the X-ray table, a contrast medium is injected into a vein in your arm. X-rays of your kidneys and ureters are taken at intervals.

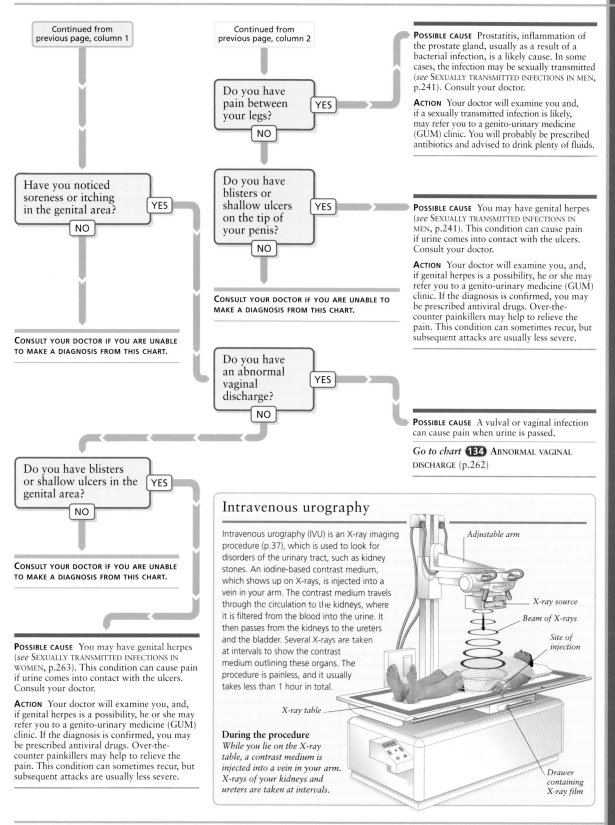

Adjustable arm

X-ray source

Beam of X-rays

Site of injection

X-ray table

Drawer containing X-ray film

110 Painful joints

For swelling of the ankles with no associated pain, see chart 115, SWOLLEN ANKLES *(p.231).*

A joint is the junction of two or more bones. Most joints are designed to allow some movement, but the range and type of movement depend on the structure of the joint. Aches and pains in joints are common and are most often the result of overuse or of a minor injury. Such symptoms are usually short-lived and do not need medical treatment. However, persistent pain in a joint implies a potentially serious underlying disorder and should be investigated. The major weight-bearing joints, such as the hips and the knees, undergo constant wear and tear and are particularly prone to disorders such as osteoarthritis. Consult this chart if you have one or more painful joints.

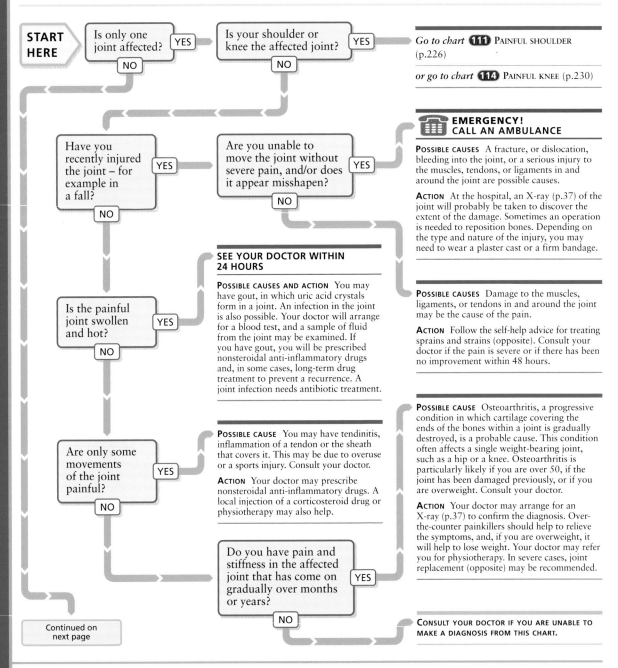

START HERE

Is only one joint affected? — NO

YES → **Is your shoulder or knee the affected joint?** — NO

YES → *Go to chart* **111** PAINFUL SHOULDER (p.226)

or go to chart **114** PAINFUL KNEE (p.230)

Have you recently injured the joint – for example in a fall? — NO

YES → **Are you unable to move the joint without severe pain, and/or does it appear misshapen?** — NO

YES →

📞 **EMERGENCY! CALL AN AMBULANCE**

POSSIBLE CAUSES A fracture, or dislocation, bleeding into the joint, or a serious injury to the muscles, tendons, or ligaments in and around the joint are possible causes.

ACTION At the hospital, an X-ray (p.37) of the joint will probably be taken to discover the extent of the damage. Sometimes an operation is needed to reposition bones. Depending on the type and nature of the injury, you may need to wear a plaster cast or a firm bandage.

SEE YOUR DOCTOR WITHIN 24 HOURS

POSSIBLE CAUSES AND ACTION You may have gout, in which uric acid crystals form in a joint. An infection in the joint is also possible. Your doctor will arrange for a blood test, and a sample of fluid from the joint may be examined. If you have gout, you will be prescribed nonsteroidal anti-inflammatory drugs and, in some cases, long-term drug treatment to prevent a recurrence. A joint infection needs antibiotic treatment.

Is the painful joint swollen and hot? — NO

YES →

POSSIBLE CAUSES Damage to the muscles, ligaments, or tendons in and around the joint may be the cause of the pain.

ACTION Follow the self-help advice for treating sprains and strains (opposite). Consult your doctor if the pain is severe or if there has been no improvement within 48 hours.

Are only some movements of the joint painful? — NO

YES →

POSSIBLE CAUSE You may have tendinitis, inflammation of a tendon or the sheath that covers it. This may be due to overuse or a sports injury. Consult your doctor.

ACTION Your doctor may prescribe nonsteroidal anti-inflammatory drugs. A local injection of a corticosteroid drug or physiotherapy may also help.

POSSIBLE CAUSE Osteoarthritis, a progressive condition in which cartilage covering the ends of the bones within a joint is gradually destroyed, is a probable cause. This condition often affects a single weight-bearing joint, such as a hip or a knee. Osteoarthritis is particularly likely if you are over 50, if the joint has been damaged previously, or if you are overweight. Consult your doctor.

ACTION Your doctor may arrange for an X-ray (p.37) to confirm the diagnosis. Over-the-counter painkillers should help to relieve the symptoms, and, if you are overweight, it will help to lose weight. Your doctor may refer you for physiotherapy. In severe cases, joint replacement (opposite) may be recommended.

Do you have pain and stiffness in the affected joint that has come on gradually over months or years? — NO

YES →

CONSULT YOUR DOCTOR IF YOU ARE UNABLE TO MAKE A DIAGNOSIS FROM THIS CHART.

Continued on next page

Continued from previous page

Are several of your joints hot and swollen? **YES**

NO

Do you have pain and stiffness in your joints that has come on gradually over several months or years? **YES**

NO

CONSULT YOUR DOCTOR IF YOU ARE UNABLE TO MAKE A DIAGNOSIS FROM THIS CHART.

POSSIBLE CAUSE Osteoarthritis, a progressive condition in which cartilage covering the ends of the bones within a joint is gradually destroyed, is a probable cause. This condition may run in families, particularly if the small joints at the ends of the fingers are affected. Consult your doctor.

ACTION Your doctor may arrange for blood tests or an X-ray (p.37) to exclude other types of arthritis. Over-the-counter painkillers should help to relieve the symptoms. Your doctor may refer you for physiotherapy.

SELF-HELP Treating sprains and strains

Treat sprains and strains by following the RICE procedure – Rest, Ice, Compression, and Elevation. Apply a cold compress or wrapped ice pack for several minutes. Then wrap a bandage firmly over a thick layer of cotton wool to provide compression. Try to rest with the injury elevated for at least 24 hours. If it is no better in 48 hours, consult your doctor.

Treating sprains
Apply an ice pack to the affected area, and keep the limb raised.

Ice pack

Have you recently had an infection such as a genital tract infection or gastroenteritis? **YES**

NO

Do you have psoriasis or an inflammatory bowel disease, such as Crohn's disease or ulcerative colitis? **YES**

NO

Do you have any of the following?
- Pain and swelling affecting the small joints of both hands
- Generalized stiffness lasting at least an hour in the morning
- Tiredness and feeling generally unwell **YES**

NO

SEE YOUR DOCTOR WITHIN 24 HOURS IF YOU ARE UNABLE TO MAKE A DIAGNOSIS FROM THIS CHART.

SEE YOUR DOCTOR WITHIN 24 HOURS

POSSIBLE CAUSE Rheumatoid arthritis, an autoimmune disorder (in which the body attacks its own tissues), is the most likely cause of your symptoms.

ACTION Your doctor may arrange for a blood test and X-rays (p.37) to confirm the diagnosis. He or she will probably prescribe nonsteroidal anti-inflammatory drugs to relieve the pain. In most cases, you will be referred to hospital for further treatment with drugs that suppress the immune system and for physiotherapy.

SEE YOUR DOCTOR WITHIN 24 HOURS

POSSIBLE CAUSE Reactive arthritis, which is inflammation of the joints in response to an infection elsewhere, may be the cause.

ACTION Your doctor may arrange for tests to confirm that the infection has cleared up. He or she will probably prescribe nonsteroidal anti-inflammatory drugs. Reactive arthritis often clears up promptly but in rare cases may persist for months or even years.

SEE YOUR DOCTOR WITHIN 24 HOURS

POSSIBLE CAUSE These conditions may be associated with psoriatic arthritis, a type of arthritis affecting the lower spine and pelvis. In many cases, other joints are also involved, such as the joints at the ends of the fingers and toes.

ACTION Further treatment of your underlying condition may improve your joint symptoms. Your doctor may prescribe nonsteroidal anti-inflammatory drugs to relieve joint pain.

Joint replacement

Joints that have been severely damaged by a disorder such as arthritis or by an injury may be surgically replaced with artificial joints made of metal, ceramic, or plastic. Joint replacement is most commonly performed for hips, knees, and shoulders, but most joints in the body can now be replaced, even tiny finger joints. During the operation, the ends of the damaged bones are removed, and the artificial components are fixed in place. The procedure usually relieves pain and increases the range of movement possible in the affected joint.

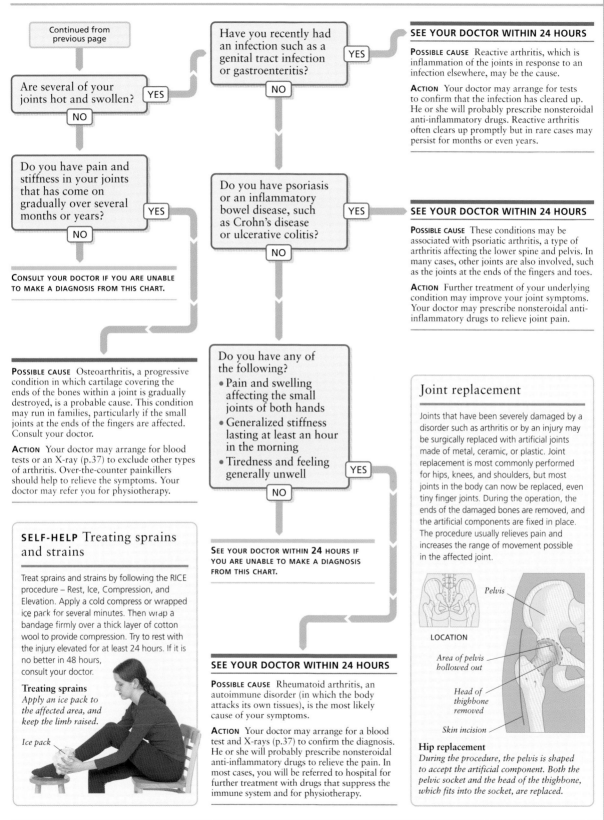

Pelvis

LOCATION

Area of pelvis hollowed out

Head of thighbone removed

Skin incision

Hip replacement
During the procedure, the pelvis is shaped to accept the artificial component. Both the pelvic socket and the head of the thighbone, which fits into the socket, are replaced.

111 Painful shoulder

The shoulder is one of the most complex joints in the body and has a very wide range of movements. If you play sports that involve strenuous arm movements, such as tennis, or regularly lift heavy weights, shoulder injuries are a risk. Shoulder pain and/or stiffness without any obvious cause occurs most commonly in elderly people.

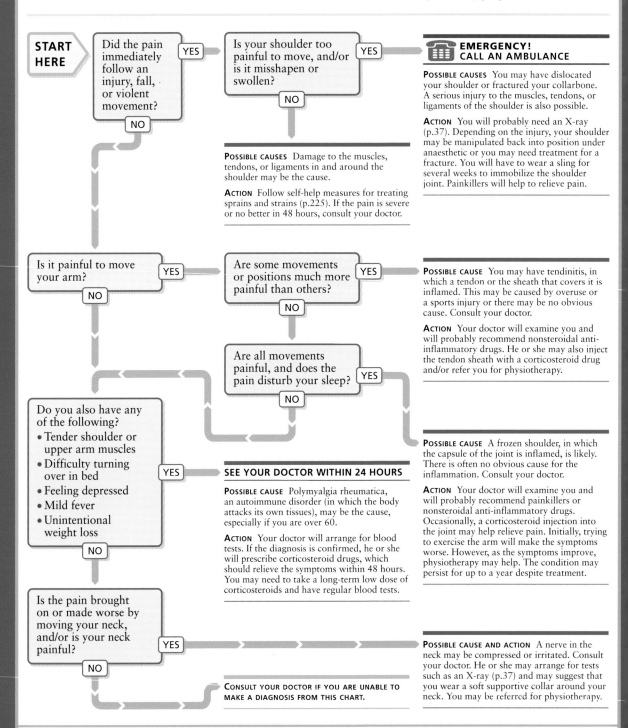

START HERE

Did the pain immediately follow an injury, fall, or violent movement?

YES →

Is your shoulder too painful to move, and/or is it misshapen or swollen?

YES →

📞 EMERGENCY! CALL AN AMBULANCE

POSSIBLE CAUSES You may have dislocated your shoulder or fractured your collarbone. A serious injury to the muscles, tendons, or ligaments of the shoulder is also possible.

ACTION You will probably need an X-ray (p.37). Depending on the injury, your shoulder may be manipulated back into position under anaesthetic or you may need treatment for a fracture. You will have to wear a sling for several weeks to immobilize the shoulder joint. Painkillers will help to relieve pain.

NO ↓

POSSIBLE CAUSES Damage to the muscles, tendons, or ligaments in and around the shoulder may be the cause.

ACTION Follow self-help measures for treating sprains and strains (p.225). If the pain is severe or no better in 48 hours, consult your doctor.

NO ↓

Is it painful to move your arm?

YES →

Are some movements or positions much more painful than others?

YES →

POSSIBLE CAUSE You may have tendinitis, in which a tendon or the sheath that covers it is inflamed. This may be caused by overuse or a sports injury or there may be no obvious cause. Consult your doctor.

ACTION Your doctor will examine you and will probably recommend nonsteroidal anti-inflammatory drugs. He or she may also inject the tendon sheath with a corticosteroid drug and/or refer you for physiotherapy.

NO ↓

Are all movements painful, and does the pain disturb your sleep?

YES →

POSSIBLE CAUSE A frozen shoulder, in which the capsule of the joint is inflamed, is likely. There is often no obvious cause for the inflammation. Consult your doctor.

ACTION Your doctor will examine you and will probably recommend painkillers or nonsteroidal anti-inflammatory drugs. Occasionally, a corticosteroid injection into the joint may help relieve pain. Initially, trying to exercise the arm will make the symptoms worse. However, as the symptoms improve, physiotherapy may help. The condition may persist for up to a year despite treatment.

NO ↓

Do you also have any of the following?
- Tender shoulder or upper arm muscles
- Difficulty turning over in bed
- Feeling depressed
- Mild fever
- Unintentional weight loss

YES →

SEE YOUR DOCTOR WITHIN 24 HOURS

POSSIBLE CAUSE Polymyalgia rheumatica, an autoimmune disorder (in which the body attacks its own tissues), may be the cause, especially if you are over 60.

ACTION Your doctor will arrange for blood tests. If the diagnosis is confirmed, he or she will prescribe corticosteroid drugs, which should relieve the symptoms within 48 hours. You may need to take a long-term low dose of corticosteroids and have regular blood tests.

NO ↓

Is the pain brought on or made worse by moving your neck, and/or is your neck painful?

YES →

POSSIBLE CAUSE AND ACTION A nerve in the neck may be compressed or irritated. Consult your doctor. He or she may arrange for tests such as an X-ray (p.37) and may suggest that you wear a soft supportive collar around your neck. You may be referred for physiotherapy.

NO ↓

CONSULT YOUR DOCTOR IF YOU ARE UNABLE TO MAKE A DIAGNOSIS FROM THIS CHART.

112 Painful arm

Pain in the arm may result from injury or straining of the muscles, tendons, or ligaments that hold the various bones and joints in place. Such injuries are particularly likely to occur after any unaccustomed, strenuous physical activity, such as playing a sport for the first time in many years. Arm pain that develops gradually may originate from problems in the neck. In some cases, pain may be related to repetitive movements such as typing or playing a musical instrument.

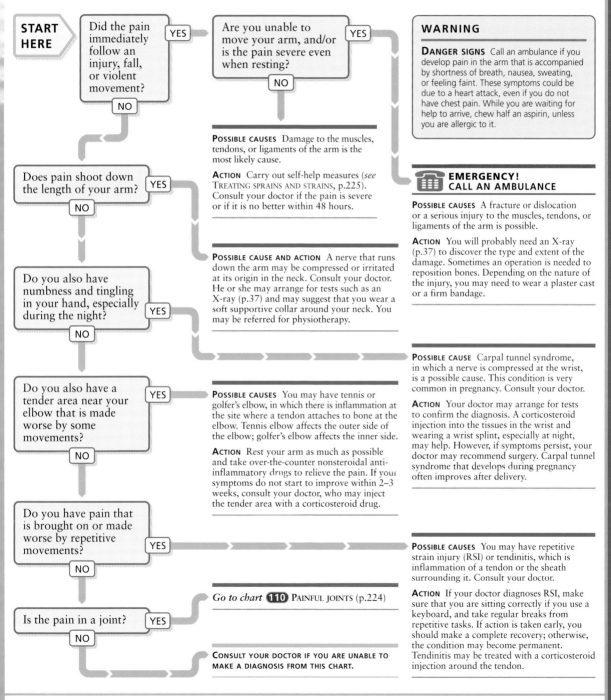

START HERE

Did the pain immediately follow an injury, fall, or violent movement? — YES → **Are you unable to move your arm, and/or is the pain severe even when resting?** — YES →

NO ↓ (from first box)

Does pain shoot down the length of your arm? — YES →

NO ↓

Do you also have numbness and tingling in your hand, especially during the night? — YES →

NO ↓

Do you also have a tender area near your elbow that is made worse by some movements? — YES →

NO ↓

Do you have pain that is brought on or made worse by repetitive movements? — YES →

NO ↓

Is the pain in a joint? — YES →

NO ↓

WARNING

DANGER SIGNS Call an ambulance if you develop pain in the arm that is accompanied by shortness of breath, nausea, sweating, or feeling faint. These symptoms could be due to a heart attack, even if you do not have chest pain. While you are waiting for help to arrive, chew half an aspirin, unless you are allergic to it.

(from "Are you unable to move your arm" NO)

POSSIBLE CAUSES Damage to the muscles, tendons, or ligaments of the arm is the most likely cause.

ACTION Carry out self-help measures (*see* TREATING SPRAINS AND STRAINS, p.225). Consult your doctor if the pain is severe or if it is no better within 48 hours.

POSSIBLE CAUSE AND ACTION A nerve that runs down the arm may be compressed or irritated at its origin in the neck. Consult your doctor. He or she may arrange for tests such as an X-ray (p.37) and may suggest that you wear a soft supportive collar around your neck. You may be referred for physiotherapy.

POSSIBLE CAUSES You may have tennis or golfer's elbow, in which there is inflammation at the site where a tendon attaches to bone at the elbow. Tennis elbow affects the outer side of the elbow; golfer's elbow affects the inner side.

ACTION Rest your arm as much as possible and take over-the-counter nonsteroidal anti-inflammatory drugs to relieve the pain. If your symptoms do not start to improve within 2–3 weeks, consult your doctor, who may inject the tender area with a corticosteroid drug.

Go to chart **110** PAINFUL JOINTS (p.224)

CONSULT YOUR DOCTOR IF YOU ARE UNABLE TO MAKE A DIAGNOSIS FROM THIS CHART.

📞 **EMERGENCY! CALL AN AMBULANCE**

POSSIBLE CAUSES A fracture or dislocation or a serious injury to the muscles, tendons, or ligaments of the arm is possible.

ACTION You will probably need an X-ray (p.37) to discover the type and extent of the damage. Sometimes an operation is needed to reposition bones. Depending on the nature of the injury, you may need to wear a plaster cast or a firm bandage.

POSSIBLE CAUSE Carpal tunnel syndrome, in which a nerve is compressed at the wrist, is a possible cause. This condition is very common in pregnancy. Consult your doctor.

ACTION Your doctor may arrange for tests to confirm the diagnosis. A corticosteroid injection into the tissues in the wrist and wearing a wrist splint, especially at night, may help. However, if symptoms persist, your doctor may recommend surgery. Carpal tunnel syndrome that develops during pregnancy often improves after delivery.

POSSIBLE CAUSES You may have repetitive strain injury (RSI) or tendinitis, which is inflammation of a tendon or the sheath surrounding it. Consult your doctor.

ACTION If your doctor diagnoses RSI, make sure that you are sitting correctly if you use a keyboard, and take regular breaks from repetitive tasks. If action is taken early, you should make a complete recovery; otherwise, the condition may become permanent. Tendinitis may be treated with a corticosteroid injection around the tendon.

113 Painful leg

For pain in the foot, see chart 116, FOOT PROBLEMS (p.232).
Pain in the leg is often the result of minor damage to muscles, tendons, or ligaments. Such injuries are likely to be the cause of pain that comes on after unaccustomed strenuous exercise or playing a sport for the first time in years. However, pain in the leg may also have a more serious cause, such as a disorder affecting the blood vessels that supply the leg. If you are in any doubt about the cause of a painful leg, consult your doctor.

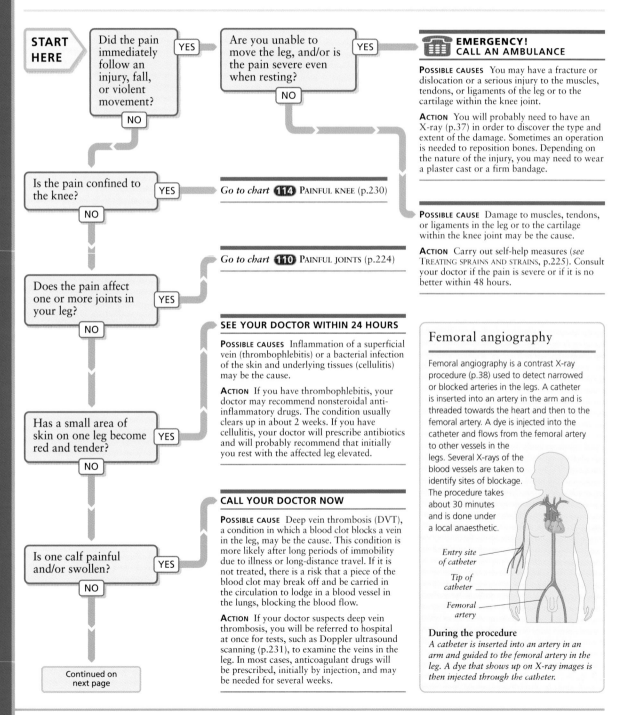

START HERE

Did the pain immediately follow an injury, fall, or violent movement? — **YES** → Are you unable to move the leg, and/or is the pain severe even when resting? — **YES** →

NO ↓ / **NO** ↓

☎ **EMERGENCY! CALL AN AMBULANCE**

POSSIBLE CAUSES You may have a fracture or dislocation or a serious injury to the muscles, tendons, or ligaments of the leg or to the cartilage within the knee joint.

ACTION You will probably need to have an X-ray (p.37) in order to discover the type and extent of the damage. Sometimes an operation is needed to reposition bones. Depending on the nature of the injury, you may need to wear a plaster cast or a firm bandage.

Is the pain confined to the knee? — **YES** → *Go to chart* **114** PAINFUL KNEE (p.230)

NO ↓

POSSIBLE CAUSE Damage to muscles, tendons, or ligaments in the leg or to the cartilage within the knee joint may be the cause.

ACTION Carry out self-help measures (*see* TREATING SPRAINS AND STRAINS, p.225). Consult your doctor if the pain is severe or if it is no better within 48 hours.

Does the pain affect one or more joints in your leg? — **YES** → *Go to chart* **110** PAINFUL JOINTS (p.224)

NO ↓

Has a small area of skin on one leg become red and tender? — **YES** →

NO ↓

SEE YOUR DOCTOR WITHIN 24 HOURS

POSSIBLE CAUSES Inflammation of a superficial vein (thrombophlebitis) or a bacterial infection of the skin and underlying tissues (cellulitis) may be the cause.

ACTION If you have thrombophlebitis, your doctor may recommend nonsteroidal anti-inflammatory drugs. The condition usually clears up in about 2 weeks. If you have cellulitis, your doctor will prescribe antibiotics and will probably recommend that initially you rest with the affected leg elevated.

Is one calf painful and/or swollen? — **YES** →

NO ↓

CALL YOUR DOCTOR NOW

POSSIBLE CAUSE Deep vein thrombosis (DVT), a condition in which a blood clot blocks a vein in the leg, may be the cause. This condition is more likely after long periods of immobility due to illness or long-distance travel. If it is not treated, there is a risk that a piece of the blood clot may break off and be carried in the circulation to lodge in a blood vessel in the lungs, blocking the blood flow.

ACTION If your doctor suspects deep vein thrombosis, you will be referred to hospital at once for tests, such as Doppler ultrasound scanning (p.231), to examine the veins in the leg. In most cases, anticoagulant drugs will be prescribed, initially by injection, and may be needed for several weeks.

Continued on next page

Femoral angiography

Femoral angiography is a contrast X-ray procedure (p.38) used to detect narrowed or blocked arteries in the legs. A catheter is inserted into an artery in the arm and is threaded towards the heart and then to the femoral artery. A dye is injected into the catheter and flows from the femoral artery to other vessels in the legs. Several X-rays of the blood vessels are taken to identify sites of blockage. The procedure takes about 30 minutes and is done under a local anaesthetic.

Entry site of catheter

Tip of catheter

Femoral artery

During the procedure
A catheter is inserted into an artery in an arm and guided to the femoral artery in the leg. A dye that shows up on X-ray images is then injected through the catheter.

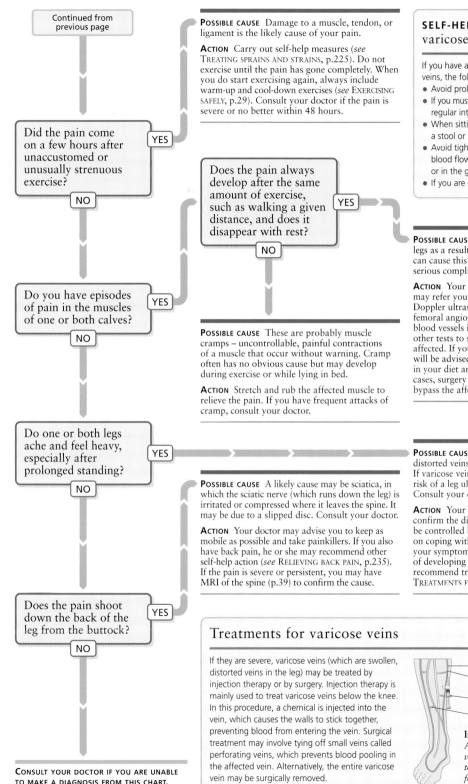

Continued from previous page

Did the pain come on a few hours after unaccustomed or unusually strenuous exercise?

YES

POSSIBLE CAUSE Damage to a muscle, tendon, or ligament is the likely cause of your pain.

ACTION Carry out self-help measures (*see* TREATING SPRAINS AND STRAINS, p.225). Do not exercise until the pain has gone completely. When you do start exercising again, always include warm-up and cool-down exercises (*see* EXERCISING SAFELY, p.29). Consult your doctor if the pain is severe or no better within 48 hours.

NO

Does the pain always develop after the same amount of exercise, such as walking a given distance, and does it disappear with rest?

YES

NO

Do you have episodes of pain in the muscles of one or both calves?

YES

POSSIBLE CAUSE These are probably muscle cramps – uncontrollable, painful contractions of a muscle that occur without warning. Cramp often has no obvious cause but may develop during exercise or while lying in bed.

ACTION Stretch and rub the affected muscle to relieve the pain. If you have frequent attacks of cramp, consult your doctor.

NO

Do one or both legs ache and feel heavy, especially after prolonged standing?

YES

NO

POSSIBLE CAUSE A likely cause may be sciatica, in which the sciatic nerve (which runs down the leg) is irritated or compressed where it leaves the spine. It may be due to a slipped disc. Consult your doctor.

ACTION Your doctor may advise you to keep as mobile as possible and take painkillers. If you also have back pain, he or she may recommend other self-help action (*see* RELIEVING BACK PAIN, p.235). If the pain is severe or persistent, you may have MRI of the spine (p.39) to confirm the cause.

Does the pain shoot down the back of the leg from the buttock?

YES

NO

CONSULT YOUR DOCTOR IF YOU ARE UNABLE TO MAKE A DIAGNOSIS FROM THIS CHART.

SELF-HELP Coping with varicose veins

If you have aching legs caused by varicose veins, the following measures may help:
- Avoid prolonged standing.
- If you must stand, move your feet and legs at regular intervals to keep the blood flowing.
- When sitting, keep your legs elevated on a stool or footrest.
- Avoid tight clothing that may restrict the blood flow in the legs either at the knee or in the groin.
- If you are overweight, try to lose weight.

POSSIBLE CAUSE Impaired blood flow to the legs as a result of narrowing of the arteries can cause this type of pain and may result in serious complications. Consult your doctor.

ACTION Your doctor will examine you and may refer you to hospital for tests such as Doppler ultrasound scanning (p.231) or femoral angiography (opposite) to assess the blood vessels in your legs. You may also need other tests to see if blood vessels elsewhere are affected. If you smoke, you should stop. You will be advised to cut down the amount of fat in your diet and take regular exercise. In some cases, surgery will be required to widen or bypass the affected arteries.

POSSIBLE CAUSE Varicose veins, swollen and distorted veins in the legs, may be the cause. If varicose veins are severe, they increase the risk of a leg ulcer developing in the future. Consult your doctor.

ACTION Your doctor will examine you to confirm the diagnosis. Symptoms can usually be controlled by following self-help advice on coping with varicose veins (above). If your symptoms are severe or you are at risk of developing a leg ulcer, your doctor may recommend treatment such as surgery (*see* TREATMENTS FOR VARICOSE VEINS, below).

Treatments for varicose veins

If they are severe, varicose veins (which are swollen, distorted veins in the leg) may be treated by injection therapy or by surgery. Injection therapy is mainly used to treat varicose veins below the knee. In this procedure, a chemical is injected into the vein, which causes the walls to stick together, preventing blood from entering the vein. Surgical treatment may involve tying off small veins called perforating veins, which prevents blood pooling in the affected vein. Alternatively, the entire varicose vein may be surgically removed.

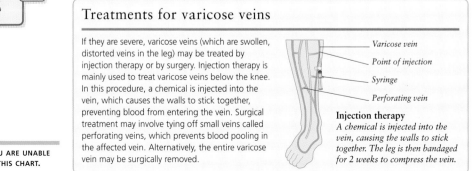

Varicose vein
Point of injection
Syringe
Perforating vein

Injection therapy
A chemical is injected into the vein, causing the walls to stick together. The leg is then bandaged for 2 weeks to compress the vein.

114 Painful knee

The knee is one of the principal weight-bearing joints in the body and is subject to much wear and tear. Its stability largely depends on the muscles and ligaments around it.

Doing work that involves a lot of bending or kneeling, or playing certain sports, increases the risk of damaging your knees. Consult this chart if one or both knees are painful.

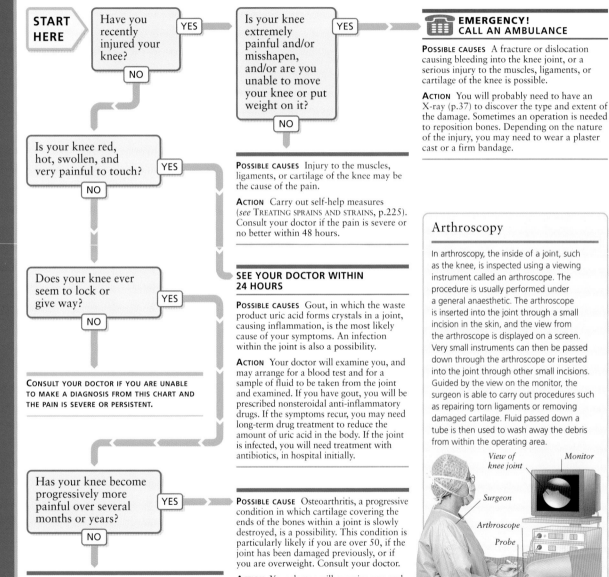

START HERE

Have you recently injured your knee?
YES → **Is your knee extremely painful and/or misshapen, and/or are you unable to move your knee or put weight on it?**

YES →

☎ **EMERGENCY! CALL AN AMBULANCE**

POSSIBLE CAUSES A fracture or dislocation causing bleeding into the knee joint, or a serious injury to the muscles, ligaments, or cartilage of the knee is possible.

ACTION You will probably need to have an X-ray (p.37) to discover the type and extent of the damage. Sometimes an operation is needed to reposition bones. Depending on the nature of the injury, you may need to wear a plaster cast or a firm bandage.

NO →

Have you recently injured your knee? NO ↓

Is your knee extremely... put weight on it? NO ↓

POSSIBLE CAUSES Injury to the muscles, ligaments, or cartilage of the knee may be the cause of the pain.

ACTION Carry out self-help measures (*see* TREATING SPRAINS AND STRAINS, p.225). Consult your doctor if the pain is severe or no better within 48 hours.

Is your knee red, hot, swollen, and very painful to touch?
YES →

SEE YOUR DOCTOR WITHIN 24 HOURS

POSSIBLE CAUSES Gout, in which the waste product uric acid forms crystals in a joint, causing inflammation, is the most likely cause of your symptoms. An infection within the joint is also a possibility.

ACTION Your doctor will examine you, and may arrange for a blood test and for a sample of fluid to be taken from the joint and examined. If you have gout, you will be prescribed nonsteroidal anti-inflammatory drugs. If the symptoms recur, you may need long-term drug treatment to reduce the amount of uric acid in the body. If the joint is infected, you will need treatment with antibiotics, in hospital initially.

NO ↓

Does your knee ever seem to lock or give way?
YES →

CONSULT YOUR DOCTOR IF YOU ARE UNABLE TO MAKE A DIAGNOSIS FROM THIS CHART AND THE PAIN IS SEVERE OR PERSISTENT.

NO ↓

Has your knee become progressively more painful over several months or years?
YES →

POSSIBLE CAUSE Osteoarthritis, a progressive condition in which cartilage covering the ends of the bones within a joint is slowly destroyed, is a possibility. This condition is particularly likely if you are over 50, if the joint has been damaged previously, or if you are overweight. Consult your doctor.

ACTION Your doctor will examine you and may arrange for you to have blood tests and an X-ray (p.37) to confirm the diagnosis. Over-the-counter painkillers should help to relieve your symptoms. If you are also overweight, it will help to lose weight. In some cases, your doctor may refer you for physiotherapy to strengthen the muscles around the joint. In severe cases, a joint replacement (p.225) may be needed.

NO ↓

POSSIBLE CAUSES A torn cartilage or damage to a ligament within the knee joint may be the cause. Such injuries are commonly caused by twisting the joint while it is supporting your weight. Consult your doctor.

ACTION You doctor may refer you to hospital for tests such as arthroscopy (right). Any damage may be repaired during the arthroscopy, or you may require surgery at a later date.

Arthroscopy

In arthroscopy, the inside of a joint, such as the knee, is inspected using a viewing instrument called an arthroscope. The procedure is usually performed under a general anaesthetic. The arthroscope is inserted into the joint through a small incision in the skin, and the view from the arthroscope is displayed on a screen. Very small instruments can then be passed down through the arthroscope or inserted into the joint through other small incisions. Guided by the view on the monitor, the surgeon is able to carry out procedures such as repairing torn ligaments or removing damaged cartilage. Fluid passed down a tube is then used to wash away the debris from within the operating area.

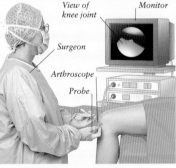

View of knee joint — *Monitor*
Surgeon
Arthroscope
Probe

During the procedure
An arthroscope and a probe are inserted into the joint, allowing the surgeon to inspect the joint. The probe can be used to manipulate the cartilage and improve the view.

115 Swollen ankles

If you are pregnant, see chart 146, SWOLLEN ANKLES IN PREGNANCY (p.279). For painful swelling of one or both ankles, see chart 110, PAINFUL JOINTS (p.224).
Painless swelling of the ankles is most often caused by fluid accumulating in the tissues after long periods of sitting or standing still. It is also common in pregnancy due to increased pressure on blood vessels in the abdomen. However, occasionally, swelling of the ankles may be due to a potentially serious heart, liver, or kidney disorder. If you frequently have swollen ankles, consult your doctor.

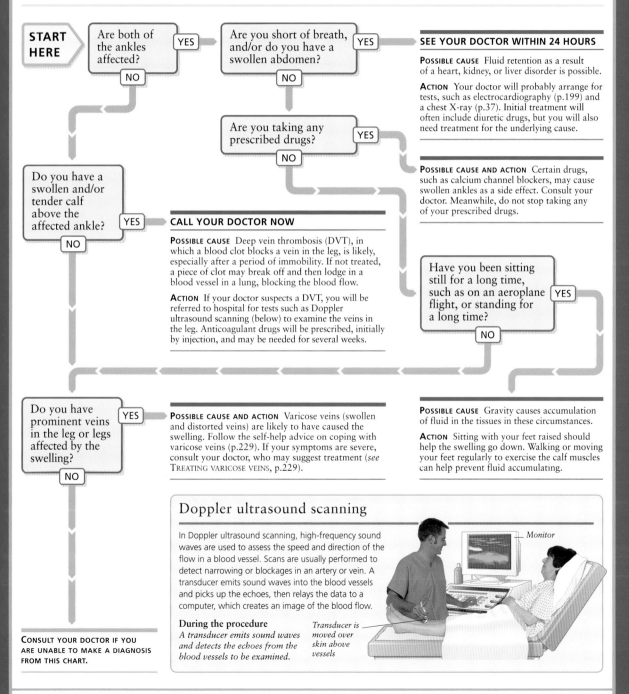

START HERE

Are both of the ankles affected? — YES → **Are you short of breath, and/or do you have a swollen abdomen?** — YES →

SEE YOUR DOCTOR WITHIN 24 HOURS

POSSIBLE CAUSE Fluid retention as a result of a heart, kidney, or liver disorder is possible.

ACTION Your doctor will probably arrange for tests, such as electrocardiography (p.199) and a chest X-ray (p.37). Initial treatment will often include diuretic drugs, but you will also need treatment for the underlying cause.

Are you short of breath, and/or do you have a swollen abdomen? — NO →

Are you taking any prescribed drugs? — YES →

POSSIBLE CAUSE AND ACTION Certain drugs, such as calcium channel blockers, may cause swollen ankles as a side effect. Consult your doctor. Meanwhile, do not stop taking any of your prescribed drugs.

Are you taking any prescribed drugs? — NO

Are both of the ankles affected? — NO

Do you have a swollen and/or tender calf above the affected ankle? — YES →

CALL YOUR DOCTOR NOW

POSSIBLE CAUSE Deep vein thrombosis (DVT), in which a blood clot blocks a vein in the leg, is likely, especially after a period of immobility. If not treated, a piece of clot may break off and then lodge in a blood vessel in a lung, blocking the blood flow.

ACTION If your doctor suspects a DVT, you will be referred to hospital for tests such as Doppler ultrasound scanning (below) to examine the veins in the leg. Anticoagulant drugs will be prescribed, initially by injection, and may be needed for several weeks.

Have you been sitting still for a long time, such as on an aeroplane flight, or standing for a long time? — YES →

POSSIBLE CAUSE Gravity causes accumulation of fluid in the tissues in these circumstances.

ACTION Sitting with your feet raised should help the swelling go down. Walking or moving your feet regularly to exercise the calf muscles can help prevent fluid accumulating.

Have you been sitting still for a long time...? — NO

Do you have a swollen and/or tender calf above the affected ankle? — NO

Do you have prominent veins in the leg or legs affected by the swelling? — YES →

POSSIBLE CAUSE AND ACTION Varicose veins (swollen and distorted veins) are likely to have caused the swelling. Follow the self-help advice on coping with varicose veins (p.229). If your symptoms are severe, consult your doctor, who may suggest treatment (*see* TREATING VARICOSE VEINS, p.229).

Do you have prominent veins in the leg or legs affected by the swelling? — NO

CONSULT YOUR DOCTOR IF YOU ARE UNABLE TO MAKE A DIAGNOSIS FROM THIS CHART.

Doppler ultrasound scanning

In Doppler ultrasound scanning, high-frequency sound waves are used to assess the speed and direction of the flow in a blood vessel. Scans are usually performed to detect narrowing or blockages in an artery or vein. A transducer emits sound waves into the blood vessels and picks up the echoes, then relays the data to a computer, which creates an image of the blood flow.

Monitor

During the procedure
A transducer emits sound waves and detects the echoes from the blood vessels to be examined.

Transducer is moved over skin above vessels

116 Foot problems

For ankles that are swollen but not painful, see chart 115, SWOLLEN ANKLES (p.231).

Most foot problems are the result of an injury or infections of the skin or nails. They are usually minor, except in people whose feet are affected by poor circulation, including those who have diabetes mellitus. Consult this chart if you have any pain, irritation, or itching in your feet or if your feet become misshapen in any way.

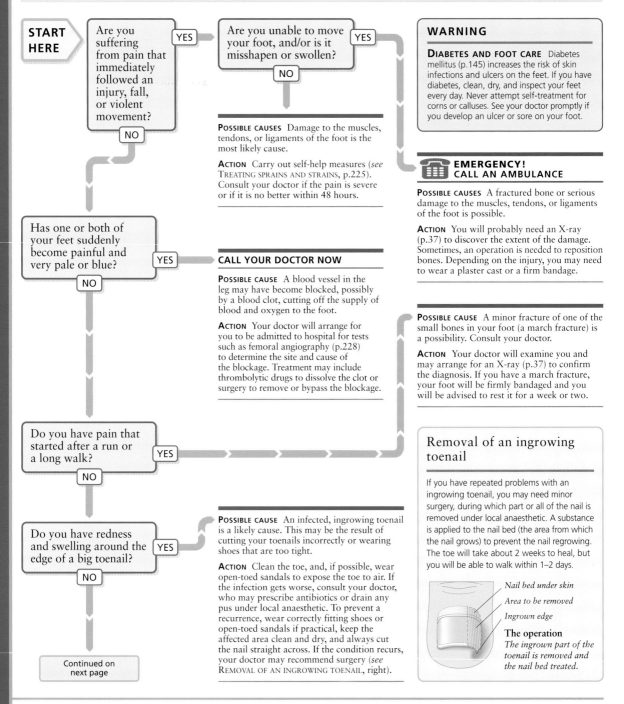

START HERE

Are you suffering from pain that immediately followed an injury, fall, or violent movement? — YES → **Are you unable to move your foot, and/or is it misshapen or swollen?** — YES →

NO ↓ (from first question)
NO ↓ (from second question)

POSSIBLE CAUSES Damage to the muscles, tendons, or ligaments of the foot is the most likely cause.

ACTION Carry out self-help measures (*see* TREATING SPRAINS AND STRAINS, p.225). Consult your doctor if the pain is severe or if it is no better within 48 hours.

Has one or both of your feet suddenly become painful and very pale or blue? — YES →

NO ↓

CALL YOUR DOCTOR NOW

POSSIBLE CAUSE A blood vessel in the leg may have become blocked, possibly by a blood clot, cutting off the supply of blood and oxygen to the foot.

ACTION Your doctor will arrange for you to be admitted to hospital for tests such as femoral angiography (p.228) to determine the site and cause of the blockage. Treatment may include thrombolytic drugs to dissolve the clot or surgery to remove or bypass the blockage.

Do you have pain that started after a run or a long walk? — YES →

NO ↓

Do you have redness and swelling around the edge of a big toenail? — YES →

NO ↓

POSSIBLE CAUSE An infected, ingrowing toenail is a likely cause. This may be the result of cutting your toenails incorrectly or wearing shoes that are too tight.

ACTION Clean the toe, and, if possible, wear open-toed sandals to expose the toe to air. If the infection gets worse, consult your doctor, who may prescribe antibiotics or drain any pus under local anaesthetic. To prevent a recurrence, wear correctly fitting shoes or open-toed sandals if practical, keep the affected area clean and dry, and always cut the nail straight across. If the condition recurs, your doctor may recommend surgery (*see* REMOVAL OF AN INGROWING TOENAIL, right).

Continued on next page

WARNING

DIABETES AND FOOT CARE Diabetes mellitus (p.145) increases the risk of skin infections and ulcers on the feet. If you have diabetes, clean, dry, and inspect your feet every day. Never attempt self-treatment for corns or calluses. See your doctor promptly if you develop an ulcer or sore on your foot.

EMERGENCY! CALL AN AMBULANCE

POSSIBLE CAUSES A fractured bone or serious damage to the muscles, tendons, or ligaments of the foot is possible.

ACTION You will probably need an X-ray (p.37) to discover the extent of the damage. Sometimes, an operation is needed to reposition bones. Depending on the injury, you may need to wear a plaster cast or a firm bandage.

POSSIBLE CAUSE A minor fracture of one of the small bones in your foot (a march fracture) is a possibility. Consult your doctor.

ACTION Your doctor will examine you and may arrange for an X-ray (p.37) to confirm the diagnosis. If you have a march fracture, your foot will be firmly bandaged and you will be advised to rest it for a week or two.

Removal of an ingrowing toenail

If you have repeated problems with an ingrowing toenail, you may need minor surgery, during which part or all of the nail is removed under local anaesthetic. A substance is applied to the nail bed (the area from which the nail grows) to prevent the nail regrowing. The toe will take about 2 weeks to heal, but you will be able to walk within 1–2 days.

Nail bed under skin

Area to be removed

Ingrown edge

The operation
The ingrown part of the toenail is removed and the nail bed treated.

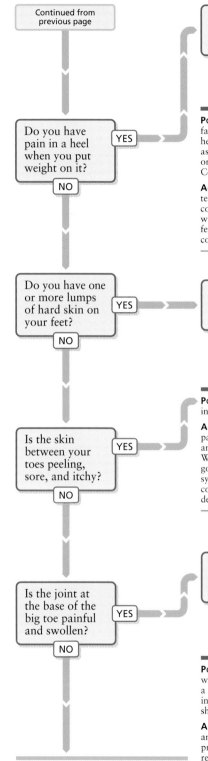

Continued from previous page

Do you have pain in a heel when you put weight on it? — YES

Is the skin of the heel thickened, and are there painful cracks? — YES

> **POSSIBLE CAUSE** Thickened skin on the heels tends to crack over time, causing pain.
>
> **ACTION** Avoid thickened skin building up by soaking your feet and then using a pumice stone or foot file on the skin. Use moisturizing cream regularly. If these measures do not help, consult your doctor or a chiropodist. If you have diabetes mellitus (p.145), consult your doctor before removing thickened skin.

NO

> **POSSIBLE CAUSE** You may have plantar fasciitis, in which fibrous tissues in the heel are inflamed. This condition may be associated with certain types of arthritis or an overgrowth of bone under the heel. Consult your doctor.
>
> **ACTION** Your doctor may arrange for blood tests or X-rays (p.37) to look for associated conditions. He or she may recommend you wear inserts in your shoes to cushion your feet. You may be given an injection of a corticosteroid drug into the heel.

NO

Do you have one or more lumps of hard skin on your feet? — YES

Are the lumps on the toes or the sides of the feet? — YES

> **POSSIBLE CAUSE** These are probably areas of abnormally thickened skin that are known as calluses (or corns if they are on a toe). Calluses and corns form to protect the foot in areas where there is excessive pressure, such as that caused by badly fitting shoes.
>
> **ACTION** Soak your feet to soften the skin, and rub the lumps with a pumice stone. Adhesive sponge padding, available over the counter, can be stuck over tender areas to protect them from pressure. If this does not help, consult your doctor or a chiropodist. If you have diabetes, consult your doctor before removing any thickened skin. To prevent a recurrence, always wear correctly fitting shoes.

NO

NO

Is the skin between your toes peeling, sore, and itchy? — YES

> **POSSIBLE CAUSE** Athlete's foot, a fungal infection, is the likeliest cause.
>
> **ACTION** Wash and dry your feet carefully, particularly between your toes, and apply an over-the-counter antifungal preparation. When indoors, wear open-toed sandals or go without shoes whenever possible. If the symptoms persist for more than 2 weeks, consult your doctor. If redness and swelling develop, see your doctor within 24 hours.

> **POSSIBLE CAUSE** A verruca, a wart caused by a viral infection of the skin, is a possibility, especially if the lump is on the sole of the foot. A verruca may be tender because it grows into the sole of the foot.
>
> **ACTION** Most verrucas disappear without treatment, but this may take months or years. Several preparations for treating verrucas are available over the counter. If a verruca persists after self-treatment and is painful, consult your doctor. He or she may destroy the verruca by freezing it with liquid nitrogen.

NO

Is the joint at the base of the big toe painful and swollen? — YES

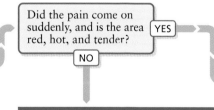

Did the pain come on suddenly, and is the area red, hot, and tender? — YES

NO

SEE YOUR DOCTOR WITHIN 24 HOURS

> **POSSIBLE CAUSES** Gout, in which uric acid accumulates in the bloodstream, causing crystals to form in the joints, is the most likely cause of these symptoms. Alternatively, you may have an infection in the joint.
>
> **ACTION** Your doctor will examine you. He or she may arrange for a blood test and may withdraw a sample of fluid from the joint for testing. If you have gout, your doctor will prescribe nonsteroidal anti-inflammatory drugs. If your symptoms recur, you may need long-term drug treatment. A joint infection usually needs to be treated in hospital.

NO

> **POSSIBLE CAUSE** You may have a bunion, in which inflamed, thickened tissue develops over a misaligned joint. The condition tends to run in families and may be made worse by wearing shoes with pointed toes.
>
> **ACTION** Although a bunion may look unsightly and cause discomfort, it is not a serious medical problem. Wearing well-fitting shoes should help reduce discomfort. If you are still concerned, consult your doctor, who may suggest surgery to correct the underlying misalignment.

CONSULT YOUR DOCTOR IF YOU ARE UNABLE TO MAKE A DIAGNOSIS FROM THIS CHART.

117 ▶ Back pain

Most people have at least one episode of back pain during their lives, and they usually recover without needing medical help. Back pain is often due to poor posture. However, it may be a sign of damage to the joints, ligaments, or discs of cartilage in the spine, in many cases as a result of tasks such as lifting excessively heavy weights. Severe back pain may be due to pressure on a nerve or, rarely, it may be due to a problem with an internal organ such as a kidney.

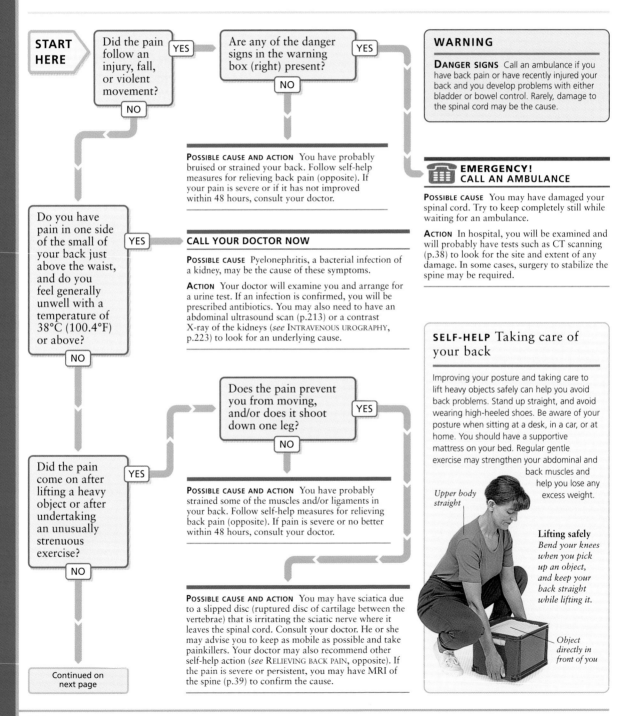

START HERE → **Did the pain follow an injury, fall, or violent movement?** —YES→ **Are any of the danger signs in the warning box (right) present?** —YES→

NO ↓

NO (from danger signs box)

POSSIBLE CAUSE AND ACTION You have probably bruised or strained your back. Follow self-help measures for relieving back pain (opposite). If your pain is severe or if it has not improved within 48 hours, consult your doctor.

Do you have pain in one side of the small of your back just above the waist, and do you feel generally unwell with a temperature of 38°C (100.4°F) or above? —YES→

NO ↓

CALL YOUR DOCTOR NOW

POSSIBLE CAUSE Pyelonephritis, a bacterial infection of a kidney, may be the cause of these symptoms.

ACTION Your doctor will examine you and arrange for a urine test. If an infection is confirmed, you will be prescribed antibiotics. You may also need to have an abdominal ultrasound scan (p.213) or a contrast X-ray of the kidneys (*see* INTRAVENOUS UROGRAPHY, p.223) to look for an underlying cause.

Does the pain prevent you from moving, and/or does it shoot down one leg? —YES→

NO ↓

Did the pain come on after lifting a heavy object or after undertaking an unusually strenuous exercise? —YES→

NO ↓

POSSIBLE CAUSE AND ACTION You have probably strained some of the muscles and/or ligaments in your back. Follow self-help measures for relieving back pain (opposite). If pain is severe or no better within 48 hours, consult your doctor.

POSSIBLE CAUSE AND ACTION You may have sciatica due to a slipped disc (ruptured disc of cartilage between the vertebrae) that is irritating the sciatic nerve where it leaves the spinal cord. Consult your doctor. He or she may advise you to keep as mobile as possible and take painkillers. Your doctor may also recommend other self-help action (*see* RELIEVING BACK PAIN, opposite). If the pain is severe or persistent, you may have MRI of the spine (p.39) to confirm the cause.

Continued on next page

WARNING

DANGER SIGNS Call an ambulance if you have back pain or have recently injured your back and you develop problems with either bladder or bowel control. Rarely, damage to the spinal cord may be the cause.

📞 EMERGENCY! CALL AN AMBULANCE

POSSIBLE CAUSE You may have damaged your spinal cord. Try to keep completely still while waiting for an ambulance.

ACTION In hospital, you will be examined and will probably have tests such as CT scanning (p.38) to look for the site and extent of any damage. In some cases, surgery to stabilize the spine may be required.

SELF-HELP Taking care of your back

Improving your posture and taking care to lift heavy objects safely can help you avoid back problems. Stand up straight, and avoid wearing high-heeled shoes. Be aware of your posture when sitting at a desk, in a car, or at home. You should have a supportive mattress on your bed. Regular gentle exercise may strengthen your abdominal and back muscles and help you lose any excess weight.

Upper body straight

Lifting safely
Bend your knees when you pick up an object, and keep your back straight while lifting it.

Object directly in front of you

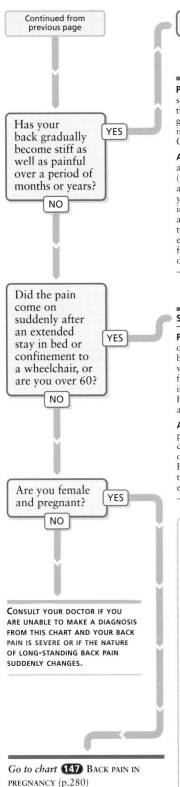

Continued from previous page

Has your back gradually become stiff as well as painful over a period of months or years?

NO / YES

Did the pain come on suddenly after an extended stay in bed or confinement to a wheelchair, or are you over 60?

NO / YES

Are you female and pregnant?

NO / YES

CONSULT YOUR DOCTOR IF YOU ARE UNABLE TO MAKE A DIAGNOSIS FROM THIS CHART AND YOUR BACK PAIN IS SEVERE OR IF THE NATURE OF LONG-STANDING BACK PAIN SUDDENLY CHANGES.

Go to chart **147** BACK PAIN IN PREGNANCY (p.280)

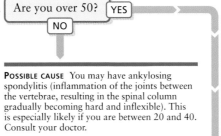

Are you over 50?

NO / YES

POSSIBLE CAUSE You may have ankylosing spondylitis (inflammation of the joints between the vertebrae, resulting in the spinal column gradually becoming hard and inflexible). This is especially likely if you are between 20 and 40. Consult your doctor.

ACTION Your doctor will examine you and arrange for you to have a blood test and X-rays (p.37) of your back and pelvic areas. If you are found to have ankylosing spondylitis, you will probably be given nonsteroidal anti-inflammatory drugs. You will also be referred to a physiotherapist, who will teach you exercises to help keep your back mobile. These mobility exercises are an essential part of the treatment for this disorder and can be supplemented by other physical activities, such as swimming.

SEE YOUR DOCTOR WITHIN 24 HOURS

POSSIBLE CAUSE You may have a crush fracture of a vertebra as a result of osteoporosis, in which bones throughout the body become thin and weak. Osteoporosis is symptomless unless a fracture occurs. The disorder is most common in women who have passed the menopause. However, a prolonged period of immobility will also lead to the development of osteoporosis.

ACTION Initial treatment for the pain is with painkillers. Your doctor may also request bone densitometry (below). Specific treatment for osteoporosis depends on the underlying cause. However, in all cases, it is important that you try to remain active and take weight-bearing exercise, such as walking.

SELF-HELP Relieving back pain

Most back pain is the result of minor sprains or strains that normally clear up on their own and can usually be helped by simple measures. Try the following:
- If possible, keep moving and carry out your normal daily activities.
- Rest in bed if the pain is severe, but do not stay in bed for more than 2 days.
- Take over-the-counter paracetamol or nonsteroidal anti-inflammatory drugs.
- Place a heating pad or wrapped hot-water bottle against the painful area.
- If heat does not provide relief, try using an ice pack (or a wrapped pack of frozen peas); place it over the painful area for 15 minutes every 2–3 hours.

If your backache is severe or is no better within 2 days, consult your doctor.

Once the pain has cleared up, follow the self-help advice for taking care of your back (opposite) to prevent a recurrence.

POSSIBLE CAUSE Osteoarthritis of the spine is probably the cause of your symptoms. In this condition, joints between the vertebrae in the spine are progressively damaged. This is particularly likely if you are over 50 and you are overweight. Consult your doctor.

ACTION Your doctor may arrange for blood tests and an X-ray (p.37) to confirm the diagnosis. Over-the-counter painkillers should help to relieve your symptoms. If you are overweight, it will help to lose weight (*see* HOW TO LOSE WEIGHT SAFELY, p.147). Your doctor may refer you for physiotherapy to help you strengthen the muscles that support the spine.

Bone densitometry

This technique uses low-intensity X-rays (p.37) to measure the density of bone. X-rays are passed through the body, and their absorption is interpreted by a computer and displayed as an image. The computer calculates the average bone density and compares it with the normal range for the person's age and sex. The procedure takes about 20 minutes and is painless.

During the procedure
The X-ray generator and detector move along the length of the spine, and information is displayed on a monitor.

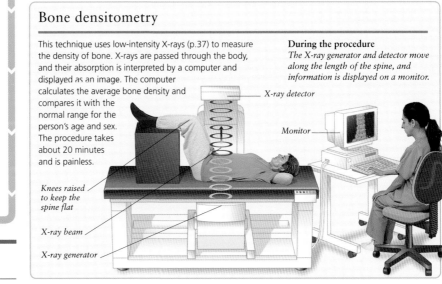

X-ray detector

Monitor

Knees raised to keep the spine flat

X-ray beam

X-ray generator

118 Painful or stiff neck

A painful or stiff neck is most often the result of a muscle spasm brought on by sitting or sleeping in an uncomfortable position or by doing unaccustomed exercise or activity.

Although the symptoms are uncomfortable, they usually improve within 48 hours without medical attention. If the pain and/or stiffness persist or become severe, consult your doctor.

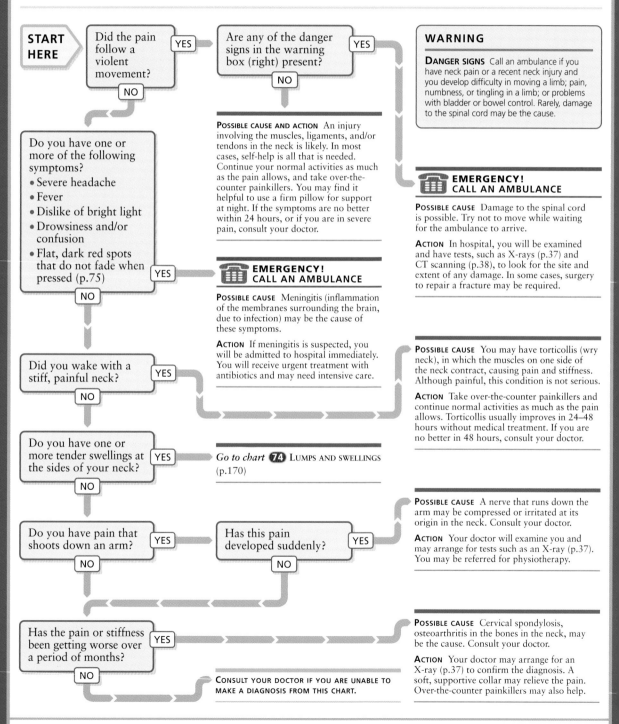

START HERE

Did the pain follow a violent movement? — YES →

Are any of the danger signs in the warning box (right) present? — YES →

NO

NO

WARNING

DANGER SIGNS Call an ambulance if you have neck pain or a recent neck injury and you develop difficulty in moving a limb; pain, numbness, or tingling in a limb; or problems with bladder or bowel control. Rarely, damage to the spinal cord may be the cause.

POSSIBLE CAUSE AND ACTION An injury involving the muscles, ligaments, and/or tendons in the neck is likely. In most cases, self-help is all that is needed. Continue your normal activities as much as the pain allows, and take over-the-counter painkillers. You may find it helpful to use a firm pillow for support at night. If the symptoms are no better within 24 hours, or if you are in severe pain, consult your doctor.

EMERGENCY! CALL AN AMBULANCE

POSSIBLE CAUSE Damage to the spinal cord is possible. Try not to move while waiting for the ambulance to arrive.

ACTION In hospital, you will be examined and have tests, such as X-rays (p.37) and CT scanning (p.38), to look for the site and extent of any damage. In some cases, surgery to repair a fracture may be required.

Do you have one or more of the following symptoms?
- Severe headache
- Fever
- Dislike of bright light
- Drowsiness and/or confusion
- Flat, dark red spots that do not fade when pressed (p.75)

— YES →

NO

EMERGENCY! CALL AN AMBULANCE

POSSIBLE CAUSE Meningitis (inflammation of the membranes surrounding the brain, due to infection) may be the cause of these symptoms.

ACTION If meningitis is suspected, you will be admitted to hospital immediately. You will receive urgent treatment with antibiotics and may need intensive care.

POSSIBLE CAUSE You may have torticollis (wry neck), in which the muscles on one side of the neck contract, causing pain and stiffness. Although painful, this condition is not serious.

ACTION Take over-the-counter painkillers and continue normal activities as much as the pain allows. Torticollis usually improves in 24–48 hours without medical treatment. If you are no better in 48 hours, consult your doctor.

Did you wake with a stiff, painful neck? — YES →

NO

Do you have one or more tender swellings at the sides of your neck? — YES →

NO

Go to chart **74** LUMPS AND SWELLINGS (p.170)

POSSIBLE CAUSE A nerve that runs down the arm may be compressed or irritated at its origin in the neck. Consult your doctor.

ACTION Your doctor will examine you and may arrange for tests such as an X-ray (p.37). You may be referred for physiotherapy.

Do you have pain that shoots down an arm? — YES →

NO

Has this pain developed suddenly? — YES →

NO

POSSIBLE CAUSE Cervical spondylosis, osteoarthritis in the bones in the neck, may be the cause. Consult your doctor.

ACTION Your doctor may arrange for an X-ray (p.37) to confirm the diagnosis. A soft, supportive collar may relieve the pain. Over-the-counter painkillers may also help.

Has the pain or stiffness been getting worse over a period of months? — YES →

NO

CONSULT YOUR DOCTOR IF YOU ARE UNABLE TO MAKE A DIAGNOSIS FROM THIS CHART.

CHARTS FOR MEN

119 Bladder control problems in men

For other urinary problems, see chart 108, GENERAL
URINARY PROBLEMS **(p.220).**
Problems with bladder control may range from a complete
inability to pass urine to incontinence, in which urine is
passed involuntarily. These problems can be due to various
underlying conditions, including an enlarged prostate gland,
which can block the outflow of urine from the bladder, and
disorders affecting the nerves that supply the bladder.

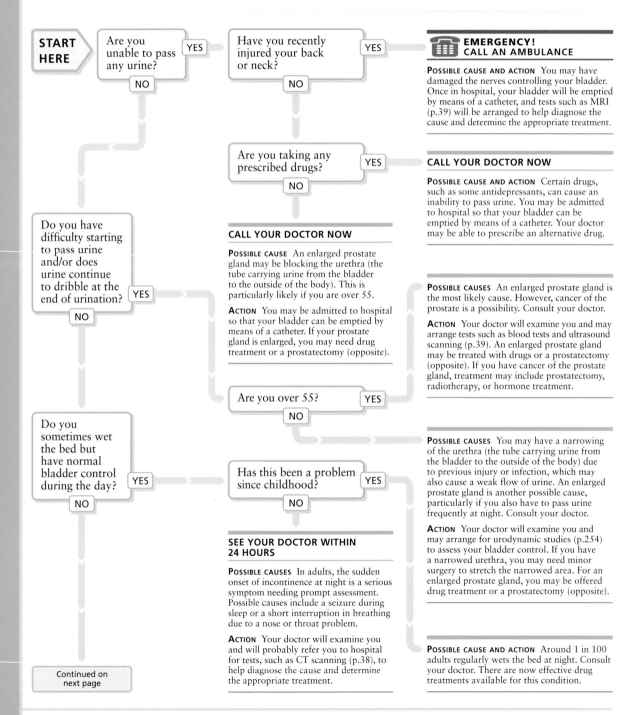

START HERE

Are you unable to pass any urine? — YES / NO

Have you recently injured your back or neck? — YES / NO

EMERGENCY! CALL AN AMBULANCE

POSSIBLE CAUSE AND ACTION You may have damaged the nerves controlling your bladder. Once in hospital, your bladder will be emptied by means of a catheter, and tests such as MRI (p.39) will be arranged to help diagnose the cause and determine the appropriate treatment.

Are you taking any prescribed drugs? — YES / NO

CALL YOUR DOCTOR NOW

POSSIBLE CAUSE AND ACTION Certain drugs, such as some antidepressants, can cause an inability to pass urine. You may be admitted to hospital so that your bladder can be emptied by means of a catheter. Your doctor may be able to prescribe an alternative drug.

Do you have difficulty starting to pass urine and/or does urine continue to dribble at the end of urination? — YES / NO

CALL YOUR DOCTOR NOW

POSSIBLE CAUSE An enlarged prostate gland may be blocking the urethra (the tube carrying urine from the bladder to the outside of the body). This is particularly likely if you are over 55.

ACTION You may be admitted to hospital so that your bladder can be emptied by means of a catheter. If your prostate gland is enlarged, you may need drug treatment or a prostatectomy (opposite).

POSSIBLE CAUSES An enlarged prostate gland is the most likely cause. However, cancer of the prostate is a possibility. Consult your doctor.

ACTION Your doctor will examine you and may arrange tests such as blood tests and ultrasound scanning (p.39). An enlarged prostate gland may be treated with drugs or a prostatectomy (opposite). If you have cancer of the prostate gland, treatment may include prostatectomy, radiotherapy, or hormone treatment.

Are you over 55? — YES / NO

Do you sometimes wet the bed but have normal bladder control during the day? — YES / NO

Has this been a problem since childhood? — YES / NO

POSSIBLE CAUSES You may have a narrowing of the urethra (the tube carrying urine from the bladder to the outside of the body) due to previous injury or infection, which may also cause a weak flow of urine. An enlarged prostate gland is another possible cause, particularly if you also have to pass urine frequently at night. Consult your doctor.

ACTION Your doctor will examine you and may arrange for urodynamic studies (p.254) to assess your bladder control. If you have a narrowed urethra, you may need minor surgery to stretch the narrowed area. For an enlarged prostate gland, you may be offered drug treatment or a prostatectomy (opposite).

SEE YOUR DOCTOR WITHIN 24 HOURS

POSSIBLE CAUSES In adults, the sudden onset of incontinence at night is a serious symptom needing prompt assessment. Possible causes include a seizure during sleep or a short interruption in breathing due to a nose or throat problem.

ACTION Your doctor will examine you and will probably refer you to hospital for tests, such as CT scanning (p.38), to help diagnose the cause and determine the appropriate treatment.

POSSIBLE CAUSE AND ACTION Around 1 in 100 adults regularly wets the bed at night. Consult your doctor. There are now effective drug treatments available for this condition.

Continued on next page

Continued from previous page

Do you have problems with incontinence during the daytime? **YES**

Do any of the following apply to you?
- You have had a stroke
- You have diabetes
- You have multiple sclerosis or another long-standing nervous system disorder

YES

POSSIBLE CAUSE In some cases, damage to the brain, spinal cord, or nerves controlling the bladder can cause continence problems. Consult your doctor.

ACTION Your doctor will examine you and may request a urine test to exclude an additional problem such as a urine infection. In some cases, drug treatment may help. Alternatively, you may be referred to a continence adviser, who will help you manage the problem.

NO

NO

CONSULT YOUR DOCTOR IF YOU ARE UNABLE TO MAKE A DIAGNOSIS FROM THIS CHART.

POSSIBLE CAUSE In some cases, constipation can prevent the bladder from emptying normally, resulting in the bladder becoming overfilled and sometimes leaking urine. Consult your doctor.

ACTION Your doctor will examine you in order to confirm the diagnosis. He or she may prescribe laxatives and may arrange for tests to investigate the cause of the constipation.

Is the incontinence associated with swelling of the abdomen, and/or do you pass only small volumes of urine when you try to empty your bladder? **YES**

Are you constipated? **YES**

NO

NO

Prostatectomy

Prostatectomy is a surgical procedure in which part or all of the prostate gland is removed. Partial prostatectomy is usually performed to relieve urinary symptoms, such as leakage of urine, caused by an enlarged prostate gland. The most common procedure is transurethral prostatectomy (TURP), in which the excess tissue is removed through the urethra. Total prostatectomy may be performed to treat prostate cancer. It involves removing the entire gland through an incision in the abdomen and requires a longer stay in hospital than TURP. Both procedures can cause fertility problems because sperm may pass into the bladder on ejaculation. Other complications, such as incontinence or erectile dysfunction, are rare with TURP but can occur after total prostatectomy.

POSSIBLE CAUSE You may have an enlarged prostate gland that is blocking the flow of urine out of the bladder. This results in the bladder becoming overfilled and possibly leaking urine. Consult your doctor.

ACTION Your doctor will examine you and may arrange for tests, including blood tests and ultrasound scanning (p.39), to establish the cause. If the blockage is due to an enlarged prostate, treatment will be with either drugs or a prostatectomy (right).

Are you taking any prescribed drugs? **YES**

NO

POSSIBLE CAUSE AND ACTION Drugs such as diuretics, which result in a sudden increase in the amount of urine produced, may cause episodes of incontinence. Consult your doctor about the problem. He or she may be able to adjust your drug treatment or give you advice on coping with the effects of the drugs.

Are you over 65, and have you become increasingly forgetful? **YES**

NO

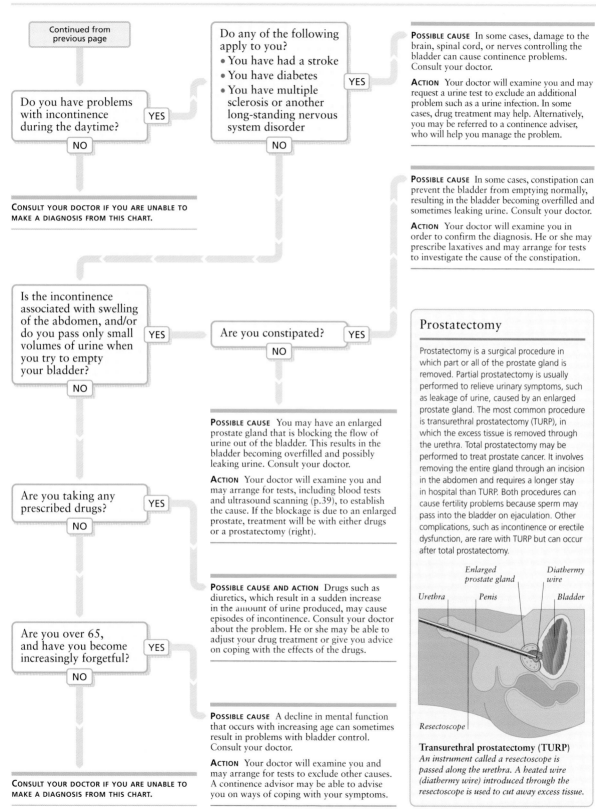

Enlarged prostate gland *Diathermy wire*

Urethra *Penis* *Bladder*

Resectoscope

Transurethral prostatectomy (TURP)
An instrument called a resectoscope is passed along the urethra. A heated wire (diathermy wire) introduced through the resectoscope is used to cut away excess tissue.

POSSIBLE CAUSE A decline in mental function that occurs with increasing age can sometimes result in problems with bladder control. Consult your doctor.

ACTION Your doctor will examine you and may arrange for tests to exclude other causes. A continence advisor may be able to advise you on ways of coping with your symptoms.

CONSULT YOUR DOCTOR IF YOU ARE UNABLE TO MAKE A DIAGNOSIS FROM THIS CHART.

120 Problems with the penis

For ejaculation problems or blood in the semen, see chart 122, Ejaculation problems *(p.243).* For pain when *passing urine, see chart 109,* Painful urination *(p.222).* Pain in the penis or soreness of the skin can signal a variety of disorders affecting the penis itself or the urinary tract.

Many painful conditions are the result of minor injuries, such as bruising or abrasion (perhaps sustained in activities such as playing sport), or are caused by infections, some of which can be sexually transmitted. Good genital hygiene is essential to avoid problems, particularly in uncircumcised men.

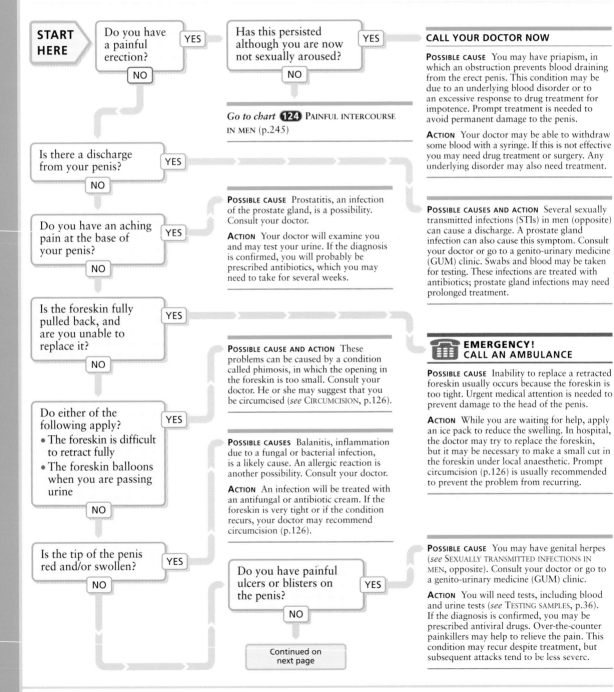

START HERE → Do you have a painful erection? — YES → Has this persisted although you are now not sexually aroused? — YES →

CALL YOUR DOCTOR NOW

POSSIBLE CAUSE You may have priapism, in which an obstruction prevents blood draining from the erect penis. This condition may be due to an underlying blood disorder or to an excessive response to drug treatment for impotence. Prompt treatment is needed to avoid permanent damage to the penis.

ACTION Your doctor may be able to withdraw some blood with a syringe. If this is not effective you may need drug treatment or surgery. Any underlying disorder may also need treatment.

Painful erection NO ↓ / *persisted* NO ↓

Go to chart **124** Painful intercourse in men *(p.245)*

Is there a discharge from your penis? — YES →

POSSIBLE CAUSE Prostatitis, an infection of the prostate gland, is a possibility. Consult your doctor.

ACTION Your doctor will examine you and may test your urine. If the diagnosis is confirmed, you will probably be prescribed antibiotics, which you may need to take for several weeks.

POSSIBLE CAUSES AND ACTION Several sexually transmitted infections (STIs) in men (opposite) can cause a discharge. A prostate gland infection can also cause this symptom. Consult your doctor or go to a genito-urinary medicine (GUM) clinic. Swabs and blood may be taken for testing. These infections are treated with antibiotics; prostate gland infections may need prolonged treatment.

NO ↓

Do you have an aching pain at the base of your penis? — YES →

NO ↓

Is the foreskin fully pulled back, and are you unable to replace it? — YES →

EMERGENCY! CALL AN AMBULANCE

POSSIBLE CAUSE Inability to replace a retracted foreskin usually occurs because the foreskin is too tight. Urgent medical attention is needed to prevent damage to the head of the penis.

ACTION While you are waiting for help, apply an ice pack to reduce the swelling. In hospital, the doctor may try to replace the foreskin, but it may be necessary to make a small cut in the foreskin under local anaesthetic. Prompt circumcision (p.126) is usually recommended to prevent the problem from recurring.

NO ↓

Do either of the following apply?
• The foreskin is difficult to retract fully
• The foreskin balloons when you are passing urine
— YES →

POSSIBLE CAUSE AND ACTION These problems can be caused by a condition called phimosis, in which the opening in the foreskin is too small. Consult your doctor. He or she may suggest that you be circumcised (*see* Circumcision, p.126).

POSSIBLE CAUSES Balanitis, inflammation due to a fungal or bacterial infection, is a likely cause. An allergic reaction is another possibility. Consult your doctor.

ACTION An infection will be treated with an antifungal or antibiotic cream. If the foreskin is very tight or if the condition recurs, your doctor may recommend circumcision (p.126).

NO ↓

Is the tip of the penis red and/or swollen? — YES →

NO ↓

Do you have painful ulcers or blisters on the penis? — YES →

POSSIBLE CAUSE You may have genital herpes (*see* Sexually transmitted infections in men, opposite). Consult your doctor or go to a genito-urinary medicine (GUM) clinic.

ACTION You will need tests, including blood and urine tests (*see* Testing samples, p.36). If the diagnosis is confirmed, you may be prescribed antiviral drugs. Over-the-counter painkillers may help to relieve the pain. This condition may recur despite treatment, but subsequent attacks tend to be less severe.

NO ↓

Continued on next page

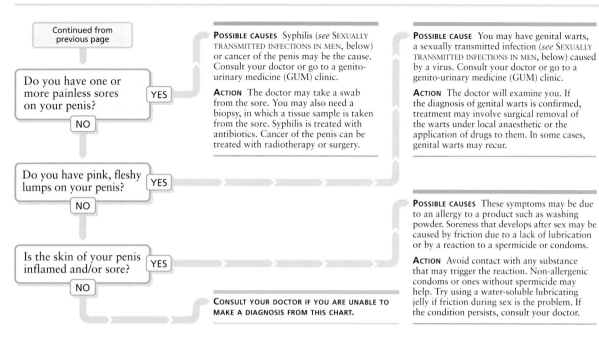

Continued from previous page

Do you have one or more painless sores on your penis? YES

NO

POSSIBLE CAUSES Syphilis (*see* SEXUALLY TRANSMITTED INFECTIONS IN MEN, below) or cancer of the penis may be the cause. Consult your doctor or go to a genito-urinary medicine (GUM) clinic.

ACTION The doctor may take a swab from the sore. You may also need a biopsy, in which a tissue sample is taken from the sore. Syphilis is treated with antibiotics. Cancer of the penis can be treated with radiotherapy or surgery.

POSSIBLE CAUSE You may have genital warts, a sexually transmitted infection (*see* SEXUALLY TRANSMITTED INFECTIONS IN MEN, below) caused by a virus. Consult your doctor or go to a genito-urinary medicine (GUM) clinic.

ACTION The doctor will examine you. If the diagnosis of genital warts is confirmed, treatment may involve surgical removal of the warts under local anaesthetic or the application of drugs to them. In some cases, genital warts may recur.

Do you have pink, fleshy lumps on your penis? YES

NO

Is the skin of your penis inflamed and/or sore? YES

NO

POSSIBLE CAUSES These symptoms may be due to an allergy to a product such as washing powder. Soreness that develops after sex may be caused by friction due to a lack of lubrication or by a reaction to a spermicide or condoms.

ACTION Avoid contact with any substance that may trigger the reaction. Non-allergenic condoms or ones without spermicide may help. Try using a water-soluble lubricating jelly if friction during sex is the problem. If the condition persists, consult your doctor.

CONSULT YOUR DOCTOR IF YOU ARE UNABLE TO MAKE A DIAGNOSIS FROM THIS CHART.

Sexually transmitted infections in men

Infections passed from one person to another during sexual intercourse (vaginal, anal, or oral) are known as sexually transmitted infections (STIs). Although these infections affect both men and women, the symptoms are often different (*see* SEXUALLY TRANSMITTED INFECTIONS IN WOMEN, p.263). The symptoms may also vary depending on the type of sexual contact you have had; for example, in homosexual men, rectal symptoms are often more common. Even if there are few symptoms, some infections can be serious

and may cause permanent damage if left untreated. If you think that you or your partner have an STI, consult your doctor or go to a genito-urinary medicine (GUM) clinic at a local hospital, where you will be treated in confidence. It is common to have more than one STI at a time, and tests will be arranged to look for several diseases. You should avoid sex until your doctor confirms that the infection has completely cleared up. The risk of contracting an STI can be reduced by practising safe sex (p.32).

Infection	Incubation period*	Symptoms in men	Diagnosis and treatment
Genital herpes	4–7 days	Initial symptoms include soreness or itching on the shaft of the penis or, in some cases, in the rectum or anus. A crop of small, painful blisters then appears. These burst to produce shallow, painful ulcers, which heal after 10–21 days. Some people may also have a fever during the attack. The condition tends to be recurrent.	The diagnosis is usually made according to the appearance of the skin. The doctor may also take a swab from one of the sores. Oral antiviral drugs taken early shorten the episodes but do not eradicate the virus. Genital herpes is most infectious while the ulcers are present, but in some cases can remain infectious after the ulcers have healed.
Genital warts	1–20 months	Pink, fleshy lumps on the penis and, in some cases, around the anus or scrotum. A rectal infection may cause pain on passing faeces.	Treatment may be by surgical removal under local anaesthetic or by applying topical drugs to the warts. In some cases, the warts may recur after treatment.
Gonorrhoea	2–10 days	There may be pain on passing urine and, in some cases, a discharge from the penis. There may also be pain in the lower abdomen and pain or tenderness in the testicles.	The doctor will take a swab from the rectum or the urethra (the tube that carries urine out of the body) to identify the infectious organism. Treatment is with antibiotics.
HIV infection	6–8 weeks	There may be no initial symptoms, but some people may have a brief flu-like illness, sometimes with a rash and swollen lymph nodes. After years without symptoms, AIDS may develop (see HIV INFECTION AND AIDS, p.144). HIV can be passed on whether or not you have symptoms.	Diagnosis is made by a blood test taken 3 or more months after the initial infection. People with HIV infection are usually referred to special centres for treatment. Combinations of antiviral drugs are given that may be effective in delaying the progression of HIV to AIDS.
Non-gonococcal urethritis	1–6 weeks	Pain on passing urine, especially first thing in the morning. There may also be a discharge from the penis.	The doctor will take a swab from the urethra (the tube that carries urine out of the body) to find the cause – often a chlamydial infection. Treatment is usually with antibiotics.
Pubic lice	0–17 days	Usually there is intense itching in the pubic region, particularly at night. Lice are 1–2 mm long and may be visible.	Treatment is with a lotion that kills the lice and their eggs. Such lotions can be bought over the counter.
Syphilis	1–12 weeks	A highly infectious, painless sore develops in the genital area, usually on the penis or in the rectum. If untreated, the condition can progress to involve internal organs, and rash, fever, and swollen lymph nodes will develop.	The disease is diagnosed by blood tests and tests on swabs taken from any sores. The usual treatment is a course of antibiotic injections.

Time between contact with the disease and the appearance of symptoms

241

121 Erection difficulties

If you have a painful erection, see chart 120, PROBLEMS
WITH THE PENIS **(p.240).**
From time to time, most men have problems with achieving
or maintaining an erection. Although distressing, occasional
erection difficulties are normal and are usually caused by
stress, tiredness, anxiety, or alcohol. If you frequently have
difficulty in achieving an erection, consult your doctor. Safe
and effective treatments are available.

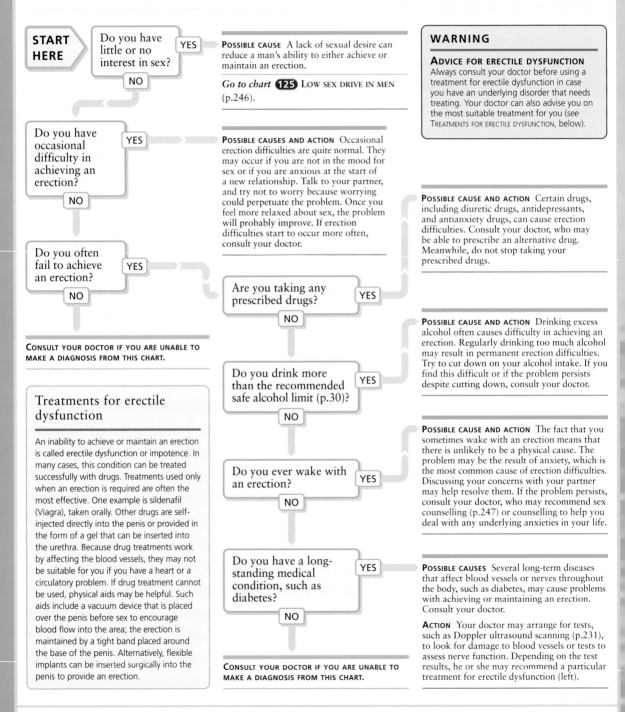

START HERE

Do you have little or no interest in sex?
YES →

NO

POSSIBLE CAUSE A lack of sexual desire can
reduce a man's ability to either achieve or
maintain an erection.

Go to chart **125** LOW SEX DRIVE IN MEN
(p.246).

Do you have occasional difficulty in achieving an erection?
YES →

NO

POSSIBLE CAUSES AND ACTION Occasional
erection difficulties are quite normal. They
may occur if you are not in the mood for
sex or if you are anxious at the start of
a new relationship. Talk to your partner,
and try not to worry because worrying
could perpetuate the problem. Once you
feel more relaxed about sex, the problem
will probably improve. If erection
difficulties start to occur more often,
consult your doctor.

Do you often fail to achieve an erection?
YES →

NO

**CONSULT YOUR DOCTOR IF YOU ARE UNABLE TO
MAKE A DIAGNOSIS FROM THIS CHART.**

WARNING

ADVICE FOR ERECTILE DYSFUNCTION
Always consult your doctor before using a
treatment for erectile dysfunction in case
you have an underlying disorder that needs
treating. Your doctor can also advise you on
the most suitable treatment for you (*see*
TREATMENTS FOR ERECTILE DYSFUNCTION, below).

Are you taking any prescribed drugs?
YES →

NO

POSSIBLE CAUSE AND ACTION Certain drugs,
including diuretic drugs, antidepressants,
and antianxiety drugs, can cause erection
difficulties. Consult your doctor, who may
be able to prescribe an alternative drug.
Meanwhile, do not stop taking your
prescribed drugs.

Do you drink more than the recommended safe alcohol limit (p.30)?
YES →

NO

POSSIBLE CAUSE AND ACTION Drinking excess
alcohol often causes difficulty in achieving an
erection. Regularly drinking too much alcohol
may result in permanent erection difficulties.
Try to cut down on your alcohol intake. If you
find this difficult or if the problem persists
despite cutting down, consult your doctor.

Do you ever wake with an erection?
YES →

NO

POSSIBLE CAUSE AND ACTION The fact that you
sometimes wake with an erection means that
there is unlikely to be a physical cause. The
problem may be the result of anxiety, which is
the most common cause of erection difficulties.
Discussing your concerns with your partner
may help resolve them. If the problem persists,
consult your doctor, who may recommend sex
counselling (p.247) or counselling to help you
deal with any underlying anxieties in your life.

Do you have a long-standing medical condition, such as diabetes?
YES →

NO

POSSIBLE CAUSES Several long-term diseases
that affect blood vessels or nerves throughout
the body, such as diabetes, may cause problems
with achieving or maintaining an erection.
Consult your doctor.

ACTION Your doctor may arrange for tests,
such as Doppler ultrasound scanning (p.231),
to look for damage to blood vessels or tests to
assess nerve function. Depending on the test
results, he or she may recommend a particular
treatment for erectile dysfunction (left).

**CONSULT YOUR DOCTOR IF YOU ARE UNABLE TO
MAKE A DIAGNOSIS FROM THIS CHART.**

Treatments for erectile dysfunction

An inability to achieve or maintain an erection
is called erectile dysfunction or impotence. In
many cases, this condition can be treated
successfully with drugs. Treatments used only
when an erection is required are often the
most effective. One example is sildenafil
(Viagra), taken orally. Other drugs are self-
injected directly into the penis or provided in
the form of a gel that can be inserted into
the urethra. Because drug treatments work
by affecting the blood vessels, they may not
be suitable for you if you have a heart or a
circulatory problem. If drug treatment cannot
be used, physical aids may be helpful. Such
aids include a vacuum device that is placed
over the penis before sex to encourage
blood flow into the area; the erection is
maintained by a tight band placed around
the base of the penis. Alternatively, flexible
implants can be inserted surgically into the
penis to provide an erection.

122 Ejaculation problems

If you are unable to achieve an erection, see chart 121, ERECTION DIFFICULTIES **(opposite).**
Consult this chart if ejaculation (the moment at which semen is released at orgasm) occurs sooner than you and your partner would like, or, if despite having a normal erection, ejaculation is delayed or does not occur. Ejaculation problems

are common and can be made worse by the resulting anxiety. Discussing your sexual needs with your partner can help relieve many of these problems. Premature ejaculation rarely has a physical cause. Absent or delayed ejaculation may result from a physical cause or an emotional problem. Orgasm without ejaculation is usually the result of previous prostate surgery.

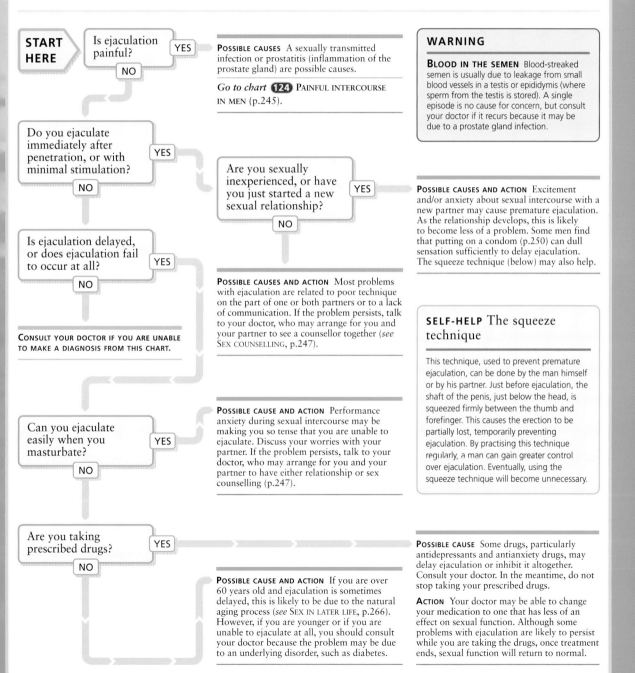

START HERE

Is ejaculation painful? — YES → **POSSIBLE CAUSES** A sexually transmitted infection or prostatitis (inflammation of the prostate gland) are possible causes.

Go to chart **124** PAINFUL INTERCOURSE IN MEN (p.245).

NO

Do you ejaculate immediately after penetration, or with minimal stimulation? — YES →

Are you sexually inexperienced, or have you just started a new sexual relationship? — YES → **POSSIBLE CAUSES AND ACTION** Excitement and/or anxiety about sexual intercourse with a new partner may cause premature ejaculation. As the relationship develops, this is likely to become less of a problem. Some men find that putting on a condom (p.250) can dull sensation sufficiently to delay ejaculation. The squeeze technique (below) may also help.

NO

NO

Is ejaculation delayed, or does ejaculation fail to occur at all? — YES → **POSSIBLE CAUSES AND ACTION** Most problems with ejaculation are related to poor technique on the part of one or both partners or to a lack of communication. If the problem persists, talk to your doctor, who may arrange for you and your partner to see a counsellor together (*see* SEX COUNSELLING, p.247).

NO

CONSULT YOUR DOCTOR IF YOU ARE UNABLE TO MAKE A DIAGNOSIS FROM THIS CHART.

Can you ejaculate easily when you masturbate? — YES → **POSSIBLE CAUSE AND ACTION** Performance anxiety during sexual intercourse may be making you so tense that you are unable to ejaculate. Discuss your worries with your partner. If the problem persists, talk to your doctor, who may arrange for you and your partner to have either relationship or sex counselling (p.247).

NO

Are you taking prescribed drugs? — YES → **POSSIBLE CAUSE** Some drugs, particularly antidepressants and antianxiety drugs, may delay ejaculation or inhibit it altogether. Consult your doctor. In the meantime, do not stop taking your prescribed drugs.

NO

POSSIBLE CAUSE AND ACTION If you are over 60 years old and ejaculation is sometimes delayed, this is likely to be due to the natural aging process (*see* SEX IN LATER LIFE, p.266). However, if you are younger or if you are unable to ejaculate at all, you should consult your doctor because the problem may be due to an underlying disorder, such as diabetes.

ACTION Your doctor may be able to change your medication to one that has less of an effect on sexual function. Although some problems with ejaculation are likely to persist while you are taking the drugs, once treatment ends, sexual function will return to normal.

WARNING

BLOOD IN THE SEMEN Blood-streaked semen is usually due to leakage from small blood vessels in a testis or epididymis (where sperm from the testis is stored). A single episode is no cause for concern, but consult your doctor if it recurs because it may be due to a prostate gland infection.

SELF-HELP The squeeze technique

This technique, used to prevent premature ejaculation, can be done by the man himself or by his partner. Just before ejaculation, the shaft of the penis, just below the head, is squeezed firmly between the thumb and forefinger. This causes the erection to be partially lost, temporarily preventing ejaculation. By practising this technique regularly, a man can gain greater control over ejaculation. Eventually, using the squeeze technique will become unnecessary.

123 Testes and scrotum problems

All men should examine their testes regularly (*see* EXAMINING THE TESTES, below) as there is a small possibility that a change could indicate cancer of the testis. Cancer treatment is most likely to be successful if the diagnosis is made early. If you have pain or notice a lump or swelling in or around the testes or elsewhere in the scrotum, consult this chart to determine how quickly you should seek medical advice. In some cases, prompt treatment is essential to preserve fertility.

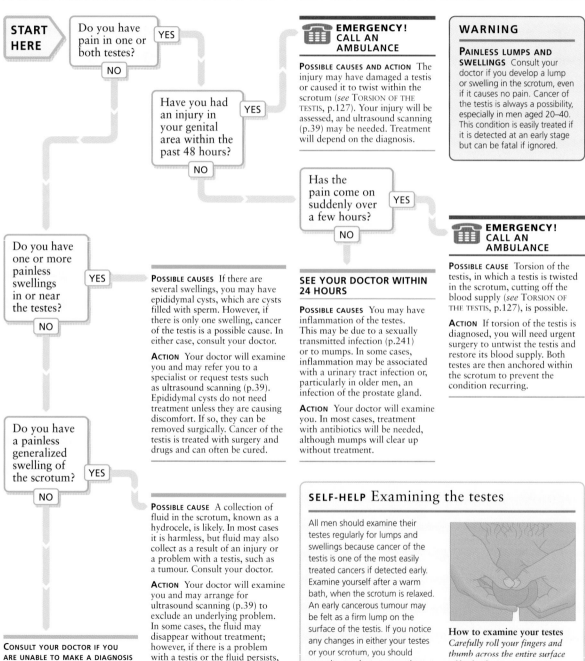

START HERE

Do you have pain in one or both testes? — YES / NO

Have you had an injury in your genital area within the past 48 hours? — YES / NO

Has the pain come on suddenly over a few hours? — YES / NO

Do you have one or more painless swellings in or near the testes? — YES / NO

Do you have a painless generalized swelling of the scrotum? — YES / NO

EMERGENCY! CALL AN AMBULANCE

POSSIBLE CAUSES AND ACTION The injury may have damaged a testis or caused it to twist within the scrotum (*see* TORSION OF THE TESTIS, p.127). Your injury will be assessed, and ultrasound scanning (p.39) may be needed. Treatment will depend on the diagnosis.

WARNING

PAINLESS LUMPS AND SWELLINGS Consult your doctor if you develop a lump or swelling in the scrotum, even if it causes no pain. Cancer of the testis is always a possibility, especially in men aged 20–40. This condition is easily treated if it is detected at an early stage but can be fatal if ignored.

POSSIBLE CAUSES If there are several swellings, you may have epididymal cysts, which are cysts filled with sperm. However, if there is only one swelling, cancer of the testis is a possible cause. In either case, consult your doctor.

ACTION Your doctor will examine you and may refer you to a specialist or request tests such as ultrasound scanning (p.39). Epididymal cysts do not need treatment unless they are causing discomfort. If so, they can be removed surgically. Cancer of the testis is treated with surgery and drugs and can often be cured.

SEE YOUR DOCTOR WITHIN 24 HOURS

POSSIBLE CAUSES You may have inflammation of the testes. This may be due to a sexually transmitted infection (p.241) or to mumps. In some cases, inflammation may be associated with a urinary tract infection or, particularly in older men, an infection of the prostate gland.

ACTION Your doctor will examine you. In most cases, treatment with antibiotics will be needed, although mumps will clear up without treatment.

EMERGENCY! CALL AN AMBULANCE

POSSIBLE CAUSE Torsion of the testis, in which a testis is twisted in the scrotum, cutting off the blood supply (*see* TORSION OF THE TESTIS, p.127), is possible.

ACTION If torsion of the testis is diagnosed, you will need urgent surgery to untwist the testis and restore its blood supply. Both testes are then anchored within the scrotum to prevent the condition recurring.

POSSIBLE CAUSE A collection of fluid in the scrotum, known as a hydrocele, is likely. In most cases it is harmless, but fluid may also collect as a result of an injury or a problem with a testis, such as a tumour. Consult your doctor.

ACTION Your doctor will examine you and may arrange for ultrasound scanning (p.39) to exclude an underlying problem. In some cases, the fluid may disappear without treatment; however, if there is a problem with a testis or the fluid persists, you may need surgery.

CONSULT YOUR DOCTOR IF YOU ARE UNABLE TO MAKE A DIAGNOSIS FROM THIS CHART.

SELF-HELP Examining the testes

All men should examine their testes regularly for lumps and swellings because cancer of the testis is one of the most easily treated cancers if detected early. Examine yourself after a warm bath, when the scrotum is relaxed. An early cancerous tumour may be felt as a firm lump on the surface of the testis. If you notice any changes in either your testes or your scrotum, you should consult your doctor promptly.

How to examine your testes
Carefully roll your fingers and thumb across the entire surface of both of your testes.

124 Painful intercourse in men

Consult this chart if sexual intercourse is painful. If the cause of the pain is not treated, erection difficulties and ejaculation problems may develop. There are several different possible causes of painful intercourse in men, including a disorder affecting the surface of the penis, a tight foreskin, an infection, or lack of lubrication.

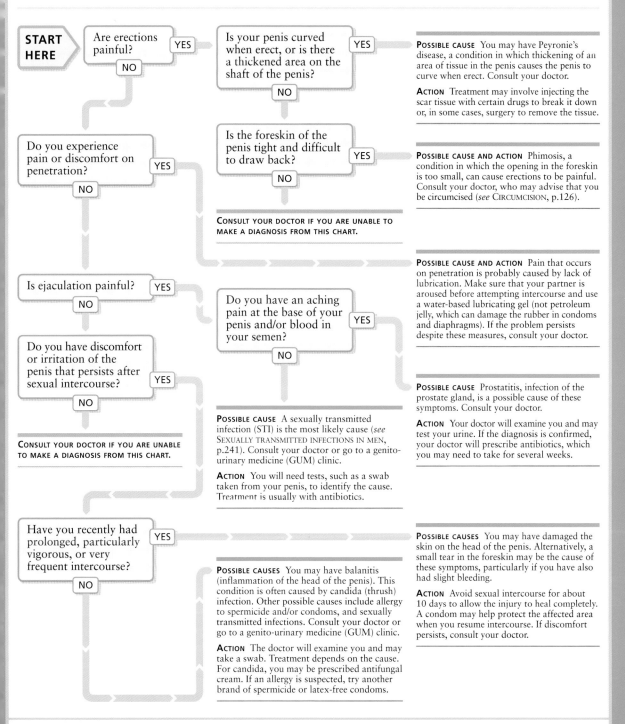

START HERE

Are erections painful? — YES → **Is your penis curved when erect, or is there a thickened area on the shaft of the penis?** — YES → **POSSIBLE CAUSE** You may have Peyronie's disease, a condition in which thickening of an area of tissue in the penis causes the penis to curve when erect. Consult your doctor.

ACTION Treatment may involve injecting the scar tissue with certain drugs to break it down or, in some cases, surgery to remove the tissue.

NO ↓ (Are erections painful?)

NO ↓ (Is your penis curved when erect...?) → **Is the foreskin of the penis tight and difficult to draw back?** — YES → **POSSIBLE CAUSE AND ACTION** Phimosis, a condition in which the opening in the foreskin is too small, can cause erections to be painful. Consult your doctor, who may advise that you be circumcised (see CIRCUMCISION, p.126).

Do you experience pain or discomfort on penetration? — YES →

NO ↓

NO ↓ (Is the foreskin tight?)

CONSULT YOUR DOCTOR IF YOU ARE UNABLE TO MAKE A DIAGNOSIS FROM THIS CHART.

POSSIBLE CAUSE AND ACTION Pain that occurs on penetration is probably caused by lack of lubrication. Make sure that your partner is aroused before attempting intercourse and use a water-based lubricating gel (not petroleum jelly, which can damage the rubber in condoms and diaphragms). If the problem persists despite these measures, consult your doctor.

Is ejaculation painful? — YES →

NO ↓

Do you have an aching pain at the base of your penis and/or blood in your semen? — YES →

NO ↓

Do you have discomfort or irritation of the penis that persists after sexual intercourse? — YES →

NO ↓

POSSIBLE CAUSE Prostatitis, infection of the prostate gland, is a possible cause of these symptoms. Consult your doctor.

ACTION Your doctor will examine you and may test your urine. If the diagnosis is confirmed, your doctor will prescribe antibiotics, which you may need to take for several weeks.

CONSULT YOUR DOCTOR IF YOU ARE UNABLE TO MAKE A DIAGNOSIS FROM THIS CHART.

POSSIBLE CAUSE A sexually transmitted infection (STI) is the most likely cause (see SEXUALLY TRANSMITTED INFECTIONS IN MEN, p.241). Consult your doctor or go to a genito-urinary medicine (GUM) clinic.

ACTION You will need tests, such as a swab taken from your penis, to identify the cause. Treatment is usually with antibiotics.

Have you recently had prolonged, particularly vigorous, or very frequent intercourse? — YES → **POSSIBLE CAUSES** You may have damaged the skin on the head of the penis. Alternatively, a small tear in the foreskin may be the cause of these symptoms, particularly if you have also had slight bleeding.

ACTION Avoid sexual intercourse for about 10 days to allow the injury to heal completely. A condom may help protect the affected area when you resume intercourse. If discomfort persists, consult your doctor.

NO ↓

POSSIBLE CAUSES You may have balanitis (inflammation of the head of the penis). This condition is often caused by candida (thrush) infection. Other possible causes include allergy to spermicide and/or condoms, and sexually transmitted infections. Consult your doctor or go to a genito-urinary medicine (GUM) clinic.

ACTION The doctor will examine you and may take a swab. Treatment depends on the cause. For candida, you may be prescribed antifungal cream. If an allergy is suspected, try another brand of spermicide or latex-free condoms.

125 Low sex drive in men

Normal levels of interest in sex vary from person to person. If you have always had little interest in a sexual relationship or rarely masturbate or feel sexually aroused, you may simply have a naturally low sex drive. Consult this chart if you are concerned about your low sex drive or if your sex drive has decreased recently. A decrease in sex drive often has a psychological cause but can also be the result of a disorder affecting levels of the sex hormone testosterone.

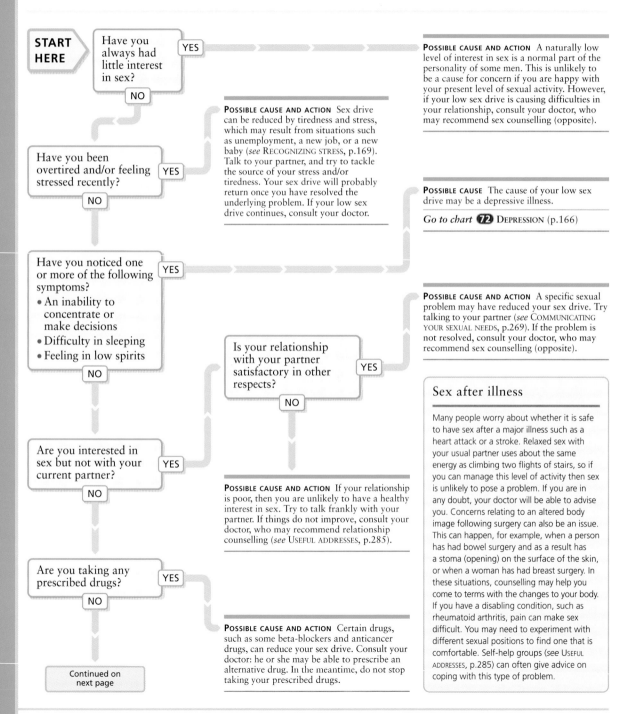

START HERE

Have you always had little interest in sex?
YES →

NO

POSSIBLE CAUSE AND ACTION A naturally low level of interest in sex is a normal part of the personality of some men. This is unlikely to be a cause for concern if you are happy with your present level of sexual activity. However, if your low sex drive is causing difficulties in your relationship, consult your doctor, who may recommend sex counselling (opposite).

Have you been overtired and/or feeling stressed recently?
YES →

NO

POSSIBLE CAUSE AND ACTION Sex drive can be reduced by tiredness and stress, which may result from situations such as unemployment, a new job, or a new baby (see RECOGNIZING STRESS, p.169). Talk to your partner, and try to tackle the source of your stress and/or tiredness. Your sex drive will probably return once you have resolved the underlying problem. If your low sex drive continues, consult your doctor.

POSSIBLE CAUSE The cause of your low sex drive may be a depressive illness.

Go to chart **72** DEPRESSION (p.166)

Have you noticed one or more of the following symptoms?
- An inability to concentrate or make decisions
- Difficulty in sleeping
- Feeling in low spirits

YES →

NO

POSSIBLE CAUSE AND ACTION A specific sexual problem may have reduced your sex drive. Try talking to your partner (see COMMUNICATING YOUR SEXUAL NEEDS, p.269). If the problem is not resolved, consult your doctor, who may recommend sex counselling (opposite).

Is your relationship with your partner satisfactory in other respects?
YES →

NO

Are you interested in sex but not with your current partner?
YES →

NO

POSSIBLE CAUSE AND ACTION If your relationship is poor, then you are unlikely to have a healthy interest in sex. Try to talk frankly with your partner. If things do not improve, consult your doctor, who may recommend relationship counselling (see USEFUL ADDRESSES, p.285).

Are you taking any prescribed drugs?
YES →

NO

POSSIBLE CAUSE AND ACTION Certain drugs, such as some beta-blockers and anticancer drugs, can reduce your sex drive. Consult your doctor: he or she may be able to prescribe an alternative drug. In the meantime, do not stop taking your prescribed drugs.

Sex after illness

Many people worry about whether it is safe to have sex after a major illness such as a heart attack or a stroke. Relaxed sex with your usual partner uses about the same energy as climbing two flights of stairs, so if you can manage this level of activity then sex is unlikely to pose a problem. If you are in any doubt, your doctor will be able to advise you. Concerns relating to an altered body image following surgery can also be an issue. This can happen, for example, when a person has had bowel surgery and as a result has a stoma (opening) on the surface of the skin, or when a woman has had breast surgery. In these situations, counselling may help you come to terms with the changes to your body. If you have a disabling condition, such as rheumatoid arthritis, pain can make sex difficult. You may need to experiment with different sexual positions to find one that is comfortable. Self-help groups (see USEFUL ADDRESSES, p.285) can often give advice on coping with this type of problem.

Continued on next page

Continued from
previous page

Have you recently
recovered from a major
illness or operation?
YES
NO

Have you noticed any
of the following?
• Loss of body hair
• Reduced testes size
• Development
of breasts
YES
NO

Do you often drink
more than the
recommended safe
alcohol limit (p.30)?
YES
NO

Are you generally
anxious, and/or do you
have specific anxieties
about sex?
YES
NO

Are you over 50?
YES
NO

CONSULT YOUR DOCTOR IF YOU ARE UNABLE TO
MAKE A DIAGNOSIS FROM THIS CHART.

Sex counselling

Counselling with a sex therapist or counsellor is often helpful when there is a psychological basis for a sexual problem. The sessions usually last about 1 hour and a course of treatment may last for several weeks or months. Both partners need to attend the therapy sessions so that the therapist can help them to understand their sexual needs and communicate them honestly. A therapist may also suggest exercises to do at home. One such exercise is a technique called sensate focus. In this exercise, a couple touch and stimulate each other's bodies but agree not to have full sexual intercourse for several weeks. Sensate focus can be helpful for problems that stem from anxiety about sexual performance.

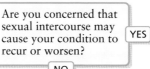

Talking therapy
A sex therapist may be able to help you and your partner develop better communication and work through sexual problems in a safe, supportive environment.

Are you concerned that
sexual intercourse may
cause your condition to
recur or worsen?
YES
NO

POSSIBLE CAUSES AND ACTION These symptoms may be caused by low levels of the male sex hormone testosterone. The problem may result from a disorder that affects the testes or an organ such as the liver, which processes hormones. Consult your doctor, who may arrange for blood tests to check your hormone levels and detect any underlying cause. Treatment may be of the underlying cause or may include hormone treatment.

POSSIBLE CAUSES AND ACTION General anxiety can reduce your sex drive. Specific concerns about sex, such as worry about contracting a sexually transmitted infection (*see* SEXUALLY TRANSMITTED INFECTIONS IN MEN, p.241) or making your partner pregnant, can also suppress sex drive. Concern about sexual orientation (right) is another possible cause. Talk to your partner, and, if you are still concerned, consult your doctor.

POSSIBLE CAUSE Sex drive may decline slightly as you get older (*see* SEX IN LATER LIFE, p.266). This need not be a problem if your needs and your partner's are compatible. If your loss of sex drive has occurred suddenly or if you are concerned, consult your doctor.

ACTION Your doctor may arrange for blood tests to check your hormone levels. Any cause will be treated, if possible, whatever your age.

POSSIBLE CAUSE AND ACTION People who have been ill or had major surgery are often concerned that sex will make their condition worse (*see* SEX AFTER ILLNESS, opposite). These concerns may lower sex drive. In most cases, after a recovery period of about 6 weeks, sex rarely causes problems; however, you should consult your doctor for advice and reassurance.

POSSIBLE CAUSE AND ACTION Serious illness or surgery can sometimes alter your perception of your body and of yourself in general (*see* SEX AFTER ILLNESS, opposite), resulting in a reduced sex drive. Consult your doctor, who may advise counselling (*see* USEFUL ADDRESSES, p.285).

POSSIBLE CAUSE AND ACTION Alcohol can reduce your sex drive and can cause erection difficulties as well as more serious health problems. Try to drink less alcohol. You should also consult your doctor so that any other causes can be excluded.

Sexual orientation

Although heterosexuality is considered the norm by some people, it is common for adolescents to go through a phase of having homosexual feelings before they become attracted to people of the opposite sex. Some people, however, remain homosexual or bisexual throughout their lives. While homosexuality and bisexuality are becoming more openly accepted, some people still have feelings of guilt associated with their sexuality or are victims of prejudice. Whatever your sexual orientation, if you have multiple partners, you are at an increased risk of sexually transmitted infections, including HIV infection and AIDS (p.144), and need to practise safe sex (*see* SEX AND HEALTH, p.32).

126 Fertility problems in men

See also chart 139, FERTILITY PROBLEMS IN WOMEN **(p.270).** Fertility problems affect 1 in 10 couples who want children, and, in many cases, a cause is not found. Failure to conceive may be the result of a problem affecting either one or both partners; this chart deals only with possible problems in men. The two main causes of infertility in men are insufficient sperm production and a blockage of the vas deferens, the tubes that transport the sperm to the penis during ejaculation.

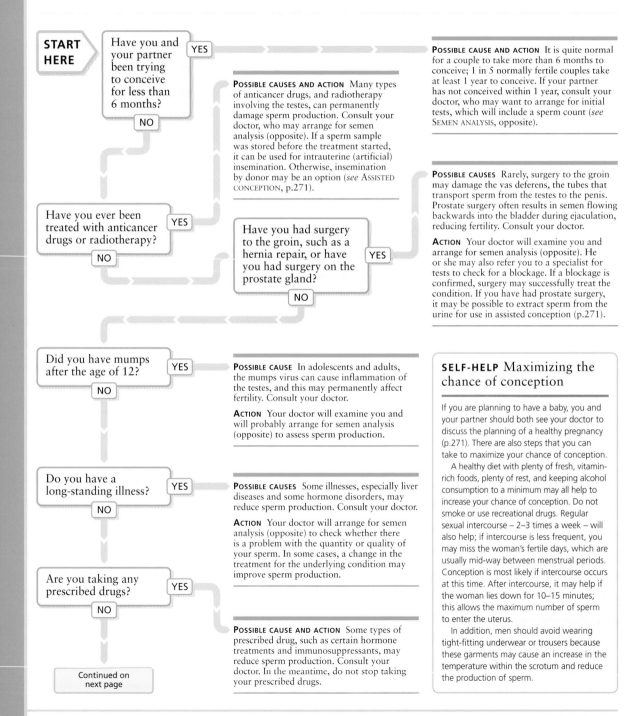

START HERE → Have you and your partner been trying to conceive for less than 6 months? — **YES**

POSSIBLE CAUSE AND ACTION It is quite normal for a couple to take more than 6 months to conceive; 1 in 5 normally fertile couples take at least 1 year to conceive. If your partner has not conceived within 1 year, consult your doctor, who may want to arrange for initial tests, which will include a sperm count (*see* SEMEN ANALYSIS, opposite).

NO ↓

Have you ever been treated with anticancer drugs or radiotherapy? — **YES**

POSSIBLE CAUSES AND ACTION Many types of anticancer drugs, and radiotherapy involving the testes, can permanently damage sperm production. Consult your doctor, who may arrange for semen analysis (opposite). If a sperm sample was stored before the treatment started, it can be used for intrauterine (artificial) insemination. Otherwise, insemination by donor may be an option (*see* ASSISTED CONCEPTION, p.271).

NO ↓

Have you had surgery to the groin, such as a hernia repair, or have you had surgery on the prostate gland? — **YES**

POSSIBLE CAUSES Rarely, surgery to the groin may damage the vas deferens, the tubes that transport sperm from the testes to the penis. Prostate surgery often results in semen flowing backwards into the bladder during ejaculation, reducing fertility. Consult your doctor.

ACTION Your doctor will examine you and arrange for semen analysis (opposite). He or she may also refer you to a specialist for tests to check for a blockage. If a blockage is confirmed, surgery may successfully treat the condition. If you have had prostate surgery, it may be possible to extract sperm from the urine for use in assisted conception (p.271).

NO ↓

Did you have mumps after the age of 12? — **YES**

POSSIBLE CAUSE In adolescents and adults, the mumps virus can cause inflammation of the testes, and this may permanently affect fertility. Consult your doctor.

ACTION Your doctor will examine you and will probably arrange for semen analysis (opposite) to assess sperm production.

NO ↓

Do you have a long-standing illness? — **YES**

POSSIBLE CAUSES Some illnesses, especially liver diseases and some hormone disorders, may reduce sperm production. Consult your doctor.

ACTION Your doctor will arrange for semen analysis (opposite) to check whether there is a problem with the quantity or quality of your sperm. In some cases, a change in the treatment for the underlying condition may improve sperm production.

NO ↓

Are you taking any prescribed drugs? — **YES**

POSSIBLE CAUSE AND ACTION Some types of prescribed drug, such as certain hormone treatments and immunosuppressants, may reduce sperm production. Consult your doctor. In the meantime, do not stop taking your prescribed drugs.

NO ↓

Continued on next page

SELF-HELP Maximizing the chance of conception

If you are planning to have a baby, you and your partner should both see your doctor to discuss the planning of a healthy pregnancy (p.271). There are also steps that you can take to maximize your chance of conception.

A healthy diet with plenty of fresh, vitamin-rich foods, plenty of rest, and keeping alcohol consumption to a minimum may all help to increase your chance of conception. Do not smoke or use recreational drugs. Regular sexual intercourse – 2–3 times a week – will also help; if intercourse is less frequent, you may miss the woman's fertile days, which are usually mid-way between menstrual periods. Conception is most likely if intercourse occurs at this time. After intercourse, it may help if the woman lies down for 10–15 minutes; this allows the maximum number of sperm to enter the uterus.

In addition, men should avoid wearing tight-fitting underwear or trousers because these garments may cause an increase in the temperature within the scrotum and reduce the production of sperm.

Continued from previous page

POSSIBLE CAUSE Sexually transmitted infections (*see* SEXUALLY TRANSMITTED INFECTIONS IN MEN, p.241) can result in a blockage of the vas deferens, the tubes that transport sperm from the testes to the penis. Consult your doctor.

ACTION Your doctor will examine you, and he or she may refer you to a specialist for tests to establish whether the tubes leading from your testes are blocked. In some cases, surgery to relieve the blockage may be possible.

Have you had a sexually transmitted infection in the past? — **YES**

NO

POSSIBLE CAUSE AND ACTION Infrequent intercourse is a common cause of failure to conceive because the chance of sperm being present to fertilize an egg when it is released is reduced. If possible, try to have intercourse with your partner more often (*see* MAXIMIZING THE CHANCE OF CONCEPTION, opposite). If your partner has still not conceived within a further 3–6 months, consult your doctor.

Do you have sex less than 2–3 times a week on average? — **YES**

NO

Do you regularly drink more than the recommended safe alcohol limit (p.30)? — **YES**

NO

Are you outside the healthy weight range for your height (*see* ASSESSING YOUR WEIGHT, p.29), or has there been a sudden change in your weight? — **YES**

NO

POSSIBLE CAUSES AND ACTION If you are substantially overweight or underweight your fertility may be reduced. Consult your doctor, who may arrange for semen analysis (above). Make sure that you eat a healthy diet. If you are overweight, you should try to lose weight (*see* HOW TO LOSE WEIGHT SAFELY, p.147). If you are underweight, follow the advice on gaining weight safely (p.145).

Do you smoke or use recreational drugs? — **YES**

NO

POSSIBLE CAUSES Smoking and/or using recreational drugs can impair sperm function or reduce the production of sperm in the testes. Consult your doctor.

ACTION Your doctor may arrange for semen analysis (above). Try to stop smoking and/or using recreational drugs.

Do you wear underpants that are tight-fitting, or do you use saunas or steam baths frequently? — **YES**

NO

CONSULT YOUR DOCTOR IF YOU ARE UNABLE TO MAKE A DIAGNOSIS FROM THIS CHART.

Semen analysis

If a couple has fertility problems, semen analysis is usually one of the first tests that is carried out. The man is asked to ejaculate into a clean container (semen collected from a condom is not suitable). The sample must then be kept at body temperature and analysed within 2 hours. The volume of semen is measured, and a sample is then viewed under a microscope to assess the shape and activity levels of the sperm and to count the number of sperm. Each millilitre of semen normally contains at least 50 million sperm, the majority of which are healthy. A low sperm count is defined as fewer than 20 million sperm per millilitre. If the test shows any abnormality, it will be repeated.

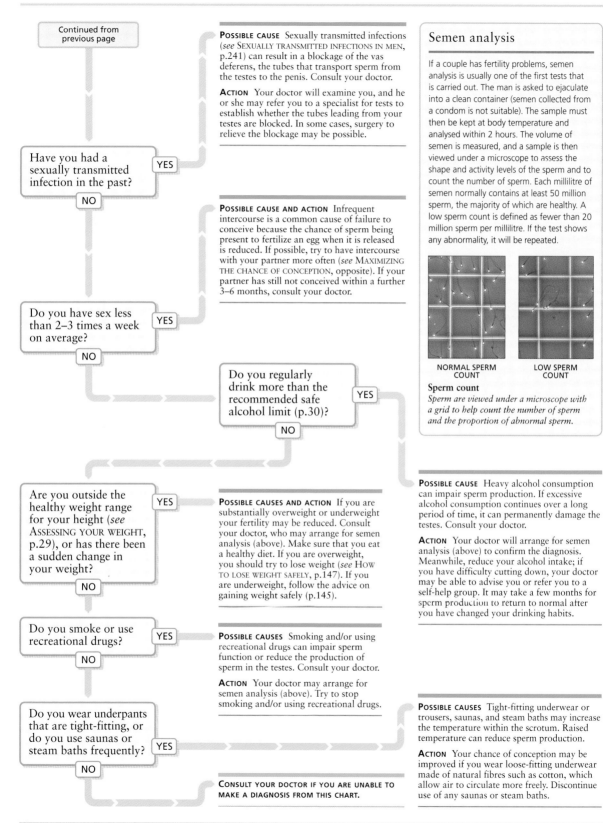

NORMAL SPERM COUNT   LOW SPERM COUNT

Sperm count
Sperm are viewed under a microscope with a grid to help count the number of sperm and the proportion of abnormal sperm.

POSSIBLE CAUSE Heavy alcohol consumption can impair sperm production. If excessive alcohol consumption continues over a long period of time, it can permanently damage the testes. Consult your doctor.

ACTION Your doctor will arrange for semen analysis (above) to confirm the diagnosis. Meanwhile, reduce your alcohol intake; if you have difficulty cutting down, your doctor may be able to advise you or refer you to a self-help group. It may take a few months for sperm production to return to normal after you have changed your drinking habits.

POSSIBLE CAUSES Tight-fitting underwear or trousers, saunas, and steam baths may increase the temperature within the scrotum. Raised temperature can reduce sperm production.

ACTION Your chance of conception may be improved if you wear loose-fitting underwear made of natural fibres such as cotton, which allow air to circulate more freely. Discontinue use of any saunas or steam baths.

127 Contraception choices for men

For women's contraception choices, see chart 140,
CONTRACEPTION CHOICES FOR WOMEN (p.272).
The two main methods of contraception currently available for men are condoms (sheaths) and vasectomy. There is no hormonal method of contraception for men. Your choice of contraceptive method will depend on various factors, including your sexual lifestyle and age. If you have a regular partner, the decision is best shared. Condoms have the advantages of being 95 per cent effective and of helping to provide protection against sexually transmitted infections for both the user and his sexual partner. Many men choose to have a vasectomy (male sterilization) when they are certain they will not want children in the future. Vasectomy is a simple procedure, but it must be considered irreversible.

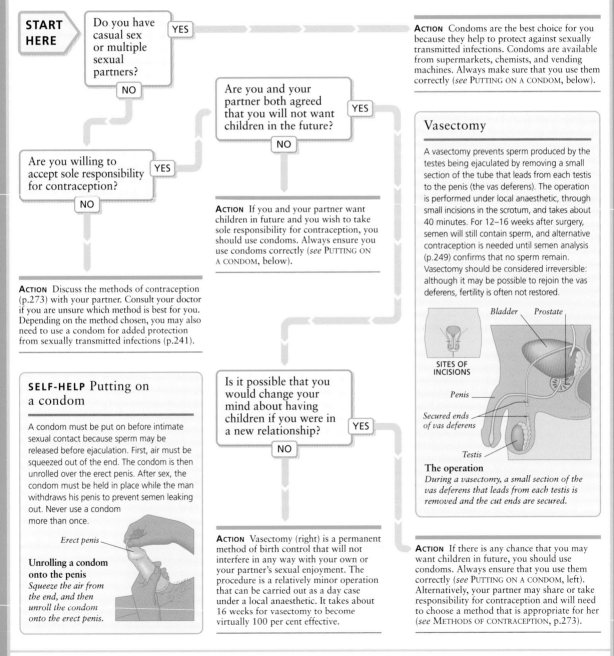

START HERE

Do you have casual sex or multiple sexual partners? — **YES**

NO

Are you willing to accept sole responsibility for contraception? — **YES**

NO

Are you and your partner both agreed that you will not want children in the future? — **YES**

NO

ACTION Condoms are the best choice for you because they help to protect against sexually transmitted infections. Condoms are available from supermarkets, chemists, and vending machines. Always make sure that you use them correctly (*see* PUTTING ON A CONDOM, below).

ACTION If you and your partner want children in future and you wish to take sole responsibility for contraception, you should use condoms. Always ensure you use condoms correctly (*see* PUTTING ON A CONDOM, below).

ACTION Discuss the methods of contraception (p.273) with your partner. Consult your doctor if you are unsure which method is best for you. Depending on the method chosen, you may also need to use a condom for added protection from sexually transmitted infections (p.241).

Is it possible that you would change your mind about having children if you were in a new relationship? — **YES**

NO

SELF-HELP Putting on a condom

A condom must be put on before intimate sexual contact because sperm may be released before ejaculation. First, air must be squeezed out of the end. The condom is then unrolled over the erect penis. After sex, the condom must be held in place while the man withdraws his penis to prevent semen leaking out. Never use a condom more than once.

Erect penis

Unrolling a condom onto the penis
Squeeze the air from the end, and then unroll the condom onto the erect penis.

ACTION Vasectomy (right) is a permanent method of birth control that will not interfere in any way with your own or your partner's sexual enjoyment. The procedure is a relatively minor operation that can be carried out as a day case under a local anaesthetic. It takes about 16 weeks for vasectomy to become virtually 100 per cent effective.

Vasectomy

A vasectomy prevents sperm produced by the testes being ejaculated by removing a small section of the tube that leads from each testis to the penis (the vas deferens). The operation is performed under local anaesthetic, through small incisions in the scrotum, and takes about 40 minutes. For 12–16 weeks after surgery, semen will still contain sperm, and alternative contraception is needed until semen analysis (p.249) confirms that no sperm remain. Vasectomy should be considered irreversible: although it may be possible to rejoin the vas deferens, fertility is often not restored.

Bladder   *Prostate*

SITES OF INCISIONS

Penis

Secured ends of vas deferens

Testis

The operation
During a vasectomy, a small section of the vas deferens that leads from each testis is removed and the cut ends are secured.

ACTION If there is any chance that you may want children in future, you should use condoms. Always ensure that you use them correctly (*see* PUTTING ON A CONDOM, left). Alternatively, your partner may share or take responsibility for contraception and will need to choose a method that is appropriate for her (*see* METHODS OF CONTRACEPTION, p.273).

CHARTS FOR

WOMEN

128 Breast problems

For breast problems during pregnancy or after giving birth, see chart 149, BREAST PROBLEMS AND PREGNANCY *(p.282).* Although the majority of breast problems are not serious, breast cancer is one of the most common cancers in women. Rarely, it also occurs in men. If diagnosed early enough, breast cancer can often be successfully treated. It is therefore important to familiarize yourself with the look and feel of your breasts (*see* BREAST AWARENESS, below) so that you will be able to detect any changes. If you do find a change in your breast, you should seek medical advice immediately.

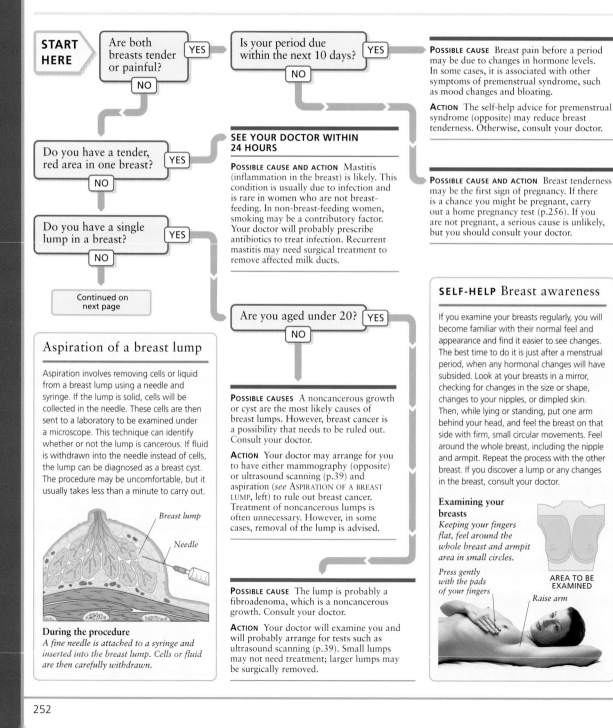

START HERE

Are both breasts tender or painful? — YES

NO

Is your period due within the next 10 days? — YES

NO

POSSIBLE CAUSE Breast pain before a period may be due to changes in hormone levels. In some cases, it is associated with other symptoms of premenstrual syndrome, such as mood changes and bloating.

ACTION The self-help advice for premenstrual syndrome (opposite) may reduce breast tenderness. Otherwise, consult your doctor.

Do you have a tender, red area in one breast? — YES

NO

SEE YOUR DOCTOR WITHIN 24 HOURS

POSSIBLE CAUSE AND ACTION Mastitis (inflammation in the breast) is likely. This condition is usually due to infection and is rare in women who are not breast-feeding. In non-breast-feeding women, smoking may be a contributory factor. Your doctor will probably prescribe antibiotics to treat infection. Recurrent mastitis may need surgical treatment to remove affected milk ducts.

POSSIBLE CAUSE AND ACTION Breast tenderness may be the first sign of pregnancy. If there is a chance you might be pregnant, carry out a home pregnancy test (p.256). If you are not pregnant, a serious cause is unlikely, but you should consult your doctor.

Do you have a single lump in a breast? — YES

NO

Continued on next page

Are you aged under 20? — YES

NO

Aspiration of a breast lump

Aspiration involves removing cells or liquid from a breast lump using a needle and syringe. If the lump is solid, cells will be collected in the needle. These cells are then sent to a laboratory to be examined under a microscope. This technique can identify whether or not the lump is cancerous. If fluid is withdrawn into the needle instead of cells, the lump can be diagnosed as a breast cyst. The procedure may be uncomfortable, but it usually takes less than a minute to carry out.

Breast lump

Needle

During the procedure
A fine needle is attached to a syringe and inserted into the breast lump. Cells or fluid are then carefully withdrawn.

POSSIBLE CAUSES A noncancerous growth or cyst are the most likely causes of breast lumps. However, breast cancer is a possibility that needs to be ruled out. Consult your doctor.

ACTION Your doctor may arrange for you to have either mammography (opposite) or ultrasound scanning (p.39) and aspiration (*see* ASPIRATION OF A BREAST LUMP, left) to rule out breast cancer. Treatment of noncancerous lumps is often unnecessary. However, in some cases, removal of the lump is advised.

POSSIBLE CAUSE The lump is probably a fibroadenoma, which is a noncancerous growth. Consult your doctor.

ACTION Your doctor will examine you and will probably arrange for tests such as ultrasound scanning (p.39). Small lumps may not need treatment; larger lumps may be surgically removed.

SELF-HELP Breast awareness

If you examine your breasts regularly, you will become familiar with their normal feel and appearance and find it easier to see changes. The best time to do it is just after a menstrual period, when any hormonal changes will have subsided. Look at your breasts in a mirror, checking for changes in the size or shape, changes to your nipples, or dimpled skin. Then, while lying or standing, put one arm behind your head, and feel the breast on that side with firm, small circular movements. Feel around the whole breast, including the nipple and armpit. Repeat the process with the other breast. If you discover a lump or any changes in the breast, consult your doctor.

Examining your breasts
Keeping your fingers flat, feel around the whole breast and armpit area in small circles.

Press gently with the pads of your fingers

AREA TO BE EXAMINED

Raise arm

Mammography

Mammography uses X-rays (p.37) to detect abnormal areas of breast tissue. It is used as a screening test to detect signs of breast cancer and is also carried out to investigate breast lumps. Mammography is offered every 3 years from age 50 to 70. The breast is positioned in the X-ray machine and compressed so that the breast tissue can be easily seen on the X-ray. Two X-rays are usually taken of each breast. The procedure is uncomfortable but lasts only a few seconds. If an abnormality is detected, you will need further tests such as aspiration (see ASPIRATION OF A BREAST LUMP, opposite) to determine the cause of the abnormality.

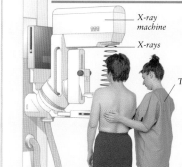

X-ray machine
X-rays
Technician

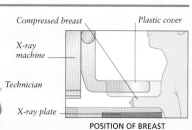

Compressed breast
Plastic cover
X-ray machine
X-ray plate

POSITION OF BREAST

During the procedure
Your breast is compressed between the plastic cover and X-ray plate. X-rays pass through the breast tissue onto the plate.

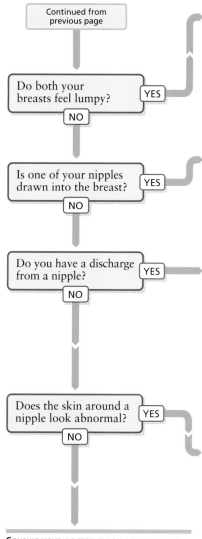

Continued from previous page

Do both your breasts feel lumpy? — YES

POSSIBLE CAUSE AND ACTION Some women have lumpier breasts than others. Lumps are usually more obvious before a period. If you are particularly worried, consult your doctor, who will examine your breasts to make sure that there are no individual lumps that require investigation. Naturally lumpy breasts do not require treatment and do not increase the risk of breast cancer.

NO

Is one of your nipples drawn into the breast? — YES

Has this developed recently? — YES

NO

NO

POSSIBLE CAUSES A change in a nipple may be a sign of breast cancer. However, normal aging may also cause a nipple to become indrawn. Consult your doctor.

ACTION Your doctor will examine your breasts and will probably arrange for tests such as mammography (above) to exclude a problem deeper in the breast.

POSSIBLE CAUSE AND ACTION If your nipple has always been drawn in, this is not a cause for concern, although it may make breast-feeding difficult. Wearing a nipple shell inside your bra during pregnancy may help to draw the nipple out in preparation for breast-feeding.

Do you have a discharge from a nipple? — YES

NO

POSSIBLE CAUSES Nipple discharge is usually due to hormone changes and is no cause for concern. In rare cases, a cancerous or noncancerous growth affecting a milk duct is the cause. Consult your doctor.

ACTION The doctor will examine your breasts and may arrange for mammography (above) to exclude an abnormality in the underlying breast tissue. Treatment is often not necessary, but occasionally affected milk ducts may need to be removed surgically.

Does the skin around a nipple look abnormal? — YES

NO

POSSIBLE CAUSES You may have a skin condition, such as eczema. However, Paget's disease, a rare form of breast cancer, is a possibility. Consult your doctor.

ACTION Your doctor will examine your breasts. If you have a skin condition, you may be prescribed corticosteroid creams. If your doctor suspects Paget's disease, you will probably be referred for tests such as mammography (above).

CONSULT YOUR DOCTOR IF YOU ARE UNABLE TO MAKE A DIAGNOSIS FROM THIS CHART.

SELF-HELP Premenstrual syndrome

Premenstrual syndrome is a group of symptoms, often including bloating, mood swings, and breast tenderness, that some women experience in the days leading up to a period. The following measures may help to prevent or relieve your symptoms:

- If possible, keep stress to a minimum.
- Try relaxation exercises (p.32) or take up an exercise such as yoga.
- Eat regularly to keep your blood sugar levels steady. Include carbohydrates such as pasta and potatoes, and eat plenty of fruit and vegetables.
- Avoid sugary snacks as they can make blood sugar levels fluctuate too strongly.
- Reduce your salt intake; instead, flavour foods with herbs and spices.
- Drink 6–8 glasses of water a day. Avoid drinks containing large amounts of caffeine, such as coffee, tea, and cola.

129 Bladder control problems in women

For other urinary problems, see chart 108, GENERAL URINARY PROBLEMS *(p.220).*
Bladder control problems affect 1 in 10 women. Incontinence, in which urine is passed involuntarily, is the most common problem. This is often related to childbirth, but it may have other causes. Many effective treatments for incontinence are now available. Inability to pass any urine is a less common problem but always needs immediate medical attention.

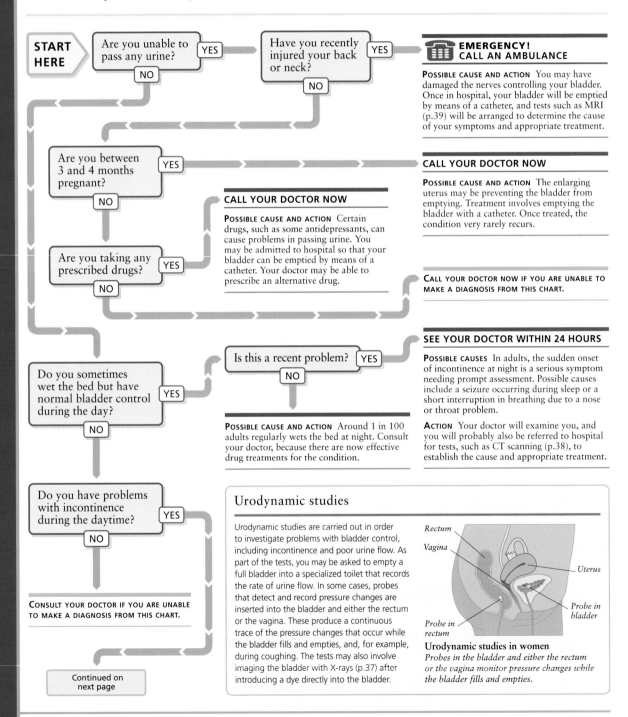

START HERE

Are you unable to pass any urine? — NO / YES

Have you recently injured your back or neck? — NO / YES

☎ **EMERGENCY! CALL AN AMBULANCE**

POSSIBLE CAUSE AND ACTION You may have damaged the nerves controlling your bladder. Once in hospital, your bladder will be emptied by means of a catheter, and tests such as MRI (p.39) will be arranged to determine the cause of your symptoms and appropriate treatment.

Are you between 3 and 4 months pregnant? — NO / YES

CALL YOUR DOCTOR NOW

POSSIBLE CAUSE AND ACTION The enlarging uterus may be preventing the bladder from emptying. Treatment involves emptying the bladder with a catheter. Once treated, the condition very rarely recurs.

Are you taking any prescribed drugs? — NO / YES

CALL YOUR DOCTOR NOW

POSSIBLE CAUSE AND ACTION Certain drugs, such as some antidepressants, can cause problems in passing urine. You may be admitted to hospital so that your bladder can be emptied by means of a catheter. Your doctor may be able to prescribe an alternative drug.

CALL YOUR DOCTOR NOW IF YOU ARE UNABLE TO MAKE A DIAGNOSIS FROM THIS CHART.

Do you sometimes wet the bed but have normal bladder control during the day? — NO / YES

Is this a recent problem? — NO / YES

SEE YOUR DOCTOR WITHIN 24 HOURS

POSSIBLE CAUSES In adults, the sudden onset of incontinence at night is a serious symptom needing prompt assessment. Possible causes include a seizure occurring during sleep or a short interruption in breathing due to a nose or throat problem.

ACTION Your doctor will examine you, and you will probably also be referred to hospital for tests, such as CT scanning (p.38), to establish the cause and appropriate treatment.

POSSIBLE CAUSE AND ACTION Around 1 in 100 adults regularly wets the bed at night. Consult your doctor, because there are now effective drug treatments for the condition.

Do you have problems with incontinence during the daytime? — NO / YES

CONSULT YOUR DOCTOR IF YOU ARE UNABLE TO MAKE A DIAGNOSIS FROM THIS CHART.

Urodynamic studies

Urodynamic studies are carried out in order to investigate problems with bladder control, including incontinence and poor urine flow. As part of the tests, you may be asked to empty a full bladder into a specialized toilet that records the rate of urine flow. In some cases, probes that detect and record pressure changes are inserted into the bladder and either the rectum or the vagina. These produce a continuous trace of the pressure changes that occur while the bladder fills and empties, and, for example, during coughing. The tests may also involve imaging the bladder with X-rays (p.37) after introducing a dye directly into the bladder.

Rectum
Vagina
Uterus
Probe in bladder
Probe in rectum

Urodynamic studies in women
Probes in the bladder and either the rectum or the vagina monitor pressure changes while the bladder fills and empties.

Continued on next page

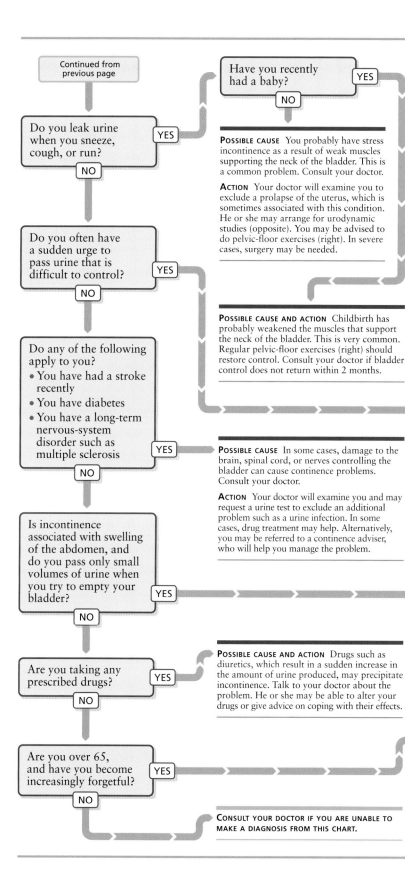

Continued from previous page

Do you leak urine when you sneeze, cough, or run?
NO / YES

Do you often have a sudden urge to pass urine that is difficult to control?
NO / YES

Do any of the following apply to you?
• You have had a stroke recently
• You have diabetes
• You have a long-term nervous-system disorder such as multiple sclerosis
NO / YES

Is incontinence associated with swelling of the abdomen, and do you pass only small volumes of urine when you try to empty your bladder?
NO / YES

Are you taking any prescribed drugs?
NO / YES

Are you over 65, and have you become increasingly forgetful?
NO / YES

Have you recently had a baby?
NO / YES

POSSIBLE CAUSE You probably have stress incontinence as a result of weak muscles supporting the neck of the bladder. This is a common problem. Consult your doctor.

ACTION Your doctor will examine you to exclude a prolapse of the uterus, which is sometimes associated with this condition. He or she may arrange for urodynamic studies (opposite). You may be advised to do pelvic-floor exercises (right). In severe cases, surgery may be needed.

POSSIBLE CAUSE AND ACTION Childbirth has probably weakened the muscles that support the neck of the bladder. This is very common. Regular pelvic-floor exercises (right) should restore control. Consult your doctor if bladder control does not return within 2 months.

POSSIBLE CAUSE In some cases, damage to the brain, spinal cord, or nerves controlling the bladder can cause continence problems. Consult your doctor.

ACTION Your doctor will examine you and may request a urine test to exclude an additional problem such as a urine infection. In some cases, drug treatment may help. Alternatively, you may be referred to a continence adviser, who will help you manage the problem.

POSSIBLE CAUSE AND ACTION Drugs such as diuretics, which result in a sudden increase in the amount of urine produced, may precipitate incontinence. Talk to your doctor about the problem. He or she may be able to alter your drugs or give advice on coping with their effects.

CONSULT YOUR DOCTOR IF YOU ARE UNABLE TO MAKE A DIAGNOSIS FROM THIS CHART.

SELF-HELP Pelvic-floor strengthening exercises

Exercises can help strengthen the pelvic-floor muscles, which support the bladder, uterus, and rectum. If done regularly, they can help prevent and treat urinary incontinence.

You can perform pelvic-floor exercises lying down, sitting, or standing. In order to identify the pelvic-floor muscles, imagine that you are passing urine and have to stop suddenly midstream. The muscles that you feel tighten around the vagina, urethra, and rectum are the pelvic-floor muscles.

To strengthen the pelvic-floor muscles, contract them and hold them contracted for 10 seconds. Then relax the muscles slowly. Repeat this contraction and relaxation cycle 10 times. Practice your pelvic-floor exercises at least every hour during the day.

If you have been doing the exercises to treat bladder control problems, you should see an improvement within 2 weeks, but you will need to continue doing the exercises regularly to maintain the improvement.

POSSIBLE CAUSE You may have an irritable bladder, in which there is a strong urge to pass urine even when the bladder contains little urine. Consult your doctor.

ACTION Your doctor will examine you and test your urine to rule out an infection, which can cause similar symptoms. He or she may also arrange for bladder function tests (see URODYNAMIC STUDIES, opposite). In most cases, drug treatment to reduce the sensitivity of the bladder, combined with exercises to increase the amount of urine that the bladder can hold without triggering the urge to pass urine, will help to improve the symptoms.

POSSIBLE CAUSE AND ACTION You may have an obstruction to the outflow of the bladder, which is preventing the bladder from emptying normally. This causes the bladder to become overfull and results in urine leaking from the bladder. Constipation is a possible cause of the obstruction. Consult your doctor, who will probably arrange for tests to determine the underlying cause. He or she may refer you to hospital so that your bladder can be drained and for treatment of the blockage.

POSSIBLE CAUSE A decline in mental function with increasing age is associated with bladder control problems in certain circumstances. Consult your doctor.

ACTION Your doctor will examine you and may arrange for tests to exclude other causes. He or she may refer you to a trained continence adviser, who can advise you on ways of coping with the problem.

130 Absent periods

Menstruation normally starts between the ages of 11 and 14, although in girls who are below average height and/or weight it may not start until some time later. Once periods start, they may be irregular for the first few years and may not settle down to a regular monthly cycle until the late teens. Once the menstrual cycle is established, it varies in length among individual women from as little as 24 days between periods to about 35 days. Absence of periods

(amenorrhoea) may occur in healthy women for several reasons, the most common of which is pregnancy. Other factors that may affect your monthly cycle include illness, stress, and strenuous physical activity. It is normal for periods to cease permanently as you approach middle age. Only rarely is absence of periods a sign of an underlying disorder. Consult this chart if you have never had a period, or if your period is more than 2 weeks late.

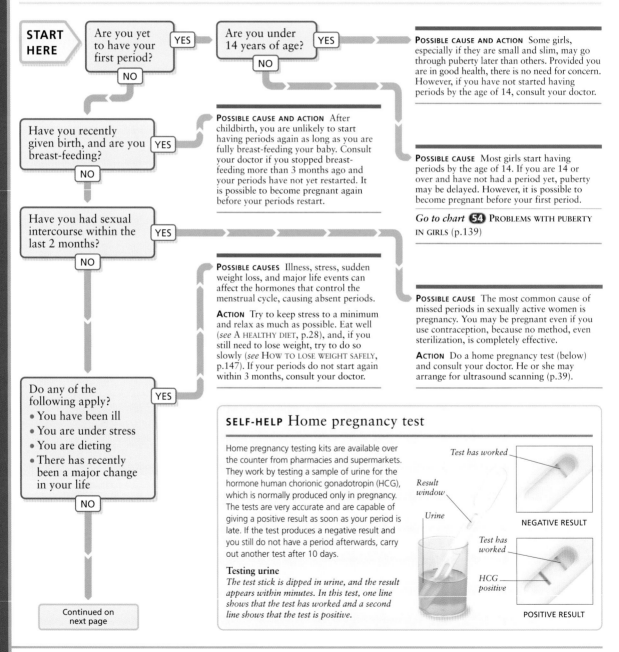

START HERE

Are you yet to have your first period? — YES → **Are you under 14 years of age?** — YES →

POSSIBLE CAUSE AND ACTION Some girls, especially if they are small and slim, may go through puberty later than others. Provided you are in good health, there is no need for concern. However, if you have not started having periods by the age of 14, consult your doctor.

NO ↓ (first period)

Are you under 14 years of age? NO →

POSSIBLE CAUSE Most girls start having periods by the age of 14. If you are 14 or over and have not had a period yet, puberty may be delayed. However, it is possible to become pregnant before your first period.

Go to chart **54** PROBLEMS WITH PUBERTY IN GIRLS (p.139)

Have you recently given birth, and are you breast-feeding? — YES →

POSSIBLE CAUSE AND ACTION After childbirth, you are unlikely to start having periods again as long as you are fully breast-feeding your baby. Consult your doctor if you stopped breast-feeding more than 3 months ago and your periods have not yet restarted. It is possible to become pregnant again before your periods restart.

NO ↓

Have you had sexual intercourse within the last 2 months? — YES →

POSSIBLE CAUSE The most common cause of missed periods in sexually active women is pregnancy. You may be pregnant even if you use contraception, because no method, even sterilization, is completely effective.

ACTION Do a home pregnancy test (below) and consult your doctor. He or she may arrange for ultrasound scanning (p.39).

NO ↓

Do any of the following apply?
- You have been ill
- You are under stress
- You are dieting
- There has recently been a major change in your life

— YES →

POSSIBLE CAUSES Illness, stress, sudden weight loss, and major life events can affect the hormones that control the menstrual cycle, causing absent periods.

ACTION Try to keep stress to a minimum and relax as much as possible. Eat well (*see* A HEALTHY DIET, p.28), and, if you still need to lose weight, try to do so slowly (*see* HOW TO LOSE WEIGHT SAFELY, p.147). If your periods do not start again within 3 months, consult your doctor.

NO ↓

Continued on next page

SELF-HELP Home pregnancy test

Home pregnancy testing kits are available over the counter from pharmacies and supermarkets. They work by testing a sample of urine for the hormone human chorionic gonadotropin (HCG), which is normally produced only in pregnancy. The tests are very accurate and are capable of giving a positive result as soon as your period is late. If the test produces a negative result and you still do not have a period afterwards, carry out another test after 10 days.

Testing urine
The test stick is dipped in urine, and the result appears within minutes. In this test, one line shows that the test has worked and a second line shows that the test is positive.

Test has worked

Result window

Urine

NEGATIVE RESULT

Test has worked

HCG positive

POSITIVE RESULT

Continued from previous page

Are you underweight (*see* ASSESSING YOUR WEIGHT, p.29), and/or do you have a rigorous exercise programme?

YES →

POSSIBLE CAUSES Being underweight and/or following a rigorous exercise programme can cause periods to stop temporarily.

ACTION Eat a healthy diet (p.28), and cut down on the amount of exercise you do. If your periods do not start again within 3 months, consult your doctor.

NO ↓

Have you recently started or stopped taking the oral contraceptive pill?

YES →

POSSIBLE CAUSE AND ACTION Oral contraceptive pills alter your normal hormone levels and may affect your periods. Some pills intentionally stop periods occurring. If your periods do not return after stopping the pill, carry out a home pregnancy test (opposite). If the result is negative and your periods have not restarted within 3 months, consult your doctor.

NO ↓

Have you recently been fitted with a progestogen intrauterine contraceptive device?

YES →

POSSIBLE CAUSE AND ACTION Progestogen intrauterine contraceptive devices can reduce the amount of bleeding during periods or stop periods altogether. Many women consider this an advantage, but if you are worried, consult your doctor. He or she may suggest an alternative method of contraception (*see* METHODS OF CONTRACEPTION, p.273).

NO ↓

Have you had chemotherapy and/or radiotherapy to the lower abdomen?

YES →

POSSIBLE CAUSES Both chemotherapy and radiotherapy may damage the ovaries, causing premature menopause and absent periods. Consult your doctor.

ACTION Your doctor may arrange for a blood test to confirm that you are menopausal. He or she may want to discuss with you the possibility of hormone replacement therapy (*see* A HEALTHY MENOPAUSE, right).

NO ↓

Are you over 45?

YES →

POSSIBLE CAUSE You may be approaching the menopause. Consult your doctor.

ACTION Your doctor may arrange for a blood test to confirm that you are menopausal. He or she may discuss hormone replacement therapy with you (*see* A HEALTHY MENOPAUSE, right).

NO ↓

Have you noticed an increase in facial or body hair and/or deepening of the voice?

YES →

POSSIBLE CAUSES You may have polycystic ovary syndrome, a condition in which there are multiple fluid-filled cysts on both of the ovaries and ovulation does not occur normally. Alternatively, a hormonal disorder is a possibility. Consult your doctor.

ACTION Your doctor will probably arrange for tests, such as blood tests to measure hormone levels and ultrasound scanning (p.39) of your pelvis to detect ovarian cysts. Treatment depends on the cause but will probably include drug treatment.

NO ↓

CONSULT YOUR DOCTOR IF YOU ARE UNABLE TO MAKE A DIAGNOSIS FROM THIS CHART.

A healthy menopause

The menopause is the stage in a woman's life when periods stop, the ovaries no longer produce eggs, and the amount of the sex hormone oestrogen declines. It normally occurs between the ages of 45 and 55. Around 8 in 10 women have mild symptoms at menopause, but some may develop more severe problems, including hot flushes, mood swings, and night sweats. The decline in oestrogen levels also increases the risk of osteoporosis and heart disease in later life.

Lifestyle changes

An adequate intake of calcium and regular weight-bearing exercise will help to reduce the risk of osteoporosis. Exercise also helps to protect against heart disease, as does stopping smoking and eating a healthy diet (p.28). If you suffer from mood swings, talk to your partner or to friends. Relaxation techniques (p.32) may also be helpful for you.

Drug treatment

Talk to your doctor about hormone replacement therapy (HRT). This drug treatment may help to relieve many of the symptoms associated with the menopause. However, HRT is usually only advised for short-term use around the menopause; long-term use is associated with an increased risk of disorders such as breast cancer and thromboembolism.

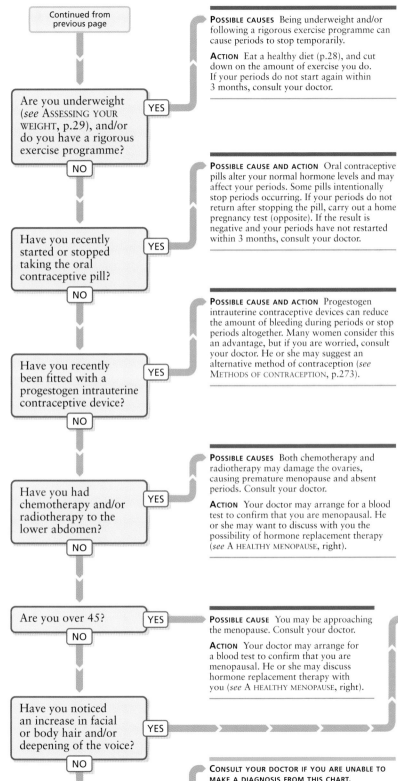

Keeping active
Weight-bearing exercise, such as jogging, can help to prevent osteoporosis after menopause. Exercise is also good for the heart and has a positive effect on mood.

131 Heavy periods

Heavy periods, also known as menorrhagia, are periods in which an excessive amount of blood is lost due to heavy or prolonged bleeding. For most women, bleeding lasts about 5 days. Consult this chart if your periods last longer than this, if normal sanitary protection is insufficient, if you pass clots, or if your periods suddenly become heavier than usual. In most cases, the cause is not serious, but heavy periods can cause iron deficiency and lead to anaemia.

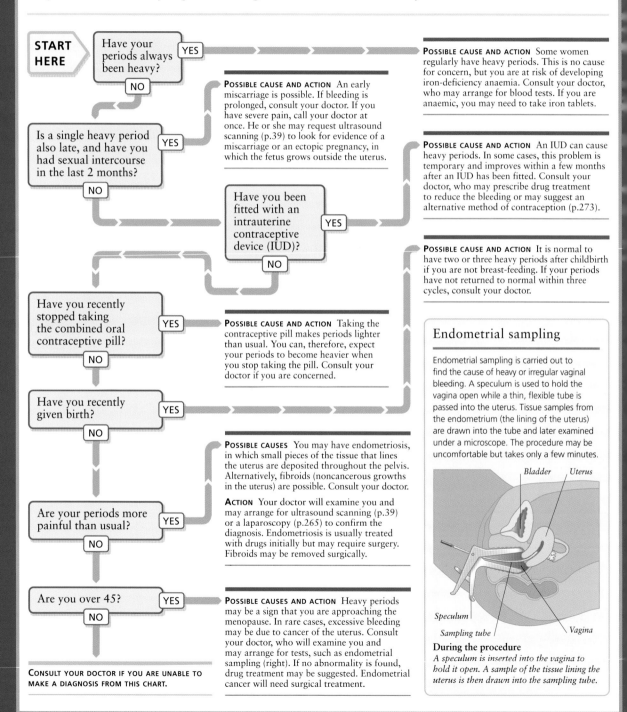

START HERE

Have your periods always been heavy? — YES → **POSSIBLE CAUSE AND ACTION** Some women regularly have heavy periods. This is no cause for concern, but you are at risk of developing iron-deficiency anaemia. Consult your doctor, who may arrange for blood tests. If you are anaemic, you may need to take iron tablets.

NO ↓

Is a single heavy period also late, and have you had sexual intercourse in the last 2 months? — YES → **POSSIBLE CAUSE AND ACTION** An early miscarriage is possible. If bleeding is prolonged, consult your doctor. If you have severe pain, call your doctor at once. He or she may request ultrasound scanning (p.39) to look for evidence of a miscarriage or an ectopic pregnancy, in which the fetus grows outside the uterus.

NO ↓

Have you been fitted with an intrauterine contraceptive device (IUD)? — YES → **POSSIBLE CAUSE AND ACTION** An IUD can cause heavy periods. In some cases, this problem is temporary and improves within a few months after an IUD has been fitted. Consult your doctor, who may prescribe drug treatment to reduce the bleeding or may suggest an alternative method of contraception (p.273).

NO ↓

Have you recently stopped taking the combined oral contraceptive pill? — YES → **POSSIBLE CAUSE AND ACTION** Taking the contraceptive pill makes periods lighter than usual. You can, therefore, expect your periods to become heavier when you stop taking the pill. Consult your doctor if you are concerned.

NO ↓

Have you recently given birth? — YES → **POSSIBLE CAUSE AND ACTION** It is normal to have two or three heavy periods after childbirth if you are not breast-feeding. If your periods have not returned to normal within three cycles, consult your doctor.

NO ↓

Are your periods more painful than usual? — YES → **POSSIBLE CAUSES** You may have endometriosis, in which small pieces of the tissue that lines the uterus are deposited throughout the pelvis. Alternatively, fibroids (noncancerous growths in the uterus) are possible. Consult your doctor.

ACTION Your doctor will examine you and may arrange for ultrasound scanning (p.39) or a laparoscopy (p.265) to confirm the diagnosis. Endometriosis is usually treated with drugs initially but may require surgery. Fibroids may be removed surgically.

NO ↓

Are you over 45? — YES → **POSSIBLE CAUSES AND ACTION** Heavy periods may be a sign that you are approaching the menopause. In rare cases, excessive bleeding may be due to cancer of the uterus. Consult your doctor, who will examine you and may arrange for tests, such as endometrial sampling (right). If no abnormality is found, drug treatment may be suggested. Endometrial cancer will need surgical treatment.

NO ↓

CONSULT YOUR DOCTOR IF YOU ARE UNABLE TO MAKE A DIAGNOSIS FROM THIS CHART.

Endometrial sampling

Endometrial sampling is carried out to find the cause of heavy or irregular vaginal bleeding. A speculum is used to hold the vagina open while a thin, flexible tube is passed into the uterus. Tissue samples from the endometrium (the lining of the uterus) are drawn into the tube and later examined under a microscope. The procedure may be uncomfortable but takes only a few minutes.

Bladder   *Uterus*

Speculum

Sampling tube   *Vagina*

During the procedure
A speculum is inserted into the vagina to hold it open. A sample of the tissue lining the uterus is then drawn into the sampling tube.

132 Painful periods

Many women experience some degree of pain or discomfort during menstrual periods. The pain – sometimes known as dysmenorrhoea – is usually cramping and is felt in the lower abdomen or back. In most cases, painful periods are not due to an underlying disorder and do not disrupt everyday activities. However, if you suffer from severe pain or if your periods suddenly become much more painful than usual, you should consult your doctor.

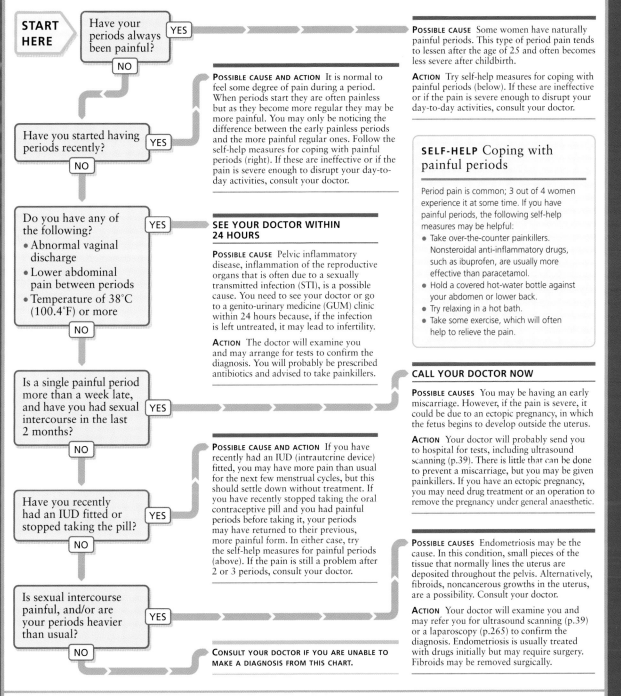

START HERE → Have your periods always been painful? **YES** →

POSSIBLE CAUSE Some women have naturally painful periods. This type of period pain tends to lessen after the age of 25 and often becomes less severe after childbirth.

ACTION Try self-help measures for coping with painful periods (below). If these are ineffective or if the pain is severe enough to disrupt your day-to-day activities, consult your doctor.

NO ↓

Have you started having periods recently? **YES** →

POSSIBLE CAUSE AND ACTION It is normal to feel some degree of pain during a period. When periods start they are often painless but as they become more regular they may be more painful. You may only be noticing the difference between the early painless periods and the more painful regular ones. Follow the self-help measures for coping with painful periods (right). If these are ineffective or if the pain is severe enough to disrupt your day-to-day activities, consult your doctor.

NO ↓

Do you have any of the following?
- Abnormal vaginal discharge
- Lower abdominal pain between periods
- Temperature of 38°C (100.4°F) or more

YES →

SEE YOUR DOCTOR WITHIN 24 HOURS

POSSIBLE CAUSE Pelvic inflammatory disease, inflammation of the reproductive organs that is often due to a sexually transmitted infection (STI), is a possible cause. You need to see your doctor or go to a genito-urinary medicine (GUM) clinic within 24 hours because, if the infection is left untreated, it may lead to infertility.

ACTION The doctor will examine you and may arrange for tests to confirm the diagnosis. You will probably be prescribed antibiotics and advised to take painkillers.

NO ↓

Is a single painful period more than a week late, and have you had sexual intercourse in the last 2 months? **YES** →

NO ↓

Have you recently had an IUD fitted or stopped taking the pill? **YES** →

POSSIBLE CAUSE AND ACTION If you have recently had an IUD (intrautcrine device) fitted, you may have more pain than usual for the next few menstrual cycles, but this should settle down without treatment. If you have recently stopped taking the oral contraceptive pill and you had painful periods before taking it, your periods may have returned to their previous, more painful form. In either case, try the self-help measures for painful periods (above). If the pain is still a problem after 2 or 3 periods, consult your doctor.

NO ↓

Is sexual intercourse painful, and/or are your periods heavier than usual? **YES** →

NO ↓

CONSULT YOUR DOCTOR IF YOU ARE UNABLE TO MAKE A DIAGNOSIS FROM THIS CHART.

SELF-HELP Coping with painful periods

Period pain is common; 3 out of 4 women experience it at some time. If you have painful periods, the following self-help measures may be helpful:
- Take over-the-counter painkillers. Nonsteroidal anti-inflammatory drugs, such as ibuprofen, are usually more effective than paracetamol.
- Hold a covered hot-water bottle against your abdomen or lower back.
- Try relaxing in a hot bath.
- Take some exercise, which will often help to relieve the pain.

CALL YOUR DOCTOR NOW

POSSIBLE CAUSES You may be having an early miscarriage. However, if the pain is severe, it could be due to an ectopic pregnancy, in which the fetus begins to develop outside the uterus.

ACTION Your doctor will probably send you to hospital for tests, including ultrasound scanning (p.39). There is little that can be done to prevent a miscarriage, but you may be given painkillers. If you have an ectopic pregnancy, you may need drug treatment or an operation to remove the pregnancy under general anaesthetic.

POSSIBLE CAUSES Endometriosis may be the cause. In this condition, small pieces of the tissue that normally lines the uterus are deposited throughout the pelvis. Alternatively, fibroids, noncancerous growths in the uterus, are a possibility. Consult your doctor.

ACTION Your doctor will examine you and may refer you for ultrasound scanning (p.39) or a laparoscopy (p.265) to confirm the diagnosis. Endometriosis is usually treated with drugs initially but may require surgery. Fibroids may be removed surgically.

133 Irregular vaginal bleeding

Irregular vaginal bleeding includes any bleeding outside the normal menstrual cycle or after the menopause. The bleeding may consist of occasional light "spotting", or it may be heavier. Although there is often a simple explanation, you should always consult your doctor if you have any abnormal vaginal bleeding. Bleeding between periods or after sexual intercourse may be a sign of a serious underlying disorder and should be investigated by your doctor.

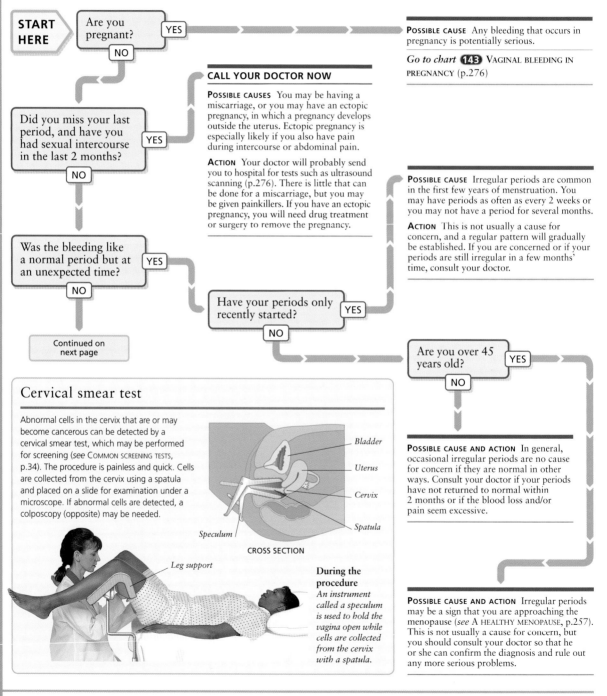

START HERE

Are you pregnant? — YES →

POSSIBLE CAUSE Any bleeding that occurs in pregnancy is potentially serious.

Go to chart **143** VAGINAL BLEEDING IN PREGNANCY (p.276)

NO ↓

Did you miss your last period, and have you had sexual intercourse in the last 2 months? — YES →

CALL YOUR DOCTOR NOW

POSSIBLE CAUSES You may be having a miscarriage, or you may have an ectopic pregnancy, in which a pregnancy develops outside the uterus. Ectopic pregnancy is especially likely if you also have pain during intercourse or abdominal pain.

ACTION Your doctor will probably send you to hospital for tests such as ultrasound scanning (p.276). There is little that can be done for a miscarriage, but you may be given painkillers. If you have an ectopic pregnancy, you will need drug treatment or surgery to remove the pregnancy.

NO ↓

Was the bleeding like a normal period but at an unexpected time? — YES →

Have your periods only recently started? — YES →

POSSIBLE CAUSE Irregular periods are common in the first few years of menstruation. You may have periods as often as every 2 weeks or you may not have a period for several months.

ACTION This is not usually a cause for concern, and a regular pattern will gradually be established. If you are concerned or if your periods are still irregular in a few months' time, consult your doctor.

NO ↓

Continued on next page

NO ↓

Are you over 45 years old? — YES →

NO ↓

Cervical smear test

Abnormal cells in the cervix that are or may become cancerous can be detected by a cervical smear test, which may be performed for screening (*see* COMMON SCREENING TESTS, p.34). The procedure is painless and quick. Cells are collected from the cervix using a spatula and placed on a slide for examination under a microscope. If abnormal cells are detected, a colposcopy (opposite) may be needed.

Bladder

Uterus

Cervix

Spatula

Speculum

CROSS SECTION

Leg support

During the procedure
An instrument called a speculum is used to hold the vagina open while cells are collected from the cervix with a spatula.

POSSIBLE CAUSE AND ACTION In general, occasional irregular periods are no cause for concern if they are normal in other ways. Consult your doctor if your periods have not returned to normal within 2 months or if the blood loss and/or pain seem excessive.

POSSIBLE CAUSE AND ACTION Irregular periods may be a sign that you are approaching the menopause (*see* A HEALTHY MENOPAUSE, p.257). This is not usually a cause for concern, but you should consult your doctor so that he or she can confirm the diagnosis and rule out any more serious problems.

Continued from
previous page

Colposcopy

A colposcope is a microscope that gives a magnified view of the cervix from outside the body. It is used if a cervical smear test (opposite) has detected abnormal cells. During the procedure, the doctor may apply a substance to the cervix that distinguishes between normal and abnormal tissue. Samples can then be taken from abnormal areas for examination in a laboratory. Various treatments can also be carried out during colposcopy. For example, abnormal tissue can be destroyed using a laser or by freezing tissue with a probe. The whole procedure usually takes less than 40 minutes.

During the procedure
The vagina is held open by a speculum, and the doctor inspects the cervix through the colposcope. A monitor may display the image.

Monitor

Colposcope

Leg support

Does the unexpected bleeding occur only in the first few hours after sexual intercourse?

YES

NO

Are you over 45, and is it more than 6 months since your last period?

YES

NO

Hysteroscopy

In hysteroscopy, a viewing instrument called a hysteroscope is used to examine the inside of the uterus and detect disorders such as uterine polyps. The hysteroscope is introduced through the vagina and cervix under local or general anaesthesia. The lining of the uterus can be inspected, and treatments such as removal of a polyp may be carried out during the procedure; it usually takes less than 15 minutes to perform.

Hysteroscope

Inflated uterus

Illuminated area

Inflated fallopian tube

During the procedure
Gas is passed through the hysteroscope to inflate the uterus and the fallopian tubes. A light illuminates the area.

POSSIBLE CAUSES Bleeding that occurs more than 6 months after the last period is known as postmenopausal bleeding. Most commonly, the bleeding is from the walls of the vagina, which become fragile in the absence of oestrogen. Less commonly, polyps inside the uterus or cancer of the uterus or cervix may be the cause. Consult your doctor.

ACTION Your doctor will examine you and carry out a cervical smear test (opposite). He or she may also refer you for tests such as hysteroscopy (left) or endometrial sampling (p.258). For bleeding from the vagina, your doctor may suggest hormone replacement therapy or local oestrogen creams. Polyps can often be removed during hysteroscopy. If cancer of the uterus or cervix is diagnosed, you will probably need a hysterectomy.

POSSIBLE CAUSES You may have cervical ectopy (also known as cervical erosion). In this condition, the delicate cells on the inner lining of the cervix extend on to its surface. Rarely, the bleeding may result from abnormal cells that are associated with cancer of the cervix. Consult your doctor.

ACTION Your doctor will examine you and may carry out a cervical smear test (opposite). Cervical ectopy may need no treatment or may be treated by freezing the cells using a probe. If abnormal cells are present, treatment will depend on the results of colposcopy (above), but may include laser surgery.

POSSIBLE CAUSES AND ACTION Some irregular bleeding may occur in the first few months after starting the oral contraceptive pill or having a progestogen intrauterine contraceptive device (IUS) fitted. Despite the bleeding, you are still protected against pregnancy. If abnormal bleeding persists for more than a few months or develops when there have previously been no problems, consult your doctor, who may suggest an alternative contraceptive method (*see* METHODS OF CONTRACEPTION, p.273).

Are you taking the oral contraceptive pill, or have you had a progestogen intrauterine contraceptive device (IUS) fitted recently?

YES

NO

CONSULT YOUR DOCTOR IF YOU ARE UNABLE TO MAKE A DIAGNOSIS FROM THIS CHART.

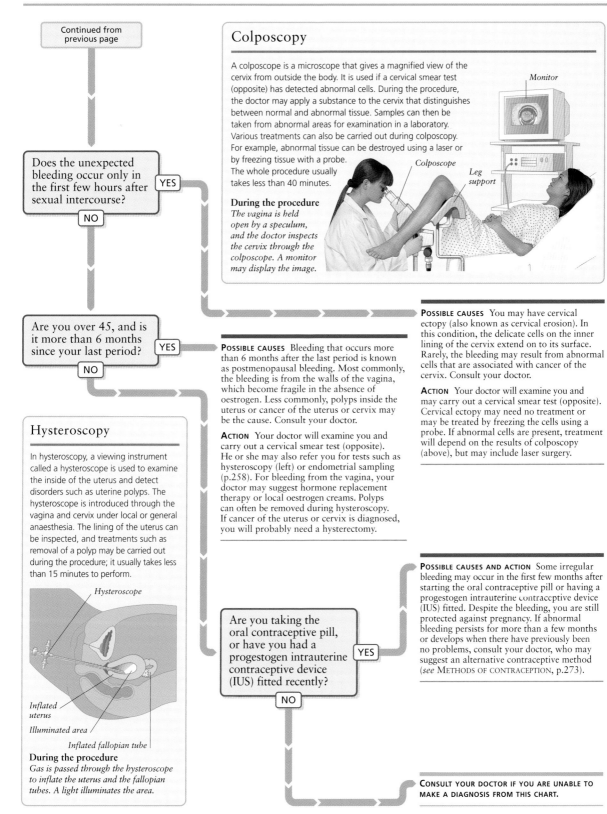

134 Abnormal vaginal discharge

Consult this chart if you notice an increase in your vaginal discharge or a change in its colour, consistency, or smell. Secretions from the walls of the vagina and the cervix keep the vagina moist and clean. The secretions usually produce a thin yellowish-white discharge that varies in quantity and consistency during the menstrual cycle. The volume of secretions increases at times of sexual arousal and during

pregnancy. This is completely normal and is no cause for concern. However, a sudden increase in the amount of vaginal discharge for no obvious reason or vaginal discharge that looks abnormal or smells unpleasant may be a sign of an infection. If the abnormal discharge is accompanied by abdominal pain and/or fever, the infection may involve the reproductive organs and needs urgent treatment.

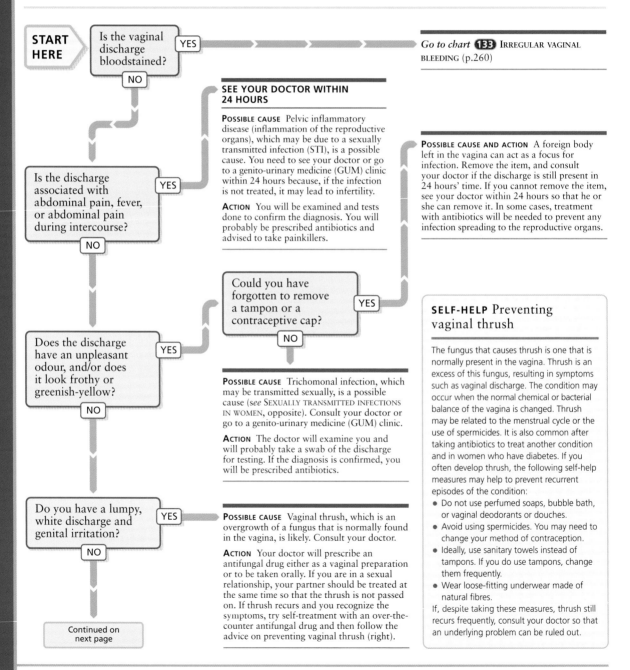

START HERE

Is the vaginal discharge bloodstained?
— YES → *Go to chart* **133** IRREGULAR VAGINAL BLEEDING (p.260)
— NO

Is the discharge associated with abdominal pain, fever, or abdominal pain during intercourse?
— YES →

SEE YOUR DOCTOR WITHIN 24 HOURS

POSSIBLE CAUSE Pelvic inflammatory disease (inflammation of the reproductive organs), which may be due to a sexually transmitted infection (STI), is a possible cause. You need to see your doctor or go to a genito-urinary medicine (GUM) clinic within 24 hours because, if the infection is not treated, it may lead to infertility.

ACTION You will be examined and tests done to confirm the diagnosis. You will probably be prescribed antibiotics and advised to take painkillers.

— NO

Could you have forgotten to remove a tampon or a contraceptive cap?
— YES →

POSSIBLE CAUSE AND ACTION A foreign body left in the vagina can act as a focus for infection. Remove the item, and consult your doctor if the discharge is still present in 24 hours' time. If you cannot remove the item, see your doctor within 24 hours so that he or she can remove it. In some cases, treatment with antibiotics will be needed to prevent any infection spreading to the reproductive organs.

— NO

Does the discharge have an unpleasant odour, and/or does it look frothy or greenish-yellow?
— YES →

POSSIBLE CAUSE Trichomonal infection, which may be transmitted sexually, is a possible cause (see SEXUALLY TRANSMITTED INFECTIONS IN WOMEN, opposite). Consult your doctor or go to a genito-urinary medicine (GUM) clinic.

ACTION The doctor will examine you and will probably take a swab of the discharge for testing. If the diagnosis is confirmed, you will be prescribed antibiotics.

— NO

Do you have a lumpy, white discharge and genital irritation?
— YES →

POSSIBLE CAUSE Vaginal thrush, which is an overgrowth of a fungus that is normally found in the vagina, is likely. Consult your doctor.

ACTION Your doctor will prescribe an antifungal drug either as a vaginal preparation or to be taken orally. If you are in a sexual relationship, your partner should be treated at the same time so that the thrush is not passed on. If thrush recurs and you recognize the symptoms, try self-treatment with an over-the-counter antifungal drug and then follow the advice on preventing vaginal thrush (right).

— NO

Continued on next page

SELF-HELP Preventing vaginal thrush

The fungus that causes thrush is one that is normally present in the vagina. Thrush is an excess of this fungus, resulting in symptoms such as vaginal discharge. The condition may occur when the normal chemical or bacterial balance of the vagina is changed. Thrush may be related to the menstrual cycle or the use of spermicides. It is also common after taking antibiotics to treat another condition and in women who have diabetes. If you often develop thrush, the following self-help measures may help to prevent recurrent episodes of the condition:

- Do not use perfumed soaps, bubble bath, or vaginal deodorants or douches.
- Avoid using spermicides. You may need to change your method of contraception.
- Ideally, use sanitary towels instead of tampons. If you do use tampons, change them frequently.
- Wear loose-fitting underwear made of natural fibres.

If, despite taking these measures, thrush still recurs frequently, consult your doctor so that an underlying problem can be ruled out.

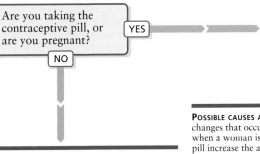

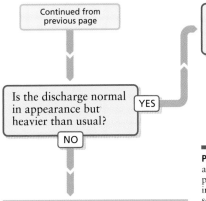

Continued from previous page

Are you taking the contraceptive pill, or are you pregnant? — YES

NO

Is the discharge normal in appearance but heavier than usual? — YES

NO

CONSULT YOUR DOCTOR IF YOU ARE UNABLE TO MAKE A DIAGNOSIS FROM THIS CHART.

POSSIBLE CAUSE AND ACTION Changes in the amount of vaginal discharge are a normal part of the menstrual cycle. Vaginal secretions increase just before a period and when you are sexually aroused. Your symptoms are unlikely to be due to a disorder, but consult your doctor if you are concerned.

POSSIBLE CAUSES AND ACTION The hormonal changes that occur during pregnancy or when a woman is taking the contraceptive pill increase the amount of vaginal secretions. There is also a possibility of cervical ectopy (also known as erosion), in which the delicate cells on the inner lining of the cervix extend on to its surface. No treatment is needed, but if you are not pregnant, your doctor may recommend a cervical smear test (p.260) to check for cervical erosion.

Sexually transmitted infections in women

Infections passed from one person to another during sexual intercourse (vaginal, anal, or oral) are known as sexually transmitted infections (STIs). Although these infections affect both men and women, the symptoms are often different (see SEXUALLY TRANSMITTED INFECTIONS IN MEN, p.241). The symptoms may also affect different areas of the body depending on which type of sexual contact you have had. Even when there are few symptoms, infection can spread from the vagina to all of the reproductive organs and may cause permanent damage if left untreated. An STI contracted during pregnancy may affect the fetus, or the baby may acquire the infection during delivery. If you think you or your partner have an STI, you should consult your doctor or go to a genito-urinary medicine (GUM) clinic at a local hospital, where you will be treated in confidence. You should avoid sex until your doctor confirms that the infection has cleared up. The risk of contracting an STI can be reduced by practising safe sex (p.32).

Infection	Incubation period*	Symptoms in women	Diagnosis and treatment
Chlamydial infection	14–21 days	Often causes few or no symptoms. There may be an abnormal vaginal discharge or pain on passing urine. If the infection affects the fallopian tubes, there may be fever, abdominal pain, or pain on intercourse.	The doctor will take a swab from the cervix to identify the infectious organism. Treatment is usually with antibiotics.
Genital herpes	4–7 days	There is usually soreness or itching in the genital area or on the thighs, followed by the appearance of a crop of small, painful blisters. The blisters burst to produce shallow ulcers, which are painful on urinating. The ulcers heal after 10–21 days. The condition may recur.	The diagnosis is usually made according to the appearance of the skin. A swab may be taken from one of the sores. Oral antiviral drugs taken early shorten episodes but do not eradicate the virus. Genital herpes is most infectious while the ulcers are present, but in some cases can remain infectious after the ulcers heal.
Genital warts	1–20 months	Pink, fleshy lumps on the vulva, and in some cases, inside the vagina, on the cervix, and around the anus. Warts may go unnoticed if they occur internally.	The doctor may treat warts by applying a chemical lotion or by freezing them off. Sometimes, surgery may be necessary. Never attempt to treat genital warts with over-the-counter wart preparations.
Gonorrhoea	7–21 days	May be symptomless in women. It may cause abnormal vaginal discharge, lower abdominal pain, and fever. Rectal infection may cause pain on passing faeces.	The doctor will take a swab from the vagina or the rectum to identify the infectious organism. Treatment is with antibiotics.
HIV infection	6–8 weeks	May be no initial symptoms, but some people may have a brief flu-like illness, sometimes with a rash and swollen lymph nodes. After years without symptoms, AIDS may develop (see HIV INFECTION AND AIDS, p.144). HIV can be passed on whether or not you have symptoms.	Diagnosis is made by a blood test taken 3 or more months after the initial infection. People with HIV infection are usually referred to special centres for treatment. Combinations of antiviral drugs are often effective in delaying the progression of HIV to AIDS.
Pubic lice	0–17 days	Usually there is intense itching in the pubic region, particularly at night. The lice are 1–2 mm long and may be visible.	Treatment is with a lotion that kills the lice and their eggs. Such lotions can be bought over the counter.
Syphilis	1–12 weeks	In the first stage, a highly infectious, painless sore called a chancre develops in the genital area or inside the vagina. In some cases, the sores go unnoticed. If the condition is left untreated, it can progress to involve internal organs, causing a rash, fever, and swollen lymph nodes.	The disease is diagnosed by blood tests and tests on swabs taken from any sores. The usual treatment is a course of antibiotic injections.
Trichomonal infection	Variable	An unpleasant-smelling, greenish-yellow discharge, with irritation and soreness around the vagina. Painful intercourse. Sometimes symptoms may go unnoticed.	The diagnosis is confirmed by examination of a sample of discharge taken from the vagina. The usual treatment is with oral antibiotics.

*Time between contact with the disease and the appearance of symptoms

135 Genital irritation

Consult this chart if you are suffering from itching and/or discomfort in the vagina or around the vulva (the external genital area). Such irritation may also cause stinging when you pass urine and may make sexual intercourse uncomfortable.

In many cases, these symptoms are the result of an infection, but an allergic reaction is another common cause. Scented soaps, vaginal deodorants, and douches can often cause irritation, and you should avoid using them.

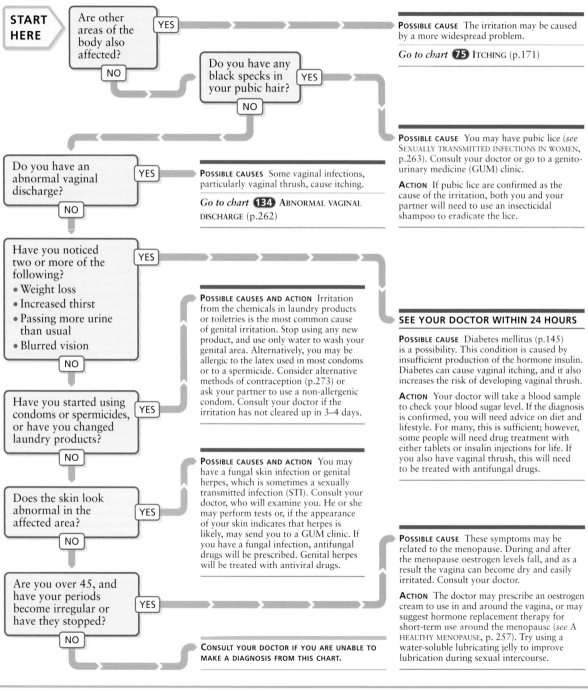

START HERE

Are other areas of the body also affected?
YES → **POSSIBLE CAUSE** The irritation may be caused by a more widespread problem.

Go to chart **75** ITCHING (p.171)

NO ↓

Do you have any black specks in your pubic hair?
YES → **POSSIBLE CAUSE** You may have pubic lice (*see* SEXUALLY TRANSMITTED INFECTIONS IN WOMEN, p.263). Consult your doctor or go to a genito-urinary medicine (GUM) clinic.

ACTION If pubic lice are confirmed as the cause of the irritation, both you and your partner will need to use an insecticidal shampoo to eradicate the lice.

NO ↓

Do you have an abnormal vaginal discharge?
YES → **POSSIBLE CAUSES** Some vaginal infections, particularly vaginal thrush, cause itching.

Go to chart **134** ABNORMAL VAGINAL DISCHARGE (p.262)

NO ↓

Have you noticed two or more of the following?
- Weight loss
- Increased thirst
- Passing more urine than usual
- Blurred vision

YES →

POSSIBLE CAUSES AND ACTION Irritation from the chemicals in laundry products or toiletries is the most common cause of genital irritation. Stop using any new product, and use only water to wash your genital area. Alternatively, you may be allergic to the latex used in most condoms or to a spermicide. Consider alternative methods of contraception (p.273) or ask your partner to use a non-allergenic condom. Consult your doctor if the irritation has not cleared up in 3–4 days.

NO ↓

Have you started using condoms or spermicides, or have you changed laundry products?
YES →

NO ↓

Does the skin look abnormal in the affected area?
YES →

POSSIBLE CAUSES AND ACTION You may have a fungal skin infection or genital herpes, which is sometimes a sexually transmitted infection (STI). Consult your doctor, who will examine you. He or she may perform tests or, if the appearance of your skin indicates that herpes is likely, may send you to a GUM clinic. If you have a fungal infection, antifungal drugs will be prescribed. Genital herpes will be treated with antiviral drugs.

NO ↓

Are you over 45, and have your periods become irregular or have they stopped?
YES →

NO ↓

CONSULT YOUR DOCTOR IF YOU ARE UNABLE TO MAKE A DIAGNOSIS FROM THIS CHART.

SEE YOUR DOCTOR WITHIN 24 HOURS

POSSIBLE CAUSE Diabetes mellitus (p.145) is a possibility. This condition is caused by insufficient production of the hormone insulin. Diabetes can cause vaginal itching, and it also increases the risk of developing vaginal thrush.

ACTION Your doctor will take a blood sample to check your blood sugar level. If the diagnosis is confirmed, you will need advice on diet and lifestyle. For many, this is sufficient; however, some people will need drug treatment with either tablets or insulin injections for life. If you also have vaginal thrush, this will need to be treated with antifungal drugs.

POSSIBLE CAUSE These symptoms may be related to the menopause. During and after the menopause oestrogen levels fall, and as a result the vagina can become dry and easily irritated. Consult your doctor.

ACTION The doctor may prescribe an oestrogen cream to use in and around the vagina, or may suggest hormone replacement therapy for short-term use around the menopause (*see* A HEALTHY MENOPAUSE, p. 257). Try using a water-soluble lubricating jelly to improve lubrication during sexual intercourse.

136 Lower abdominal pain in women

Consult this chart only after reading chart 100,
Abdominal pain (p.210).
Disorders affecting the urinary tract or the intestine may cause abdominal pain in both men and women but there are also several disorders causing lower abdominal pain that are specific to women. These disorders affect the female reproductive organs, such as the ovaries, uterus, and the fallopian tubes. Some of them may need medical attention.

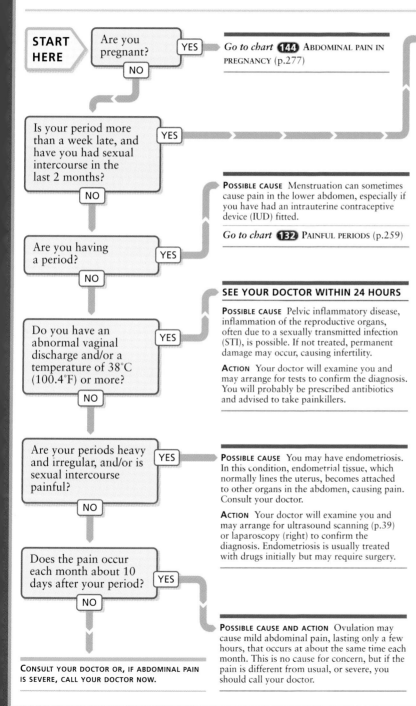

START HERE → Are you pregnant? — **YES** → *Go to chart* 144 Abdominal pain in pregnancy (p.277)

NO ↓

Is your period more than a week late, and have you had sexual intercourse in the last 2 months? — **YES** →

NO ↓

Are you having a period? — **YES** →

POSSIBLE CAUSE Menstruation can sometimes cause pain in the lower abdomen, especially if you have had an intrauterine contraceptive device (IUD) fitted.

Go to chart 132 Painful periods (p.259)

NO ↓

Do you have an abnormal vaginal discharge and/or a temperature of 38°C (100.4°F) or more? — **YES** →

NO ↓

Are your periods heavy and irregular, and/or is sexual intercourse painful? — **YES** →

NO ↓

Does the pain occur each month about 10 days after your period? — **YES** →

NO ↓

CONSULT YOUR DOCTOR OR, IF ABDOMINAL PAIN IS SEVERE, CALL YOUR DOCTOR NOW.

CALL YOUR DOCTOR NOW

POSSIBLE CAUSES You may be pregnant and having a miscarriage, or you may have an ectopic pregnancy, in which a pregnancy develops outside the uterus.

ACTION Your doctor will probably send you to hospital for ultrasound scanning (p.39). There is little that can be done to prevent a miscarriage, but you may be given painkillers. If you have an ectopic pregnancy, you may need drug treatment or an operation under general anaesthetic.

SEE YOUR DOCTOR WITHIN 24 HOURS

POSSIBLE CAUSE Pelvic inflammatory disease, inflammation of the reproductive organs, often due to a sexually transmitted infection (STI), is possible. If not treated, permanent damage may occur, causing infertility.

ACTION Your doctor will examine you and may arrange for tests to confirm the diagnosis. You will probably be prescribed antibiotics and advised to take painkillers.

POSSIBLE CAUSE You may have endometriosis. In this condition, endometrial tissue, which normally lines the uterus, becomes attached to other organs in the abdomen, causing pain. Consult your doctor.

ACTION Your doctor will examine you and may arrange for ultrasound scanning (p.39) or laparoscopy (right) to confirm the diagnosis. Endometriosis is usually treated with drugs initially but may require surgery.

POSSIBLE CAUSE AND ACTION Ovulation may cause mild abdominal pain, lasting only a few hours, that occurs at about the same time each month. This is no cause for concern, but if the pain is different from usual, or severe, you should call your doctor.

Laparoscopy

Laparoscopy is a procedure in which a rigid, tube-like viewing instrument is introduced into the abdomen through a small incision. It may be performed to look for disorders of the female reproductive organs, such as endometriosis, or to investigate other abdominal disorders, such as appendicitis; it is also used to take tissue samples or carry out surgery. Before the laparoscope is inserted, gas is pumped through the incision to make viewing easier. Tools for performing procedures may be introduced through another small incision in the abdomen or through the vagina. The procedure is done under general anaesthetic.

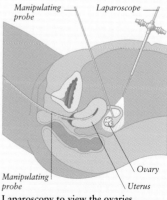

Laparoscopy to view the ovaries
The laparoscope is inserted through a small incision to give an illuminated view of the ovaries. Probes are used to move organs or manipulate the ovaries for better viewing.

137 Painful intercourse in women

Consult this chart if sexual intercourse is painful. Feeling pain or discomfort in or around the vagina at the time of penetration or during or following intercourse is a relatively common problem in women. It may occur for a variety of physical or emotional reasons. Whatever the reason, you should seek medical advice, because persistent pain during intercourse will affect your desire for sex and may damage your relationship with your partner.

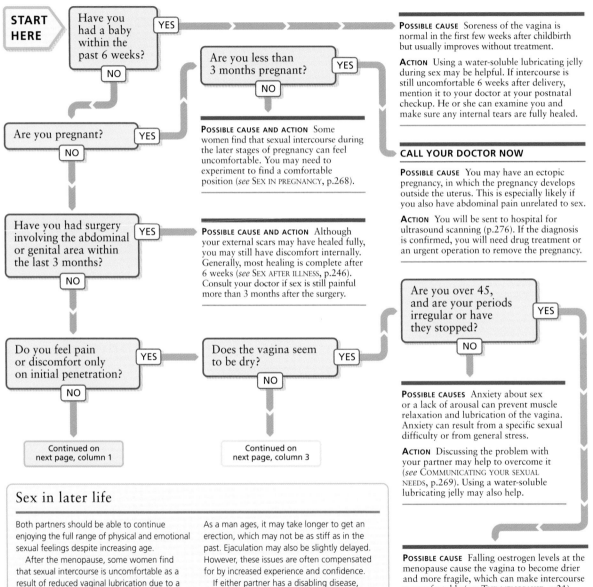

START HERE

Have you had a baby within the past 6 weeks? — NO / YES

Are you pregnant? — NO / YES

Are you less than 3 months pregnant? — NO / YES

Have you had surgery involving the abdominal or genital area within the last 3 months? — NO / YES

Do you feel pain or discomfort only on initial penetration? — NO / YES

Does the vagina seem to be dry? — NO / YES

Are you over 45, and are your periods irregular or have they stopped? — NO / YES

POSSIBLE CAUSE Soreness of the vagina is normal in the first few weeks after childbirth but usually improves without treatment.

ACTION Using a water-soluble lubricating jelly during sex may be helpful. If intercourse is still uncomfortable 6 weeks after delivery, mention it to your doctor at your postnatal checkup. He or she can examine you and make sure any internal tears are fully healed.

POSSIBLE CAUSE AND ACTION Some women find that sexual intercourse during the later stages of pregnancy can feel uncomfortable. You may need to experiment to find a comfortable position (*see* SEX IN PREGNANCY, p.268).

CALL YOUR DOCTOR NOW

POSSIBLE CAUSE You may have an ectopic pregnancy, in which the pregnancy develops outside the uterus. This is especially likely if you also have abdominal pain unrelated to sex.

ACTION You will be sent to hospital for ultrasound scanning (p.276). If the diagnosis is confirmed, you will need drug treatment or an urgent operation to remove the pregnancy.

POSSIBLE CAUSE AND ACTION Although your external scars may have healed fully, you may still have discomfort internally. Generally, most healing is complete after 6 weeks (*see* SEX AFTER ILLNESS, p.246). Consult your doctor if sex is still painful more than 3 months after the surgery.

POSSIBLE CAUSES Anxiety about sex or a lack of arousal can prevent muscle relaxation and lubrication of the vagina. Anxiety can result from a specific sexual difficulty or from general stress.

ACTION Discussing the problem with your partner may help to overcome it (*see* COMMUNICATING YOUR SEXUAL NEEDS, p.269). Using a water-soluble lubricating jelly may also help.

POSSIBLE CAUSE Falling oestrogen levels at the menopause cause the vagina to become drier and more fragile, which can make intercourse uncomfortable (*see* THE MENOPAUSE, p.21). Consult your doctor to exclude other causes.

ACTION Your doctor may recommend a water-soluble lubricating jelly and may discuss with you the pros and cons of hormone replacement therapy (*see* A HEALTHY MENOPAUSE, p.257), which can help to relieve the symptoms.

Continued on next page, column 1

Continued on next page, column 3

Sex in later life

Both partners should be able to continue enjoying the full range of physical and emotional sexual feelings despite increasing age.

After the menopause, some women find that sexual intercourse is uncomfortable as a result of reduced vaginal lubrication due to a fall in levels of oestrogen. In the short term, using a water-soluble lubricant jelly and adapting sexual techniques are often the best solutions. In the long term, vaginal dryness can sometimes be helped by hormone replacement therapy (*see* A HEALTHY MENOPAUSE, p.257).

As a man ages, it may take longer to get an erection, which may not be as stiff as in the past. Ejaculation may also be slightly delayed. However, these issues are often compensated for by increased experience and confidence.

If either partner has a disabling disease, experimenting with different positions and forms of sexual contact may help. Some people who have had sexual problems in the past use age as an excuse to avoid sex, but it is never too late to seek counselling for a problem and age is not a bar to receiving treatment.

Continued from previous page, column 1

Do you have a fever and/or an abnormal vaginal discharge? **YES**

NO

Are your periods irregular, heavy, and/or painful? **YES**

NO

Do you feel pain only when having intercourse in certain positions? **YES**

NO

CONSULT YOUR DOCTOR IF YOU ARE UNABLE TO MAKE A DIAGNOSIS FROM THIS CHART.

SEE YOUR DOCTOR WITHIN 24 HOURS

POSSIBLE CAUSE You may have pelvic inflammatory disease, inflammation of the reproductive organs due to an infection.

ACTION Your doctor will examine you and may arrange for tests to confirm the diagnosis. You will probably be prescribed antibiotics and advised to take painkillers.

POSSIBLE CAUSE You may have endometriosis, in which small pieces of the tissue normally lining the uterus become attached to organs in the pelvic cavity. Consult your doctor.

ACTION Your doctor will examine you and may arrange for a laparoscopy (p.265) to confirm the diagnosis. Treatment is usually with drugs and/or surgery.

POSSIBLE CAUSES The pain may be caused by pressure on an ovary during intercourse. However, an ovarian cyst is also a possibility. Consult your doctor.

ACTION Your doctor will examine you and may arrange for you to have ultrasound scanning (p.39) or a laparoscopy (p.265), which will determine what treatment, if any, you will need.

Continued from previous page, column 2

Do you have vaginal irritation with or without a discharge? **YES**

NO

Have you just had sexual intercourse for the first time? **YES**

NO

Have you had prolonged, particularly vigorous, or very frequent intercourse? **YES**

NO

Is penetration too painful for sexual intercourse to occur at all? **YES**

NO

CONSULT YOUR DOCTOR IF YOU ARE UNABLE TO MAKE A DIAGNOSIS FROM THIS CHART.

POSSIBLE CAUSES You may have a vaginal infection, such as thrush or a sexually transmitted infection (p.263). Consult your doctor.

ACTION Your doctor will examine you. If you have thrush, you will be prescribed an antifungal drug and advised on measures for preventing vaginal thrush (p.262). If a sexually transmitted infection (STI) is possible, your doctor may refer you to a genito-urinary medicine (GUM) clinic for tests and appropriate treatment.

POSSIBLE CAUSE It is relatively common for women to feel some pain when they first have sexual intercourse. This is especially likely if the hymen, the membrane that partially covers the opening to the vagina, is still intact.

ACTION Try using a water-soluble lubricating jelly before intercourse. Sex should become less painful on subsequent occasions.

POSSIBLE CAUSE AND ACTION Soreness of the genital area may occur after very frequent sex and is sometimes associated with urinary symptoms. This is usually no cause for concern. If soreness is severe, abstaining from sex for a few days should help.

POSSIBLE CAUSE You may have vaginismus, a condition in which the muscles around the vagina go into spasm, making intercourse painful or impossible. It is usually caused by anxieties relating to sexual issues or, occasionally, by a physical disorder, in which the vagina is abnormally narrowed. Consult your doctor.

ACTION Your doctor will look for any physical problems that could be making sexual intercourse painful. If no physical problems can be found, your doctor will probably refer you to a specialist for treatment (*see* TREATMENTS FOR VAGINISMUS, left).

Treatments for vaginismus

Vaginismus is a condition in which the muscles around the vagina go into spasm, preventing penetration. In one method of treatment, the woman inserts dilators of gradually increasing diameter into her vagina. This can help to allay fears about the ability of the vagina to stretch sufficiently to allow penetration. Vaginismus and some other sexual problems that affect women often have a psychological basis. Sexual counselling can often help to resolve fears or unreconciled past sexual traumas and so treat the condition.

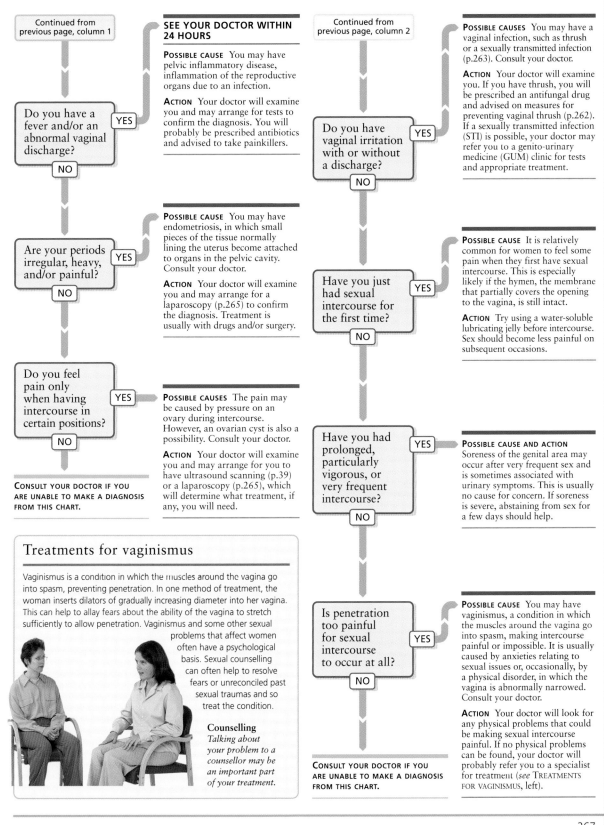

Counselling
Talking about your problem to a counsellor may be an important part of your treatment.

267

138 Low sex drive in women

Some women feel the need for sex once or twice a week or less, others every day. All points in this range are normal. However, a sudden decrease in your normal level of sexual desire may be a sign of a problem. There may be a physical cause – for example, an infection that makes intercourse uncomfortable can reduce your sex drive. In many cases,

low sex drive has a psychological cause, such as stress, depression, or anxiety about a specific sexual difficulty. Consult this chart if you are concerned that your interest in sex is abnormally low or you notice that you are not as easily aroused as you used to be. A delay in seeking help could damage the relationship with your partner.

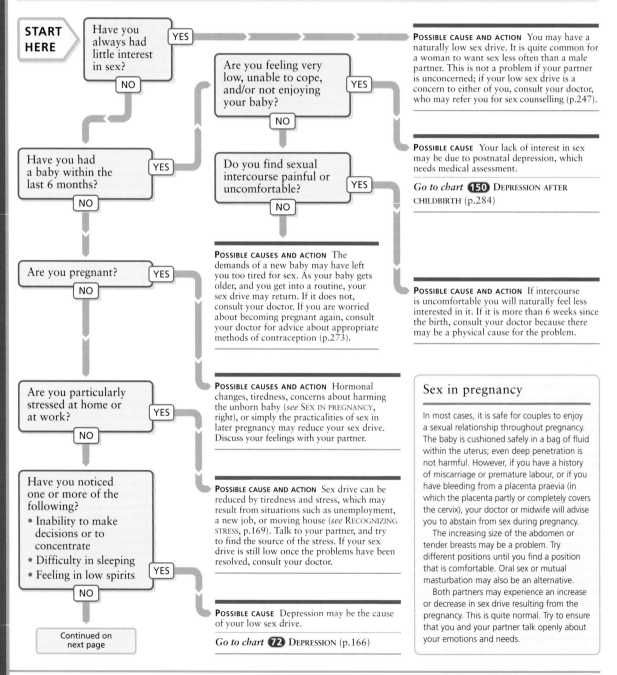

START HERE

Have you always had little interest in sex? — YES →

POSSIBLE CAUSE AND ACTION You may have a naturally low sex drive. It is quite common for a woman to want sex less often than a male partner. This is not a problem if your partner is unconcerned; if your low sex drive is a concern to either of you, consult your doctor, who may refer you for sex counselling (p.247).

NO ↓

Have you had a baby within the last 6 months? — YES →

Are you feeling very low, unable to cope, and/or not enjoying your baby? — YES →

POSSIBLE CAUSE Your lack of interest in sex may be due to postnatal depression, which needs medical assessment.

Go to chart **150** DEPRESSION AFTER CHILDBIRTH (p.284)

NO ↓

Do you find sexual intercourse painful or uncomfortable? — YES →

POSSIBLE CAUSE AND ACTION If intercourse is uncomfortable you will naturally feel less interested in it. If it is more than 6 weeks since the birth, consult your doctor because there may be a physical cause for the problem.

NO ↓

POSSIBLE CAUSES AND ACTION The demands of a new baby may have left you too tired for sex. As your baby gets older, and you get into a routine, your sex drive may return. If it does not, consult your doctor. If you are worried about becoming pregnant again, consult your doctor for advice about appropriate methods of contraception (p.273).

NO ↓

Are you pregnant? — YES →

POSSIBLE CAUSES AND ACTION Hormonal changes, tiredness, concerns about harming the unborn baby (*see* SEX IN PREGNANCY, right), or simply the practicalities of sex in later pregnancy may reduce your sex drive. Discuss your feelings with your partner.

NO ↓

Are you particularly stressed at home or at work? — YES →

POSSIBLE CAUSE AND ACTION Sex drive can be reduced by tiredness and stress, which may result from situations such as unemployment, a new job, or moving house (*see* RECOGNIZING STRESS, p.169). Talk to your partner, and try to find the source of the stress. If your sex drive is still low once the problems have been resolved, consult your doctor.

NO ↓

Have you noticed one or more of the following?
- **Inability to make decisions or to concentrate**
- **Difficulty in sleeping**
- **Feeling in low spirits** — YES →

POSSIBLE CAUSE Depression may be the cause of your low sex drive.

Go to chart **72** DEPRESSION (p.166)

NO ↓

Continued on next page

Sex in pregnancy

In most cases, it is safe for couples to enjoy a sexual relationship throughout pregnancy. The baby is cushioned safely in a bag of fluid within the uterus; even deep penetration is not harmful. However, if you have a history of miscarriage or premature labour, or if you have bleeding from a placenta praevia (in which the placenta partly or completely covers the cervix), your doctor or midwife will advise you to abstain from sex during pregnancy.

The increasing size of the abdomen or tender breasts may be a problem. Try different positions until you find a position that is comfortable. Oral sex or mutual masturbation may also be an alternative.

Both partners may experience an increase or decrease in sex drive resulting from the pregnancy. This is quite normal. Try to ensure that you and your partner talk openly about your emotions and needs.

Continued from previous page

Is your relationship with your partner satisfactory in other respects? **YES**

NO

POSSIBLE CAUSE AND ACTION If you or your partner have a specific sexual problem, concern about it may have reduced your sex drive. Try to talk frankly with your partner (*see* COMMUNICATING YOUR SEXUAL NEEDS, below). If the problem is not resolved, consult your doctor, who may recommend sex counselling (p.247).

Is your lack of interest in sex only with your current partner? **YES**

NO

POSSIBLE CAUSE AND ACTION If the relationship is poor, then you are unlikely to have a healthy interest in sex. Try to talk frankly with your partner. If things do not improve, consult your doctor, who may recommend relationship counselling (*see* USEFUL ADDRESSES, p.285).

Have you recently recovered from a major illness or operation? **YES**

NO

Are you concerned that sexual intercourse may cause your condition to recur or worsen? **YES**

NO

> ### SELF-HELP Communicating your sexual needs
>
> Many people feel that the sexual side of their relationship could be improved but find it difficult to discuss their sexual needs with their partner. The following suggestions may help to improve communication and mutual understanding with your partner, which are the keys to a better sex life.
> - Think carefully about the timing of discussions with your partner. Avoid sounding hostile or critical.
> - Talk about the positive aspects of your sex life, as well as problems.
> - Suggest sexual activities that you would like to do or to spend more time on.
> - Keep your comments open and your suggestions positive.
> - Listen to what your partner says.
> - Create an action plan together and include the points that you would both like to work on.

Are you taking any prescribed drugs? **YES**

NO

POSSIBLE CAUSE AND ACTION Serious illness or surgery can sometimes alter your perception of your body and of yourself in general (*see* SEX AFTER ILLNESS, p.246), resulting in a reduced sex drive. Consult your doctor, who may advise counselling (*see* USEFUL ADDRESSES, p.285).

POSSIBLE CAUSE AND ACTION People who have been ill or had major surgery are often concerned that sex will make their condition worse (*see* SEX AFTER ILLNESS, p.246). These concerns may lower sex drive. In most cases, after a recovery period of about 6 weeks, sex rarely causes problems; however, you should consult your doctor for advice and reassurance.

Are you generally anxious, and/or do you have specific anxieties about sex? **YES**

NO

POSSIBLE CAUSE AND ACTION Sex drive can be reduced by general anxiety or by specific sexual concerns, such as fear of pregnancy or of contracting a sexually transmitted infection (*see* SEXUALLY TRANSMITTED INFECTIONS IN WOMEN, p.263). Concern about your sexual orientation (p.247) is another possible cause. Talk to your partner, and if you are still concerned, consult your doctor.

POSSIBLE CAUSE AND ACTION Certain drugs, such as some beta-blockers and anticancer drugs, can affect hormone levels, reducing sex drive. Consult your doctor. He or she may be able to prescribe an alternative drug. In the meantime, do not stop taking your prescribed drugs.

Are you over 50? **YES**

NO

POSSIBLE CAUSE Sex drive may decline slightly as you get older (*see* SEX IN LATER LIFE, p.266). This need not be a problem as long as your needs and your partner's are compatible. If your loss of sex drive has occurred suddenly, or if you are concerned, consult your doctor.

ACTION Your doctor may arrange for tests to check your hormone levels. Any cause will be treated, if possible, whatever your age.

CONSULT YOUR DOCTOR IF YOU ARE UNABLE TO MAKE A DIAGNOSIS FROM THIS CHART.

139 Fertility problems in women

See also chart 126, FERTILITY PROBLEMS IN MEN **(p.248).**
Fertility problems affect about 1 in 10 couples, and in about one-third of cases no cause is found. Failure to conceive may be the result of a problem affecting either one or both partners. This chart deals only with possible problems in women that may be responsible for a failure to conceive. How soon you should consult your doctor depends to some extent on your age, as fertility begins to fall after age 35.

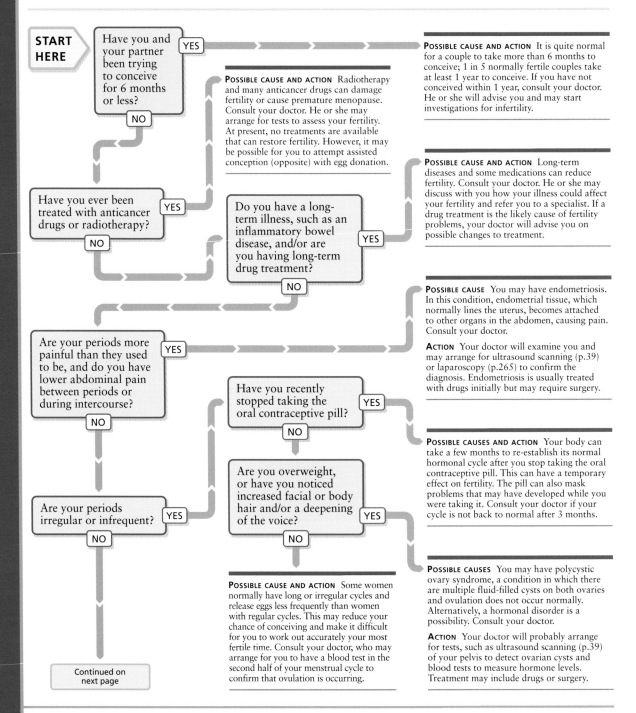

START HERE

Have you and your partner been trying to conceive for 6 months or less? — YES

POSSIBLE CAUSE AND ACTION It is quite normal for a couple to take more than 6 months to conceive; 1 in 5 normally fertile couples take at least 1 year to conceive. If you have not conceived within 1 year, consult your doctor. He or she will advise you and may start investigations for infertility.

NO

Have you ever been treated with anticancer drugs or radiotherapy? — YES

POSSIBLE CAUSE AND ACTION Radiotherapy and many anticancer drugs can damage fertility or cause premature menopause. Consult your doctor. He or she may arrange for tests to assess your fertility. At present, no treatments are available that can restore fertility. However, it may be possible for you to attempt assisted conception (opposite) with egg donation.

NO

Do you have a long-term illness, such as an inflammatory bowel disease, and/or are you having long-term drug treatment? — YES

POSSIBLE CAUSE AND ACTION Long-term diseases and some medications can reduce fertility. Consult your doctor. He or she may discuss with you how your illness could affect your fertility and refer you to a specialist. If a drug treatment is the likely cause of fertility problems, your doctor will advise you on possible changes to treatment.

NO

Are your periods more painful than they used to be, and do you have lower abdominal pain between periods or during intercourse? — YES

POSSIBLE CAUSE You may have endometriosis. In this condition, endometrial tissue, which normally lines the uterus, becomes attached to other organs in the abdomen, causing pain. Consult your doctor.

ACTION Your doctor will examine you and may arrange for ultrasound scanning (p.39) or laparoscopy (p.265) to confirm the diagnosis. Endometriosis is usually treated with drugs initially but may require surgery.

NO

Have you recently stopped taking the oral contraceptive pill? — YES

POSSIBLE CAUSES AND ACTION Your body can take a few months to re-establish its normal hormonal cycle after you stop taking the oral contraceptive pill. This can have a temporary effect on fertility. The pill can also mask problems that may have developed while you were taking it. Consult your doctor if your cycle is not back to normal after 3 months.

NO

Are you overweight, or have you noticed increased facial or body hair and/or a deepening of the voice? — YES

POSSIBLE CAUSES You may have polycystic ovary syndrome, a condition in which there are multiple fluid-filled cysts on both ovaries and ovulation does not occur normally. Alternatively, a hormonal disorder is a possibility. Consult your doctor.

ACTION Your doctor will probably arrange for tests, such as ultrasound scanning (p.39) of your pelvis to detect ovarian cysts and blood tests to measure hormone levels. Treatment may include drugs or surgery.

NO

Are your periods irregular or infrequent? — YES

POSSIBLE CAUSE AND ACTION Some women normally have long or irregular cycles and release eggs less frequently than women with regular cycles. This may reduce your chance of conceiving and make it difficult for you to work out accurately your most fertile time. Consult your doctor, who may arrange for you to have a blood test in the second half of your menstrual cycle to confirm that ovulation is occurring.

NO

Continued on next page

Continued from previous page

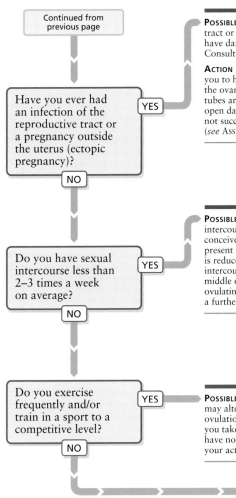

Have you ever had an infection of the reproductive tract or a pregnancy outside the uterus (ectopic pregnancy)?   **YES**

NO

POSSIBLE CAUSES Infection of the reproductive tract or a previous ectopic pregnancy may have damaged or blocked the fallopian tubes. Consult your doctor.

ACTION Your doctor will probably arrange for you to have a laparoscopy (p.265) to inspect the ovaries and establish whether the fallopian tubes are healthy. Surgery may be done to open damaged fallopian tubes. If surgery is not successful, you may be referred for IVF (*see* ASSISTED CONCEPTION, below).

Do you have sexual intercourse less than 2–3 times a week on average?   **YES**

NO

POSSIBLE CAUSE AND ACTION Infrequent sexual intercourse is a common cause of failure to conceive because the chance of sperm being present to fertilize an egg when it is released is reduced. If possible, try to have sexual intercourse at your most fertile time: in the middle of your menstrual cycle, when you are ovulating. If you have still not conceived within a further 3–6 months, consult your doctor.

Do you exercise frequently and/or train in a sport to a competitive level?   **YES**

NO

POSSIBLE CAUSE AND ACTION Vigorous training may alter your hormone levels, affecting ovulation. Reducing the amount of exercise you take may improve your fertility. If you have not conceived 3–6 months after lowering your activity level, consult your doctor.

Planning for a healthy pregnancy

Whether or not you are having problems conceiving, it is worth taking steps to ensure that if or when you do conceive, you have the best chance of a healthy pregnancy. Ideally, you and your partner should see your doctor at least 3 months before you start trying to conceive so that any problems can be dealt with in advance. Your doctor will probably do the following:

- Ensure that any pre-existing disease, such as diabetes, is well controlled.
- Review prescription drugs to avoid potential harm to the fetus.
- Ask about inherited conditions in your and your partner's families so that genetic counselling can be arranged if needed.
- Check that you are immune to rubella (German measles), which if contracted in early pregnancy can cause birth defects.
- Advise you to take a daily supplement of 400 micrograms of folic acid, starting at least 3 months before trying to conceive, to reduce the risk of neural tube defects such as spina bifida.
- Give you and your partner general health advice about factors that could affect fertility such as diet, smoking, and alcohol consumption (*see* MAXIMIZING THE CHANCE OF CONCEPTION, p.248).

Are you underweight (*see* ASSESSING YOUR WEIGHT, p.29), or have you recently lost a lot of weight?   **YES**

NO

CONSULT YOUR DOCTOR IF YOU ARE UNABLE TO MAKE A DIAGNOSIS FROM THIS CHART.

Assisted conception

The most common techniques that are used to aid conception are intrauterine (artificial) insemination (IUI) and in vitro fertilization (IVF). IUI is the simplest technique. In this procedure, timed to coincide with ovulation, semen from the partner or a donor is introduced into the uterus through a flexible tube passed through the vagina and cervix. IVF involves combining eggs and sperm outside the body and can be done using donated eggs and/or sperm if necessary. Drugs are given to stimulate the ovary to produce several eggs, which are then collected during laparoscopy (p.265). In the laboratory, sperm are combined with the eggs to allow fertilization to take place. Two or three fertilized eggs are introduced into the uterus in order to ensure the best chance of successful implantation into the uterus. The success rate of assisted conception is variable; on average, one in five attempts results in a pregnancy.

In vitro fertilization
In IVF, fertilization occurs in a laboratory. Two or three fertilized eggs are introduced into the uterus via a thin tube passed through the cervix.

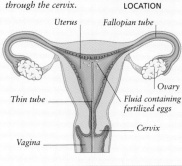

LOCATION

Uterus   Fallopian tube

Thin tube

Ovary

Fluid containing fertilized eggs

Cervix

Vagina

POSSIBLE CAUSES AND ACTION Being below a healthy weight for your height or losing weight rapidly can affect the menstrual cycle and reduce fertility. Try to eat sensibly; if you are trying to lose weight, aim to lose no more than 0.5 kg (1 lb) per week. If you are worried about your weight, consult your doctor.

140 Contraception choices for women

For contraception choices for men, see chart 127,
CONTRACEPTION CHOICES FOR MEN (p.250).
Deciding which method of contraception to use is partly a
matter of personal choice; your age, lifestyle, state of health,
and personal beliefs will all affect your choice. If you have
a regular partner, the decision is best shared. This chart is
intended as a guide to help you work out which methods
might be most suitable for you, so that you will be able to

discuss them with your usual doctor or a family-planning
clinic doctor (*see also* USEFUL ADDRESSES, p.285). If you have
had unprotected sex within the last 5 days, this chart will
advise you on the actions you can take to reduce the risk
of becoming pregnant. Most methods of contraception do
not provide you with protection from sexually transmitted
infections (STIs); however, male and female condoms are
thought to be 95 per cent effective.

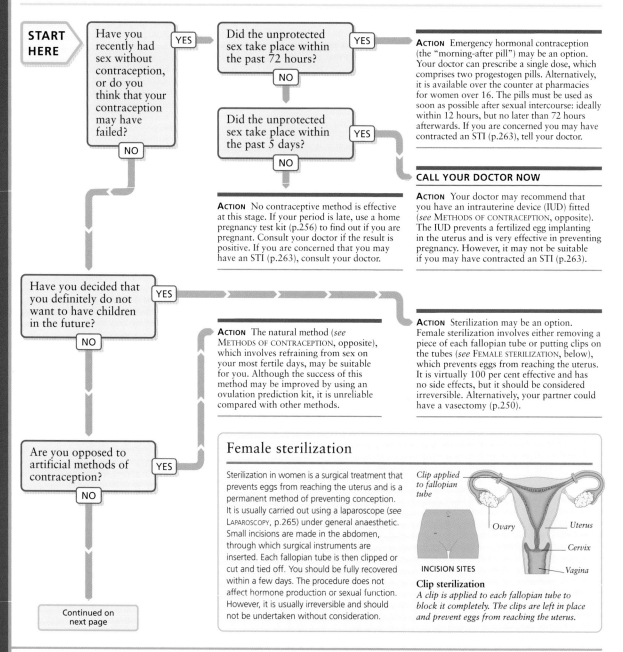

START HERE

Have you recently had sex without contraception, or do you think that your contraception may have failed? — YES → **Did the unprotected sex take place within the past 72 hours?** — YES → **ACTION** Emergency hormonal contraception (the "morning-after pill") may be an option. Your doctor can prescribe a single dose, which comprises two progestogen pills. Alternatively, it is available over the counter at pharmacies for women over 16. The pills must be used as soon as possible after sexual intercourse: ideally within 12 hours, but no later than 72 hours afterwards. If you are concerned you may have contracted an STI (p.263), tell your doctor.

Did the unprotected sex take place within the past 72 hours? — NO ↓

Did the unprotected sex take place within the past 5 days? — YES → **CALL YOUR DOCTOR NOW**

ACTION Your doctor may recommend that you have an intrauterine device (IUD) fitted (*see* METHODS OF CONTRACEPTION, opposite). The IUD prevents a fertilized egg implanting in the uterus and is very effective in preventing pregnancy. However, it may not be suitable if you may have contracted an STI (p.263).

Did the unprotected sex take place within the past 5 days? — NO ↓

ACTION No contraceptive method is effective at this stage. If your period is late, use a home pregnancy test kit (p.256) to find out if you are pregnant. Consult your doctor if the result is positive. If you are concerned that you may have an STI (p.263), consult your doctor.

Have you decided that you definitely do not want to have children in the future? — YES →

ACTION Sterilization may be an option. Female sterilization involves either removing a piece of each fallopian tube or putting clips on the tubes (*see* FEMALE STERILIZATION, below), which prevents eggs from reaching the uterus. It is virtually 100 per cent effective and has no side effects, but it should be considered irreversible. Alternatively, your partner could have a vasectomy (p.250).

Have you decided that you definitely do not want to have children in the future? — NO ↓

ACTION The natural method (*see* METHODS OF CONTRACEPTION, opposite), which involves refraining from sex on your most fertile days, may be suitable for you. Although the success of this method may be improved by using an ovulation prediction kit, it is unreliable compared with other methods.

Are you opposed to artificial methods of contraception? — YES ↑

Are you opposed to artificial methods of contraception? — NO ↓

Female sterilization

Sterilization in women is a surgical treatment that prevents eggs from reaching the uterus and is a permanent method of preventing conception. It is usually carried out using a laparoscope (*see* LAPAROSCOPY, p.265) under general anaesthetic. Small incisions are made in the abdomen, through which surgical instruments are inserted. Each fallopian tube is then clipped or cut and tied off. You should be fully recovered within a few days. The procedure does not affect hormone production or sexual function. However, it is usually irreversible and should not be undertaken without consideration.

Clip applied to fallopian tube

INCISION SITES

Ovary — Uterus — Cervix — Vagina

Clip sterilization
A clip is applied to each fallopian tube to block it completely. The clips are left in place and prevent eggs from reaching the uterus.

Continued on next page

Methods of contraception

A wide choice of contraceptive methods is available, although the majority are for use by the woman. Choose a method that is safe and effective for you and also suits your lifestyle and preferences. If you have decided you definitely do not want children in the future, male sterilization (*see* VASECTOMY, p.250) or female sterilization (opposite) may be suitable.

Barrier methods
These methods prevent sperm entering the uterus. They include the cervical cap, the diaphragm (right), and male and female condoms. Barrier methods are more effective when used with a spermicide, already present in many condoms.

Hormonal methods
The combined oral contraceptive pill (COCP) contains the hormones oestrogen and progestogen. It prevents the release of eggs. COCPs are effective and safe in women who do not have risk factors such as smoking, obesity, or a history of blood clots. The progestogen-only pill (POP) acts mainly by thickening the mucus at the entrance to the cervix, so sperm cannot enter the uterus, and is suitable for most women. To be effective, most POPs must be taken at or around the same time each day. A new form of POP is available that acts by inhibiting ovulation; this form is therefore more effective than traditional types. Progestogens can also be given as 3-monthly injections or as an implant lasting 3 years.

Mechanical methods
The intrauterine device, or IUD, (right) is placed in the uterus by a doctor to prevent fertilized eggs implanting. It stays in place for 3–10 years. The intrauterine system (IUS), a progestogen-releasing IUD, also reduces blood loss and pain during periods.

Natural method
The most commonly used natural method involves monitoring body temperature and mucus from the cervix in order to predict ovulation. Sex is then avoided around this time.

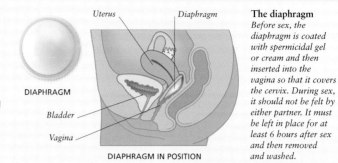

DIAPHRAGM

Uterus — *Diaphragm*

Bladder

Vagina

DIAPHRAGM IN POSITION

The diaphragm
Before sex, the diaphragm is coated with spermicidal gel or cream and then inserted into the vagina so that it covers the cervix. During sex, it should not be felt by either partner. It must be left in place for at least 6 hours after sex and then removed and washed.

Combined oral contraceptive pills
These pills contain the hormones oestrogen and progestogen. They are usually taken, one a day, for 21 days, followed by 7 pill-free days, during which you will have your period. On the 29th day, you begin another pack.

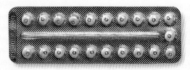

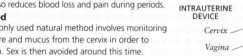

Copper wire

Threads extend through cervix

INTRAUTERINE DEVICE

Cervix

Vagina

Uterus — IUD — *Ovary*

IUD IN POSITION

The intrauterine device (IUD)
IUDs stop fertilized eggs implanting in the uterus. Some contain copper, which kills sperm. The intrauterine system (IUS) releases progestogen, which thins the uterus lining and thickens cervical mucus. IUDs last for 3–10 years.

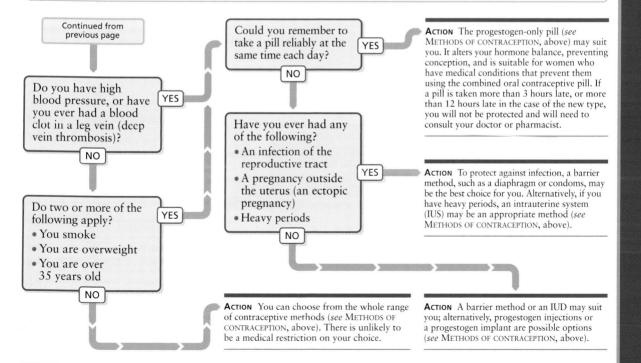

Continued from previous page

Do you have high blood pressure, or have you ever had a blood clot in a leg vein (deep vein thrombosis)?
NO / YES

Do two or more of the following apply?
- You smoke
- You are overweight
- You are over 35 years old

YES / NO

Could you remember to take a pill reliably at the same time each day?
YES / NO

Have you ever had any of the following?
- An infection of the reproductive tract
- A pregnancy outside the uterus (an ectopic pregnancy)
- Heavy periods

YES / NO

ACTION The progestogen-only pill (*see* METHODS OF CONTRACEPTION, above) may suit you. It alters your hormone balance, preventing conception, and is suitable for women who have medical conditions that prevent them using the combined oral contraceptive pill. If a pill is taken more than 3 hours late, or more than 12 hours late in the case of the new type, you will not be protected and will need to consult your doctor or pharmacist.

ACTION To protect against infection, a barrier method, such as a diaphragm or condoms, may be the best choice for you. Alternatively, if you have heavy periods, an intrauterine system (IUS) may be an appropriate method (*see* METHODS OF CONTRACEPTION, above).

ACTION You can choose from the whole range of contraceptive methods (*see* METHODS OF CONTRACEPTION, above). There is unlikely to be a medical restriction on your choice.

ACTION A barrier method or an IUD may suit you; alternatively, progestogen injections or a progestogen implant are possible options (*see* METHODS OF CONTRACEPTION, above).

143 Vaginal bleeding in pregnancy

If you have any vaginal bleeding during pregnancy, consult this chart to determine how quickly you should seek medical advice. While in most cases there is no danger to you or the fetus, this is a potentially serious symptom and should always receive medical attention whether you have only slight spotting or more profuse blood loss. If the bleeding is from the placenta, emergency treatment will be necessary. In other cases, rest and regular monitoring may be all that is needed.

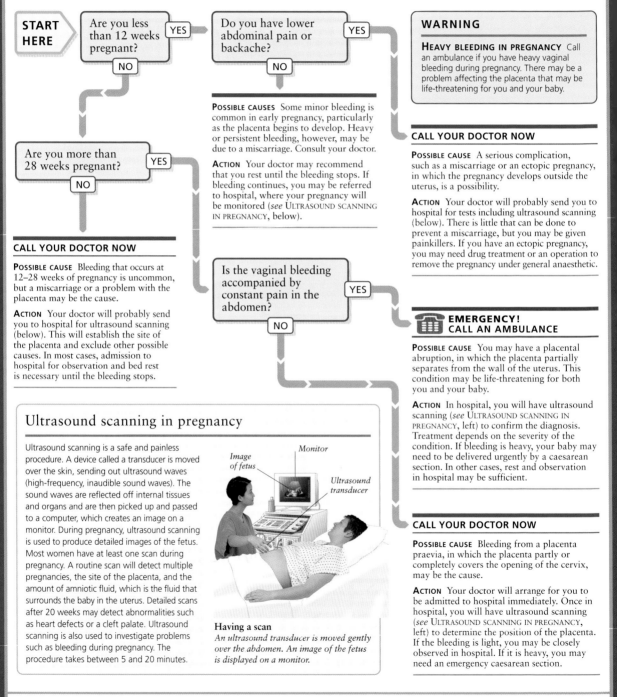

START HERE

Are you less than 12 weeks pregnant? — YES → **Do you have lower abdominal pain or backache?**

NO ↓

Are you more than 28 weeks pregnant? — YES →

NO ↓

Do you have lower abdominal pain or backache? — YES →

NO ↓

POSSIBLE CAUSES Some minor bleeding is common in early pregnancy, particularly as the placenta begins to develop. Heavy or persistent bleeding, however, may be due to a miscarriage. Consult your doctor.

ACTION Your doctor may recommend that you rest until the bleeding stops. If bleeding continues, you may be referred to hospital, where your pregnancy will be monitored (*see* ULTRASOUND SCANNING IN PREGNANCY, below).

Is the vaginal bleeding accompanied by constant pain in the abdomen? — YES →

NO ↓

WARNING

HEAVY BLEEDING IN PREGNANCY Call an ambulance if you have heavy vaginal bleeding during pregnancy. There may be a problem affecting the placenta that may be life-threatening for you and your baby.

CALL YOUR DOCTOR NOW

POSSIBLE CAUSE A serious complication, such as a miscarriage or an ectopic pregnancy, in which the pregnancy develops outside the uterus, is a possibility.

ACTION Your doctor will probably send you to hospital for tests including ultrasound scanning (below). There is little that can be done to prevent a miscarriage, but you may be given painkillers. If you have an ectopic pregnancy, you may need drug treatment or an operation to remove the pregnancy under general anaesthetic.

CALL YOUR DOCTOR NOW

POSSIBLE CAUSE Bleeding that occurs at 12–28 weeks of pregnancy is uncommon, but a miscarriage or a problem with the placenta may be the cause.

ACTION Your doctor will probably send you to hospital for ultrasound scanning (below). This will establish the site of the placenta and exclude other possible causes. In most cases, admission to hospital for observation and bed rest is necessary until the bleeding stops.

EMERGENCY! CALL AN AMBULANCE

POSSIBLE CAUSE You may have a placental abruption, in which the placenta partially separates from the wall of the uterus. This condition may be life-threatening for both you and your baby.

ACTION In hospital, you will have ultrasound scanning (*see* ULTRASOUND SCANNING IN PREGNANCY, left) to confirm the diagnosis. Treatment depends on the severity of the condition. If bleeding is heavy, your baby may need to be delivered urgently by a caesarean section. In other cases, rest and observation in hospital may be sufficient.

Ultrasound scanning in pregnancy

Ultrasound scanning is a safe and painless procedure. A device called a transducer is moved over the skin, sending out ultrasound waves (high-frequency, inaudible sound waves). The sound waves are reflected off internal tissues and organs and are then picked up and passed to a computer, which creates an image on a monitor. During pregnancy, ultrasound scanning is used to produce detailed images of the fetus. Most women have at least one scan during pregnancy. A routine scan will detect multiple pregnancies, the site of the placenta, and the amount of amniotic fluid, which is the fluid that surrounds the baby in the uterus. Detailed scans after 20 weeks may detect abnormalities such as heart defects or a cleft palate. Ultrasound scanning is also used to investigate problems such as bleeding during pregnancy. The procedure takes between 5 and 20 minutes.

Image of fetus — *Monitor* — *Ultrasound transducer*

Having a scan
An ultrasound transducer is moved gently over the abdomen. An image of the fetus is displayed on a monitor.

CALL YOUR DOCTOR NOW

POSSIBLE CAUSE Bleeding from a placenta praevia, in which the placenta partly or completely covers the opening of the cervix, may be the cause.

ACTION Your doctor will arrange for you to be admitted to hospital immediately. Once in hospital, you will have ultrasound scanning (*see* ULTRASOUND SCANNING IN PREGNANCY, left) to determine the position of the placenta. If the bleeding is light, you may be closely observed in hospital. If it is heavy, you may need an emergency caesarean section.

144 Abdominal pain in pregnancy

Consult this chart only after reading chart 100,
ABDOMINAL PAIN (p.210).
Conditions that cause abdominal pain in non-pregnant
women, such as appendicitis, can also occur during pregnancy.

However, conditions specific to pregnancy can also cause
abdominal pain. These may be the result of compression of
the internal organs by the growing baby, hormone changes,
or problems with the placenta or the uterus.

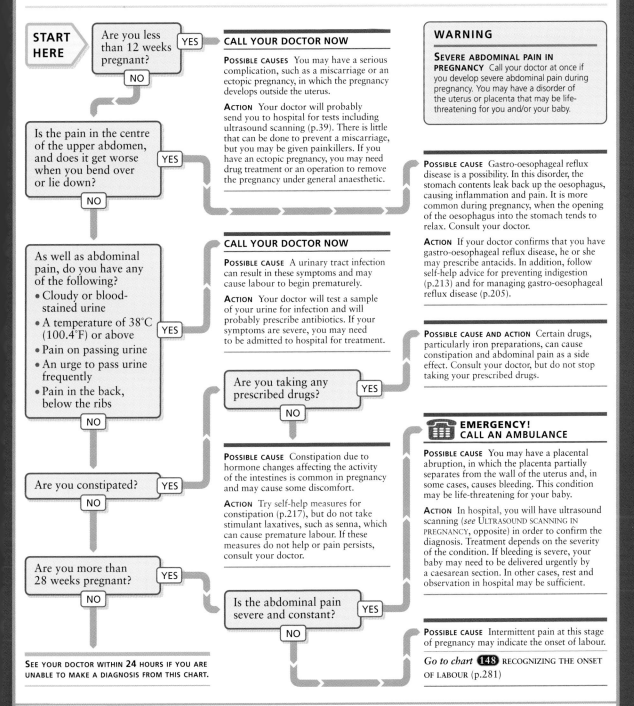

START HERE

Are you less than 12 weeks pregnant? — YES

CALL YOUR DOCTOR NOW

POSSIBLE CAUSES You may have a serious complication, such as a miscarriage or an ectopic pregnancy, in which the pregnancy develops outside the uterus.

ACTION Your doctor will probably send you to hospital for tests including ultrasound scanning (p.39). There is little that can be done to prevent a miscarriage, but you may be given painkillers. If you have an ectopic pregnancy, you may need drug treatment or an operation to remove the pregnancy under general anaesthetic.

NO

Is the pain in the centre of the upper abdomen, and does it get worse when you bend over or lie down? — YES

NO

As well as abdominal pain, do you have any of the following?
- Cloudy or blood-stained urine
- A temperature of 38°C (100.4°F) or above
- Pain on passing urine
- An urge to pass urine frequently
- Pain in the back, below the ribs

— YES

CALL YOUR DOCTOR NOW

POSSIBLE CAUSE A urinary tract infection can result in these symptoms and may cause labour to begin prematurely.

ACTION Your doctor will test a sample of your urine for infection and will probably prescribe antibiotics. If your symptoms are severe, you may need to be admitted to hospital for treatment.

NO

Are you constipated? — YES

NO

Are you taking any prescribed drugs? — YES

NO

POSSIBLE CAUSE Constipation due to hormone changes affecting the activity of the intestines is common in pregnancy and may cause some discomfort.

ACTION Try self-help measures for constipation (p.217), but do not take stimulant laxatives, such as senna, which can cause premature labour. If these measures do not help or pain persists, consult your doctor.

Are you more than 28 weeks pregnant? — YES

NO

Is the abdominal pain severe and constant? — YES

NO

WARNING

SEVERE ABDOMINAL PAIN IN PREGNANCY Call your doctor at once if you develop severe abdominal pain during pregnancy. You may have a disorder of the uterus or placenta that may be life-threatening for you and/or your baby.

POSSIBLE CAUSE Gastro-oesophageal reflux disease is a possibility. In this disorder, the stomach contents leak back up the oesophagus, causing inflammation and pain. It is more common during pregnancy, when the opening of the oesophagus into the stomach tends to relax. Consult your doctor.

ACTION If your doctor confirms that you have gastro-oesophageal reflux disease, he or she may prescribe antacids. In addition, follow self-help advice for preventing indigestion (p.213) and for managing gastro-oesophageal reflux disease (p.205).

POSSIBLE CAUSE AND ACTION Certain drugs, particularly iron preparations, can cause constipation and abdominal pain as a side effect. Consult your doctor, but do not stop taking your prescribed drugs.

📞 EMERGENCY! CALL AN AMBULANCE

POSSIBLE CAUSE You may have a placental abruption, in which the placenta partially separates from the wall of the uterus and, in some cases, causes bleeding. This condition may be life-threatening for your baby.

ACTION In hospital, you will have ultrasound scanning (*see* ULTRASOUND SCANNING IN PREGNANCY, opposite) in order to confirm the diagnosis. Treatment depends on the severity of the condition. If bleeding is severe, your baby may need to be delivered urgently by a caesarean section. In other cases, rest and observation in hospital may be sufficient.

POSSIBLE CAUSE Intermittent pain at this stage of pregnancy may indicate the onset of labour.

Go to chart **148** RECOGNIZING THE ONSET OF LABOUR (p.281)

SEE YOUR DOCTOR WITHIN **24** HOURS IF YOU ARE UNABLE TO MAKE A DIAGNOSIS FROM THIS CHART.

145 Skin changes in pregnancy

Hormone changes during pregnancy may affect the skin in a variety of ways. Most women find that their skin becomes more oily, but others may find it becomes drier. The skin often becomes darker due to an increase in pigment. If you had a skin condition before you became pregnant you may find that it improves during pregnancy but gets worse again after delivery. The exact effects of pregnancy on the skin depend on the woman's individual hormone balance and skin type.

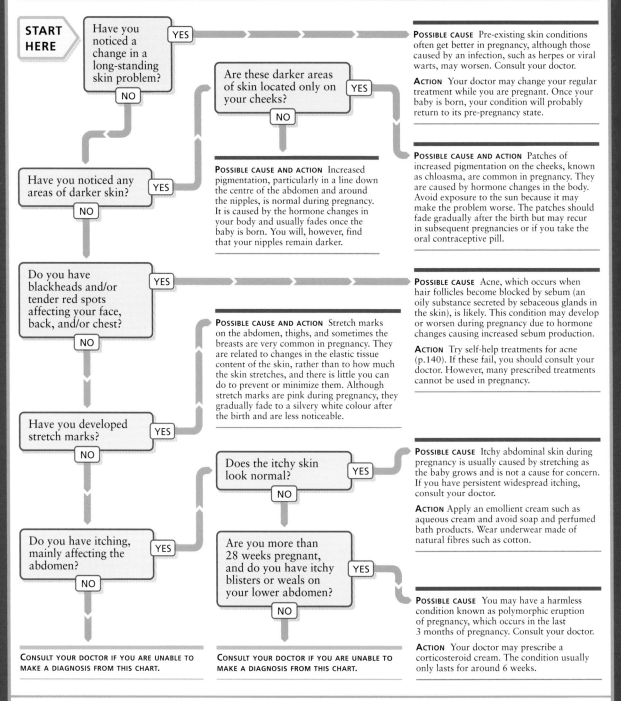

START HERE

Have you noticed a change in a long-standing skin problem? — YES → **POSSIBLE CAUSE** Pre-existing skin conditions often get better in pregnancy, although those caused by an infection, such as herpes or viral warts, may worsen. Consult your doctor.

ACTION Your doctor may change your regular treatment while you are pregnant. Once your baby is born, your condition will probably return to its pre-pregnancy state.

NO

Are these darker areas of skin located only on your cheeks? — YES → **POSSIBLE CAUSE AND ACTION** Patches of increased pigmentation on the cheeks, known as chloasma, are common in pregnancy. They are caused by hormone changes in the body. Avoid exposure to the sun because it may make the problem worse. The patches should fade gradually after the birth but may recur in subsequent pregnancies or if you take the oral contraceptive pill.

NO

POSSIBLE CAUSE AND ACTION Increased pigmentation, particularly in a line down the centre of the abdomen and around the nipples, is normal during pregnancy. It is caused by the hormone changes in your body and usually fades once the baby is born. You will, however, find that your nipples remain darker.

Have you noticed any areas of darker skin? — YES

NO

Do you have blackheads and/or tender red spots affecting your face, back, and/or chest? — YES → **POSSIBLE CAUSE** Acne, which occurs when hair follicles become blocked by sebum (an oily substance secreted by sebaceous glands in the skin), is likely. This condition may develop or worsen during pregnancy due to hormone changes causing increased sebum production.

ACTION Try self-help treatments for acne (p.140). If these fail, you should consult your doctor. However, many prescribed treatments cannot be used in pregnancy.

NO

POSSIBLE CAUSE AND ACTION Stretch marks on the abdomen, thighs, and sometimes the breasts are very common in pregnancy. They are related to changes in the elastic tissue content of the skin, rather than to how much the skin stretches, and there is little you can do to prevent or minimize them. Although stretch marks are pink during pregnancy, they gradually fade to a silvery white colour after the birth and are less noticeable.

Have you developed stretch marks? — YES

NO

Does the itchy skin look normal? — YES → **POSSIBLE CAUSE** Itchy abdominal skin during pregnancy is usually caused by stretching as the baby grows and is not a cause for concern. If you have persistent widespread itching, consult your doctor.

ACTION Apply an emollient cream such as aqueous cream and avoid soap and perfumed bath products. Wear underwear made of natural fibres such as cotton.

NO

Do you have itching, mainly affecting the abdomen? — YES

NO

Are you more than 28 weeks pregnant, and do you have itchy blisters or weals on your lower abdomen? — YES → **POSSIBLE CAUSE** You may have a harmless condition known as polymorphic eruption of pregnancy, which occurs in the last 3 months of pregnancy. Consult your doctor.

ACTION Your doctor may prescribe a corticosteroid cream. The condition usually only lasts for around 6 weeks.

NO

CONSULT YOUR DOCTOR IF YOU ARE UNABLE TO MAKE A DIAGNOSIS FROM THIS CHART.

CONSULT YOUR DOCTOR IF YOU ARE UNABLE TO MAKE A DIAGNOSIS FROM THIS CHART.

146 Swollen ankles in pregnancy

Swollen ankles are very common in pregnancy, particularly during hot weather or in the later stages of pregnancy, when excess fluid tends to accumulate. Mild swelling of the ankles is usually not a cause for concern. Elevating your ankles, preferably to the same level as your hips, whenever possible and wearing support tights may ease the swelling. Your ankles may be checked, along with your blood pressure and urine, at each antenatal visit (*see* ROUTINE ANTENATAL CARE, below). However, swelling confined to only one ankle should always be brought to your doctor's attention immediately.

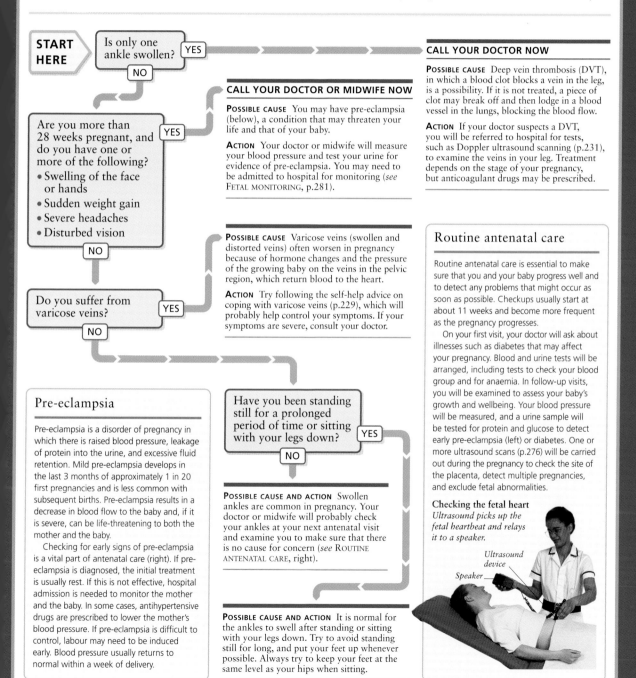

START HERE

Is only one ankle swollen? — **YES**

NO

Are you more than 28 weeks pregnant, and do you have one or more of the following?
- Swelling of the face or hands
- Sudden weight gain
- Severe headaches
- Disturbed vision

YES

NO

Do you suffer from varicose veins? — **YES**

NO

Have you been standing still for a prolonged period of time or sitting with your legs down? — **YES**

NO

CALL YOUR DOCTOR OR MIDWIFE NOW

POSSIBLE CAUSE You may have pre-eclampsia (below), a condition that may threaten your life and that of your baby.

ACTION Your doctor or midwife will measure your blood pressure and test your urine for evidence of pre-eclampsia. You may need to be admitted to hospital for monitoring (*see* FETAL MONITORING, p.281).

POSSIBLE CAUSE Varicose veins (swollen and distorted veins) often worsen in pregnancy because of hormone changes and the pressure of the growing baby on the veins in the pelvic region, which return blood to the heart.

ACTION Try following the self-help advice on coping with varicose veins (p.229), which will probably help control your symptoms. If your symptoms are severe, consult your doctor.

CALL YOUR DOCTOR NOW

POSSIBLE CAUSE Deep vein thrombosis (DVT), in which a blood clot blocks a vein in the leg, is a possibility. If it is not treated, a piece of clot may break off and then lodge in a blood vessel in the lungs, blocking the blood flow.

ACTION If your doctor suspects a DVT, you will be referred to hospital for tests, such as Doppler ultrasound scanning (p.231), to examine the veins in your leg. Treatment depends on the stage of your pregnancy, but anticoagulant drugs may be prescribed.

Routine antenatal care

Routine antenatal care is essential to make sure that you and your baby progress well and to detect any problems that might occur as soon as possible. Checkups usually start at about 11 weeks and become more frequent as the pregnancy progresses.

On your first visit, your doctor will ask about illnesses such as diabetes that may affect your pregnancy. Blood and urine tests will be arranged, including tests to check your blood group and for anaemia. In follow-up visits, you will be examined to assess your baby's growth and wellbeing. Your blood pressure will be measured, and a urine sample will be tested for protein and glucose to detect early pre-eclampsia (left) or diabetes. One or more ultrasound scans (p.276) will be carried out during the pregnancy to check the site of the placenta, detect multiple pregnancies, and exclude fetal abnormalities.

Checking the fetal heart
Ultrasound picks up the fetal heartbeat and relays it to a speaker.

Ultrasound device

Speaker

Pre-eclampsia

Pre-eclampsia is a disorder of pregnancy in which there is raised blood pressure, leakage of protein into the urine, and excessive fluid retention. Mild pre-eclampsia develops in the last 3 months of approximately 1 in 20 first pregnancies and is less common with subsequent births. Pre-eclampsia results in a decrease in blood flow to the baby and, if it is severe, can be life-threatening to both the mother and the baby.

Checking for early signs of pre-eclampsia is a vital part of antenatal care (right). If pre-eclampsia is diagnosed, the initial treatment is usually rest. If this is not effective, hospital admission is needed to monitor the mother and the baby. In some cases, antihypertensive drugs are prescribed to lower the mother's blood pressure. If pre-eclampsia is difficult to control, labour may need to be induced early. Blood pressure usually returns to normal within a week of delivery.

POSSIBLE CAUSE AND ACTION Swollen ankles are common in pregnancy. Your doctor or midwife will probably check your ankles at your next antenatal visit and examine you to make sure that there is no cause for concern (*see* ROUTINE ANTENATAL CARE, right).

POSSIBLE CAUSE AND ACTION It is normal for the ankles to swell after standing or sitting with your legs down. Try to avoid standing still for long, and put your feet up whenever possible. Always try to keep your feet at the same level as your hips when sitting.

147 Back pain in pregnancy

Consult this chart only after first consulting chart 117,
BACK PAIN (p.234).

Pain and aching in the middle and lower back are common during pregnancy. They are usually caused by the effects of hormones that soften the ligaments supporting the spine and by difficulty in maintaining good posture as a result of the weight of the growing fetus. Backache tends to get worse as pregnancy progresses and may make it difficult to get up from a sitting or lying position. Although backache in pregnancy is not usually a cause for concern, if it develops suddenly you should contact your doctor, as it may indicate a miscarriage in early pregnancy or the onset of labour in late pregnancy.

START HERE

Are you less than 12 weeks pregnant, and do you have cramping abdominal pain and/or vaginal bleeding? → YES

NO

Do you have a temperature of 38°C (100.4°F) or above and/or any of the following?
- Pain on passing urine
- Cloudy urine
- A frequent urge to pass urine

YES

NO

Are you more than 28 weeks pregnant, is the pain different from previous back pain, and does the pain stay the same when you change position? → YES

NO

Do you have a shooting pain and/or pins and needles down the back of one leg? → YES

NO

CALL YOUR DOCTOR NOW

POSSIBLE CAUSE Pyelonephritis, inflammation of a kidney due to a bacterial infection, can result in severe back pain and may cause labour to begin prematurely.

ACTION Your doctor will test a sample of your urine for signs of infection and will probably prescribe antibiotics. In some cases, you may need to be admitted to hospital.

CALL YOUR DOCTOR NOW

POSSIBLE CAUSES A serious complication, such as a miscarriage or an ectopic pregnancy, in which the pregnancy develops outside the uterus, is a possibility.

ACTION Your doctor will probably refer you to hospital for ultrasound scanning (p.276) so that your pregnancy can be assessed. There is little that can be done for a miscarriage, although you may be given painkillers. If the cause is an ectopic pregnancy, you will need drug treatment or an operation under a general anaesthetic to remove the pregnancy.

POSSIBLE CAUSE This type of backache may be an indication of the onset of labour. You should check to see whether you have other signs that labour has started.

Go to chart **148** RECOGNIZING THE ONSET OF LABOUR (opposite)

POSSIBLE CAUSE Even in early pregnancy, hormone changes can soften the ligaments supporting the spine, leading to backache.

ACTION Follow the advice on looking after your back in pregnancy (left). Consult your doctor if the pain becomes severe enough to restrict your activities.

POSSIBLE CAUSE Sciatica, in which the sciatic nerve is compressed at the point where it leaves the spine, may be the cause. In pregnancy, this condition is due to hormone changes softening the ligaments supporting the spine.

ACTION Follow the self-help advice for looking after your back in pregnancy (left). Consult your doctor if the pain becomes severe enough to restrict your daily activities.

SELF-HELP Looking after your back in pregnancy

Your back is especially vulnerable during pregnancy because ligaments around the spine soften and because the enlarging abdomen may lead to poor posture. The following measures will protect your back and help to prevent back pain:
- Adopt a good posture when you are standing: your back should be kept straight and your buttocks tucked in.
- Wear flat shoes rather than high heels.
- Use a chair with good back support.
- Sleep on a firm mattress.
- Try gentle stretching exercises for the lower back.
- Make sure you lift small children and heavy objects safely.

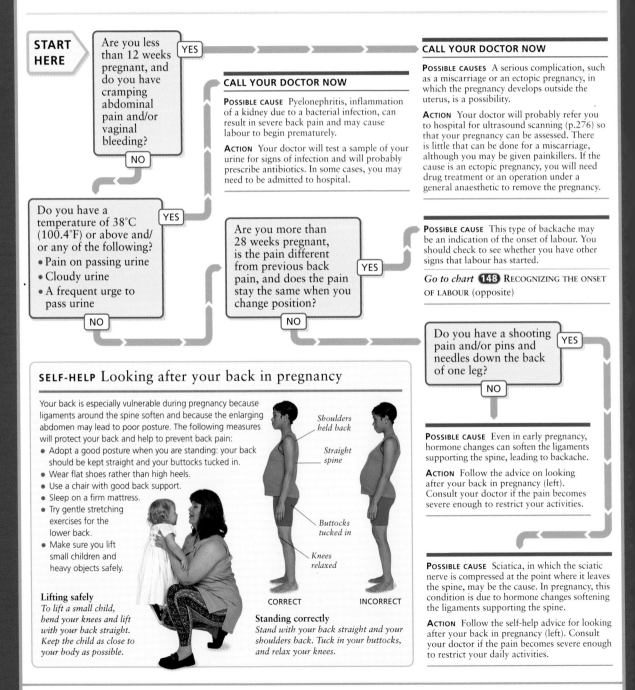

Lifting safely
To lift a small child, bend your knees and lift with your back straight. Keep the child as close to your body as possible.

Shoulders held back

Straight spine

Buttocks tucked in

Knees relaxed

CORRECT   INCORRECT

Standing correctly
Stand with your back straight and your shoulders back. Tuck in your buttocks, and relax your knees.

148 Recognizing the onset of labour

On average, pregnancy lasts for 40 weeks. However, it is quite normal for a baby to be born as early as 37 weeks or as late as 42 weeks. During labour – the series of events leading to the delivery of your baby – you experience regular contractions that dilate your cervix. Whether or not your cervix is dilating can be determined only by an internal examination. The onset of labour may be heralded by a number of different signs, including the passage of a plug of thick, perhaps bloodstained mucus (a "show"), abdominal or lower back pains, and the waters breaking (rupture of the membranes). These signs of labour vary from woman to woman. This chart is designed to help you determine whether labour may have started and how urgently you should contact your doctor or midwife for further advice.

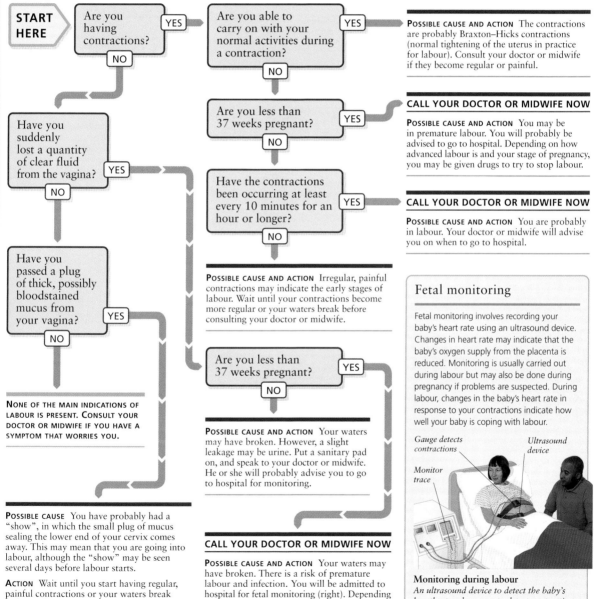

START HERE

Are you having contractions? — YES → **Are you able to carry on with your normal activities during a contraction?** — YES → **POSSIBLE CAUSE AND ACTION** The contractions are probably Braxton–Hicks contractions (normal tightening of the uterus in practice for labour). Consult your doctor or midwife if they become regular or painful.

NO ↓ (Are you having contractions?)

NO ↓ (Are you able to carry on...)

Have you suddenly lost a quantity of clear fluid from the vagina? — YES →

NO ↓

Are you less than 37 weeks pregnant? — YES → **CALL YOUR DOCTOR OR MIDWIFE NOW**
POSSIBLE CAUSE AND ACTION You may be in premature labour. You will probably be advised to go to hospital. Depending on how advanced labour is and your stage of pregnancy, you may be given drugs to try to stop labour.

NO ↓

Have the contractions been occurring at least every 10 minutes for an hour or longer? — YES → **CALL YOUR DOCTOR OR MIDWIFE NOW**
POSSIBLE CAUSE AND ACTION You are probably in labour. Your doctor or midwife will advise you on when to go to hospital.

NO ↓

POSSIBLE CAUSE AND ACTION Irregular, painful contractions may indicate the early stages of labour. Wait until your contractions become more regular or your waters break before consulting your doctor or midwife.

Have you passed a plug of thick, possibly bloodstained mucus from your vagina? — YES →

NO ↓

Are you less than 37 weeks pregnant? — YES →

NO ↓

POSSIBLE CAUSE AND ACTION Your waters may have broken. However, a slight leakage may be urine. Put a sanitary pad on, and speak to your doctor or midwife. He or she will probably advise you to go to hospital for monitoring.

NONE OF THE MAIN INDICATIONS OF LABOUR IS PRESENT. CONSULT YOUR DOCTOR OR MIDWIFE IF YOU HAVE A SYMPTOM THAT WORRIES YOU.

POSSIBLE CAUSE You have probably had a "show", in which the small plug of mucus sealing the lower end of your cervix comes away. This may mean that you are going into labour, although the "show" may be seen several days before labour starts.

ACTION Wait until you start having regular, painful contractions or your waters break before calling your doctor or midwife. He or she will advise you on when to go to hospital.

CALL YOUR DOCTOR OR MIDWIFE NOW

POSSIBLE CAUSE AND ACTION Your waters may have broken. There is a risk of premature labour and infection. You will be admitted to hospital for fetal monitoring (right). Depending on the stage of pregnancy, your doctor may try to delay labour or let labour progress.

Fetal monitoring

Fetal monitoring involves recording your baby's heart rate using an ultrasound device. Changes in heart rate may indicate that the baby's oxygen supply from the placenta is reduced. Monitoring is usually carried out during labour but may also be done during pregnancy if problems are suspected. During labour, changes in the baby's heart rate in response to your contractions indicate how well your baby is coping with labour.

Gauge detects contractions

Ultrasound device

Monitor trace

Monitoring during labour
An ultrasound device to detect the baby's heartbeat and a gauge to detect contractions are strapped to the abdomen.

149 Breast problems and pregnancy

Breast problems are common during and immediately after pregnancy but are usually easy to treat. During pregnancy, hormones cause changes in the breasts: the milk-producing glands become larger and increase in number, and the breasts may become tender. After the baby is born, the breasts can produce about 1 litre (2 pints) of milk per day. Problems soon after childbirth are often associated with establishing breast-feeding. However, these problems are usually short-lived. In most cases, breast-feeding is still possible and is the best option for the baby (*see* FEEDING YOUR BABY, below).

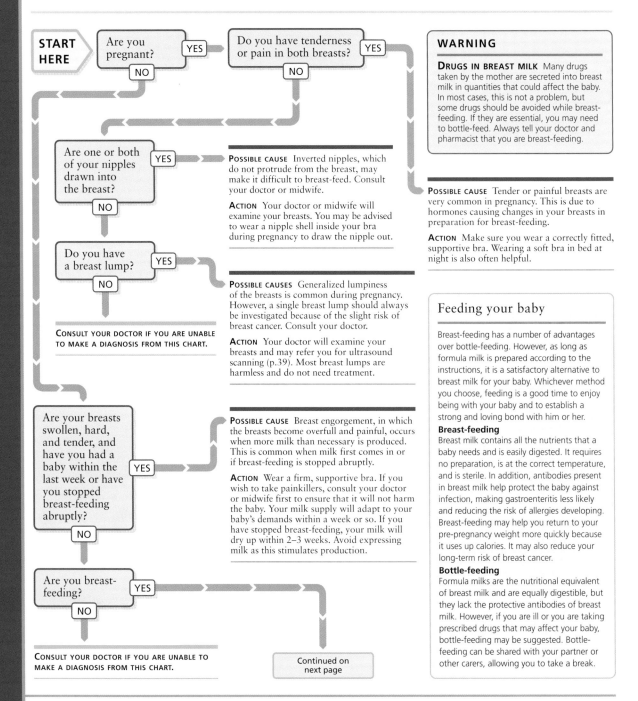

START HERE

Are you pregnant? — YES → **Do you have tenderness or pain in both breasts?** — YES →

NO / NO

Are one or both of your nipples drawn into the breast? — YES →

POSSIBLE CAUSE Inverted nipples, which do not protrude from the breast, may make it difficult to breast-feed. Consult your doctor or midwife.

ACTION Your doctor or midwife will examine your breasts. You may be advised to wear a nipple shell inside your bra during pregnancy to draw the nipple out.

NO

Do you have a breast lump? — YES →

POSSIBLE CAUSES Generalized lumpiness of the breasts is common during pregnancy. However, a single breast lump should always be investigated because of the slight risk of breast cancer. Consult your doctor.

ACTION Your doctor will examine your breasts and may refer you for ultrasound scanning (p.39). Most breast lumps are harmless and do not need treatment.

NO

CONSULT YOUR DOCTOR IF YOU ARE UNABLE TO MAKE A DIAGNOSIS FROM THIS CHART.

Are your breasts swollen, hard, and tender, and have you had a baby within the last week or have you stopped breast-feeding abruptly? — YES →

POSSIBLE CAUSE Breast engorgement, in which the breasts become overfull and painful, occurs when more milk than necessary is produced. This is common when milk first comes in or if breast-feeding is stopped abruptly.

ACTION Wear a firm, supportive bra. If you wish to take painkillers, consult your doctor or midwife first to ensure that it will not harm the baby. Your milk supply will adapt to your baby's demands within a week or so. If you have stopped breast-feeding, your milk will dry up within 2–3 weeks. Avoid expressing milk as this stimulates production.

NO

Are you breast-feeding? — YES →

NO

CONSULT YOUR DOCTOR IF YOU ARE UNABLE TO MAKE A DIAGNOSIS FROM THIS CHART.

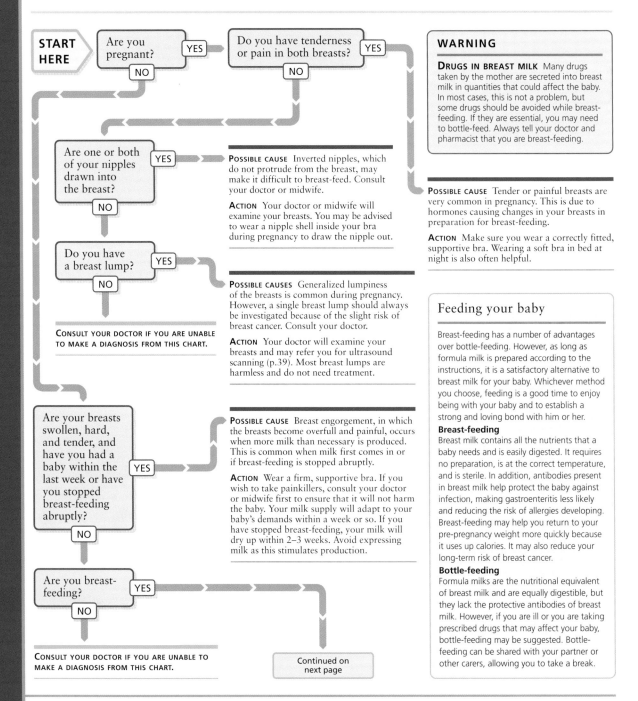
Continued on next page

WARNING

DRUGS IN BREAST MILK Many drugs taken by the mother are secreted into breast milk in quantities that could affect the baby. In most cases, this is not a problem, but some drugs should be avoided while breast-feeding. If they are essential, you may need to bottle-feed. Always tell your doctor and pharmacist that you are breast-feeding.

POSSIBLE CAUSE Tender or painful breasts are very common in pregnancy. This is due to hormones causing changes in your breasts in preparation for breast-feeding.

ACTION Make sure you wear a correctly fitted, supportive bra. Wearing a soft bra in bed at night is also often helpful.

Feeding your baby

Breast-feeding has a number of advantages over bottle-feeding. However, as long as formula milk is prepared according to the instructions, it is a satisfactory alternative to breast milk for your baby. Whichever method you choose, feeding is a good time to enjoy being with your baby and to establish a strong and loving bond with him or her.

Breast-feeding
Breast milk contains all the nutrients that a baby needs and is easily digested. It requires no preparation, is at the correct temperature, and is sterile. In addition, antibodies present in breast milk help protect the baby against infection, making gastroenteritis less likely and reducing the risk of allergies developing. Breast-feeding may help you return to your pre-pregnancy weight more quickly because it uses up calories. It may also reduce your long-term risk of breast cancer.

Bottle-feeding
Formula milks are the nutritional equivalent of breast milk and are equally digestible, but they lack the protective antibodies of breast milk. However, if you are ill or you are taking prescribed drugs that may affect your baby, bottle-feeding may be suggested. Bottle-feeding can be shared with your partner or other carers, allowing you to take a break.

Continued from previous page

SELF-HELP Avoiding cracked nipples

Cracked nipples are common at the start of breast-feeding. They usually occur because the baby has not latched on properly. To prevent your baby from tugging on your nipple, hold his or her tummy against yours and cradle the head and bottom securely. Alternatively, support your baby with a pillow and tuck his or her bottom under your arm (like holding a rugby ball). Make sure your baby takes the entire nipple and most of the areola (the darker area around it) into his or her mouth. Dry your nipples thoroughly after each feed. Use absorbent breast pads and change them frequently. Ask your midwife for lanolin cream designed to soothe sore nipples.

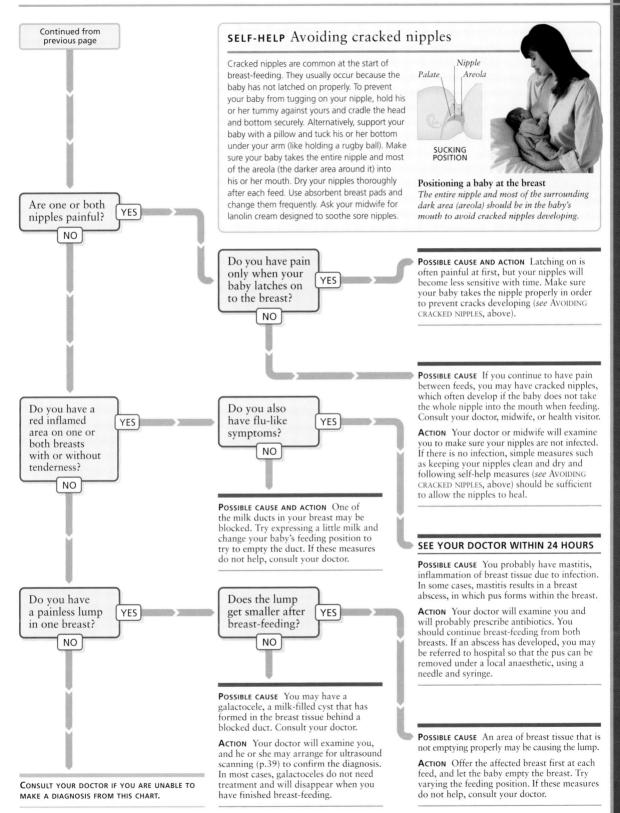

Nipple
Palate   Areola

SUCKING POSITION

Positioning a baby at the breast
The entire nipple and most of the surrounding dark area (areola) should be in the baby's mouth to avoid cracked nipples developing.

Are one or both nipples painful? YES / NO

Do you have pain only when your baby latches on to the breast? YES / NO

POSSIBLE CAUSE AND ACTION Latching on is often painful at first, but your nipples will become less sensitive with time. Make sure your baby takes the nipple properly in order to prevent cracks developing (*see* AVOIDING CRACKED NIPPLES, above).

POSSIBLE CAUSE If you continue to have pain between feeds, you may have cracked nipples, which often develop if the baby does not take the whole nipple into the mouth when feeding. Consult your doctor, midwife, or health visitor.

ACTION Your doctor or midwife will examine you to make sure your nipples are not infected. If there is no infection, simple measures such as keeping your nipples clean and dry and following self-help measures (*see* AVOIDING CRACKED NIPPLES, above) should be sufficient to allow the nipples to heal.

Do you have a red inflamed area on one or both breasts with or without tenderness? YES / NO

Do you also have flu-like symptoms? YES / NO

POSSIBLE CAUSE AND ACTION One of the milk ducts in your breast may be blocked. Try expressing a little milk and change your baby's feeding position to try to empty the duct. If these measures do not help, consult your doctor.

SEE YOUR DOCTOR WITHIN 24 HOURS

POSSIBLE CAUSE You probably have mastitis, inflammation of breast tissue due to infection. In some cases, mastitis results in a breast abscess, in which pus forms within the breast.

ACTION Your doctor will examine you and will probably prescribe antibiotics. You should continue breast-feeding from both breasts. If an abscess has developed, you may be referred to hospital so that the pus can be removed under a local anaesthetic, using a needle and syringe.

Do you have a painless lump in one breast? YES / NO

Does the lump get smaller after breast-feeding? YES / NO

POSSIBLE CAUSE You may have a galactocele, a milk-filled cyst that has formed in the breast tissue behind a blocked duct. Consult your doctor.

ACTION Your doctor will examine you, and he or she may arrange for ultrasound scanning (p.39) to confirm the diagnosis. In most cases, galactoceles do not need treatment and will disappear when you have finished breast-feeding.

POSSIBLE CAUSE An area of breast tissue that is not emptying properly may be causing the lump.

ACTION Offer the affected breast first at each feed, and let the baby empty the breast. Try varying the feeding position. If these measures do not help, consult your doctor.

CONSULT YOUR DOCTOR IF YOU ARE UNABLE TO MAKE A DIAGNOSIS FROM THIS CHART.

150 Depression after childbirth

Childbirth is followed by a dramatic alteration in the body's hormones as you begin to adjust to no longer being pregnant. Your emotions are also likely to be in turmoil – a new baby brings huge changes to your lifestyle, and you may not find it easy to come to terms with the reality of motherhood and the demands that your baby makes on you.

Friends and family may be willing to help but will tend to direct all their attention towards the new baby rather than you, a huge switch from the time when you were pregnant. Around 8 out of every 10 women suffer from "baby blues" soon after giving birth. Some 1 in 10 women develop a much more severe, longer-term postnatal depression.

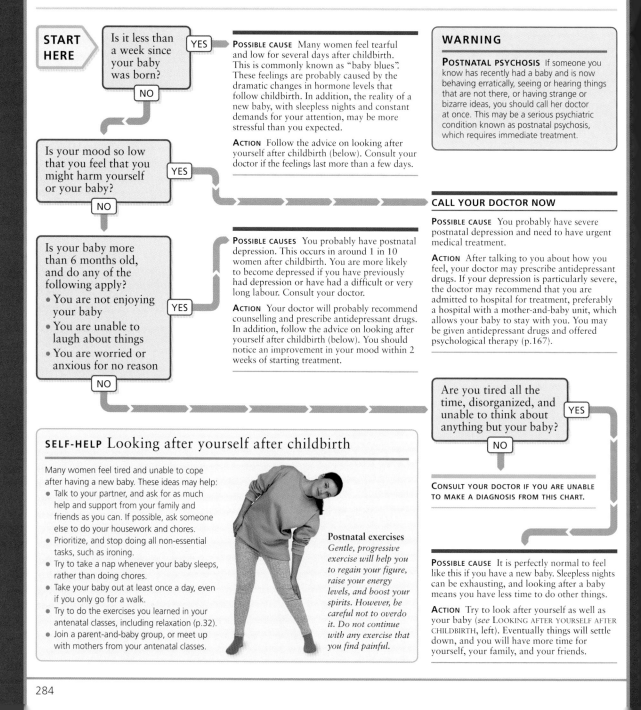

START HERE

Is it less than a week since your baby was born? — YES →

POSSIBLE CAUSE Many women feel tearful and low for several days after childbirth. This is commonly known as "baby blues". These feelings are probably caused by the dramatic changes in hormone levels that follow childbirth. In addition, the reality of a new baby, with sleepless nights and constant demands for your attention, may be more stressful than you expected.

ACTION Follow the advice on looking after yourself after childbirth (below). Consult your doctor if the feelings last more than a few days.

NO ↓

Is your mood so low that you feel that you might harm yourself or your baby? — YES →

NO ↓

Is your baby more than 6 months old, and do any of the following apply?
- You are not enjoying your baby
- You are unable to laugh about things
- You are worried or anxious for no reason

— YES →

POSSIBLE CAUSES You probably have postnatal depression. This occurs in around 1 in 10 women after childbirth. You are more likely to become depressed if you have previously had depression or have had a difficult or very long labour. Consult your doctor.

ACTION Your doctor will probably recommend counselling and prescribe antidepressant drugs. In addition, follow the advice on looking after yourself after childbirth (below). You should notice an improvement in your mood within 2 weeks of starting treatment.

NO ↓

WARNING

POSTNATAL PSYCHOSIS If someone you know has recently had a baby and is now behaving erratically, seeing or hearing things that are not there, or having strange or bizarre ideas, you should call her doctor at once. This may be a serious psychiatric condition known as postnatal psychosis, which requires immediate treatment.

CALL YOUR DOCTOR NOW

POSSIBLE CAUSE You probably have severe postnatal depression and need to have urgent medical treatment.

ACTION After talking to you about how you feel, your doctor may prescribe antidepressant drugs. If your depression is particularly severe, the doctor may recommend that you are admitted to hospital for treatment, preferably a hospital with a mother-and-baby unit, which allows your baby to stay with you. You may be given antidepressant drugs and offered psychological therapy (p.167).

Are you tired all the time, disorganized, and unable to think about anything but your baby? — YES →

NO ↓

CONSULT YOUR DOCTOR IF YOU ARE UNABLE TO MAKE A DIAGNOSIS FROM THIS CHART.

POSSIBLE CAUSE It is perfectly normal to feel like this if you have a new baby. Sleepless nights can be exhausting, and looking after a baby means you have less time to do other things.

ACTION Try to look after yourself as well as your baby (see LOOKING AFTER YOURSELF AFTER CHILDBIRTH, left). Eventually things will settle down, and you will have more time for yourself, your family, and your friends.

SELF-HELP Looking after yourself after childbirth

Many women feel tired and unable to cope after having a new baby. These ideas may help:
- Talk to your partner, and ask for as much help and support from your family and friends as you can. If possible, ask someone else to do your housework and chores.
- Prioritize, and stop doing all non-essential tasks, such as ironing.
- Try to take a nap whenever your baby sleeps, rather than doing chores.
- Take your baby out at least once a day, even if you only go for a walk.
- Try to do the exercises you learned in your antenatal classes, including relaxation (p.32).
- Join a parent-and-baby group, or meet up with mothers from your antenatal classes.

Postnatal exercises
Gentle, progressive exercise will help you to regain your figure, raise your energy levels, and boost your spirits. However, be careful not to overdo it. Do not continue with any exercise that you find painful.

USEFUL

ADDRESSES

In order to learn more about a particular
health issue, you may wish to contact a
specialist organization or look on the internet.
This final section comprises a basic list of
official bodies, charities, and self-help groups
that provide information and support for a
range of health concerns. Contact details,
including website and e-mail addresses, are
given for each entry. In some cases, brief
descriptions of the organizations' work
are also provided.

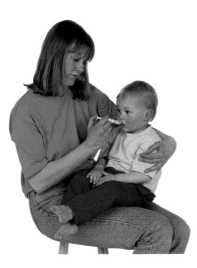

USEFUL ADDRESSES

Throughout the UK, hundreds of organizations, from government agencies such as the Department of Health to nonprofit organizations such as the Red Cross, are dedicated to helping people deal with most conditions.

This list is a limited sample of such organizations, but further information is available from local libraries, hospitals, and GP or health clinics. Most organizations provide information about resources for specific medical or emotional conditions, and many have support groups or can provide information about groups in your area.

No responsibility for information provided by the organizations or online sites listed here can be accepted by the British Medical Association (BMA). The inclusion of an organization or online site in this list does not indicate endorsement by the BMA, and you are advised always to consult your doctor on personal health matters.

Acne Support Group
PO Box 9
Newquay, Cornwall TR9 6WG
Tel: 0870 870 2263
Online: www.m2w3.com/acne

Action for ME
Campaign to improve the lives of people with myalgic encephalomyelitis
PO Box 1302
Wells, Somerset BA5 1YE
Tel: (01749) 670799
E-mail: admin@afme.org.uk
Online: www.afme.org.uk

Action on Smoking and Health
102 Clifton Street
London EC2A 4HW
Tel: (020) 7739 5902
E-mail: enquiries@ash.org.uk
Online: www.ash.org.uk

Addiction Recovery Foundation
122A Wilton Road
London SW1V 1JZ
Tel: (020) 7233 5333
E-mail: enquiries@addictiontoday.co.uk
Online: www.addictiontoday.co.uk

Age Concern
1268 London Road
London SW16 4ER
Tel: (020) 8765 7200
E-mail: ace@ace.org.uk
Online: www.ace.org.uk

Alcoholics Anonymous
PO Box 1, Stonebow House
Stonebow Road, York YO1 7NJ
Helpline: 0845 769 7555
Tel: (01904) 644026
Online: www.alcoholics-anonymous.org.uk

Allergy UK (British Allergy Foundation)
3 White Oak Square, London Road
Swanley, Kent BR8 7AG
Helpline: (01322) 619864
Tel: (01322) 619898
Online: www.allergyuk.org

Alzheimer's Society
Provides information and support for people with dementia and carers
10 Greencoat Place
London SW1P 1PH
Helpline: 0845 300 0336
Tel: (020) 7306 0606
Online: www.alzheimers.org.uk

Anthony Nolan Trust
National register for bone marrow and stem cell donors
The Royal Free Hospital
Hampstead, London NW3 2QG
Tel: (020) 7284 1234
Online: www.anthonynolan.org.uk

Arthritis Care
18 Stephenson Way
London NW1 2HD
Tel: (020) 7380 6500
Online: www.arthritiscare.org.uk

Arthritis Research Campaign
Copeman House, St. Mary's Court
St. Mary's Gate, Chesterfield
Derbyshire S41 7TD
Tel: (01246) 558033
Online: www.arc.org.uk

Asthma UK (National Asthma Campaign)
Providence House
Providence Place, London N1 0NT
Helpline: 0845 701 0203
Tel: (020) 7226 2260
Online: www.asthma.org.uk

BackCare
16 Elmtree Road, Teddington,
Middlesex TW11 8ST
Tel: (020) 8977 5474
Online: www.backcare.org.uk

BBC Online Health
Online: www.bbc.co.uk/health

Brain and Spine Foundation
7 Winchester House, Cranmer Road
Kennington Park, London SW9 6EJ
Helpline: 0808 808 1000
Tel: (020) 7793 5900
Online: www.bbsf.org.uk

Breast Cancer Campaign
110 Clifton Street
London EC2A 4HT
Tel: (020) 7749 3700
Online: www.bcc-uk.org

Breast Cancer Care
Kiln House, 210 New Kings Road
London SW6 4NZ
Helpline: 0808 800 6000
Tel: (020) 7384 2984
E-mail: info@breastcancercare.org.uk
Online: www.breastcancercare.org.uk

Breastfeeding Network
PO Box 11126
Paisley PA2 8YB
Helpline: 0870 900 8787
Online: www.breastfeedingnetwork.org.uk

British Association for Counselling and Psychotherapy
BACP House
35–37 Albert Street
Rugby
Warwickshire CV21 2SG
Tel: 0870 443 5252
E-mail: bacp@bacp.co.uk
Online: www.bacp.co.uk

British Association for Sexual and Relationship Therapy
PO Box 13686
London SW20 9ZH
Tel: (020) 8543 2707
E-mail: info@basrt.org.uk
Online: www.basrt.org.uk

British Chiropractic Association
Blagrave House
17 Blagrave Street
Reading
Berkshire RG1 1QB
Tel: (0118) 950 5950
E-mail: enquiries@chiropractic-uk.co.uk
Online: www.chiropractic-uk.co.uk

British Colostomy Association
15 Station Road
Reading
Berkshire RG1 1LG
Helpline: 0800 328 4257
Tel: (0118) 939 1537
Online: www.bcass.org.uk

British Dental Health Foundation
Smile House
2 East Union Street
Rugby
Warwickshire CV22 6AJ
Helpline: 0845 063 1188
Tel: 0870 770 4000
E-mail: mail@dentalhealth.org.uk
Online: www.dentalhealth.org.uk

British Dyslexia Association
98 London Road
Reading RG1 5AU
Helpline: (0118) 966 8271
Tel: (0118) 966 2677
E-mail: info@dyslexiahelp-bda.demon.co.uk
Online: www.bda-dyslexia.org.uk

British Heart Foundation
14 Fitzhardinge Street
London W1H 6DH
Helpline: 0845 070 8070
Tel: (020) 7935 0185
Online: www.bhf.org.uk

British Kidney Patient Association (BKPA)
Oakhanger Place
Bordon
Hampshire GU35 9JZ
Tel: (01420) 472021
Online: www.britishkidney-pa.co.uk

British Liver Trust
Portman House, 44 High Street
Ringwood
Hampshire BH24 1AG
Tel: (01425) 463080
E-mail: info@britishlivertrust.org.uk
Online: www.britishlivertrust.org.uk

British Lung Foundation

73–75 Goswell Road
London EC1V 7ER

Tel: (020) 7688 5555
E-mail: enquiries@blf-uk.org
Online: www.lunguk.org

British Medical Acupuncture Society

BMAS House
3 Winnington Court
Northwich
Cheshire CW8 1AQ

Tel: (01606) 786782
E-mail: Admin@medical-acupuncture.org.uk
Online: www.medical-acupuncture.co.uk

British Medical Association

BMA House
Tavistock Square
London WC1H 9JP

Tel: (0205) 7387 4499
E-mail: info.web@bma.org.uk
Online: www.bma.org.uk

British Osteopathic Association

Langham House West, Mill Street
Luton, Bedfordshire LU1 2NA

Tel: (01582) 488455
E-mail: enquiries@osteopathy.org
Online: www.osteopathy.org

British Pregnancy Advisory Service

Service for people wishing to prevent or end an unwanted pregnancy

Austy Manor
Wootton Warren
Solihull
West Midlands B95 6BX

Helpline: 0845 730 4030
Tel: (01564) 793225
Online: www.bpas.org

British Red Cross Society

9 Grosvenor Crescent
London SW1X 7EJ

Tel: (020) 7235 5454
Online: www.redcross.org.uk

British Snoring and Sleep Apnoea Association

2nd floor suite
52 Albert Road North
Reigate, Surrey RH2 9EL

Tel: (01737) 245638
E-mail: info@britishsnoring.co.uk
Online: www.britishsnoring.co.uk

British Stammering Association

15 Old Ford Road
London E2 9PJ

Helpline: 0845 603 2001
Tel: (020) 8983 1003
E-mail: mail@stammering.org
Online: www.stammering.org

British Tinnitus Association

Ground floor
Unit 5, Acorn Business Park
Woodseats Close
Sheffield S8 0TB

Tel: 0800 018 0527
E-mail: info@tinnitus.org.uk
Online: www.tinnitus.org.uk

CancerBACUP

3 Bath Place, Rivington Street
London EC2A 3JR

Helpline: 0800 800 1234
Tel: (020) 7696 9003
E-mail: info@cancerbacup.org
Online: www.cancerbacup.org.uk

Cancer and Leukaemia in Childhood (CLIC)

Abbey Wood Business Park
Filton, Bristol BS34 7JU

Tel: 0845 301 0031
Online: www.clic.org.uk

Cancer Research UK

formerly Imperial Cancer Research Fund/Cancer Research Campaign

PO Box 123, Lincoln's Inn Fields
London WC2A 3PX

Tel: (020) 7242 0200
Online: www.cancer.org.uk

Careline

Helpline for young people and adults facing emotional crises

Helpline: (020) 8514 1177

Carers UK

20–25 Glasshouse Yard
London EC1A 4JT

Helpline: 0345 573369
Tel: (020) 7490 8818
Online: www.carersuk.org

ChildLine

Helpline: 0800 1111
Online: www.childline.org.uk

Coeliac UK (the Coeliac Society)

PO Box 220, High Wycombe
Buckinghamshire HP11 2HY

Helpline: 0870 444 8804
Tel: (01494) 437278
Online: www.coeliac.co.uk

Colon Cancer Concern

7 Rickett Street, London SW6 1RU

Helpline: 08708 506050
Tel: (020) 7381 9711
Online: www.coloncancer.org.uk

The Continence Foundation

307 Hatton Square
16 Baldwins Gardens
London EC1N 7RJ

Helpline: 0845 345 0165
Tel: (020) 7404 6875
Online: www.continence-foundation.org.uk

CRUSE Bereavement Care

CRUSE House
126 Sheen Road
Richmond
Surrey TW9 1UR

Helpline: 0870 167 1677
Tel: (020) 8939 9530
Online: www.crusebereavementcare.org.uk

Cystic Fibrosis Trust

11 London Road
Bromley
Kent BR1 1BY

Helpline: 0845 859 1000
Tel: (020) 8464 7211
E-mail: enquiries@cftrust.org.uk
Online: www.cftrust.org.uk

Cystitis and Overactive Bladder Foundation (Interstitial Cystitis Support Group)

76 High Street
Stony Stratford
Buckinghamshire MK11 1AH

Tel: (01908) 569169
E-mail: info@cobfoundation.org
Online: www.interstitialcystitis.co.uk

Depression Alliance

35 Westminster Bridge Road
London SE1 7JB

Tel: 0845 123 2320
Online: www.depressionalliance.org

Diabetes UK (British Diabetic Association)

10 Parkway
London NW1 7AA

Helpline: 0845 120 2960
Tel: (020) 7424 1000
E-mail: info@diabetes.org.uk
Online: www.diabetes.org.uk

Digestive Disorders Foundation (CORE)

3 St Andrews Place
London NW1 4LB

Tel: (020) 7486 0341
Online: www.digestivedisorders.org.uk

Dyspraxia Foundation

8 West Alley
Hitchin
Hertfordshire SG5 1EG

Helpline: (01462) 454986
Online: www.dyspraxiafoundation.org.uk

Eating Disorders Association

1st floor
Wensum House
103 Prince of Wales Road
Norwich NR1 1DW

Helpline: 0845 634 1414
Youth helpline: 0845 634 7650
E-mail: helpmail@edauk.com
Online: www.edauk.com

Epilepsy Action (British Epilepsy Association)

New Anstey House
Gate Way Drive
Yeadon
Leeds LS19 7XY

Helpline: 0808 800 5050
Tel: (0113) 210 8800
E-mail: epilepsy@epilepsy.org.uk
Online: www.epilepsy.org.uk

Family Planning Association

2–12 Pentonville Road
London N1 9FP

Helpline: 0845 310 1334
Tel: (020) 7837 5432
Online: www.fpa.org.uk

Gamblers Anonymous

PO Box 88, London SW10 0EU

Helpline: 0870 050 8880
Tel: (020) 7384 3040
Online: www.gamblersanonymous.org.uk

Healthnet

Heart care information

Online: www.healthnet.org.uk

High Blood Pressure Foundation

Department of Medical Sciences
Western General Hospital
Edinburgh EH4 2XU

Tel: (0131) 332 9211
E-mail: hbpf@hbpf.org.uk
Online: www.hbpf.org.uk

Homoeopathic Medical Association UK

6 Livingstone Road, Gravesend
Kent DA12 5DZ

Tel: (01474) 560336
Online: www.the-hma.org

Infertility Network UK

formerly ISSUE and CHILD

Charter House
43 St Leonard's Road
Bexhill on Sea
East Sussex TN40 1JA

Tel: 0870 118 8088
Online: www.infertilitynetworkuk.com

International Glaucoma Association

108C Warner Road
London SE5 9HQ

Tel: (020) 7737 3265
E-mail: info@iga.org.uk
Online: www.iga.org.uk

Juvenile Diabetes Research Foundation

19 Angel Gate, City Road
London EC1V 2PT

Tel: (020) 7713 2030
E-mail: info@jdrf.org.uk
Online: www.jdrf.org.uk

Leukaemia Research Fund

43 Great Ormond Street
London WC1N 3JJ

Tel: (020) 7405 0101
E-mail: info@lrf.org.uk
Online: www.lrf.org.uk

Macmillan Cancer Relief

89 Albert Embankment
London SE1 7UQ

Helpline: 0808 808 2020
Tel: (020) 7840 7840
E-mail: cancerline@
macmillan.org.uk
Online: www.macmillan.org.uk

Medical Advisory Service for Travellers Abroad

Travellers' Health Line:
0906 550 1402

Online: www.masta.org

Medic Alert Foundation

*For people with hidden medical
conditions; provides tags carrying
information in case of emergencies*

1 Bridge Wharf
156 Caledonian Road
London N1 9UU

Tel: (020) 7833 3034
Freephone: 0800 581420
Online: www.medicalert.co.uk

MENCAP

MENCAP National Centre,
123 Golden Lane
London EC1Y 0RT

Helpline: 0800 808 1111
Tel: (020) 7454 0454
Online: www.mencap.org.uk

Mental Health Foundation

83 Victoria Street
London SW1H 0HW

Tel: (020) 7802 0300
E-mail: mhf@mhf.org.uk
Online: www.mentalhealth.org.uk

Migraine Action Association

Unit 6
Oakley Hay Lodge Business Park
Great Folds Road, Great Oakley
Northamptonshire NN18 9AS

Tel: (01536) 461333
E-mail: info@migraine.org.uk
Online: www.migraine.org.uk

MIND

15–19 Broadway, London E15 4BQ

Helpline: 0845 766 0163
Online: www.mind.org.uk

Miscarriage Association

c/o Clayton Hospital, Northgate
Wakefield, West Yorkshire WF1 3JS

Helpline: (01924) 200799
Tel: (01924) 200795
Online:
www.miscarriageassociation.org.uk

Multiple Sclerosis Society

MS National Centre
372 Edgware Road
London NW2 6ND

Helpline: 0808 800 8000
Tel: (020) 8438 0700
Online: www.mssociety.org.uk

National Association for Colitis and Crohn's Disease

4 Beaumont House, Sutton Road
St Albans, Herts AL1 5HH

Tel: 0845 130 2233
E-mail: nacc@nacc.org.uk
Online: www.nacc.org.uk

National Association for Premenstrual Syndrome

41 Old Road, East Peckham
Kent TN12 5AP

Helpline: 0870 777 2177
Tel: 0870 777 2178
Online: www.pms.org.uk

National Childbirth Trust

Alexandra House, Oldham Terrace
Acton, London W3 6NH

Tel: 0870 444 8707
Online:
www.nctpregnancyandbabycare.com

National Drugs Helpline

Tel: 0800 776600

National Eczema Society

Hill House, Highgate Hill
London N19 5NA

Helpline: 0870 241 3604
Tel: (020) 7281 3553
Online: www.eczema.org

National Endometriosis Society

50 Westminster Palace Gardens
Artillery Row
London SW1P 1RR

Helpline: 0808 808 2227
Tel: (020) 7222 2781
Online: www.endo.org.uk

National Osteoporosis Society

Camerton, Bath BA2 0PJ

Helpline: 0845 450 0230
Tel: (01761) 471771
E-mail: info@nos.org.uk
Online: www.nos.org.uk

NHS Direct

*Helpline for health problems and
provides links to other sites*

Helpline: 0845 4647
Online: www.nhsdirect.nhs.uk

NSPCC

42 Curtain Road
London EC2A 3NH

Helpline: 0808 800 5000
Textphone: 0800 056 0566
Tel: (020) 7825 2500
E-mail: help@nspcc.org.uk
Online: www.nspcc.org.uk

Orchid Cancer Appeal

*Provides information about cancers
of the penis, testis, and prostate*

St Bartholomew's Hospital
London EC1A 7BE

Tel: (020) 7601 7808
Online: www.orchid-cancer.org.uk

Pain Relief Foundation

Clinical Sciences Centre
University Hospital Aintree
Lower Lane, Liverpool L9 7AL

Tel: (0151) 529 5820
Online:
www.painrelieffoundation.org.uk

Parentline Plus

*Provides support and information
on parenting issues*

520 Highgate Studios
53–79 Highgate Road
London NW5 1TL

Helpline: 0808 800 2222
Online: www.parentlineplus.org.uk

Parkinson's Disease Society

215 Vauxhall Bridge Road
London SW1V 1EJ

Helpline: 0808 800 0303
Tel: (020) 7931 8080
E-mail: info@parkinsons.org.uk
Online: www.parkinsons.org.uk

Patient UK

*Directory of websites providing
information on health issues*

Online: www.patient.co.uk

Psoriasis Association

Milton House, 7 Milton Street
Northampton NN2 7JG

Tel: 0845 676 0076
Online: www.psoriasis-
association.org.uk

Quit

Charity helping people stop smoking

Ground floor, 211 Old Street
London EC1V 9NR

Helpline: 0800 002200
Tel: (020) 7251 1551
Online: www.quit.org.uk

RELATE

*Provides support for people who
wish to improve their relationships*

Herbert Gray College
Little Church Street
Rugby, Warwickshire CV21 3AP

Tel: (01788) 573241
Online: www.relate.org.uk

Royal National Institute for the Blind

105 Judd Street
London WC1H 9NE

Helpline: 0845 766 9999
Tel: (020) 7388 1266
Online: www.rnib.org.uk

Royal National Institute for Deaf People

19–23 Featherstone Street
London EC1Y 8SL

Tel: 0808 808 0123
Textphone: 0808 808 9000
Online: www.rnid.org.uk

St. Andrew's Ambulance Association

St. Andrew's House
48 Milton Street, Glasgow G4 0HR

Tel: (0141) 332 4031
Online: www.firstaid.org.uk

St. John Ambulance

Edwina Mountbatten House
63 York Street, London W1H 1PS

Tel: (020) 7258 3456
Online: www.sja.org.uk

The Samaritans

The Upper Mill, Kingston Road
Ewell, Surrey KT17 2AF

Helpline: 0845 790 9090
Tel: (020) 8394 8300
E-mail: jo@samaritans.org
Online: www.samaritans.org.uk

SANDS: Stillbirth and Neonatal Death Society

28 Portland Place, London W1B 1LY

Helpline: (020) 7436 5881
Tel: (020) 7436 7940
E-mail: support@uk-sands.org
Online: www.uk-sands.org

Self Help UK

Database of self-help organizations

Online: www.self-help.org.uk

The Stress Management Society (Stress UK)

PO Box 193, Harrow
Middlesex HA1 3ZE

Tel: 0870 199 3260
Online: www.stress.org.uk

The Stroke Association

240 City Road, London EC1V 2PR

Helpline: 0845 303 3100
Tel: (020) 7566 0300
Online: www.stroke.org.uk

Terrence Higgins Trust

*Provides support and information
for people with HIV and AIDS*

52–54 Grays Inn Road
London WC1X 8JU

Helpline: 0845 122 1200
Tel: (020) 7831 0330
Online: www.tht.org.uk

Women's Nationwide Cancer Control Campaign

128–130 Curtain Road
London EC2A 3AQ

Helpline: (020) 7729 2299
Tel: (020) 7729 4688

INDEX

This index gives entries for the major symptoms covered in the book as well as entries for many of the diseases and disorders that may be the cause of symptoms. There are also entries for parts of human anatomy, and for issues covered in the first part of the book. However, as with any index, it cannot be comprehensive. Page numbers that appear in **bold** indicate a reference to an entire symptom chart. Page numbers that appear in *italics* indicate a reference to an illustration. For detailed advice on how to use the 150 charts, see pp.42–43. In addition to this index, the chartfinder on p.44, which gives page references for all the symptoms covered in the book, can also be used to help find the particular charts you need.

ACKNOWLEDGMENTS

PICTURE CREDITS
Abbreviations: t = top; c = centre; b = bottom; l = left; r = right
Biofotos: 11tr; **Robert Harding Picture Library:** Front jacket bc, 12tr;
National Meningitis Trust: 75br; **Philips PR Dept:** 39tr; **Dr Janet Page:**
13tr, 13cr, 37c, 38tl; **Science Photo Library:** Front jacket bl, 15cl, 40br;
CNRI 38cr, 39cr; **Dr Robert Friedland:** 40tl; Gca - CNRI: 38br;
James King-Holmes: 249tr, 249tr2; Petit Format/CSI: 21tr;
Professor P. Motta/Dept. of Anatomy/University "La Sapienza" Rome:
21bl; Secchi, Lecaque, Roussel, UCLAF, CNRI: 19br; **St John's Institute
of Dermatology:** 179br.

PREVIOUS EDITIONS
MEDICAL EDITORS Dr Tony Smith, Dr Sue Davidson
MEDICAL CONSULTANTS Sir Peter Beale, Dr Peter Cantillon, Dr Mark
Furman, Dr Stephen Hughes, Dr Warren Hyer, Dr S M M Kinder, Dr
Penny Preston, Dr T J L Richards, Dr Andrew Shennan, Dr H B Valman,
Dr Frances Williams

EDITORIAL DIRECTOR Amy Carroll
ART DIRECTORS Chez Picthall, Bryn Walls
SENIOR MANAGING EDITOR Martyn Page
EDITORIAL MANAGER Andrea Bagg
SENIOR EDITORS Mary Atkinson, Nicki Lampon, Andrew Macintyre
PROJECT EDITORS Cathy Meeus, Christine Murdoch
EDITORS Jillian Agar, Candace Burch, Jane Farrell, Jolyon Goddard, Katie
John, Janet Mohun, Terence Monaighan, Teresa Pritlove, Hazel Richardson
ADDITIONAL EDITORIAL ASSISTANCE Ann Baggaley, Alyson Lacewing
EDITORIAL ADVISER Donald Berwick
MANAGING ART EDITOR Louise Dick
SENIOR ART EDITOR Marianne Markham
ART EDITORS Janice English, Dinah Lone, Chris Walker
DESIGN ASSISTANCE Peter Cross, Simone End, Sara Freeman, Sarah Ponder,
Sally Powell, Jane Tetzlaff, Ellen Woodward

ADDITIONAL DESIGN AND DTP ASSISTANCE Chloe Burnett, Kirsten Cashman,
Julian Dams, John Goldsmid, Jason Little, Andrew Nash, Louise Paddick,
Schermuly Design Company
PICTURE RESEARCH ASSISTANT Marie Osborn
PHOTOGRAPHERS Steve Bartholomew, Andy Crawford, Jo Foord, Steve
Gorton, Dave King, Ranald Mckechnie, Tracy Morgan, Gary Ombler,
Susanna Price, Tim Ridley, Jules Selmes, Steve Shott, Debi Treloar
ILLUSTRATORS Evi Antoniou, Joanna Cameron, Gary Cross, John Egan,
Mick Gillah, Debbie Maizels, Patrick Mulrey, Peter Ruane, Richard
Tibbits, Halli Verrinder, Philip Wilson, Deborah Woodward
PRODUCTION MANAGER Michelle Thomas
OUT-OF-HOUSE TECHNICAL SERVICES MANAGER Nicola Erdpresser
PROJECT ADMINISTRATION Joanna Benwell, Delyth Hughes
INDEXER Julie Rimington

PREVIOUS EDITIONS: DK INDIA
HEAD OF PUBLISHING Anita Roy
MANAGING EDITOR Prita Maitra
MANAGING ART EDITOR Shuka Jain
PROJECT EDITOR Atanu Raychaudhuri
EDITORS Chandana Chandra, Sudhanshu Gupta
PROJECT DESIGNER Sabyasachi Kundu
DESIGNER Sukanto Bhattacharjya
DTP COORDINATOR AND SOFTWARE TRAINER Jacob Joshua
DTP DESIGNER Shailesh Sharma